niversity
7688 7555

COMPREHENSIVE TEXTBOOK OF SUICIDOLOGY

COMPREHENSIVE TEXTBOOK OF SUICIDOLOGY

Ronald W. Maris
Alan L. Berman
Morton M. Silverman

with contributions by

Bruce Bongar and Associates
Norman L. Farberow
Mark J. Goldblatt
David A. Jobes and Associates
David Lester
Paul A. Nisbet
Robert Plutchik
Steven Stack
Bryan L. Tanney
Anton J. L. van Hooff

Foreword by Robert D. Goldney

THE GUILFORD PRESS
New York   London

© 2000 The Guilford Press
A Division of Guilford Publications, Inc.
72 Spring Street, New York, NY 10012
www.guilford.com

Printed in the United States of America

This book is printed on acid-free paper.

Last digit is print number: 9   8   7   6   5   4   3   2   1

Library of Congress Cataloging-in-Publication Data

Maris, Ronald W.
 Comprehensive textbook of suicidology / Ronald W. Maris,
  Alan L. Berman, Morton M. Silverman ; with contributions
  by Bruce Bongar . . . [et al.]
   p. cm.
 Includes bibliographical references and index.
 ISBN 1-57230-541-X
  1. Suicide. I. Berman, Alan L. (Alan Lee), 1943–   . II.
Silverman, Morton M. III. Bongar, Bruce Michael.
IV. Title.

RC569.M37 2000
616.85′8455—dc21   00-037640

"Resume," on page 288, copyright 1926, 1928, renewed 1954, (c) 1956 by Dorothy Parker, from
The Portable Dorothy Parker by Dorothy Parker. Used by permission of Viking Penguin, a division
of Penguin Putnam Inc.

*To all who died unnecessarily
and prematurely, and
those who loved them*

About the Primary Authors

Ronald W. Maris, PhD, is Director of the Center for the Study of Suicide and Professor of Psychiatry at the University of South Carolina. He is a past president of the American Association of Suicidology (receiving its Shneidman and Dublin awards) and Editor Emeritus of the journal *Suicide and Life-Threatening Behavior*, and has authored or edited 18 books on suicide (the latest of which is *Review of Suicidology, 2000*). He has received National Institute of Mental Health, National Science Foundation, and private research grants to study suicide. Dr. Maris is an active forensic suicidologist, consulting on numerous medical malpractice, product liability, contested life insurance, workers' compensation, and jail/prison suicide cases. He is a Fellow in the American Academy of Forensic Sciences and is board-certified in the American College of Forensic Examiners.

Alan L. Berman, PhD, is Executive Director of the American Association of Suicidology and maintains a private practice in psychotherapy and psychological and forensic consultation at the Washington Psychological Center, P.C., in Washington, DC. Formerly, he was Director of the National Center for the Study and Prevention of Suicide at the Washington School of Psychiatry, and Professor of Psychology at the American University. He is a Diplomate in Clinical Psychology of the American Board of Professional Psychology and a Fellow of both the American Psychological Association and the International Academy of Suicide Research. Dr. Berman is the author or editor of seven books (the latest of which is *Risk Management with Suicidal Patients*, 1998) and more than 80 book chapters and articles; in additon, he is a consulting editor of three professional journals. He is a past president of the American Association of Suicidology and recipient of their Shneidman Award for outstanding contributions to research.

Morton M. Silverman, MD, a psychiatrist trained at the University of Chicago, is currently Associate Professor of Psychiatry at the Pritzker School of Medicine and Director of its Student Counseling and Resource Service, and Editor-in-Chief of the journal *Suicide and Life-Threatening Behavior*. He is a Fellow of the American Psychiatric Association and a temporary advisor to the World Health Orgnization. Formerly, Dr. Silverman was Chief of the Center for Prevention Research of the National Institute of Mental Health and Associate Administrator for Prevention in the Alcohol, Drug Abuse, and Mental Health Administration. He has published a number of books and articles, especially on suicide prevention and treatment. He was recently chair of a national suicide prevention advisory committee, which made recommendations to U.S. Surgeon General David Satcher about developing a national suicide prevention strategy.

About the Contributing Authors

Bruce Bongar, PhD, ABPP, is the Calvin Professor of Psychology at the Pacific Graduate School of Psychology, a consulting professor of psychiatry and the behavioral sciences at Stanford University School of Medicine, and director of the combined JD/PhD program in clinical psychology and the law at the Golden Gate University School of Law.

Kaprice Brown, MA, is a graduate student in the combined JD/PhD program in clinical psychology and the law at the Pacific Graduate School of Psychology and Golden Gate University School of Law.

Karin Cleary, BA, is a graduate student in Clinical Psychology at the Pacific Graduate School of Psychology.

Norman L. Farberow, PhD, is a cofounder and was the director of the Los Angeles Suicide Prevention Center. He is a past president of both the American Association of Suicidology and the International Association of Suicide Prevention and the recipient of numerous awards for his research and contributions in suicide prevention.

Laura Goldberg, PhD, received her doctoral degree from the Pacific Graduate School of Psychology.

Mark J. Goldblatt, MD, is a clinical instructor in psychiatry at Harvard Medical School and an attending psychiatrist at McLean Hospital, Belmont, Massachusetts. He is also a consulting editor of *Suicide and Life-Threatening Behavior*, as well as a coeditor of *Essential Papers on Suicide*.

Lisa Anne T. Hustead, MA, is in the clinical psychology doctoral program at The Catholic University of America. Her clinical and research interests include suicide, child abuse, and child/adolescent issues.

David A. Jobes, PhD, is an associate professor of psychology at The Catholic University of America and maintains a private practice at the Washington Psychological Center (P.C.) in Washington, DC. He is a former president of the American Association of Suicidology. His research, writing, consulting, and training interests are in suicidology, with a particular interest in clinical suicidology.

David Lester, PhD, has doctoral degrees from Brandeis University (psychology) and Cambridge University (social and political science). He is a professor of psychology at The Richard Stockton College of New Jersey and former president of the International Association for Suicide Prevention.

Jason B. Luoma, MA, is a doctoral student in clinical psychology at The Catholic University of America, with research interests in clinical suicidology and the role of autobiographical memory in personality.

Rachel E. Mann, MA, is a doctoral candidate in clinical psychology at The Catholic University of America. She has pursued research in the area of suicide since 1994.

Paul A. Nisbet, PhD, is a National Institute of Mental Health National Service Research Award Postdoctoral Fellow in the Department of Psychiatry at the University of Rochester School of Medicine, where he works in the Center for the Study and Prevention of Suicide. His current research focuses on social determinants of violence, with a particular emphasis on suicide and homicide among minority populations.

Robert Plutchik, PhD, is currently Professor Emeritus at the Albert Einstein College of Medicine and an adjunct professor at the University of South Florida. He is a former associate chairman of the Psychiatry Department at Jacoby Hospital in the Bronx, New York. He is the author or coauthor of six books and 260 articles, and has edited seven books.

Steven Stack, PhD, has published over one hundred articles and book chapters on various aspects of the sociology of suicide. His articles on the subject include ones in the *American Sociological Review*, *Social Forces*, *Journal of Marriage and the Family*, and *Social Science Quarterly*. In 1985 he received the Shneidman Award from the American Association of Suicidology for excellence in research. A four-year grant from the National Institute of Mental Health funded his project on mass media or copycat effects on suicide. He has served as Secretary of the American Association of Suicidology. Currently he is Professor and Chairperson of the Department of Criminal Justice at Wayne State University.

Bryan L. Tanney, BSc, MD, FRCP(C), is a profesor of psychiatry at the University of Calgary in Calgary, Alberta, Canada. His career interest is in suicidal acts and in particular the competencies of caregivers and communities in responding to these distressing and turbulent problems. As part of LivingWorks Education, Inc., he has developed and disseminated the most widely used suicide intervention learning experience in the world. In 1996 he coedited the United Nations/WHO guidelines for the formulation and implementation of national strategies for suicide prevention.

Anton J. L. van Hooff, PhD, is a senior lecturer in ancient history and teacher training in classics at Nijmegen University, the Netherlands. He was president of the Association of Classicists in the Netherlands from 1988 to 1994 and secretary of Euroclassica, the European Federation of Associations of Classical Teachers from 1991 to 1995. He has published several books and numerous articles on Roman imperialism, Caesar, Polybius, ancient bandits, old age in antiquity, Greco-Roman self-killing (*From Autothanasia to Suicide*, 1990), and the Spartacus tradition (in Dutch, *De vonk van Spartacus*, 1993; an English version, *Spark of Spartacus*, is in preparation). He is the coauthor of numerous textbooks on history, ancient culture, and Latin.

Foreword

There have been a number of landmarks in the study of suicide and its prevention in the last hundred years. These include the 1910 psychoanalytic conference in Vienna that addressed youth suicide; the establishment of international and national organizations devoted to suicide prevention; and the publication of such seminal works as Ruth Cavan's *Suicide* in 1928, Karl Menninger's *Man against Himself* in 1938, the English translation of Emile Durkheim's *Le Suicide* in 1951, and *The Cry for Help*, edited by Norman L. Farberow and Edwin S. Shneidman in 1961. These landmarks established the foundations for the scientific examination of suicidal behavior, and 40 years ago the triumvirate of Shneidman, Farberow, and Robert Litman was seen as the driving force in the then newly named discipline of suicidology.

Since that time there has been an exponential growth in research and clinical publications. This burgeoning of information presents serious obstacles to the individual clinician, researcher, volunteer, or interested lay person seeking to gain either a concise overview of the topic or an authoritative view on particular aspects of suicidal behavior. It is fair to note that in the last two decades there have been attempts to collate this information, and several of these books are referred to in the introductory chapter of this book. However, none have provided the breadth of coverage or the cohesive style of the present work. Indeed, that is precisely the reason this *Comprehensive Textbook of Suicidology* is so welcome, and why it will undoubtedly become another significant landmark in the field.

Within this one volume is a distillation of knowledge, with appropriate wisdom, that is second to none. Due regard is given to our expanding awareness of the biological correlates of suicide, and that is integrated well with conventional sociological and psychological theories and practice. Furthermore, rather than simply being provided with lists of sometimes conflicting and ambiguous data about specific topics, it is a relief to be presented with critically assessed studies and stores of data followed by logically argued conclusions, pragmatic management recommendations, engaging clinical vignettes (often with a literary basis), and suggestions for further reading. Because of this, the book will be valued not only by various groups of professionals to whom such books have traditionally been targeted, but also by the broader range of counselors and volunteers who are now acknowledged as having an important role in the challenging task of suicide prevention.

That the authors have achieved this is not unexpected, bearing in mind their individual track records. In fact, although they have utilized the expertise of distinguished colleagues, this work is essentially that of a new triumvirate, Ronald W. Maris, Alan L. Berman and Morton M. Silverman, who with this landmark publication can be seen to be leading suicidology into the 21st century.

ROBERT D. GOLDNEY
Past President, International Association for Suicide Prevention
Professor of Psychiatry, University of Adelaide, South Australia

Preface

In spite of the ubiquity and devastating toll of self-destructive behaviors, until now there really has been no comprehensive textbook on suicidology, that is, on the scientific study, treatment, and prevention of suicidal, life-threatening, and self-injurious behavior. This volume attempts to address that need.

Suicide has been called the leading cause of unnecessary, premature death. In the United States, suicide affects many more than the 30,000 to 31,000 Americans who die each year and also more than the estimated annual 775,000 who make nonfatal suicide attempts. If every suicide intimately affects at least six family members or friends (a conservative number, at best), then every year in the United States there would be about 186,000 new survivors. If so, from 1971 to 1996 alone there would be roughly 4.5 million survivors of suicide (McIntosh, 1998).

On Wednesday, July 28, 1999, U.S. Surgeon General David Satcher (accompanied by Tipper Gore, wife of Vice President Al Gore; Harry Reid, U.S. Senator from Nevada; and John Lewis, Congressman from Georgia) declared that the national suicide rate must be reduced and that suicide poses a "serious public health problem" (suicide in 1999 was the eighth leading cause of death for all Americans). Surgeon General Satcher singled out the high suicide rate of older men as deserving special attention. This textbook discusses most of the 15 recommendations contained in his "Call to Action to Prevent Suicide 1999."

There have been other attempts at basic suicide books (see Chapter 1), but they have not been comprehensive suicidology textbooks. Our objectives and goals in writing the *Comprehensive Textbook of Suicidology* (hereafter CTS) were specific.

Edwin S. Shneidman reminds us that suicide is a multidimensional malaise in needful individuals who perceive suicide as the solution to their problems. Thus, any worthy suicidology textbook must be both comprehensive and multidisciplinary.

CTS considers both theory and methods; history and art; psychological, biological, and social factors; ethics and philosophy; indirect self-destructive behaviors; and treatment, prevention, and survivors. Chapters are relevant to psychiatry, nursing, psychology, the social and behavioral sciences, biology, psychopharmacology, the brain and neurotransmitters, and criminal justice. The three primary authors (Maris, Berman, and Silverman) come from different professional backgrounds (the social and behavioral sciences, psychology, and medicine), which ensures a comprehensive perspective.

One key focus in CTS is suicide intervention, treatment, and prevention (and thus the book is a companion volume to the 1992 Guilford Press publication, *Assessment and Prediction of Suicide*). Most chapters contain boxed text relating to the implications of the chapter subject for suicide prevention. Our textbook was also envisioned as a handbook or reference work for use in applied, clinical settings: emergency rooms, suicide prevention and crisis centers, psychiatry and psychology clinics, by emergency medical treatment (EMT) teams, the police, in jails and prisons, and so on.

CTS is grounded in the primary authors' combined 80 years of clinical experience in treating and managing suicidal clients, and is case focused. We must remember that the vast majority of suicides are associated with treatable mental disorders. Suicidal individuals die one at a time. Case presentations illustrate both general principles and the idiosyncrasies of each suicidal person. Implicit in the cases presented in each chapter is the treatment question: "How would one manage this particular case of self-destructive behavior?"

As any scientific volume should be, CTS is empirically based on relevant facts (i.e., it is data based), with specialized information being provided on subtopics by invited leading suicide experts (e.g., van Hooff, Stack, Tanney, Bongar, Goldblatt, Lester, Plutchik, Farberow, and Jobes). Chapters have ample tables, figures, graphs, and scales to emphasize the scientific knowledge base of the field of suicidology. Highlighted are Aaron Beck's depression inventory, suicide ideation, and hopelessness scales; various lethality scales (e.g., Smith et al.'s); selections from Cull and Gill's suicide probability scale; the Minnesota Multiphasic Personality Inventory; mental status tests; Motto's scale to estimate suicide risk; Maris's suicide classification scheme; and Maris et al.'s 15 predictors of suicide.

We have found that most of the earlier suicide reference books lose the reader in a sea of inconsistent, inconclusive, even contradictory, research results. We have tried to summarize our best guesses as to which conclusions about suicidal behaviors seem most credible to us at this time through "box scores" of research findings (see Chapter 13), as well as a summary and conclusion section at the end of each chapter.

CTS is guided by theory (see especially Chapter 2). Most suicide books provide readers with endless disjointed lists of factual claims or research results with no effort made to integrate these "facts." CTS starts out with careful definitions of its subject matter, proceeds to nomenclature and classification, states explicit hypotheses when possible, and even considers how discrete hypotheses might be related in more "grand theory" or causal models of suicide.

One of the unique features of CTS is its boxed text focusing on current controversies. For example, do selective serotonin reuptake inhibitors (SSRIs) cause suicide? Is suicide ever rational? Is suicide mainly a mind or body problem? Which types of treatment modalities work best for which types of suicides under which circumstances? Can the suicide rate be lowered and, if so, how?

We have tried to be pedagogical, to make CTS learner-friendly. For example, chapters pose relevant student discussion questions (see Chapter 22), and there is an expanded four-chapter introduction to the theory, methods, and history of the study of suicide. At the book's end, there are extensive references and both name and subject indices. So as not to "lose the forest for the suicidological trees" or be overwhelmed by citations, each chapter concludes with just a few key recommendations for further reading.

Unlike most suicide books, which are disjointed and fragmented, CTS presents its materials primarily in the writing style and format of its primary coauthors, Ronald Maris, Alan Berman, and Morton Silverman, who standardized, read, critiqued, and edited every chapter. Ideally, the result will be a more integrated and readable textbook with a consistent style.

Originally, the plan was to avoid an edited volume entirely and to have the three primary authors write the entire textbook. This strategy had a certain appeal and rationale. We concluded that some special suicide topics required invited experts if the text had any hope of being "state of the art."

CTS has five parts. Part I is an expanded four-chapter introduction, which includes a general introduction to suicidology, theory, methods, and a history of suicide. Part II examines special topics in the study of suicide, such as age, sex/gender, race, work, marriage and family, social relations, suicide notes, and suicide attempts and methods. Part III is primarily medical and psychiatric, including chapters on mental disorders, physical illness, alcoholism and substance abuse, biological factors, and aggression and violence. Part IV considers important related issues, such as indirect self-destructive behaviors; ethical, religious, and philosophical aspects of suicide; and suicide and the law. CTS concludes with an examination of treatment, prevention, postvention, and survivor issues. Detailed author responsibilities for the chapters in the text's five parts are specified in the remainder of this Preface and the Table of Contents, as well as repeated at the end of Chapter 1.

Part I is a unique feature of CTS, usually missing from most suicide books but, we believe, essential to any comprehensive textbook. Chapters 1 through 4 constitute a prologue to the scientific study of suicide. Chapter 1 asks, Why study suicide?, and then provides several justifications. Next, the scope of the suicide problem (largely in the United States) is surveyed by considering overview data on the incidence and prevalence of self-destructive behaviors. Treatment and suicide prevention problems are then examined. A third major section outlines the continuum of types of self-destructive behaviors: completed suicides, nonfatal attempted suicides, suicide ideators, indirect self-destructive behaviors, parasuicides, and mixed types. Chapter 1 concludes with a summary, plan, and organization for the entire text (which embellishes on material in this Preface).

Chapter 2 reviews the theoretical component in suicidology. Most suicide books lack systematic theory and, at best, posit isolated research hypotheses. A truly systematic theory is more general than hypothesis or model testing and, if done well, assists in suicide prediction. Some of the essential building blocks of suicide theory are definitions, major orienting concepts (e.g., lethality, motive, intent, and suicidal careers), hypotheses, causal models, and research results.

Chapter 3, in a sense, is the mirror image of Chapter 2; it looks at the factual or data foundations of suicidology. Some of the data of suicide include vital statistics, treatment records, surveys, experiments, first-person documents, and art or history. This chapter also provides a brief review of the basic rates of suicide (which are examined in greater detail in Part II). Next, the chapter considers major predictors of suicide, scales that assess and predict, and risk and protective factors in suicide. Chapter 3 concludes with a general discussion of research methods, design, and statistics.

Chapter 4 is the first of CTS's commissioned chapters. Because CTS concentrates on contemporary U.S. suicide, we felt it important to provide readers with the full (largely non-American) historical context for contemporary suicide, complete with illustrations. Anton J. L. van Hooff from the Netherlands has comprehensively surveyed Roman and Greek suicides (e.g., Ajax falling on his sword), suicide in the Middle Ages, early modern suicides (16th and 17th centuries), and suicides in the 18th and 19th centuries.

Part II considers some of the epidemiological "nuts and bolts" of suicidological science. Chapter 5 (coauthored with Paul A. Nisbet) notes the well-documented trend for suicide rates to increase with age, especially among white males. This chapter acknowledges many life stages in the human lifespan, but concentrates on four, that is, suicide among (1) children, (2) adolescents and young adults, (3) those in midlife, and (4) the elderly. By far the most significant association between age and suicide rates is found among the elderly. However, it is also noted that from the 1950s to the late 1970s the adolescent suicide rate tripled, and Chapter 5 explores possible explanations for this rate increase. Not only are suicide rates disproportionately high among the elderly, this increase is especially high among males.

Chapter 6 observes that it is not clear how much of this male excess suicide rate is gender related (e.g., to socialization and culture) versus sexually related (to testosterone, other hormones, biologically based aggression, etc.). Males tend to have higher death rates from most causes and shorter lifespans than do females. For suicide rates the male-to-female ratio is about 4 to 1. In Chapter 6 we note also that although men have greater access to, and familiarity with, lethal methods (e.g., guns), paradoxically women have depressive disorder rates about twice as high as men do. Probably, females have greater or extra suicide protective factors than do males (family ties, sociability, motherhood, religion, etc.). Chapter 6 also considers the role of sexual deviations/variations, sexual abuse, autoerotic asphyxias, and confused gender identity and suicide.

Chapter 7 adds a third major epidemiological "nut and bolt" in the construction of suicide outcomes: race and ethnicity. In the United States, suicide rates are especially high among Caucasians. About 90% of all U.S. suicides are by whites. White males have suicide rates about 10 times higher than those of black females. Rates are particularly high among white ethnics whose country of origin is Hungary, Germany, Lithuania, Austria, or the countries of Scandinavia. Chapter 7 explores the relationships of these ethnic identities to suicide in detail. In general African Americans (notably black women) tend to have low suicide rates. Suicide rates among Asian Americans are not especially high. Internationally, only Japan, at 12th worldwide, ranks near the top. Furthermore, Asian suicides have several unique traits (age reversals, female–male reversals, cultural variations, different methods, and different suicide types—e.g., more altruistic suicides). Chapter 7 ends with an examination of suicides among different cultures, such as Eskimos, Tikopians, South Americans, and Native Americans in the United States.

Chapter 8 features the work of another invited expert, Steven Stack, who provides a wealth of empirical data on suicide, work, and the economy. Stack cautions us that the research results in this area are often inconclusive and that associations can be confounded by additional variables, such as divorce or unemployment. With these caveats, he then addresses several subtopics. Suicide rates tend to be higher in lower socioeconomic groups, although divorce can confound this association. There can be both high and low suicide rates in the same socioeconomic strata (e.g., among professionals). As a rule, unemployment tends to be related positively to suicide rates.

Although occupational data on suicide rates are complex, we often see higher suicide rates among artists and the police. Reviewing business cycles, it is observed that suicide rates tend to be elevated during economic depressions (which may in part just be the result of heightened unemployment). Larger cohort sizes tend to result in increased suicide rates. Work mobility studies of suicide are inconclusive, but suicides tend to have downward mobility, erratic work histories, and higher unemployment rates. Finally, Stack looks at professional and executive suicides, especially higher suicide rate trends among physicians, nurses, and dentists.

Bruce Bongar and colleagues, in Chapter 9, observe the elevated suicide rates among the widowed, divorced, and single or never-married compared to the married and married with children. Starting with a family systems perspective, the authors examine the relationship between suicidal behavior and interpersonal difficulties. Certainly, suicides not only result from but also cause such interpersonal problems as grief, anger, rage, and guilt. Suicidal families tend to be less cohesive, less expressive, more conflictual, and more rigid. Scapegoating and double binding are common features of suicidal families. Suicidal families tend to have histories with more divorce, parental separation, family discord, abuse, unemployment, and psychiatric disorders. Because suicide almost never occurs in an interpersonal vacuum, in most cases treatment should include the entire family. Multiple family therapy modalities (such as those of Richman and Motto) are reviewed.

Chapter 10 notes that suicides tend either to be socially isolated or to have negative social interactions. Indicators of social isolation that are reviewed include being single, divorced, or widowed; living alone; having no or minimal family relations or social support; or having few, if any, close friends. Social forces that tend to drive one to suicide might include absent or abusive parenting early in life or involvement with groups that condone or even promote suicide (e.g., Jonestown). The history of the sociology of suicide from Durkheim to Pescosolido (including Henry and Short, Gibbs and Martin, Douglas, Maris, Phillips, and Stack) is reviewed, with some focus on egoistic, altruistic, and fatalistic suicides; anomie; status integration; contagion; and suicide clusters. Finally, Chapter 10 examines stress, negative life events, and suicide outcomes. Although there is some evidence that suicides are triggered by recent stress or life events, chronic factors are probably more important in producing suicides.

Chapter 11 asks whether suicide notes' "last words" are windows to the mind or soul of the decedent. Surely, if anyone knows why a suicide occurred, it would be the one who suicides. But there are problems here. For one, only a minority of suicides (approximately 15–30%) even leave notes. Also, suicide notes often tend to be matter-of-fact, terse, and not particularly insightful. Genuine and faked or simulated notes are distinguished, a content analysis of suicide notes is presented, motives for suicide are revealed in actual, cited suicide notes (rescue, reunion, revenge, escape, self-punishment, etc.), and a discussion of suicide notes in the context of life history is offered (in which the last written communication of Vincent Foster is examined).

Part II concludes with Chapter 12, on suicide attempts and methods. Nonfatal suicide attempters have about a 10–15% lifetime completion rate, and an annual rate of about 1% after the nonfatal attempt. However, the chapter also notes that 88% of Chicago white males over age 45 died the *first* time they attempted suicide. Most suicides are by firearms (60–65% among men), with females being much more likely to overdose. Chapter 12 reviews methods of suicide from 1960 to 1996, controlling for sex and race.

The chapter concludes that suicide prevention may rest significantly on controlling access to firearms. Availability of any method to suicide is a relevant concern. For example, 40% of all New York City suicides occur by jumping from high places. Suicide methods often have symbolic import. The chapter asks, Why do women tend to use lower lethality methods? Special chapter foci include firearms as a suicide method (e.g., body location of the wounds, proximity [contact or not?], accessibility of the site, handedness [left vs. right], trace metal residue analysis, the number of wounds, and clothing removal) versus firearm-involved homicides or accidents and other major suicide methods (such as drugs, hanging, jumping, gases [e.g., carbon monoxide], cutting, drowning, burning, and vehicles [especially cars]).

Part III examines psychiatric, medical, and biological factors in suicide outcome. It considers some of the strongest known predictors of suicide outcome, such as major depressive disorder and substance abuse. Chapter 13 (by Bryan L. Tanney) considers mental and personality disorders and diagnoses. Research study after research study finds that depressive disorder is one of the most powerful predictors of suicide. Tanney reports that the overall risk of suicide for persons with active mental disorders is 7 to 10 times that of the general population. Comorbid major depression and substance abuse represent a lethal combination. Mental disorders may be either direct or indirect links to suicide. Also, mental disorders may be necessary but not sufficient to produce suicide and should be understood as part of an intrapersonal infrastructure.

Chapter 14 (coauthored with Mark J. Goldblatt) considers physical illness and suicide. Although physical illness is a risk factor for suicide, the relationships between the two are complex and are usually contingent upon other traits. For example, it is obvious that most patients with acute or chronic illness do *not* suicide. However, some medical conditions have an associated suicide risk. For example, in one study the risk of suicide in patients undergoing kidney dialysis was found to be increased 14.5 times, 11.4 times for patients with malignant neoplasms of the head and neck, and 6.6 times for HIV/AIDS patients. The chapter reviews associations between physical illnesses (e.g., multiple sclerosis, epilepsy, cancer, spinal cord injury, HIV/AIDS, peptic ulcer disease, autoimmune disorders, and terminal illness) and suicide. The chapter also considers characteristics of physical illnesses that may predispose one to suicide.

After depressive disorders, alcoholism and other substance abuse disorders are probably the second most powerful single predictor of suicide outcomes. In Chapter 15 David Lester reviews research on both alcoholism and substance abuse as they relate to suicide attempts and completions. He notes (following Menninger) that substance abuse itself may be partially self-destructive—perhaps even a slow, chronic suicide. Substance abuse has many potentially confounding, interactive effects with suicide, such as the physiologically depressing consequences of alcoholism, cognitive effects (e.g., impulsivity) of substance abuse, and the relation of substance abuse to brain neurotransmitter changes.

Most of the substance abuse research (whether on the individual or societal level) has followed alcohol abuse. Some of the predictors of completed suicide among alcohol abusers include being male, older, white, in the later stages of alcoholism, and with more affective disorder and hopelessness, more broken homes, and more prior suicidal behavior. Many suicides consume alcohol just before killing themselves and as many as 18% of all alcoholics eventually die by suicide.

Predictors of suicide in drug abusers in general include more psychiatric disturbances in their families, more concomitant alcohol abuse, less intravenous drug use, and more prison sentences. In spite of the emphasis on the importance of substance abuse in determining suicide outcome, Lester concludes that there are not many useful, reliable alcohol or drug abuse predictors of suicide. Furthermore, many of the suicide prediction scales (such as Lettieri's) do not even include substance abuse as a measure.

Chapter 16 emphasizes that low 5-HT (serotonin) and its metabolite, 5-HIAA, are probably the best documented biological markers of suicide outcome. Research on suicides suggests that there is deregulation of central nervous system adrenergic function and of the hypothalamic–pituitary–adrenal axis. Decreased brain serotonergic function may be related to aggression, violence, and increased impulsivity, and may be independent of psychiatric diagnosis. Chapter 16 reviews (1) the genetics of suicidal behavior, twin studies, and adoption studies; (2) biochemical investigations (especially, of dopamine, neuroendocrine measures, norepinephrine and 3-methoxy-4-hydroxyphenolglycol, low 5-HIAA in violent suicides, and postmortem studies); (3) psychopharmacology of suicidal behavior and medications for the treatment of suicidal individuals (especially the SSRIs and electroconvulsive therapy); (4) special cases and combined psychopharmacological therapies; and (5) implications for suicide prevention.

In Chapter 17, Robert Plutchik, one of a team of violence and aggression experts from the Albert Einstein College of Medicine, was invited to relate general violence to the subject of suicide. The chapter attempts to delineate (although there is some obvious overlap) risk and protective factors in violence toward self versus toward others. Risk factors are outlined for suicidal behaviors versus violent nonsuicidal behaviors, as well as quantitative weights (i.e., partial correlations) for the relative strengths of these risk factors. Plutchik discusses "amplifier" versus "attenuator" variables and an interesting class of new drugs he calls "serenics," designed particularly to reduce aggressive behaviors, as opposed to a prior focus on antidepressant medications to treat suicide-related mental conditions. The chapter closes with an outline of the Einstein theoretical model of the relationships of suicide and violence.

Part IV of CTS addresses ancillary, related issues and topics that are nonetheless important in suicidology. For example, not all suicidal behavior is explicitly self-destructive, nor is the individual's intention clearly to die. Here we might think of risky sports activities, unprotected sex, driving while intoxicated, or gambling. For example, consider a case in which a young man had a blood alcohol of .4 and had used cocaine, then played Russian Roulette and died. Was this a case of suicide? Because the man had a 5/6 chance to survive, perhaps he intended to live?

Chapter 18 (coauthored with Norman L. Farberow) defines "indirect self-destructive behavior" (and distinguishes it from risk taking), discusses relevant theories, and then examines high-risk sports, pathological gambling, self-mutilation, unprotected sex, prostitution, simulated risk taking in lab situations, motor vehicle accidents, driving under the influence of substances, mountain climbing, Russian roulette, and autoerotic asphyxia—all amply illustrated by case examples.

Chapter 19 discusses ethical, religious, and philosophical issues in suicide. For example, is suicide *ever* the right thing to do? Can suicide be rational, or is "rational suicide" an oxymoron? If suicide is sometimes an appropriate death, then under what circumstances? The case of Dutch suicide Nico Spijer is presented. Should physicians help their patients die? The work of Dr. Jack Kevorkian and Derek Humphry (*Final Exit*) is reviewed, as are the types of euthanasia and the right-to-die legislation.

Generally, religion is a protective factor for suicide, except in some suicide cults (such as Heaven's Gate or Jonestown). The philosophy of suicide takes two basic positions: (1) the Kantian, which maintains that suicides depart from some ideal and are seldom, if ever, right; and (2) the utilitarian, which asks whether a suicide would produce happiness or beneficent consequences, and for whom. Finally, Chapter 19 asks, Whose life is it? Can we do anything we want to with our own bodies?

Chapter 20 observes that suicide is not now illegal (some history of suicide and the law is outlined; cf. Chapter 4), but assisted suicide tends to be illegal in most states. At the very least, suicide has serious legal consequences. For example, life insurance taken out within 2 years can be contested and payment denied (these are usually equivocal manner-of-death issues); psychological and medical caregivers can be sued for malpractice (negligence issues from standard care are involved); institutions such as jails, prisons, schools, drug companies, or hospitals can be sued for substandard care (including architectural faults) or faulty products (including the failure to warn); and there can be compensation to a worker's survivors if one's job is found to be a proximate cause of his/her suicide.

This chapter defines and reviews standard-of-care issues and threats of various treatment failures, suicide proofing at institutions, and suicide watches and security measures, among other issues—all with case illustrations.

Chapter 21 focuses on treatment, usually after the onset of "disease" (here, of suicide), and on prevention (usually before the onset and often population based). It is insufficient just to understand self-destructive behaviors. Most suicides (as we noted in the opening to this Preface) are needless, premature deaths that deserve intervention, treatment, and (if possible) prevention (first-class treatment does not guarantee suicide prevention). Treatment and prevention of suicide can be at either the individual or the population level.

At the individual level, the chapter discusses problems of compliance, transference, countertransference, assessment, inpatient versus outpatient treatment (including when to hospitalize), crisis intervention, cognitive and dialectical therapies, psychoanalytic therapy, electroconvulsive therapy, psychopharmacological treatment (cf. Chapter 16), social system interventions, and special groups (such as the aged patient).

At the institutional prevention level, Chapter 21 reviews conceptual models of prevention; distinguishes primary, secondary, and tertiary prevention; considers school suicide prevention programs; and then concludes with the July 1999 U.S. Surgeon General's "Call to Action" national suicide prevention recommendations.

Of course, suicide may end the troubled individual's problems, but it also creates serious problems for survivors of suicide (for children, spouses, parents, friends, etc.). Invited authors David A. Jobes and colleagues note in the text's concluding chapter, Chapter 22, that suicides rarely occur in an interpersonal vacuum. We estimated previously that on average each suicide affects at least six survivors. Questions often abound after a suicide: Could I have prevented this? Was I responsible for the suicide? Will my children inherit any biological or genetic predisposition to suicide themselves? Why did this suicide happen? How could he/she have done this to me (i.e., there is anger and frustration)?

This chapter provides a brief history of the survivor movement. Questions like, How is suicide survivor grief unique? are asked and answered. Research on this topic is surveyed. Chapter 22 also asks how suicide survivors can be helped and notes that clinicians who lose patients are survivors too. In a section that mirrors Chapter 10, the chapter inquires whether suicides are destined to be copied, modeled, or imitated by survivors. Chapter 22 concludes with a discussion of "postvention" (i.e., of helpful, healing acts after a suicide) and of school-based prevention programs.

We now invite readers to reflect on this overview. We would like to know what our readers think. We are hopeful that CTS will have several editions and we can incorporate our readers' feedback in subsequent editions.

To be sure, we could have done some things differently. Others might have accentuated some parts of this text and deemphasized others. One always wonders when to stop and commit the work to print. Please note that in 1998–1999, when the bulk of the writing and revision was done, 1996 vital statistics on suicide were the most recent data available.

We would like to acknowledge the unflinching support of the Guilford staff, who nonetheless managed to remind us what was possible and wise—especially Editor-in-Chief, Seymour Weingarten and our tireless Production Editor, William Meyer, who had incredible patience and good nature. Special thanks is also due to Adnan Omar, Dr. Maris's graduate assistant, who secured the majority of the permissions, and Gabriella Maris, who typed a great many of the references. Of course, without the indulgence, encouragement, and comforting of our spouses, families, and institutions, this textbook might never have been finished. Heartfelt thanks to you all.

One parting thought: In a very real sense this textbook is offered as a partial settlement of the immense intellectual and spiritual debt that we all owe our mentors and friends, including, but not limited to, Robert E. Litman, Seymour Perlin, Jerome A. Motto, Norman L. Farberow, and maybe most of all to Edwin S. Shneidman, who had the original vision for suicidology as a distinct professional and clinical subdiscipline. We hope they taught us well!

RONALD W. MARIS, PhD
ALAN L. BERMAN, PhD
MORTON M. SILVERMAN, MD

Contents

PART I

FOUNDATIONS OF SUICIDOLOGY

1

Introduction to the Study of Suicide

> No one ever lacks a good reason to suicide.
> —CESARE PAVESE

This textbook provides a systematic introduction to the scientific study of suicide (i.e., "suicidology") and to suicide prevention. It aims to be comprehensive, academically sound, and clinically relevant. Suicidal behaviors are complex and multifaceted. Their richness, diversity, and stubborn persistence transculturally throughout recorded human history are stiff challenges to those of us who would understand, predict, and intervene in them.

WHY STUDY SUICIDE?

On the most fundamental existential level we pay attention to suicide because it is there, has a kind of riveting compulsion to it, and is an unavoidable, sometimes devastating, life issue. The French philosopher/novelist Albert Camus (1945) has written eloquently about this essential, compelling aspect of suicides. Whether one can live or chooses to live is the only truly serious philosophical problem, according to Camus. Camus claims that man invented God in order to be able to live without killing himself and that the only human liberty is to come to terms with death. "Suicide," Camus writes, "is prepared within the silence of the heart, as is a great work of art" (Camus, 1945).

Sigmund Freud as well saw life-and-death wishes as inextricably intertwined (see Gay, 1988, Chs. 8 and 9). Freud argued, "Life is impoverished, it loses its interest, when the highest stake in the game of living, life itself, cannot be risked" (quoted in Alvarez, 1970). Early on Freud saw aggression as a product of frustration of sexual impulses and, indeed, tended to see all life energy as sexual energy. However, after witnessing the carnage of World War I Freud decided there were two opposing basic instincts: life (*eros*) and death (*thanatos*) drives. All instincts sought tension reduction.

To illustrate, libido sought to reduce sexual tensions, whereas the death instinct sought the elimination of the tension of life itself. Basically, life sought the peace of death or, as Freud put it, the universal goal of all living substances was to "return to the quiesence of the inorganic world." Freud contended that much external aggression against others was necessary to avoid self-destruction. In discussing melancholia (depression) Freud felt that people did not find the energy to kill themselves unless they were first killing an internalized object previously identified with and then turned this prior external death wish against a fragment of their own ego ("ego splitting"; see Litman, 1967). Freud also believed that suicide is more likely in advanced civilizations requiring greater repression of sexual and aggressive energy.

Second, in a sense one also studies suicide and death in order to live better. Suicidology is not necessarily a morbid, ghoulish preoccupation, as we might naively imagine. One could argue that the cloud of a shortish, finite lifespan tends to cast a pall over all of our lives, and this can lead to a pervasive underlying mild functional depression (a kind of low-ebb dysthymia), a lack of hope about life's ultimate worthwhileness, or even despair (Becker, 1973; Brown, 1959). Some suicides may be seen as rational when, in spite of considerable effort to live better (often including repeated psychotherapy and pharmacological treatment), our lives are still insufficiently pleasurable or meaningful (Maris, 1981).

As Camus suggested, religion is part and parcel of suicidal thoughts and actions. For example, do our lives have some ultimate purpose such that we are morally obligated to live them out, even with suffering and pain to rival that of Job? Perhaps the basic societal repulsion to suicide is not that someone dies but, rather, the hubris of men and women who would take their lives into their own hands and out of the hands of God? However, one could argue convincingly that suicides more often than not have failed troubled lives and relative biological unfitness and usually find a premature, perhaps unnecessary resolution to their life problems. That is, suicide is often a kind of Darwinian inability to live at all or to live well enough to survive.

Third, what is it that we are proposing to study? Although a complete answer to this question will be deferred until Chapter 2, "suicidology" can be defined as "the scientific study of suicide and suicide prevention" (Shneidman, quoted in Maris, 1993). "Suicidology" is similar to "psychology." That is, suicidology is the science of self-destructive behaviors, thoughts, feelings, and so on in the same way that psychology is the science dealing with the mind and mental processes, feelings, desires, and so on. No doubt, "suicidology" sounds alien to many, but no doubt so did "psychology" and "psychiatry" at first. Suicidology is unlike the other behavioral sciences in that it has usually included not just the study of suicide but also its prevention. In a sense suicidology is like internal medicine. An internist might well say, "You have a lump in your breast" or "You have a mass in your prostate,"—"a surgeon ought to take a look at it." Not to add the suggested clinical intervention seems highly inappropriate (E. Shneidman, personal communication, 1992). Nevertheless, there are some suicidologists who claim that the concept of suicidology does not logically entail suicide prevention (Battin, 1996; Humphry, 1996).

Suicidology includes not only completed suicide and nonfatal attempted suicide but also partial self-destruction, suicidal gestures and ideation, parasuicide (Kreitman, 1977), deliberate self-harm, self-mutilation, and a panorama of related self-destructive behaviors and attitudes (Maris 1992d). As we shall see shortly, completed suicide is a relatively rare behavior—occurring at a rate of 1 to 3 per 10,000 per year in the general population. However, completed suicide is just the tip of the proverbial self-destructive iceberg. One must always consider the full range of a subject's dependent variable (in this case, suicide). Of course, we also have to be careful not to make our dependent variable overly broad. We do not want to have too many diverse outcomes all being designated "suicidal." Not all behaviors and attitudes are self-destructive. If we have many different self-destructive outcomes, they likely will have somewhat unique, specific explanations. Because suicide is not one thing but many related overlapping phenomena, it follows that neither does it have one cause or etiology.

An absolutely fundamental distinction is between completed suicides and nonfatal suicide attempts (Maris, 1992e). By definition "suicide" implies a death whereas a suicide attempt does not necessarily. Suicide attempters and completers are overlapping populations, but one should never forget that about 85 percent of suicide attempters eventually die a natural death. Clinicians need to be extremely careful not to generalize inappropriately from their partially self-destructive patients to completed suicides (as Freud did). How many scientific journal articles and research monographs have we all seen titled "Suicide . . . ," even though not a single case in their samples actually died? There are many important differences between completed suicides and nonfatal suicide attempts. Some of these differences include the method used, the number of suicide attempts, sex, age, the site of the self-injury, interpersonal dynamics, leaving a suicide note, physical health, and social isolation—just to mention a few. The psychodynamics, motivation, and intent, for example, of fatal and nonfatal suicide attempts are often quite different. As this is a textbook about suicide and suicide prevention, we need to be certain that our data base includes actual completed suicides (i.e., dead people). We return to this critical and complex distinction later on (in this chapter and again in Chapter 12).

Not only is the focus here be on completed suicide, it is on the treatment of suicidal *individuals*, as well. We should not forget that suicides tend to die one at a time and have their own unique life histories. High-risk groups, profiles according to the Minnesota Multiphasic Personality Inventory (MMPI) depressives, alcoholics, and so on, never kill themselves—individual people do. This should suggest to clinicians that suicide treatment plans and suicide prevention and intervention strategies need to be tailored to fit the special needs, pain, situations, and biology of a particular individual.

Furthermore, this text has a major focus on the the treatment, intervention, and prevention of individual suicides. For example, most chapters present suicide cases. The clinical management (including psychotherapies and pharmacotherapies) *of suicidal individuals* is one of our key objectives. We hope that this text can become a handbook for those faced with the daily self-destructive crises and clinical exigencies of psychiatric hospitals, emergency rooms, outpatient mental health centers, suicide prevention and crisis intervention centers, and the like.

Fourth, to study suicide we need proper textbooks, reference books, and handbooks. Currently serious *lacunae* exist for those who wish to study self-destructive behaviors or treat suicidal individuals. Put simply, there really is no basic suicidology textbook, for example, like *Comprehensive Textbook of Psychiatry* (Kaplan & Sadock, 1995) or *Introductory Textbook of Psychiatry* (Andreasen & Black, 1995). A few physicians and behavioral scientists have tried to fill this gap in the study of suicide. For example, in 1975 Perlin edited an excellent book titled *A Handbook for the Study of Suicide* based on the Johns Hopkins Medical School's postgraduate suicidology training program (see Maris, 1993). Although it was an outstanding collection of essays by distinguished authors, the *Handbook* was not a true textbook; it tended to focus on disciplines rather than on suicide topics or suicidal individuals, had little empirical information (e.g., there were almost no tables), and was not very comprehensive.

A more recent effort to produce a suicide text is *Suicide Over the Life Cycle: Risk Factors, Assessment, and Treatment of Suicidal Patients* (Blumenthal & Kupfer, 1990). This book is indeed more comprehensive, does focus on suicidal patients, and has much useful clinical information, scales, and data. Its biggest drawback is that it is also an edited volume with no consistent, integrated argument or perspective. As in most edited books, some chapters are strong while others are not as strong. Also, some chapters are highly repetitious. More important, Blumenthal and Kupfer fail to give the clinician much advice as to which of the reviewed studies, research findings, suicide prevention techniques, and so on, are recommended, preferred, or most likely to be true. One feels at sea in an ocean of suicidological alternative explanations. Both the harried clinician and the serious suicide scholar deserve more guidance than they receive from Blumenthal and Kupfer.

There have been other efforts at suicide texts (e.g., Jacobs & Brown, 1989; Jacobs, Jacobs, and Bongar, 1992), but for their considerable merits they tend to be subject to the same problems as the Perlin and Blumenthal and Kupfer books.

Clinicians in applied settings (hospital emergency rooms, crisis intervention or suicide prevention centers, community mental health centers, etc.) also need a basic suicidological reference book. For example, which specific psychotropic medications are recommended for reducing suicidal ideation or behavior and which drugs may even exacerbate it? What are the major specific alternative therapies for which type of self-destructive behaviors? How does suicide treatment vary by age, sex, race, marital status, occupation, and so on? What should one do after a suicide occurs in a hospital or clinic? How is self-destructive behavior managed differentially in various settings (jails and prisons, at home, psychiatric hospitals, seclusion rooms, outpatient clinics, schools, hotels, bridges, etc.)? What does one do exactly to treat various kinds of overdoses? The list goes on and on. Those of us who work in applied settings with suicidal individuals need such information in one convenient resource or reference book.

For a long time there was little possibility of textual codification of the study of suicide because suicidology was a relatively new subdiscipline. Much of the scientific groundwork simply had not been done. However, now a reasonably mature textbook on suicidology and suicide prevention can be written. For example, since the 1960s the National Institute of Mental Health has been funding basic research on suicide and the results have begun to accumulate. Indeed, one important service of any textbook to to consolidate and integrate research findings scattered in various scientific journals from diverse disciplines. In part the *Comprehensive Textbook of Suicidology* is being written now because it can be done and needs to be done to further the scientific study of suicide.

Finally, the study and prevention of suicide are interdependent. Understanding logically precedes intervention and control. Without a solid scientific foundation suicide prevention is doomed to be ineffective. Thus, another reason why we study suicide is to be able to intervene effectively in self-destructive behaviors. Although one could understand suicide without preventing it, almost no one studies suicide to be better able to promote or assist it (however, see Humphry, 1996; Kevorkian, 1991). Individuals who are in pain, hopeless, depressed, anxious, psychotic, and so on, have a right to relief short of irreversible cessation of their consciousness (i.e., death).

Accordingly, this textbook has an unabashed pragmatic, intervention, case-focused, clinical treatment approach. For example, each chapter includes boxed asides considering assessment, treatment, and management of specific suicidal individuals. In these boxed asides clinicians discuss the concrete practicalities of suicide prevention for actual cases.

Also, there are two suicide treatment and prevention chapters near the end of the text that address general suicide issues such as assessment tools and procedures, drug treatments, different therapeutic modalities, physical examinations and tests, the various settings of suicide intervention, primary versus secondary and tertiary suicide prevention, transference problems, and much more. The prevention of suicide deserves its science. Suicide prevention cannot be founded solely on anecdotes, visceral impressions, magic, intuition, and subjective clinical judgments—as important as these sometimes are. Having briefly reviewed why one studies suicide, let us now examine in more detail the scope of suicidal problems.

SCOPE OF THE PROBLEM

Incidence and Prevalence of Self-Destructive Behaviors

In a sense, it is misleading to speak of "the" problem of suicide or suicide prevention because suicide is not one thing or problem but is in fact many different overlapping yet somewhat distinct problems. In fact the success or failure of suicidological science depends in large measure on how carefully we specify and operationally define our dependent variables. Also, broad epidemiological or socio-demographic problems of suicide are quite different from individual suicide case treatment problems.

As Table 1.1 illustrates, suicide is relatively rare in the general population, occurring at a rate of about 11 to 12 per 100,000 or 1 to 2 per 10,000 in the United States. Even though suicide is rare we have to take it seriously, because it is a premature, fatal outcome—often with devastating interpersonal and economic consequences. Annually suicides account for under 1½% of all deaths. In the most recent year for which data were available (1996) there were 30,903 suicidal deaths in the United States (although given the stigma of suicide, 30,903 is probably an undercount). This made suicide the 9th leading cause of death, ranking ahead of liver and kidney disease deaths and just behind pneumonia, diabetes, and HIV deaths. Recent data (July 29, 1999) rank suicide as the 8th leading cause of death, HIV deaths having dropped to 15th).

When we examine causes of death over four decades (1950–1990; see Table 1.2) some interesting patterns emerge. Except for a slight peak in the 1970s (reflecting mainly increased rates for young white males) the suicide rate has been relatively constant. At the same time heart disease death rates basically have declined (from a 1950 rate of 307 to 156 in 1989), as have pneumonia and flu death rates. One consequence is that in this century suicide has moved up in the rankings of leading causes of death (as have homicide and death rates related to cigarette smoking and air pollution—like emphysema and respiratory cancers). Medical technology and improved public health apparently have lowered the rates of many leading causes of natural death (although note some recent pattern reversals in Table 1.1), but not violent death rates such as suicide and homicide.

Suicide is especially a problem for white males, who commit roughly 73% of all suicides (cf., Table 3.2). If we add white females, who commit 17% of all suicides, then it is obvious that suicide occurs primarily among whites in the United States (viz., 90% of all suicides). When we move from percentages to suicide rates by sex and race (1996 vital sta-

TABLE 1.1. **Mortality from 10 Leading Causes of Death (Rates per 100,000), United States, 1996**

Cause of death and rank order	Rate	% of total deaths
All causes	872.5	100.0
1. Diseases of the heart	276.4	31.7
2. Malignant neoplasms	203.4	23.3
3. Cerebrovascular diseases	60.3	6.9
4. Chronic obstructive pulmonary diseases	40.0	4.5
5. Accidents	35.8	4.1
6. Pneumonia and influenza	31.6	3.6
7. Diabetes mellitus	23.3	2.7
8. HIV infection	11.7	1.4
9. Suicide	**11.6**	**1.3**
10. Chronic liver disease and cirrhosis	9.4	1.1
All other causes	169.0	19.4

Source: National Center for Health Statistics (1998), *Vital Statistics of the United States, 1996: Vol. II. Mortality, Part A.* Washington, DC: U.S. Government Printing Office.

TABLE 1.2. Age-Adjusted Death Rates (per 100,000 Resident Population) for Selected Causes of Death, United States, Selected Years, 1950–1990

Cause of death	1950[a]	1960[a]	1970	1980	1990
All causes	840.5	760.9	714.3	585.8	520.2
Natural causes	766.6	695.2	636.9	519.7	465.1
Disease of heart	307.2	286.2	253.6	202.0	152.0
Ischemic heart disease	—	—	—	149.8	102.6
Cerebrovascular disease	88.6	79.7	66.3	40.8	27.7
Malignant neoplasms	125.3	125.8	129.8	132.8	135.0
Respiratory system	12.8	19.2	28.4	36.4	41.4
Colorectal	19.0	17.7	16.8	15.5	13.6
Prostate	13.4	13.1	13.3	14.4	16.7
Breast	22.2	22.3	23.1	22.7	23.1
Chronic obstructive pulmonary diseases	4.4	8.2	13.2	15.9	19.7
Pneumonia and influenza	26.2	28.0	22.1	12.9	14.0
Chronic liver disease and cirrhosis	8.5	10.5	14.7	12.2	8.6
Diabetes mellitus	14.3	13.6	14.1	10.1	11.7
Nephritis, nephrotic syndrome, and nephrosis	—	—	—	4.5	4.3
Septicemia	—	—	—	2.6	4.1
Altheroscierosis	—	—	—	5.7	2.7
Human immunodeficiency virus infection	—	—	—	—	9.8
External causes	73.9	65.7	77.4	66.1	55.1
Accident and adverse effects	57.5	49.9	53.7	42.3	32.5
Motor vehicle accidents	23.3	22.5	27.4	22.9	18~
Suicide	11.0	10.6	11.8	11.4	11.5
Homicide and legal intervention	5.4	5.2	9.1	10.8	10.2
Drug-induced causes	—	—	—	3.0	3.6
Alcohol-induced causes	—	—	—	8.4	7.2

[a]Includes deaths of nonresidents of the United States.
Note. Data are based on the National Vital Statistics System. For data years shown, the code numbers for cause of death are based on the then current International Classification of Diseases, which are described in that book's Appendix II, Tables IV and V. Categories for the coding and classification of human immunodeficiency virus infection were introduced in the United States beginning with mortality data for 1987.
Sources: National Center for Health Statistics (1968), Vital Statistics Rates in the United States, 1940–1960, by R. D. Grove & A. M. Hetzel (DHEW Pub. No. [PHS] 1677). Washington, DC: U.S. Government Printing Office; unpublished data from the Division of Vital Statistics; National Center for Health Statistics, Vital Statistics of the United States: Vol. II. Mortality, Part A, for data years 1950–1989. Washington, DC: U.S. Government Printing Office; data computed by the Division of Analysis from data compiled by the Division of Vital Statistics.

tistics; see McIntosh, 1998), white males have the highest rates (20.9 per 100,000), followed by nonwhite males (11.3), white females (4.8), and nonwhite females (2.5) (see Table 1.3; cf. Garrison, 1992: 487, and McIntosh, 1998). Male suicide rates exceed female suicide rates usually by a ratio of 4 or 5 to 1, while white suicide rates are typically a little over twice those of blacks.

Generally as we age our suicide potential also rises. Especially for white males, suicide rates are highest in the oldest age groups (e.g., 72 per 100,000 for white males 85 years old and older; see Leenaars, Maris, McIntosh, & Richman, 1992). Female suicide rates usually peak in the 45–54 age group, then drop slightly in older age groups. One striking age and suicide rate variation between 1950 and 1990 (actually the peak occurred in about 1977) occurred among young people 15–24 years old, whose suicide rate more than tripled (from 6.6 to 23.2 in white males). The relationships of suicide rates to other important predictor variables (marital status, occupation, mental disorder diagnosis, alco-

TABLE 1.3. **Death Rates for Suicide According to Sex, Race, and Age, United States, Selected Years, 1950–1996**

Sex, race and age	1950[a]	1960[a]	1970	1980	1990	1996
All races						
All ages, age adjusted	11.0	10.6	11.8	11.4	11.5	10.8
All ages, crude	11.4	10.6	11.6	11.9	12.04	11.6
Under 1 year	—	—	—	—	—	—
1–4 years	—	—	—	—	—	—
5–14 years	0.2	0.5	0.5	0.4	0.8	0.8
15–24 years	4.5	5.2	1.0	12.3	13.2	12.0
25–34 years	0.3	30.0	14.1	16.0	35.2	14.3
35–44 years	14.2	14.2	16.9	15.4	13.3	15.5
45–54 years	20.9	20.7	20.0	15.9	14.1	14.9
55–64 years	27.0	22.7	23.4	15.9	16.0	13.7
65–74 years	29.2	22.0	20.3	16.9	17.9	35.0
75–84 years	31.1	27.9	23.2	39.3	24.9	20.0
85 years and over	28.8	26.0	19.0	19.2	22.2	20.2
White male						
All ages, age adjusted	18.1	17.5	18.2	18.9	20.1	19.1
All ages, crude	19.0	17.6	18.0	19.9	22.0	21.2
Under 1 year	—	—	—	—	—	—
1–4 years	—	—	—	—	—	—
5–14 years	0.2	0.5	0.5	0.7	3.3	2.3
15–24 years	4.6	3.6	13.9	23.4	22.2	20.9
25–34 years	32.3	34.9	19.9	25.4	25.6	25.1
35–44 years	22.4	20.9	22.2	22.5	25.3	25.7
45–54 years	24.3	22.7	29.5	24.2	24.3	24.9
55–64 years	45.9	40.2	35.0	22.1	27.3	24.9
65–74 years	55.2	42.0	30.7	32.5	34.2	29.6
75–84 years	61.9	55.7	455	43.3	60.2	46.3
85 years and over	61.9	63.2	45.3	52.1	70.3	65.4
Black male						
All ages, age adjusted	7.0	7.8	9.9	11.1	12.4	11.8
All ages, crude	6.2	6.4	3.0	10.3	12.0	11.4
Under 1 year	—	—	—	—	—	—
1–4 years	—	—	—	—	—	—
5–14 years	*—	*—	*—	0.9	0.8	0.9
15–24 years	4.9	4.1	10.5	12.3	15.1	16.7
25–34 years	9.3	12.4	19.2	21.5	21.9	17.8
35–44 years	10.4	12.8	12.6	15.6	16.9	17.8
45–54 years	10.4	10.8	13.8	12.0	14.8	11.8
55–64 years	16.5	16.2	10.6	11.7	10.8	11.8
65–74 years	10.0	11.3	8.7	11.1	14.7	12.7
75–84 years	—	6.6	8.9	30.5	14.4	12.5
85 years and over	—	6.9	*8.7	*18.9	*19.6	—

(cont.)

TABLE 1.3. (*cont.*)

Sex, race and age	1950[a]	1960[a]	1970	1980	1990	1996
White female						
All ages, age adjusted	5.3	3.3	7.2	5.7	6.3	4.4
All ages, crude	3.5	5.2	7.3	5.9	5.3	4.8
Under 1 year	—	—	—	—	—	—
1–4 years	—	—	—	—	—	—
5–14 years	*0.1	*0.1	0.1	0.2	0.4	—
15–24 years	2.7	2.3	4.2	4.6	4.2	3.8
25–34 years	5.2	5.3	9.0	7.3	6.0	6.4
35–44 years	1.2	3.3	13.0	9.3	7.4	6.4
45–54 years	10.5	10.9	13.5	10.2	7.3	7.0
55–64 years	10.7	10.9	12.3	9.3	3.0	7.0
65–74 years	10.6	3.3	9.6	7.0	7.2	5.0
75–84 years	8.4	9.2	7.2	5.7	6.7	—
85 years and over	8.9	6.1	5.8	5.8	5.4	*—
Black female						
All ages, age adjusted	1.7	1.9	2.9	2.4	2.4	2.0
All ages, crude	1.3	1.6	2.6	2.2	2.3	2.0
Under 1 year	—	—	—	—	—	—
1–4 years	—	—	—	—	—	—
5–14 years	*—	*0.0	0.2	*0.1	*0.3	—
15–24 years	*1.8	*1.3	3.8	2.3	2.3	2.3
25–34 years	2.6	3.0	5.7	4.1	3.7	2.9
35–44 years	2.0	3.0	3.7	4.6	4.0	2.9
45–54 years	3.5	3.1	3.7	2.8	3.2	2.3
55–64 years	*1.1	3.0	*2.0	2.3	2.6	2.3
65–74 years	*1.9	*2.3	*2.9	*1.7	2.6	2.3
75–84 years	—	*1.3	*1.7	*1.4	*0.6	—
85 years and over	—	*—	*2.8	*—	*2.6	—

*Based on fewer than 20 deaths.
Note. Data are based on the National Vital Statistics System. For years shown, the code numbers for cause of death are based on the then current *International Classification of Diseases*, which are described in that book's Appendix II, Tables IV and V.
[a]Include deaths of nonresidents of the United States.

hol and substance abuse, methods of attempting suicide, etc.) are elaborated on in subsequent chapters.

Readers need to be aware (*caveat emptor*) that this textbook focuses on current *United States* suicidal behaviors. But clearly the incidence, prevalence, epidemiology, and etiology, of suicide and suicide rates vary by race, nation, culture, and special groups (see especially Chapter 7). For example, in some cultures or racial and ethnic groups suicide is virtually nonexistent (e.g., among the Tiv of Nigeria, the Andaman Islanders, and the Yahgans of Tierra del Fuego; see Evans & Farberow, 1988). Suicide is present in other groups but the rates are extremely low (e.g., among black American females, Irish Catholics, Mexicans, or Muslims in such countries as Egypt).

At the opposite extreme some countries have suicide rates so perennially high that they are almost part of the national character. Among these high-suicide-rate countries are Hungary, Germany, Austria, Czechoslovakia, Japan, and Finland (see Schmidtke, 1997; Diekstra, 1990; Kushner, 1991). One needs to remember these important variations in incidence and prevalence rates of suicide and self-destructive behaviors. Although suicide tends to exist in all places at all times and in all peoples, suicide is still by no means universal and its epidemiology and dynamics vary considerably. One striking example of this variation is the predominant use of guns to suicide in the United States but hanging in most of Europe.

Another caveat is that the suicide problems reflected in rates, social and economic trends, demographic groups, and countries are all very different from the problems of individual suicides. Science, including suicidology, tends to be grounded in large, random samples or empirical groups analyzed statistically and mathematically to generate confirmed hypotheses, causal models, generic research results, and, ideally, some law-like propositions related systematically in theories of suicide (e.g., Beck's cognitive theory). However, ultimately suicidology is concerned with the problems of assessing, predicting, and preventing small numbers of suicide often one at a time (although, of course, one could do broad primary prevention of suicide as well; see Felner, 1995). Clinical suicidology has special needs that, for example, public health suicidology does not. All the suicide rates, statistics, psychological tests, hypotheses, data sets, and research findings are not worth much to the front-line suicide prevention clinician if they do not speak to the pain, suffering, and needs of ad hoc, ad hominem, individual would-be suicides.

Finally, in addition to the routine problems of suicidology suggested by the table of contents of this textbook (age, sex, race, work, mental and physical illness, social relations, biology, alcoholism, etc.) the full scope of suicidology and suicide prevention also encompasses several related special problems. These special problems include the current worldwide AIDS epidemic, gun control, norms condoning violence, suicide rate surges (like that of 15- to 24-year-olds in the United States between 1950 and 1977), problems of chronic suicidality versus emergency medicine and crisis intervention, maleness and suicide, elderly suicide, assisted suicide, and many more. Often these special suicide problems are considered throughout this text in topical asides, sometimes in a "pro/con" polemical format.

Therapy and Treatment Problems

Because this text will have an individual case treatment focus, any consideration of the scope of the suicide problems must inquire about patient, client, and emergency room visits that involve suicide-related problems. Are suicide, self-destructive behavior, and suicide ideation common treatment problems? We know from studies by Chemtob, Hamada, Bauer, Kinney, and Torigoe (1988) and Bongar (1992) that the lifetime risk of a psychologist losing a patient to suicide is about 20% and the same risk for a psychiatrist is up to 50%. When Rich, Young, and Fowler (1986b) investigated completed suicides in San Diego, they concluded that about 25% of all suicides were in treatment at the time they killed themselves. In an early study by Litman (1982) it was estimated that 1% of all suicides occur in psychiatric hospitals. Jacobs (Jacobs & Brown, 1989) claims that when we move to the hospital emergency room, about 15% of all emergency room visits concern suicide or suicide ideation (cf. Doyle, 1990).

Thus, it can be concluded that suicide and self-destruction are fairly common problems among psychological or psychiatric patients—and when suicide does occur, it may lead to malpractice litigation. The most common psychiatric diagnoses associated with suicide outcome of patients are the affective or mood disorders (especially, major depressive episode), the schizophrenias, substance abuse, and some Axis II personality disorders (especially borderline and antisocial personalities, although nonfatal suicide attempts are much more common with most personality disorders; see Tanney, 1992, and Chapter 13).

Even though self-destructive behaviors are fairly common in patient populations, effective treatment depends on suicide risk assessment and prediction *before* the fact of suicide (Maris et al., 1992). Some critical questions facing suicide prevention workers are: which individuals are at risk of suicide? How high is their risk? When and under what circumstances is the suicide event likely to occur? Even in depressed psychiatric hospital patient populations, completed suicide is still relatively rare. As with any rare event, when one attempts to predict the outcome the tendency is to get false positives—here the misidentification of patients as suicides when they are not. For example, psychiatrist Alex Pokorny (1983), using the best predictive tools available, misidentified about 30% of his psychiatric inpatient sample as suicides when they were actually nonsuicides (cf. Pokorny, 1993). Ironically with rare events such as suicide, if one predicted "no suicide" every time, he or she would almost always be right. See Chapter 21 for more about this important problem.

Some psychiatrists (e.g., Motto, 1992) argue that "suicide prediction" is an impossible task if we mean a high suicide probability of a particular individual suiciding within a short time frame. Usually the best we can do is an assessment of *group* suicide risk over periods of about 5–10 years. The so-called high suicide risk groups turn out to be not high risk at all. For example, we often hear that depressed psychiatric inpatients have a 15% chance of sui- ciding (Guze & Robins, 1970; cf. Black & Winokur, 1990). But this means that 85% of them will *never* suicide and that the 15% who do suicide will do so only over usually some 35 to 50 years. Thus, the suicide rate of depressed patients is never more than about 1% in any given year. A related assessment issue is what tools, standardized scales, questionnaires, and interview techniques do clinicians have at their disposal to help assess suicide risk in clients. Several helpful standardized suicide assessment and prediction scales have been re- viewed in detail elsewhere (see Rothberg & Geer-Williams, 1992). Therapists need to use subjective clinical judgment as well as objective tests and measurements when attempting to assess the suicide potential of individuals.

Another therapy or treatment problem concerns *training and education* of suicidolo- gists. How does one become a competent suicide interventionist? How can patients and their families locate qualified physicians, psychologists, nurses, social workers, and pastoral counselors, for example, specializing in suicide prevention and treatment? We know from Bongar (1992) that only 35–40% of doctoral programs in psychology offer any suicide pre- vention or suicidology training. The psychiatry department of the Johns Hopkins University Medical School used to give full-year National Institute of Mental Health (NIMH) funded postdoctoral fellowship (Perlin, 1975).

However, currently there are no postdoctoral professional suicidology training pro- grams (although some individual fellowships are offered) and no professional board certifi- cation in suicidology. If suicide prevention is ever going to mature and develop as a medical or psychological specialty, then training programs like the Johns Hopkins fellowship have to be reinstituted by the federal government. For a more detailed examination of training problems in suicide prevention see Maris (1993).

Because suicide is not a mental disorder or a psychiatric diagnostic category, much of the treatment of suicidal behaviors and ideation is of depressive illness (and other affective or mood disorders, alcoholism and substance abuse, anxiety and panic disorders, the schiz- ophrenias, and some personality disorders). After ruling out organic causes through a thor- ough physical examination and history taking, the backbone of the treatment of most suici- dal individuals is *polydrug therapies, especially antidepressant medications,* combined with psychotherapy. The pharmacological tools of medicine used to treat depressed suicidal pa- tients are legion and new antidepressants seem to appear on the market almost every week.

The list includes sertraline, paroxetine, fluoxetine, nortriptyline, imipramine, clomipramine, amitriptyline, amoxapine, desipramine, maprotiline, trazodone, bupropion, citalopram, venlafaxine, nefazodone, some of the benzodiazepines (e.g., alprazolam), and many others (cf. Goldblatt & Schatzberg, 1990; Chapter 16, this volume). (For a fuller discussion of the scope of treatment of suicidal individuals, readers are referred to Chapter 21 and the special boxed treatment asides throughout this textbook.)

As important as the biological treatment of suicidal depression is, any treatment of a suicidal patient that relies solely on impersonal therapies (e.g., psychoactive medication, seclusion, restraint, and 15-minute checks) may be second rate (J. T. Maltsberger, personal communication, 1992). Many psychiatrists argue that the heart of the treatment of suicidal individuals is the relationship of the therapist and the patient (see Maris et al., 1992: 666), including the issues of transference, and countertransference, and social support (see comments on the mind–body suicide debate; Shneidman, 1993). Furthermore, some of the antidepressant medications have been thought to actually provoke suicidal behaviors or ideation in some individuals (see Box 1.1; however, see *Forsyth v. Eli Lilly*, 1999).

Because suicide is a multidimensional behavior evolving over long complex "suicidal careers" (often over 30 to 60 years) (Maris, 1981a), it follows that the treatment of suicidal problems is itself complex, varied, and specific to individual patients. The panorama of therapies for suicidal clients involves drug and biological treatment (including electroconvulsive therapy), cognitive therapy, crisis intervention and brief psychotherapy, milieu and sociotherapy, behavioral modification and learning therapy, psychoanalytical treatment,

---

**BOX 1.1. Can Fluoxetine (Prozac) Antidepressant Pharmacology
Cause Suicidal Ideation or Suicidal Behavior?**

Yes: Teicher, Glod, and Cole (1990).
No: Mann and Kapur (1991).

Issue Summary:

Yes: "Five depressed outpatients and one inpatient (five females and one male 19–62 years of age) developed intense suicidal thoughts a mean of 26 days (range was 12–50 days) after the initiation of fluoxetine treatment. Upon discontinuing fluoxetine the self-destructive thoughts faded after about 27 days (range 3–49 days). Four patients were receiving 60–80 mg of fluoxetine each day and two received 20–40 mg/day. No patient was actively suicidal at the time fluoxetine treatment began. Fluoxetine is known to be a potent and selective serotonergic uptake inhibitor. Serotonin may well be related to violent suicidal ideation or action and to obsessional thinking . . . fluoxetine may exert a paradoxical response in some patients (e.g., akathisia or motor restlessness, anxiety, nervousness, and insomnia might be special problems with fluoxetine treatment of some patients)."

No: "The hypothesized association [of fluoxetine and suicidal ideation or acts] is surprising because there is considerable evidence of serotonin deficiency in patients who attempt or complete suicide and fluoxetine selectively enhances serotonergic transmission. . . . In cases like Teicher's the presence of comorbid disorders, previous suicidal tendencies or attempts, and a highly variable time interval between the development of suicidal ideation and the initiation of fluoxetine treatment . . . make it difficult to draw any clear conclusions. . . . If suicidal ideation or behavior emerges with fluoxetine administration, it is not simply a complication of higher doses of fluoxetine. . . . One hypothesis is that increased suicidality is secondary to the disorganization of certain vulnerable individuals in response to drug-induced activation and akathisia . . . the emergence of intensification of suicidal ideation and behavior. . . has not been proven to be associated with any specific type of antidepressant."

and many others. The context or setting of treatment can be individual or group, inpatient or outpatient, suicide prevention centers, hospital ERs, and so on.

Other key treatment issues include whether or not to hospitalize a patient; no-suicide contracts; treatment teams; stress and anxiety management; comorbidity; special treatment for schizophrenics; adolescent versus elderly suicides; white, black, and other ethnic suicides; treatment of survivors of suicides; primary, secondary, and tertiary suicide prevention; treatment of suicidal inmates in jails and prisons; school suicide prevention; and much more (Silverman & Maris, 1995; Maris, Berman, & Maltsberger, 1992: 660–667).

It is worth emphasizing that the full scope of treatment of suicides includes therapy for the *survivors* of suicide (see Chapter 22). Suicide may resolve the life problems of the suicidal individual, but it certainly creates lifelong problems for the suicide's family (including especially the spouse, children, and parents of the suicide), friends, and professional caretakers (see Dunne, McIntosh, & Dunne-Maxim, 1987). Suicide is still a highly stigimatized, sudden, unnatural death that requires considerable coping and adjustment by those left behind—usually over a period of years.

Life insurance and other financial benefits may be revoked by a suicide, children and the surviving parent may fear a genetic component to their family member's suicide, survivors may feel guilty for not having been able to prevent a suicide, survivors may experience intense anger for the narcissism of the suicide and for the many adjustments that are required after a suicide, there may be a profound need to understand the "whys" of a suicide, and social support may be desperately needed but in fact absent.

If a physician, therapist, or family member is involved with the suicide, a malpractice suit or other legal action can be taken against them. Therapists are often sued when their clients die, whether or not they were in fact at fault (Maris, 1992b). With the recent increase of so-called rational suicides and assisted suicides (see Humphry, 1996; Kevorkian, 1991; Werth, 1996), survivors are more likely to be damaged by a family member's or friend's suicide. Part of the backlash to Dr. Kevorkian's assisted-suicide activities is that a number of states are now passing laws that make assisting a suicide a felony subject to both fine and imprisonment. The state may not be able to effectively punish a suicide cadaver, but it certainly can make life difficult for the survivors of suicide.

VARIETIES OF SELF-DESTRUCTIVE BEHAVIORS

Earlier we made an initial effort to say what suicidology and by implication this textbook was about. At first blush suicide seems simple and clear. Some pained individual ends their own life—period. However, upon reflection it becomes apparent that suicide is not that simple. For example, suicide is not one thing but many. Already we have seen that our suicidological subject matter can be divided at least into completed suicides, nonfatal suicide attempts, suicidal ideation, and indirect self-destructive behaviors. In Chapter 2 we complicate matters even more by specifying basic subtypes of completers, attempters, ideators, and so on. It will turn out that suicide has great variety. Like much in life, what at first seemed simple is in fact more complex.

Note some of the implications of the variety of suicide and self-destructive behaviors. It is vital that any science specify, define, and operationalize the full range of its dependent variable. Which outcome *exactly* is it that suicidology wishes to predict, assess, intervene in, treat or prevent? It is likely that the dynamics, variables, models, and explanations of different types of suicides, attempts, risk taking, and ideation will themselves be somewhat unique. Thus, unless one examines and describes carefully the full range of suicidological phenomena, suicidology has little hope of being precise, effective, or for that matter, scientific at all. With this in mind a brief overview of a variety of suicidology's major dependent variables follows (for subtypes and more detailed classifications, readers are referred to Chapter 2).

Completed Suicides

A major focus of this textbook is on completed suicides. Suicides are individuals who have actually *died* by their own hand; have been sent to a morgue, funeral home, burial plot, or crematory; and are beyond any therapy. As we noted earlier, many clinicians treat relatively low lethality suicide attempters (e.g., Freud did) and, thus, base their suicidological research and writing not on completed suicides at all. Minimally suicidology must at least start with dead people and their brains (see research at the New York Psychiatric Institute by John Mann and colleagues).

The typical suicide is an older white male who is depressed, maybe alcoholic; lives alone or is socially isolated; uses a highly lethal irreversible method (most often a gunshot to the head); dies after his first suicide attempt; has grown increasingly hopeless and cognitively rigid, may have some debilitating, nagging physical illnesses; has recurring work, sexual, and marital problems; has experienced a series of stressful, negative life events; in some cases has had a prior suicide in his family; and often sees suicide as the only permanent resolution to his persistent life problems (cf. Maris, 1981) concept of a "suicidal career." The rates and prevalence of completed suicides were reviewed previously and need not be repeated here.

In many ways Ernest Hemingway, the famous novelist, was a typical completed suicide (see Case 1.1). He was 61 years old when he shot himself in Ketchum, Idaho. Hemingway's physician father had also suicided (as well as a brother, sister, and granddaughter; see Maris, 1997). In fact, Hemingway's mother later sent him the pistol with which his father had shot himself—as a Christmas present! Hemingway had been depressed ("black assed," as he called it) much of his adult life and was being treated at the Mayo Clinic in Rochester, Minnesota (including electroconvulsive therapy), at the time of his death.

He also drank to excess repeatedly, until it ruined his liver. Hemingway had had multiple (especially head) injuries and illnesses over a long period (including hypertension and a chronic bad back; near the end he had to write standing up). He had been married four times and had numerous love affairs. Hemingway's writing (which he prized above all else) was going poorly and he became acutely paranoid (thinking the FBI and IRS were after him). Although surrounded by people, most of them were sycophants. In his last days Hemingway was preoccupied with thoughts of suicide.

Of course, not all suicides are like Hemingway or have all of the traits in the typical completed suicide profile. For example, although about 77–79% of all U.S. suicides are male, there are some female suicides (17–18%, almost all white; see Garrison, 1992: 487; McIntosh, 1998). And, although about 90–92% of all U.S. suicides are white, there are some nonwhite suicides (mainly males). Although the oldest white males tend to have suicide rate three times higher than younger white males, there are some adolescent suicide completers. The broad category of completed suicide includes probably 4 to 12 major subtypes (see Chapter 2 and Maris, 1992d).

One fairly straightforward way to arrive at major subtypes of suicide is to calculate the cross-classifications of sociodemographic traits and motives of suicides (see Maris, 1992d: 80–83). For example, suicides can be subdivided into younger and older white males, white females, black (African American) males, and black females (ignoring other racial or ethnic groups for the moment). If we assume basic motivations to suicide of escape, revenge, altruism, and risk taking, we could further specify suicide subtypes. To illustrate, Hemingway

CASE 1.1. ERNEST HEMINGWAY'S SUICIDAL CAREER

> On July 2, 1961, a writer whom many critics call the greatest writer of this century, a man who had a zest for life and adventure as big as his genius, a winner of the Nobel Prize and the Pulitzer Prize, a soldier of fortune with a home in Idaho's Sawtooth Mountains, where he hunted in the winter, an apartment in New York, a specially rigged yacht to fish the Gulf Stream, an available apartment at the Ritz in Paris and the Gritti in Venice, a solid marriage, no serious physical ills, good friends everywhere—on that July day, that man, the envy of other men, put a shotgun to his head and killed himself. How did this come to pass? (Hotchner, 1966: ix)

Like Sylvia Plath, *Ernest Hemingway* was a "gifted suicide" whose work and sad death are widely known. Hemingway's life exemplifies many of the traits of suicidal careers discussed throughout this book, especially the role of work problems in self-destruction among males. Accordingly, we depart from our customary consideration of our own individual cases and turn instead to the highlights of the life and death of Ernest Hemingway. Hemingway was born in Oak Park, Illinois, in 1899. His early years do not appear to have been very happy, although Hemingway denied this. Hemingway's physician-father suicided. His mother later sent Hemingway the pistol with which his father shot himself, as a "Christmas present":

> My father died in 1928—shot himself—and left me fifty thousand dollars. . . . When I asked my mother for my inheritance, she said she had already spent it on me . . . on my travel and education. . . . My mother was a music nut, a frustrated singer, and she gave musicales every week in my fifty-thousand dollar music room. . . . Several years later, at Christmas time, I received a package from my mother. It contained the revolver with which my father had killed himself. There was a card that said she thought I'd like to have it. (Hotchner, 1966: 115–116)

It would be exaggerating to conclude that Hemingway experienced some relatively early trauma. Although it might be bold to assume that Hemingway's problems with his mother were *the* cause, it is also well-known that he was married four times and had numerous affairs. His relationships with women often seemed to be explosive, compartmentalized, somewhat distant, and not altogether satisfying. However, it may be that Hemingway, like Plath, simply had great difficulty being very close to anyone over long periods of time, regardless of their sex.

Hemingway was an active, physical man who loved professional football, boxing, circuses, bullfighting, horse racing, hunting, and fishing. He once remarked to Eva Gardner: ". . . I spend a hell of a lot of time killing animals and fish so I won't kill myself. When a man is in rebellion against death, as I am in rebellion against death, he gets pleasure out of taking to himself one of the godlike attributes, that of giving it" (Hotchner, 1966: 139). For an artist, Hemingway had surprisingly little use for the arts. He did not like theater, opera, or ballet, and rarely attended musical concerts. Of course, these preferences may have been related to his avoidance of people rather than to an active dislike of some of the things people do. Hemingway went to great pains at times to avoid "the public," and one gets the unmistakable impression that most of those who did surround him on a semiregular basis ("disciples," party-attenders, etc.) were, for the most part, unabashed sycophants. As a consequence Hemingway

CASE 1.1. (*cont.*)

was often alone in the midst of a group of people and experienced what we have called, perhaps a little too blandly, "negative interaction." It might be noted that Karl Menninger has claimed that the ego suffers in direct proportion to the amount of externally directed aggression. If so, Hemingway's paranoia, anxiety, and depression may have been related to his aggressive physical behavior earlier in life. For example, Hemingway comments: "In Chicago, where you only used fists, there was this guy pulled a shiv—. . . a knife, and cut me up. We caught him and broke both his arms at the wrists by twisting till they snapped" (Hotchner, 1966: 179).

Being a very physical man, Hemingway did not tolerate illness well, although paradoxically his life style seemed to invite poor health and frequent injury. For years Hemingway had trouble with his weight, high blood pressure, a high cholesterol level, a chronic bad back, and other ailments. Yet he drank heavily, often did not watch his diet, and continued to be injured, most notably in two small aircraft crashes in Africa in 1953. One result was that he was less able to work and increasingly could not use alcohol for relief. After one particularly bad head injury on his fishing boat in the spring of 1951 (in fact, he suffered several head injuries), Hemingway started talking for the first time of being "Black Ass" or depressed. Like most depressions, Hemingway's recurred periodically throughout his life. They were associated with traits that can probably be described as paranoid schizophrenia (Hotchner, 1966: 239), rigid thinking, and suicidal thoughts. In December, 1960) Hemingway had eleven shock treatments ("ECTs") to help combat his depression and suicidal preoccupation. Subsequently, there were other ECT treatments. What seemed to trouble Hemingway the most was his inability to work. A series of statements made to Hotchner indicate the crucial importance of work for Hemingway:

> . . . writing is the only thing that makes me feel that I'm not wasting my time sticking around. (1966: 144)

> . . . when you're the champ, it's better to step down on the best day you've had than to wait until it's starting to leave you and everybody notices it. (1966: 262)

> Hotch, if I can't exist on my own terms, then existence is impossible. Do you understand? That is how I've lived, and that is how I *must* live—or not live . . . . Because—look, it doesn't matter that I don't write for a day or a year or ten years as long as the knowledge that I can write is solid inside of me. But a day without that knowledge, or not being sure of it, is eternity. (1966: 297–298).

> The worst death for anyone is to lose the center of his being, the thing he really is. Retirement is the filthiest word in the language. (1966: 228)

Near the end of his life Hemingway was increasingly unable to work. As in our group data, his career dipped at the end, he was developmentally stagnated, frustrated in maintaining achievement in his major life aspiration of writing, and was hopelessly dissatisfied. It seems that his inability to work and his eventual suicide were products of an insidious interactive effect of his early trauma; basic values of violence and aggression; high aspirations and expectations based on past actual performances; an inability to compromise and be flexible as life events demand-

ed it; aging and failing physical health; social isolation and negative interaction; recurring depressions; hopelessness (Hotchner, 1966:27 2); paranoia, delusions, and confused, chaotic thought processes; the actual failure (at least bad reviews) of a major novel; and his recent losses and
preoccupation with suicide (for which he was well equipped in terms of
knowledge, means, and the will to execute).

> Basically, Ernest's ability to work had deteriorated to the point where he
> spent endless hours with the manuscript of *A Moveable Feast* but he was un-
> able to really work on it. Besides his inability to write, Ernest was terribly de-
> pressed over the loss of the *finca* . . . his talk about destroying himself had be-
> come more frequent, and he would sometimes stand at the gun rack, holding
> one of the guns, staring out the window at the distant mountains. (Hotchner,
> 1966: 274)

Finally, in Ketchum, Idaho, in 1961, just after returning from the Mayo
Clinic, Hemingway killed himself with a shotgun in the early morning.
Hotchner remarked that Hemingway had once commented to him that a
man can be destroyed but not defeated.

Source: Maris (1981: 165–168). Copyright 1981 by Johns Hopkins University Press. Reprinted
by permission.

can be thought of as an older white male escape suicide. It might also be useful to differentiate outpatient suicides from suicides in the general population that have never been treated. Some of the complexities of the permutations and combinations of suicidal subtypes are
considered in the next chapter.

Nonfatal Suicide Attempters

A nonfatal suicide attempter is someone who intentionally injures him or herself but does
not die and is, thus, available for treatment (cf. O'Carroll et al., 1996). A typical nonfatal
suicide attempter is a younger white female who uses less "lethal" methods (i.e., the method
has a lower medical certainty of resulting in death) to attempt suicide (such as an overdose,
other "poisoning," or cutting) and is perhaps more ambivalent about dying, is often motivated by interpersonal dynamics including revenge or change in an important relationship
(and, thus, like Mark Twain's Huckleberry Finn, may want to be around to see the results
or even "be present at their own funeral"), may be more impulsive, and whose problems
can be related to anxiety or panic disorders and other Axis II personality disorders (although nonfatal suicide attempters, like completed suicides, also tend to be depressed and
abuse alcohol and other substances; see Black & Winokur, 1990; Adam, 1990).

It is well known that nonfatal suicide attempts outnumber completed suicides but the exact ratio is speculative, as no national suicide attempt data are compiled in the United States.
Stengel (1964) first estimated that nonfatal suicide attempters outnumbered completers by a
ratio of 6–8:1. McIntosh (1998) argues that the ratio is even larger (8–25:1). Among the
young the ratio of nonfatal attempts to completions may be as high as 100–200:1. Assuming
about 30,000 suicides each year in the United States (the actual number is a little higher, closer to 31,000) and using the conservative ratio of 8:1, there are roughly at least 240,000
(775,000, if we use the highest rate) nonfatal suicide attempts in the United States annually.

A related issue is what is the relationship of the subtypes of suicidal behaviors. For example, are ideators, attempters, and completers one population on a single continuum dif-

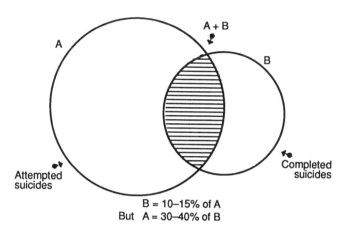

FIGURE 1.1 Relationship of attempted suicide to completed suicide. *Source:* Maris (1981: 266). Copyright 1981 by Johns Hopkins University Press. Reprinted by permission.

ferentiated, say, by seriousness of intent? Or are various types of self-destructive behaviors distinct but overlapping populations, sharing some traits but not others? Stengel (1964) contended that attempted suicides and completers overlapped and that only about 10–15% of suicide attempters ever completed suicide (put differently, 85–90% of suicide attempters eventually die mainly natural deaths; see Figure 1.1; cf. Maris, 1992e). Linehan (1986), following Kreitman (1977), also contends that suicide subtypes are distinct but overlapping populations, although she calls suicides attempters "parasuicides" (which means deliberate self-harmers regardless of suicidal intent) and adds the very large category of suicide ideators; see Figure 1.2 and the next section of this chapter).

One should also inquire about multiple versus single suicide attempts. Usually 35–40

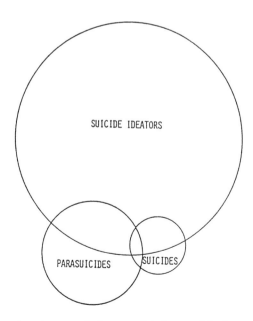

FIGURE 1.2 Linehan's overlapping populations model. *Source:* Linehan (1986: 21). Copyright 1986 by Annals of the New York Academy of Sciences. Reprinted by permission.

years after the first suicide attempt the 10% or so of nonfatal suicide attempters that will eventually suicide have completed suicide, at a rate of about 1% per year initially and somewhat less thereafter (Maris, 1992e). What is not widely known is that multiple suicide attempters among eventual completers are fairly rare. For example, in a Chicago survey (Maris, 1981: 267) found that 88% of older white male completers (the prototypical suicide) died the first time they attempted suicide (mainly because they shot themselves in the head). Among eventual suicide completers only 3% made five or more suicide attempts and those were mainly by younger women.

An important methodological conclusion is that suicidology cannot just study nonfatal attempters because it is convenient; for example, they are alive, are readily available in our clinics and hospitals, and can be given standard psychological or mental disorder diagnostic tests and scales in person. Suicidology needs to be solidly based in prospective, longitudinal studies of suicide attempters who eventually suicide (of course, with appropriate control or comparison groups). Even so, we must realize that a very large percentage of completed suicides never make nonfatal attempts, are never treated, never present at a clinic or hospital, and can only be investigated by special research projects on large random samples of the total population of completed suicides.

Suicide Ideators

Suicide ideators are individuals who think about or form an intent to suicide of varying degrees of seriousness but do not make an explicit suicide attempt or complete suicide. Brent and Kolko (1990) suggest that suicide ideas can vary from nonspecific (e.g., "Life is not worth living"), specific ("I wish I was dead"), ideas with intent ("I am going to kill myself"), to ideas with a plan ("I am going to kill myself with a gun"). As suggested by Figure 1.2, suicide ideators are a large group vis-à-vis suicide attempters and completers. For example, Linehan (1982) has estimated that 31% of the clinical population and 24% of the general population have considered suicide at some time in their lives. Pfeffer (1986) contends that 7–12% of children and adolescents have some serious suicidal ideation at some time in their lives.

Suicide ideation is probably most closely associated with depressive disorders. de Catanzaro (1992) found that between 67 and 84% of the variance in suicidal ideation in his research subjects was explained by social relationships and opposite-sex relationships—especially loneliness and being burdensome to one's family. Elsewhere we have explored suicidal ideas and their meanings in some depth and we refer the reader to those elaborations (see especially Maltsberger, 1992, and Shneidman, 1992). Two of the more common suicidal ideas or motivations are to escape from one's life problems and to get revenge on others (Maris, 1981: 258). Hillman (1977) and Lifton (1983) also argue that much of suicidal ideas concern changing one's life (what they call "tranformation drives"), not necessarily a wish to die.

One of the pioneers in the study of suicide ideation has been Aaron Beck (see Beck, Brown, Steer, Dahlgaard, & Grisham, 1999). His popular Scale for Suicide Ideation (see Figure 1.3) assesses the degree to which someone is presently suicidal. Beck's scale measures intention, lethality of the comtemplated method, availability of the method, and the presence of deterrents (protective factors) to suicide attempts. The Beck scale varies from a low of 0 to a high of 38 and is related to other scales by Beck concerning hopelessness, depression, and sucide intent (cf. Rothberg & Geer-Williams, 1992: 202–217).

Intention to suicide is a crucial component in suicidal ideas; however, it is also one of the most difficult suicidological concepts to measure—especially after the fact of completed suicide. Most suicides are expected to have both motive and intent to suicide before they

Name _____ Date _____

Day of
Interview

Time of Crisis/Most
Severe Point of Illness

Characteristics of Attitude Toward Living/Dying

( )   1. Wish to Live   ( )
            0. Moderate to strong
            1. Weak
            2. None

Characteristics of Suicide Ideation/Wish

( )   6. Time Dimension: Duration   ( )
            0. Brief, fleeting periods
            1. Longer periods
            2. Continuous (chronic), or almost continuous

FIGURE 1.3 Selections from Beck's Scale for Suicide Ideation (for Ideators). *Source:* Beck, Kovacs, & Weissman (1979). Copyright 1978 by Aaron T. Beck. Reproduced by permission of the publisher, The Psychological Corporation, a Harcourt Assessment Company. All rights reserved.

can be properly classified as a suicide. Jobes, Berman, and Josselman (1987) have listed a dozen or so operational criteria for evidence of suicidal intent (explicit verbal statments, previous suicide attempts, preparations for death, hopelessness, etc.).

Finally, suicidal ideas may come from imitation or contagion (see Diekstra, Maris, Platt, Schmidtke, & Sonneck, 1989; cf. Phillips, Lesyna, & Paight, 1992: 499–519). This is an area of suicide research deserving of special consideration. Accordingly, the topic of contagion or modeling is elaborated in Chapter 10.

Indirect Self-Destructive Behaviors and Parasuicides

Not all self-destructive behaviors are overt, explicit, or intentional. In fact, probably the majority of self-destructive actions are partial, chronic, long-term, and even unconscious. Farberow, following Menninger (1938) and Freud, calls behavior in which there is neither suicidal intention nor awareness or expectation of any suicidal outcome "indirect self-destructive behavior" (ISDB; Farberow, 1980: 4). Ignoring some important subtleties of classification, ISDBs include excessive smoking, alcoholism, risky sports, stress seeking, dangerous occupations, some sexual disorders, eating disorders, medical noncompliance, polysurgery, compulsive gambling, psychosomatic illnesses, self-mutilation, drug addiction, accident proneness, Buerger's disease, asceticism, and even chronic overwork (Cf., Chapter 18).

Of course, we need to be careful not to see *all* human behaviors as self-destructive. On the other hand, neither can we afford to neglect the chronic, cumulative, partially self-destructive behaviors in which many of us seem to engage. Freud thought there was a death instinct (*thanatos*) that compromised our life instinct (*eros*; Gay, 1988: Ch. 9). Often even those of us who do not make explicit suicide attempts nevertheless manage not to live as well or as long as we probably could have. It is as if we were chronically depressed and felt that we deserved punishment or pain for our real or imagined transgressions.

Kreitman (1977) observed that there can be self-harm even though there is not a clear intent to suicide. In many cases suicide intent cannot be documented and may not even be present. For example, with most nonfatal drug overdoses it is routinely not clear that a suicidal outcome was intended. Such self-harming actions may be the result of impulse, stress, confusion, anger, panic, anxiety, and depression. Kreitman (1977) calls these actions parasuicide. More precisely a "parasuicide" is a nonfatal act in which an individual deliberately causes self-injury or ingests a substance in excess of any prescribed or generally recognized dosage (Kreitman, 1977: 3). To the end of completely specifying the full range of our dependent variable, any suicidology text should discuss indirect self-destructive and parasuicidal behaviors.

Mixed Types

Of course, it is far too simple to suggest that one suicides, makes a nonfatal attempt, thinks about suicide, or indirectly shortens his or her life. Alfred North Whitehead once said, "Seek simplicity and distrust it." As we demonstrate in the next chapter, there are in fact many types of suicide, each with their own etiologies, causal models, and treatments. Suicides and self-destructive behaviors tend to share some traits and states but not others. They constitute mutually overlapping subsets which have both unique and common characteristics. Figure 1.4 provides a crude example which shows the similarities and differences of three hypothetical suicides.

Elsewhere (Maris, 1992d: 82, Table 4.7) we have attempted to give a multiaxial classification of self-destructive behaviors and ideation. We elaborate on it later on in this text (see Chapter 2). For now suffice it to note that completers, attempters, and ideators have to be differentiated, that each have at least four to six major subtypes, that there are also indirect self-destructive behaviors, and that there are mixed types of suicide behaviors (cf. Durkheim, quoted in Maris, 1969: 40).

Any classification of self-destructive behaviors has to specify interaction effects and comorbidity. Strictly speaking comorbidity indicates the occurrence of multiple DSM-IV diagnostic categories or conditions in the same patient at the same time. For example, a patient could be diagnosed with both a major depression (296.33) and alcohol dependence (303.90). Suicide itself is not a mental disorder but is often associated with major depression, borderline personality disorder, panic disorder, and some schizophrenic disorders (see Tanney, 1992; Chapter 13).

This is not the place to go into great detail about the mixed types of self-destructive behaviors or interactions of suicidal types. The main point is that real cases of suicide are

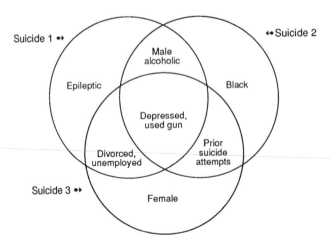

FIGURE 1.4 Overlap of traits of three hypothetical suicide cases. *Source:* Maris (1992d: 67). Copyright 1992 by The Guilford Press. Reprinted by permission.

complex and accuracy in prediction and intervention often turns on specifying the type of suicidal behavior or individual case characteristics. For example, we often simply do not know whether a decedent was a homicide or a suicide, an accident or a suicide, a natural death or a suicide. We also need to pay attention to the mix of nonfatal suicide attempts and completions (Maris, 1992d, 1992e). Some suicides involve multiple nonfatal attempts; others make only a single fatal attempt. Most suicide attempters (perhaps about 85%) never complete suicide. Still another important typology mix concerns the relative escape, revenge, risk taking, and altruistic components in a suicide. The next chapter has much more to say about types of self-destructive behaviors.

SUMMARY, PLAN, AND ORGANIZATION

There is currently no comprehensive textbook on suicidology or suicide prevention. Other related books tend to be edited, have no single author or editor, and, thus, lack integration and consistency of style. One of the best suicidology books, *Suicide Over the Life Cycle* (Blumenthal & Kupfer, 1990) is edited, has much overlap in coverage, is not case centered, and consists mainly of summaries of discrepant research findings. *Suicide Over the Life Cycle* is not comprehensive and reflects primarily a psychiatric perspective. For example, Blumenthal and Kupfer have relatively little to say about concepts, theories, data, or history and have no chapters solely dedicated to age, sexuality, race, work, suicide methods, family, physical illness, suicide notes, aggression, indirect self-destruction, religion, or suicide survivors.

Other strong books, *Suicide: Understanding and Responding* (Jacobs & Brown, 1989) and *Suicide Assessment and Intervention* (Jacobs, 1999) do have chapters on theory, survivors, and philosophical and ethical issues, but they also have significant substantive omissions. These books are primarily collections of essays originally presented in separate conferences over several years, and do not seem to be systematic, preplanned textbooks. They are also edited and not well integrated.

Aim, Purpose, Unique Features

The *Comprehensive Textbook of Suicidology* aims to be substantively comprehensive, consistent in style, original in scholarship and writing, pragmatic in focus, centered on individual case management and suicide prevention and to report the most recent suicidological scientific results (with our best guess as to the most viable, therapeutically relevant ones) and be an up-to-date reference book for clinicians. Throughout the text there is a focus on suicide intervention, prevention, and treatment. The latest research findings are applied to various treatment modalities (cognitive therapy, psychopharmacology, crisis intervention, etc.). Generous case examples of individual clinical management are incorporated in each chapter (see, e.g., Case 1.1). Treatment of suicidal individuals also receives an in-depth expanded consideration in the last two chapters of the text.

This textbook is entirely original writing and scholarship primarily by Drs. Maris (a medical social psychologist), Silverman (a psychiatrist), and Berman (a clinical psychologist). All the authors have had major federal- and state-funded suicide research grants and publications spanning many years. To ensure integration, continuity of writing style, and synthesis of individual chapters, Maris, Berman, and Silverman edited and proofed all the chapters. Ideally the end result will be a readable text with a relatively consistent style.

In an effort to avoid the customary endless lists of contradictory and inconsistent suicide research findings, an effort is made in each chapter to arrive at summary judgments, reported in a "box score" format (see, e.g., Tanney, 1992, and Chapter 13), of our best guesses as to the most probable conclusions for each topic, issue, or intervention at this point in time. Not all alternatives are equally viable and clinicians cannot afford to hide behind the skirts of the need for "further, better, larger, future research"—especially when confronted with a potential life-and-death case management situation.

It is expected that the *Comprehensive Textbook of Suicidology* will serve as a basic suicidological reference book in applied suicide treatment settings as well as in university classrooms. There is generous use of the best available and most recent suicide data in the form of relevant tables, figures, scales, graphs, standardized tests, indices, and cases. The text is based on clinical and classroom testing and experimentation with the materials over many years by the authors. Each chapter concludes with six especially relevant annotated further readings in addition to the detailed references listed at the end of the book.

Contents, Division of Labor

The text is organized into five major parts. Part I (Chapters 1–4) starts out with definitions, concepts, and theories. There is a brief review of suicide throughout history, with special attention to art, humor, and culture (by Dr. van Hooff). Part I has a chapter (3) on research and data, including discussion of prediction, scales, statistics, models, epidemiology, the psychological autopsy, and the clinical interview.

Part II (Chapters 5–12) addresses basic social, economic, epidemiologic, and sociobiological factors in suicides. These include age, sex and gender, race and ethnicity, work and economy, methods of suicide, suicide attempts, marriage and family, social relations, and suicide notes. The chapter on age is by Nisbet, the one on work is by Stack, and the one on marriage and the family is by Bongar and associates.

Part III (Chapters 13–17) is dedicated mainly to medical, psychiatric, and biological topics. Dr. Silverman is the primary author of this section. There are chapters on mental disorders (by Tanney) and personality, physical disorders, alcohol and substance abuse (by Lester), psychopharmacology, biological markers, and aggression and violence (by Plutchik).

Part IV (Chapters 18–21) is concerned with indirect self-destructive behaviors, ethical issues, religion, philosophy, and legal issues. The text concludes (Part V, Chapters 21 and 22) with chapters on treatment, prevention, postvention, and survivors (Chapter 22 by Jobes and associates).

In the next two chapters we expound on the theoretical (Chapter 2) and empirical (Chapter 3) components of suicidology. The theory chapter considers definitions of "suicide," basic suicidological concepts (e.g., lethality, motive, intent, and suicidal careers), hypotheses, causal models, and research results. Next we examine what suicides have in common and then how suicides are different (including types of suicides and classification schema). Finally, we conclude with a discussion of systematic theory of suicide.

FURTHER READING

Blumenthal, S. J., & Kupfer, D. J. (Eds.). (1990). *Suicide over the life cycle: Risk factors, assessment, and treatment of suicidal patients.* Washington, DC: American Psychiatric Press. An overview of risk factors, assessment and management of suicidal patients, special issues (e.g., suicide clusters, international variations, minority groups, suicide among physicians, and ethics and law), and a synopsis. Focuses on relative contributions of specific risk factors at different stages of the life cycle. Includes appendices of suicide scales and legal aspects of suicide.

Bongar, B. (Ed.). (1992). *Suicide: Guidelines for assessment, management, and treatment.* New York: Oxford University Press. A pragmatic, clinical focus on assessment and treatment of suicidal patients. Also considers special age groups, suicide prevention training, and legal issues.

Jacobs, D. (Ed.). (1992). *Suicide and clinical practice.* Washington, DC: American Psychiatric Press. This volume in the American Psychiatric Association (APA) clinical practice series seeks to present a practical clinical approach to psychiatry and suicide, thorough up-to-date literature reviews, and an emphasis on the latest assessment and treatment methods. Excellent chapters on medications, suicide among schizophrenics, and liability after a suicide. Cf. Jacobs, D. (Ed.). (1999). Suicide assessment and intervention,. San Franciso: Jossey-Bass.

Jacobs, D., & Brown, H. N. (Eds.). (1989). *Suicide: Understanding and responding—Harvard Medical School perspectives.* Madison, CT: International Universities Press. Originally most of the materials in this edited volume were presented as a series of lectures at Harvard University. The scope is comprehensive, including chapters on subdisciplinary foundations, assessment in special populations, treatment (including various settings and the aftermath of a suicide), as well as larger philosophical and ethical issues.

Maris, R. W., Berman, A. L., Maltsberger, J. T., & Yufit, R. I. (Eds.). (1992). *Assessment and prediction of suicide.* New York: Guilford Press. A comprehensive text on problems of suicide assessment and prediction. Unique features include chapters on theory, methods, and quantification, applications to five common cases, a review of the latest information on specific predictors of suicide in special populations, and a conceptual and empirical synthesis of major results.

Perlin, S. (1975). *A handbook for the study of suicide.* New York: Oxford University Press. A text growing out of the Johns Hopkins University Medical School's National Institute of Mental Health postdoctoral fellowship in suicidology and suicide prevention. Chapters are organized around basic academic disciplines and how they view suicide. Has unusual chapters on suicide and history, literature, and philosophy. One of the early texts on suicidology.

2

The Theoretical Component in Suicidology

There may not be anything as practical as a good theory.
—EDWIN S. SHNEIDMAN

The great, enduring suicidologists have all had theoretical biases. Emile Durkheim saw suicide as an external and constraining social fact independent of individual psychopathology. Sigmund Freud and Karl Menninger considered suicide a murderous death wish that was turned back (or "retroflexed") upon one's own self. Edwin Shneidman conceives of suicide as "psychache" or intolerable psychological pain. Psychiatrist John Mann tends to think of suicide as reflecting brain neurotransmitter abnormalities or deficiencies (especially of the serotonergic system).

Theory is usually contrasted with practice. The suspicion (perhaps especially within medicine) often is that theory is secondary to practice and at worst that theoreticians are only web spinning, impractical dilettantes who really lack the skills to be able to do much of anything (e.g., they cannot prevent a suicide). Practical suicidologists (so the story goes) should pay attention to biological facts (sleep patterns, diet, age, sex, etc.), brain chemistry, psychotropic medications, and the like.

Yet, as Shneidman argues in the tease to Chapter 2, theory is eminently practical (see Shneidman, 1993). Theory is both a way of seeing and a way of not seeing. Without a theory one does not even know what facts to pay attention to. Not everything is equally important or attentionworthy. Our theoretical assumptions (usually unstated and often unrecognized) influence what we attend to as well as what we neglect.

Webster's dictionary defines "*theory*" as contemplation, an idea or mental plan of the way to do something, a systematic statement of principles involved, a formulation of apparent relationships or underlying principles of observed phenomena which has been verified to some degree (as opposed to a "*hypothesis*," which implies an inadequacy of evidence in support of an explanation, a need for a systematic test), "pure" as opposed to applied.

More formally, a "*theory*" can be thought of as a set of laws, assumptions, and definitions that are deductively interrelated. Figure 2.1 presents one (ambitious) model for constructing systematic theory (for our purposes, of suicidal behaviors, ideas, etc.). Usually a suicidologist starts out with a hypothesis or causal model of suicidal behavior. This model is then tested statistically in the context of a research or experimental design (see Chapter 3).

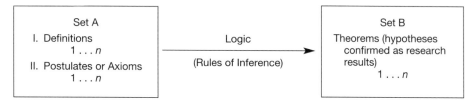

FIGURE 2.1. A model for constructing systematic theory.

Sample size, comparison and control groups, false positives, power equations, and so on, are all important considerations in this research process (Schlesselman, 1982: 144).

If we do our research carefully, we end up with probability estimates that our hypotheses or models are "true" (i.e., different from chance associations) under specified, limited circumstances. Hypotheses or models that receive this contingent empirical support are often designated as "research results" or "research findings."

However, this is only the beginning theoretically, not the stopping point. As Figure 2.1 suggests, research results themselves need to be related to each other and to our definitions, postulates, laws, and axioms concerning suicide by the use of logic (rules of inference) or mathematics. Put another way, theory building or theory construction transcends model or hypothesis testing. When research results are inferred deductively (one *could* proceed backward; i.e., inductively) from sets (see Figure 2.1, set A) of definitions, postulates, axioms, or laws using standard rules of inference, they can become "theorems" in a systematic theory. Unfortunately for the study of suicide, few suicidologists have ever attempted to construct formal theories of suicide. Later on in this chapter, after defining core elements in suicide theories, we give one example of a formal suicide theory or explanation sketch.

Set B (Figure 2.1) type research results are fairly straightforward and self-explanatory. But what do we mean by the so-called set A propositions? For the most part set A statements concern the assumptions, definitions, and laws or lawlike propositions of our disciplinary approaches or subdisciplinary perspectives. Broadly speaking, set A propositions involve overlapping domains (e.g., biology, psychiatric disorders, family history and genetics, personality, psychosocial life events, and chronic medical illness) thought to be related to suicidal behavior, such as those depicted by Blumenthal and Kupfer (1990) in Figure 2.2. Often set A propositions derive mainly from our academic disciplines; such as psychology, psychiatry, sociology, biology, and economics.

Some (not all) of the major sets of disciplinary domain assumptions, definitions, and lawlike propositions that have been applied to suicidal behaviors include the following:

Cognitive theory (Weishaar & Beck, 1992).
Psychopharmacology (Mann & Kapur, 1991).
Developmental psychology (Leenaars, 1991; Maris, 1981).
Epidemiology (Garrison, 1992).
Psychoanalytic theory (Maltsberger, 1992).
Aggression theory (van Praag, Plutchik, & Apter, 1990).
Sociobiology (de Catanzaro, 1992).
Behaviorism (Skinner, 1953).
Psychological mentalism (Shneidman, 1993).
Economics (Wasserman, 1992a).

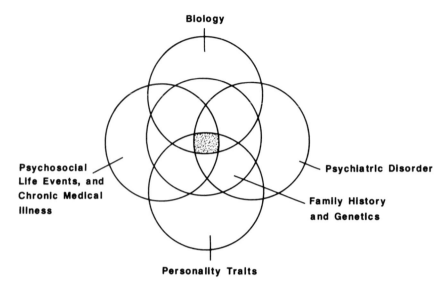

Biology

Psychosocial
Life Events, and
Chronic Medical
Illness

Psychiatric Disorder

Family History
and Genetics

Personality Traits

FIGURE 2.2. Overlap model for understanding suicidal behavior. *Source:* Blumenthal & Kupfer (1990: 693). Copyright 1990 by American Psychiatric Press. Reprinted by permission.

Our disciplinary domain assumptions are of enormous importance in determining how we approach the study of suicide and suicide prevention. While suicidologists give lip service to the multidisciplinary study of suicide, in actual fact most of us have very narrow and specialized domain assumptions—usually those related to our professional training and subdisciplinary paradigms. For example, Edwin Shneidman argues (1993), in essence suicide is primarily a product of what he now calls "psychache" or intolerable psychological or mental pain. Shneidman believes that suicide springs from an individual's psychic pain, stress, and general agitated ennui (or as he puts it alliteratively, from "pain, press, and perturbation," i.e., from the *mind*).

Contrast this theoretical perspective with that of research psychiatrist (psychopharmacologist) John Mann. Unlike Shneidman, Mann (1991) tends to see the etiology of suicide in the *brain*, most likely in dysfunctions of the serotonergic system (especially low 5-HIAA levels, postsynaptic receptors, and related biological markers). While Mann is collecting, freezing, and examining the brains of suicides and controls in a state-of-the-art biomedical laboratory in New York City, Shneidman is reading Melville's *Moby Dick*, the *Oxford English Dictionary*, and is interviewing acutely suicidal individuals in Los Angeles. These two highly divergent, almost diametrically opposed, approaches to the study and prevention of suicide grow out of fundamental theoretical differences.

Let us provide one more example of the role of theory in suicidology (Chapter 19 has more examples). In Box 2.1, philosopher Peggy Battin contends that in some circumstances suicide is rational and suicidologists, doctors, nurses, and mental health professionals should assist some patients to suicide—not try to prevent their suicides. But clinical psychologist Joseph Richman counters that "rational suicide" is an oxymoron (he apparently believes all suicide is irrational) and is almost never justified, and that health professionals should help suicidal patients resolve their life crises in such a way that excludes their resorting to suicide.

Without oversimplifying this complex debate or taking sides, note some of the obvious

---

BOX 2.1. Is Suicide Ever Rational?

Yes: Battin (1991).
No: Richman (1992a).

Issue Summary:

Yes: "How ought a mental health professional respond to a request for help in suicide when that request comes from a person contemplating suicide because of terminal illness, severe permanent disability, or advanced old age? To disregard the request or to attempt to prevent the suicide is simply to assume . . . that there can be no such thing as 'rational suicide' under these conditions, but standard clinical practices may not provide adequate ways of responding to such requests either. To put it bluntly, the mental health profession, in its clinical and counseling services; currently fails to serve an enormous clientele often much in need of help. . . . The issue of how to respond to a request for help in what may be rational suicide in these circumstances is not arcane, but of central social importance."

No: "Derek Humphry's book *Final Exit* was a challenge to review because I am opposed to physician-assisted suicide and see no basic difference between 'emotional' and 'rational' suicide. . . . The book is filled with misleading oversimplifications and an ignorance of the basic principles of psychiatry, psychology, and suicidology. For example, Humphry's list of rational determinants includes 'losing the will to live,' 'being dependent upon others,' and anticipatory anxiety. For these reasons he defends the suicide of Janet Adkins, assisted by Jack Kevorkian, although she was only in her 50s. . . . Humphry only approves of negative anticipation, while positive anticipation . . . is rejected. He fails to recognize that illness is a crisis, one that involves the family, and that the solution is crisis intervention, not death."

---

differences in theoretical assumptions between Battin and Richman. Battin is a university-based (Utah) philosophy professor; Richman is a hospital-based (New York City) psychotherapist who works with the elderly and with families. It is easy to imagine a philosopher (sometimes parodied as having a cold, logical, unemotional approach to problems) concluding that if an aged individual's suicide did not have net negative (especially, social) consequences and resolved the individual's own painful, hopeless, terminal illness, then it might "make sense" or be rational. Conversely, one can just as easily imagine a beneficent, positive-thinking psychotherapist always seeing his patients as depressed, irrational, falsely hopeless, and treatable short of suicide. Battin apparently emphasizes individual rights and self-determination, whereas Richman seems to stress social and familial responsibilities. The point here is that much of the debate about rational suicide *does not seem to turn on* facts, data, evidence, and research *but, rather, on* differences related to theory, training, disciplinary perspectives, assumptions, values, and postulates.

BUILDING BLOCKS AND THEORETICAL ELEMENTS

Now we turn to a description of the basic building blocks or elements of a systematic theory of suicide—to definitions, major concepts, hypotheses, models, and empirical research results. After discussing each theoretical element in some detail and reviewing commonalities and differences among suicides, the chapter closes with an example of systematic suicide theory construction.

Definitions

What is it exactly that we are studying in this textbook or attempting to prevent? What is our dependent variable whose variance we wish to explain? The answer seems obvious; *suicide is intentional self-murder* (Maris, 1991, 1993), or as Rosenberg et al. (1988) put it, suicide is "death arising from an act inflicted upon oneself with the intention to kill oneself." The word "suicide" derives from the Latin *sui* (of oneself) and *cide or cidium* (a killing). In German suicide is literally self-murder (i.e., *selbstmord*). The actual word "suicide" was probably first used around 1651 (*Oxford English Dictionary*; cf. Barraclough & Shepard, 1994). Table 2.1 provides several basic definitions of "suicide" from different theoretical perspectives or disciplinary perspectives. An elaboration of the major similarities and differences of these definitions follows.

Medically and legally it is useful in clarifying the definition of "suicide" to think of the categories or "manners" of death routinely available on death certificates to classify deaths. Forensically, all deaths are seen as natural, accidental, suicidal, or homicidal (forming the useful acronym "NASH"), although a few deaths in fact are classified as "pending, "undetermined," or (less commonly) "equivocal" (e.g., "suicide-accident" or some other combination). The first point to note about the definition of suicide *is that it is a death*. A death

TABLE 2.1. Definitions of Suicide

Definitions	Source	Year	Page
Suicide is applied to all cases of death resulting directly or indirectly from a positive or negative act of the victim himself, which he knows will produce this result. [Sociological]	Emile Durkheim	1951 (1897)	44
Currently in the Western world suicide is a conscious act of self-induced annihilation, best understood as a multidimensional malaise in a needful individual who defines an issue for which suicide is perceived as the best solution. [Psychological]	Edwin S. Shneidinan	1985	203
The definition of suicide has four elements: (1) a suicide has taken place only if a death occurs, (2) it must be of one's own doing, (3) the agency of suicide can be active or passive, and (4) implies intentionally ending one's own life. [Philosophical]	David J. Mayo	1992	92, 95
Suicide is (1) a murder (*selbstmord*) (involving hatred or the wish-to-kill), (2) a murder by the self (often involving guilt or the wish-to-be-killed), and (3) the wish-to-die (involving hopelessness). [Psychiatric/Psychoanalytic]	Karl Menninger	1938	23–73
Suicide denotes all behavior that seeks and finds the solution to an existential problem by making an attempt on the life of the subject. [Existential]	Jean Baechler	1979 (1975)	11
A suicide is a fatal willful self-inflicted life-threatening act without apparent desire to live; implicit are two basic components lethality and intent. [Legal]	Joseph H. Davis	1988	38

certificate has been filled out. Suicidology is *not* primarily the science of nonfatal suicide attempts, ideas of suicide, self-mutilations, and self-destructive gestures. It is amazing how many scientific papers and books have been written about "suicide . . ." but have samples with not a single completed suicide in them!

Second, *suicide is intended.* Suicide is not unintentional and it is usually not subintentional (i.e., accidental deaths generally are not seen as suicides; see the fourth definition below). Methodologically (see Jobes, Berman, & Josselson, 1987) intention is a problematic concept, especially after the fact of death (e.g., only 15–30% of all suicides leave notes). Freud claimed that we all have *both* life and death wishes (1917/1963). Also, many suicides seem to be ambivalent about suiciding; that is, their intention to die is not constant. An important question here is, "How high does one's suicide or death wish have to be vis-à-vis one's life wish for a death outcome to be classified as a suicide" (100–0%, 75–25%, 60–40%, 51–49%)? In fact, intentions or wishes to die can be episodic and impulsive (Brent & Kolko, 1990).

Third, *suicide is done by oneself and to oneself.* If someone else kills you, even if you want them to, it is usually defined as murder (as Dr. Jack Kevorkian discovered in 1999). If a virus, bacteria, or disease process kills you, it is ordinarily a natural death.

Fourth, *suicide can be indirect or passive* (See Farberow, 1980; Chapter 18). For example, not taking life-preserving medicine or intentionally not moving from the path of an oncoming train is often suicidal. In Chapter 1 we reviewed various indirect self-destructive behaviors and will not elaborate them here again. Generally, the more indirect a causal sequence is and the less certain the sequence will lead to death, the more likely a death outcome will be classified as nonsuicidal. For example, in most circumstances overeating, cigarette smoking, promiscuity, reckless driving, and so on, that results in deaths are usually not called suicides.

Suicidal behaviors and ideas are in fact complex, varied, subtle, and panoramic. Figure 2.3 illustrates one possible continuum of suicidality (clearly there are many others). Note that suicide is not one thing but a "multidisciplinary malaise," as Shneidman's definition re-

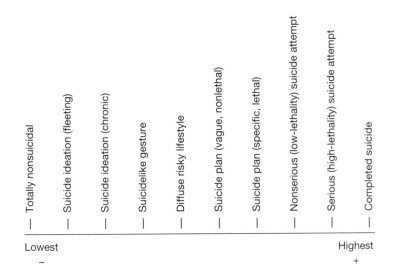

FIGURE 2.3. A continuum of suicidality.

minds us (see Table 2.1). It is imperative in suicidology that we make every effort to be clear and consistent about our outcome (dependent) variable. Explanations and predictors will vary as our dependent variable changes. Even among completed suicides, attempted suicides, and suicide ideators, there are various subtypes (as we shall see later).

This textbook discusses primarily *completed suicides*. As noted in Chapter 1, roughly 85% of all suicide attempters do not die from suicide (Maris et al., 1992, Ch. 17). Thus, any research based solely on nonfatal suicide attempters (regardless of how tempting it is to have "first-person" data) is of questionable value in predicting and preventing completed suicide. Furthermore, *the prototypical suicide* is an older white male who is often depressed, alcoholic, socially isolated, cognitively rigid, failing in physical health, and increasingly hopeless (as in Case, 1.1), *not* a young adolescent schoolgirl. However, it is useful at least to consider other aspects of suicidality on the continuum depicted in Figure 2.3, as nonfatal suicide attempts, ideas about suicide, and risk taking are all related to eventual suicidal outcomes. But they themselves are not what this text is primarily concerned with.

Without going into exquisite detail *a few general observations about definitions* are in order (see Copi, 1994):

1. The symbol or word being defined is the *definiendum* (e.g., "suicide"); the symbols or words being used to explain the meaning of the definiendum are the *definiens* (e.g., "intentional self-murder").
2. There are many types of definitions but two in particular are relevant to our purposes: *theoretical* and precising or *operational* definitions. Theoretical definitions in effect posit a theory (here of suicide; see, e.g., Shneidman's definition in Table 2.1). One has to be careful with such definitions. A definition should not be an explanation. Saying what a symbol or word is is not the same as saying why the symbol, word, or behavior exists or what causes it. Operational definitions suggest how the symbol or word should be measured. Several of the definitions in Table 2.1 (especially Mayo's) suggest that suicidologists should examine only completed suicides (perhaps only those deaths checked as suicides on death certificates by medical examiners and coroners), should think of suicide as life problem resolutions and the product of frustrated psychological needs (for love, self-esteem, security, hope, etc.), and should involve hate, guilt, and hopelessness.
3. In symbolic logic, definitions tend to be formally stated as equivalence propositions. This may seem like a trivial point but it will be relevant at the end of Chapter 2, when we attempt to sketch a formal theory of suicidal behaviors.

Basic Concepts

In this section we examine the concepts of lethality, motive and intent, and suicidal careers. Later on in this chapter and also in Chapter 3 we also consider other basic suicidological concepts (depression, hopelessness, suicide attempts, alcohol abuse, etc.) under the rubrics of common elements in and predictors of suicide. These basic concepts are our building blocks, if you will, for constructing theories of suicide.

Lethality

Clearly some suicide attempts are more serious or life-threatening than others. Lethality refers to the probability or medical certainty that an action, method, or condition will in fact kill you, that is, lead to a fatal outcome. For example, a high-caliber handgun (e.g., a

.357 magnum or .45 caliber) shot to the brainstem has almost 100% lethality. On the other hand, trying to hold your breath until you die has virtually a zero lethality. It is likely *mutatis mutandis* that the great excess of male suicide rates to female suicide rates (3 or 4:1; cf. Chapter 6) turns on males' much greater preference for firearms and head shot sites. Women tend to use a greater variety of suicide attempt methods than do men, tend to use less lethal methods, and may be more likely to shoot themselves in the chest than are men (however, see Stone, 1987).

Although lethality is not restricted to methods of suicide attempts (see Chapter 12), some interesting research has been done on this topic. In 1974 Card estimated that the most to the least lethal suicide methods (other things being equal) were:

Most lethal (+)	gunshot
	carbon monoxide
	hanging
	drowning
	plastic bag over the head
	impact
	fire
	poison
	drugs
	gas
Least lethal (−)	cutting

Beck was one of the first suicidologists to attempt to measure lethality. A committee he chaired in the early 1970s for the National Institute of Mental Health defined "lethality" as the medical certainty of death (see Weishaar & Beck, 1992: 78). Beck scored lethality as "zero, low, medium, or high." This simple lethality scale is still in use today. However, some suicide scholars believe that we need a lethality scale with 9 or 10 points (not 4) and better operational definitions and scaling techniques (Leenaars, 1992: 347). Others argue that lethality is a function not just of risk factors but also of protective factors interacting with risk factors.

Figure 2.4 (Smith, Conroy, & Ehler, 1984) is an example of one of the best available lethality scales. It features 11 anchor points and precise operational definitions complete with clinical examples and a detailed drug chart (*which now needs updating*). On the Smith et al. scale, anchor point "0" indicates that death is impossible and "10" indicates that death is almost certain. The Smith scale has been rigorously constructed and various psychometric properties are known. Readers are invited to study Figure 2.4 and to try to apply it to the clinical cases presented in boxes throughout this text (e.g., Case 1.1 and others).

A lethality scale that assesses both risk and rescue (or protective) factors was created by Weisman and Worden (1974: 193–213) at Harvard. It is aptly designated the "Risk–Rescue Rating Scale." Risk and rescue scores are calculated by assessing the following factors:

Risk factors (A)	Rescue factors (B)
1. Agent or method	1. Location
2. Impaired consciousness	2. Key person
3. Lesions/toxicity	3. Probability of discovery
4. Reversibility	4. Accessibility
5. Treatment required	5. Delay to discovery

0.0 DEATH IS AN IMPOSSIBLE *RESULT OF THE "SUICIDAL" BEHAVIOR*

Cutting: Light scratches that do not break the skin; usually done with pop can "pull tabs," broken plastic, pins, paper clips; reopening old wounds also is included at this level. Wounds requiring sutures must be rated at a higher level.

Ingestion: This includes mild overdoses and the swallowing of objects such as money, paper clips, and disposable thermometers. Ten or fewer ASA, Tylenol®, "cold pills," laxatives, or other over-the-counter drugs; mild doses of tranquilizers or prescribed medications (usually fewer than 10 pills). Putting broken glass into one's mouth but not swallowing would be rated in this category.

Other. Clearly ineffective acts which are usually shown by the patient to staff or others (e.g., going outside in cold weather with only a nightgown on after telling parents she was going to commit suicide by "freezing myself to death").

1.0 DEATH IS VERY HIGHLY IMPROBABLE. *IF IT OCCURS IT WOULD BE A RESULT OF SECONDARY COMPLICATION, AN ACCIDENT, OR HIGHLY UNUSUAL CIRCUMSTANCES.*

Cutting: Shallow cuts without tendon, nerve, or vessel damage. These wounds may require some very minor suturing. Cutting is often done with something sharp such as a razor. Very little blood loss. Scratches (as opposed to cuts) to the neck are first rated here.

Ingestion: Relatively mild overdoses or swallowing of non-sharp glass or ceramics, events usually brought by the patient to staff attention. Twenty or fewer ASA, laxatives, and/or over-the-counter meds (e.g., Sominex, Nytol®. 15 or fewer Tylenol). Small doses of potentially lethal medications (e.g., six Tuinal, four Seconal) are also common; fewer than 20 (10 mg.) Thorazine tablets.

Other: Tying a thread, string, or yarn around neck and then showing to staff.

2.0 DEATH IS IMPROBABLE *AS AN OUTCOME OF THE ACT: IF IT OCCURS IT IS PROBABLY DUE TO UNFORESEEN SECONDARY EFFECTS. FREQUENTLY THE ACT IS DONE IN A PUBLIC SETTING OR IS REPORTED BY THE PERSON OR BY OTHERS. WHILE MEDICAL AID MAY BE WARRANTED, IT IS NOT REQUIRED FOR SURVIVAL.*

Cutting: May receive but does not usually *require* medical intervention to survive.

> *Examples:* Relatively superficial cuts with a sharp instrument that may involve slight tendon damage. Cuts to the arms, legs, and wrists will require suturing. Cuts to the side of the neck are first rated in this category and should not require suturing.

Ingestion: May receive but does not usually *require* medical intervention to survive.

> *Examples:* Thirty or fewer ASA and/or other over-the-counter pills; fewer than 100 laxatives; twenty-five or fewer Regular Strength Tylenol; drinking of toxic liquids (12 ounces or less), shampoo or astringent (e.g., Ten.O.Six® Lotion), lighter fluid or other petroleum-based products (less than two ounces). Small doses of potentially lethal medications (e.g., 21 65-mg. Darvon, 12 tablets of Fiorinal, "overdosed on phenobarbital but only enough to make him very drowsy," 10–15 50-mg. Thorazine tablets), greater quantities of aspiring might be taken when staff is notified within minutes by the patient. Fourteen or fewer lithium carbonate tablets. The patient may swallow small quantities of cleaning compounds or fluids such as Comet® cleanser (less than four tablespoons).

Other: Nonlethal, usually impulsive and ineffective methods.

> *Examples:* Inhaling deodorant without respiratory distress occurring, swallowing several pieces of sharp glass, evidence of failed attempt to choke self with a piece of pillowcase (e.g., rash-type abrasions).

3.5 DEATH IS IMPROBABLE *SO LONG AS FIRST AID IS ADMINISTERED BY VICTIM OR OTHER AGENT. VICTIM USUALLY MAKES A COMMUNICATION OR COMMITS THE ACT IN A PUBLIC WAY OR TAKES NO MEASURES TO HIDE SELF OR INJURY.*

Cutting: Deep cuts involving tendon damage (or severing) and possible vessel, and artery damage: cuts to the neck will require sutures but no major vessels were severed. Blood loss is generally less than 100 cc. Cuts to neck go beyond scratching but do not actually sever main veins or arteries.

Ingestion: This is a significant overdose and may correspond to the lower part of the LD_{50} range.

> *Examples:* Fewer than 60 ASA or other over-the-counter pills. Higher doses may be taken but patient insures intervention (e.g., 64 Sominex). Over 100 laxatives; 50 or fewer Tylenol. Potentially lethal overdoses (e.g., 60 Dilantin capsules plus half a fifth of rum) but done in such a way as to insure intervention (e.g., in front of nursing staff, telling someone within 1 hour). Signs of physiological distress may be present such as nausea, elevated blood pressure, respiratory changes, convulsions, and altered consciousness stopping short of coma. Lighter fluid (three or more ounces); 15–20 lithium carbonate tablets.

Other: Possibly serious actions that are quickly brought by the patient to staff's attention (e.g., tied a shoelace tightly around neck but came to staff immediately).

FIGURE 2.4. Anchor points for Smith's Suicide Attempt Lethality Scale. *Source:* Smith, Conroy, & Ehler (1984: 237–241). Copyright 1984 by The Guilford Press. Reprinted by permission.

5.0 DEATH IS A FIFTY-FIFTY PROBABILITY *DIRECTLY OR INDIRECTLY, OR IN THE OPINION OF THE AVERAGE PERSON, THE CHOSEN METHOD HAS AN EQUIVOCAL OUTCOME. USE THIS RATING ONLY WHEN:*
  (1) DETAILS ARE VAGUE;
  (2) A CASE CANNOT BE MADE FOR RATING EITHER A 3.5 OR 7.0.

Cutting: Severe cutting resulting in sizable blood loss (more than 100 cc) with some chance of death. Cutting may be accompanied by alcohol or drugs, which may cloud the issue.

Ingestion: Reports of vague but possibly significant quantities of lethal medications. Unknown quantities of drugs that are lethal in small dosages (those with an * in Table 1) also belong here.
  Examples: "Take a large number of chloral hydrate and Doriden"; "took 60 ASA and an undetermined amount of other medications."

Other: Potentially lethal acts.
  Examples: Trying to put two bare wires into an electrical outlet with a nurse present in the room; jumping headfirst from a car driven by staff going 30 miles an hour; unscrewing a light bulb in the lounge and putting finger in socket with patients around.

7.0 DEATH IS THE PROBABLE OUTCOME *UNLESS THERE IS "IMMEDIATE" AND "VIGOROUS" FIRST AID OR MEDICAL ATTENTION BY VICTIM OR OTHER AGENT. ONE OR BOTH OF THE FOLLOWING ARE ALSO TRUE:*
  (1) MAKES COMMUNICATION (DIRECTLY OR INDIRECTLY);
  (2) PERFORMS ACT IN PUBLIC WHERE HE IS LIKELY TO BE HELPED OR DISCOVERED.

Cutting: Cuts are severe.
  Examples: Eloping and "slashing neck with razor" (including severing jugular) but returning to hospital on own and asking for help; while alone cut head with shard of glass and "almost bled to death"—called doctor after cutting. Eloping and very severely cutting self in a public restroom or motel—cuts led to hemorrhagic shock with vascular collapse—patient makes direct request for help after cutting.

Ingestion: Potentially lethal medications and quantities. This would involve a dose which, without medical intervention, would kill most people (usually at the upper end of the LD_{50} range or beyond).
  Examples: Eloping and ingesting approximately two bottles of ASA and then returning to the hospital; 50 Extra-Strength Tylenol, eloping to motel and ingesting large quantities of Inderal, Dalmane, Mellaril, and three quarters of a fifth of bourbon, then making indirect communication of distress; took 23 100-mg tablets of phenobarbital but told roommate immediately who told staff; 16–18 capsules of Nembutal—left note with a friend who missed the note resulting in the patient almost dying.

Other: Lethal actions performed in a way that maximizes chances of intervention.
  Examples: Tied towel tightly around neck—airway cut off—tried to untie it but passed out on floor—found, cyanotic and in respiratory arrest—had seen staff making rounds before attempt; string wrapped several times around neck and tied to bed—face flushed when found.

8.0 DEATH WOULD ORDINARILY BE CONSIDERED THE OUTCOME TO THE SUICIDAL ACT, UNLESS SAVED BY ANOTHER AGENT IN A "CALCULATED" RISK (e.g., NURSING ROUNDS OR EXPECTING A ROOMMATE OR SPOUSE AT A CERTAIN TIME). ONE OR BOTH OF THE FOLLOWING ARE TRUE:
  (1) MAKES NO DIRECT COMMUNICATION;
  (2) TAKES ACTION IN PRIVATE.

Cutting: Severe gashes with major and quick blood loss. May be partially hidden from staff, spouse, or friends.
  Examples: Patient went into the bathroom of his room, left the door open and severely cut one wrist resulting in major blood loss; death would have occurred had he not been found 30 minutes later by nursing staff on rounds.

Ingestion: Clearly lethal doses and no communication is made.
  Examples: Taking a lethal overdose of barbiturates but vomiting before going into a coma; overdosed on 900 mg Stelazine in apartment alone; overdosed on phenobarbital plus alcohol, found comatose in her bed. Took 20 Tuinal and became very sleepy while visiting friends—the friends became suspicious and took her to emergency room—in coma for 36 hours; took 15 Tuinal—found unconscious at home in tub of warm water.

Other: Most common here are hangings and suffocations which may or may not succeed but are performed so that a calculated chance of intervention could interrupt.
  Examples: Tying belt very tightly around neck and strangling self in shower; tied shoelace lightly around neck and going to bed—found at rounds to be cyanotic; blocked airways with plastic and had tied a stocking tightly around neck—found on top of her bed gurgling and pale but not cyanotic; elopes and attempts to drown self in nearby pond but in broad daylight; jumps in front of fast-moving car (over 30 mph); plastic bag over head—found deeply cyanotic; played Russian roulette and drew a "pass."

FIGURE 2.4. (*cont.*)

9.0 DEATH IS A HIGHLY PROBABLE OUTCOME: "CHANCE" INTERVENTION AND/OR UNFORESEEN CIR-CUMSTANCES MAY SAVE VICTIM. TWO OF THE FOLLOWING CONDITIONS ALSO EXIST:
(1) NO COMMUNICATION IS MADE;
(2) EFFORT IS PUT FORTH TO OBSCURE ACT FROM HELPERS' ATTENTION;
(3) PRECAUTIONS AGAINST BEING FOUND ARE INSTITUTED (e.g., ELOPING).

Cutting: Severe, usually multiple cuts involving severe blood loss.
    Examples: Severely cutting arm with razor and bleeding into wastebasket then got into bed (it was bedtime so being in bed did not arouse suspicion)— found unconscious and in shock: savagely biting a 2-cm piece of skin out of wrist, losing four pints of blood and found in shock under bed covers; cut neck in arts and crafts bathroom (when shop was closed) with three-inch blade, found unconscious; severely cut throat with a broken pop bottle in unit shower—this was done when most patients were away from the unit—difficulty breathing when found: cut neck and wrist in bathtub at home—died by drowning—had "hoped" husband would happen by to discover.
Ingestion: Clearly lethal doses.
    Examples: Drinking several ounces of nail polish remover—found covered in bed gagging, pale with large amount of foaming exudate coming from mouth—mildly comatose; took 30 500-mg Doriden tablets right before bedtime—in bed, appeared to be asleep but was actually unconscious in a deep coma.
Other: Highly lethal means employed.
    Examples: Plastic bag over head tied tightly with a scarf—found unconscious with head in toilet: drove head on into a gasoline truck but survived with minor scratches and bruises; stuffed plastic in both nostrils and oral pharynx, completely closing airways—she appeared to be sleeping in bed under covers; eloped to another city in car, tied plastic hose to exhaust and suffocated in parking lot; hanged self in closet with door closed—not breathing when cut down; jumped from 90-foot bridge into water—was unconscious when found. Gunshot to chest area (if shotgun used, rate 10.0); jumped headfirst from three-story building.

10.0 DEATH IS ALMOST A CERTAINTY REGARDLESS OF THE CIRCUMSTANCES OR INTERVENTIONS BY AN OUTSIDE AGENT. MOST OF THE PEOPLE AT THIS LEVEL DIE QUICKLY AFTER THE ATTEMPT. A VERY FEW SURVIVE THROUGH NO FAULT OF THEIR OWN.

Cutting: Just cuts as severe as in 9.0, except that the likelihood for intervention is even more remote. Blood loss is severe and quick.
    Examples: Eloping to an empty house and severely cutting wrists and neck with razor—when a policeman happened by the patient was sitting in a large pool of blood, warded off the policeman with the razor.
Ingestion: Because of the time usually involved before a toxin can take effect there are very few instances of overdosing that can be considered this serious.
    Examples: Some that have been serious are: ingesting furniture polish, paint thinner, and many prescription medications while alone in the house with no one expected by; overdose on large quantities of Dalmane and barbiturates with husband out of town and no children or other live-in companions in the household; ingested 60 Nembutal, went into secluded, wooded area in mid-winter, covered self with leaves which caused him not to be found for several days.
Other: These are the most common types of attempts at this level.
    Examples: Jumping off a tall building (four or more floors); jumping in front of cars on a freeway and being hit: eloping and hanging self in gym locker building at night; secretly eloping and drowning self in lake at a time when there was no activity in the lake area and when he would not be expected to be on the unit; gunshot to the head and any effort involving a shotgun.

FIGURE 2.4. (*cont.*)

Each of the five risk items is rated from 1 to 3 in severity, and rescue factors are rated 3 to 1 according to the strength of the rescue factor. Both totals are then converted to a score of 1 to 5 (total 5–6 = 1; 13–15 = 5, etc.) for A and B. The lethality score itself is then calculated by the formula $A/(A + B) \times 100$. Risk–rescue score varies from a low of 17 (high rescue–low risk) to a high of 83 (high risk–low rescue).

A case example will perhaps make the risk–rescue scale scoring clearer. A 36-year-old woman had been drinking heavily and arguing with her husband. She went into her bathroom and ingested 25–90 mg of secobarbital, as her husband was leaving for the evening. Upon noting the drugging effect, she went outside and managed to hail a taxi and delivered herself to the emergency room. Twenty minutes later she lapsed into a deep coma, was sent to the intensive care unit and later transferred to the general hospital for an anticipated stay of more than a week.

Scoring: Risk score = 5
Rescue score = 5
Risk–rescue rating = 50

Her suicide potential was moderate because although her behavior was risky (every item but Agent or Method was rated 3), her rescue or protective factors were also high (self-rescue is automatically a rescue score of 5). If the Smith lethality scale is applied to this case, the most probable score would be 7.0 because the attempter was drinking heavily and took a potentially lethal overdose of barbiturates but also took a taxi directly to the emergency room.

Finally, we need to differentiate acute and chronic lethality (Maris, 1992f: 12). "Acute lethality" refers to the short-term probability of suicidal death (e.g., the probability of suicide tonight, this weekend, if released from the hospital, or if not hospitalized). "Chronic lethality" is the long-term probability of suicidal death and is related to what Maris (1981; see later) calls a suicidal career. One well-known example of chronic lethality is the claim by Guze and Robins (1970) that there is a 15% lifetime suicide probability of depressed psychiatric hospital patients.

Motive and Intent

As we saw in our consideration of the definition of suicide, suicide is not only self-inflicted, self-murder but also intentional. In ordinary English, "*motive*" refers to one's presumed reasons for suicide (depression, divorce, hopelessness, terminal physical illness, shame, guilt, loss, etc.). In suicidology, both motive (especially) and intent are primarily legal concepts (see Black, 1979; Davis's definition of "suicide" in Table 2.1). In the law, "motive" is the cause or reason that moves the will and induces action. Motive is that which incites or stimulates a person (e.g., major depressive illness) to do an act (e.g., suicide) or to produce a result.

"Intent" is the purpose a person has in using a particular means (e.g., suicide) to effect a result (e.g., death). "Suicidal intent" usually indicates that the individual understood the physical nature and consequences of the self-destructive act (Nolan, 1988: 53–55) (e.g., "If I put this revolver in my mouth and pull the trigger, I will most likely die."). In the law in some states an individual is still thought to be able to form a suicidal intent whether he or she is "sane or insane" (see Amchin, Wettstein, & Roth, 1990: 775). Indeed, most suicide exclusion clauses in life insurance policies start out: "Whether sane or insane . . ." In other states (i.e., California, Florida, Kansas, Kentucky, Michigan, Ohio, Oklahoma, Tennessee, and Wisconsin) proof of suicidal intent is required (see Blumenthal & Kupfer, 1990: 775–777).

But how does one *know* the individual's motives or intention, especially *after the fact* of a completed suicide? If the suicide attempt is not fatal and the attempter is available for interview, standardized suicide intent scales can be administered. One of the best known such scales is Beck's Suicide Intent Scale (Beck, 1990). In an effort to determine suicidal intent the Beck scale investigates such objective circumstances as isolation, timing, precautions against discovery, acts to get help, final acts, preparations for the suicide attempt, whether a suicide note was left, and communication of intent to others. In addition, self-reports (i.e., by the attempter) of purpose, expected fatality, the lethality of method used, seriousness of the suicide attempt, attitude toward dying, rescuability, and degrees of premeditation are surveyed. Finally, the clinician also measures the attempter's reaction to the attempt, his or her vision of death, the number of prior suicide attempts, and the involvement of alcohol and other drugs.

If the individual is dead, then Jobes et al. (1987) have created a retrospective index for operationally classifying a death as a suicide. These criteria include not only prior explicit expressions of intent to kill one's self (e.g., a suicide note) but also several indirect indicators of suicidal intent. Among these are preparations for death; expressions of farewell, hopelessness, and emotional or physical pain; efforts to procure or learn about means to death (e.g., buying the book *Final Exit* or joining the organization Hemlock), precautions to avoid rescue, using lethal means to attempt, prior suicide attempts or threats, serious depression, and major life stressors.

Suicidal Careers

Suicides do not usually happen out of the blue, solely as the product of intolerable acute stressors. Almost all suicides have relevant biopsychosocial life histories that make them variously vulnerable to or protected from suicidal crises. Earlier Maris designated these suicide-prone biopsychosocial histories suicidal careers. For example, he wrote in *Pathways to Suicide* (Maris, 1981):

> The concept of suicidal careers is central. . . . No one suicides in a biographical vacuum; life histories are always relevant to the final act of suicide. Suicidal decisions develop over time and against certain social, psychological, and genetic (or biological) backdrops; they are never completely explained by acute, situational factors. (xvii)

This is still sound advice for suicidologists today, namely, seek out the relevant biopsychosocial life history of the actuely suicidal patient before you.

Later on, in an edited book by Leenaars titled *Life-Span Perspectives of Suicide* (1991), Maris expanded on this basic concept of suicidal careers:

> It is argued here that we are particularly vulnerable to suicide when death, decay, and destruction, and the terror or anxiety that can accompany them, break through our defenses in systematic patterned ways over a lifetime and dilute our will and ability to continue living, what I have designated elsewhere as *suicidal careers* (Maris, 1981). There are several separate but overlapping notions in the concept of a suicidal career. *First*, it is predicted that profiles of models for completed suicides, nonfatal suicide attempters, natural deaths, living normals, and so on will differ on given sets of variables—such as depressive illness, alcoholism, suicidal ideation, use of lethal methods, and social isolation. *Second*, the concept of suicidal careers implies that it is necessary to conceive of life-threatening behaviors as having relevant histories. Usually only a time-of-death profile is assumed, since the U.S. death registration system focuses on the situation at the time of death or the few weeks or months just before death. *Third*, suicidal deaths are never entirely reactive to present stressors. There is always a relevant set of biographies or "career contingencies" that mediate reaction to stress and help specify which individuals in so-called "high-risk" groups will be most likely to repsond to life stress or negative life events with self-destructive behaviors. *Fourth*, it follows that suicide lethality can either be acute (the short-term probability of suicide) or *chronic* (the long-term probability of suicide) and that these types of lethality may be negatively associated. For example, an individual . . . may have high acute lethality and low chronic lethality at the same time. *Fifth*, self-destructive behaviors need to be cast into causal models that span suicidal subjects' lives from birth to death (Mann and Stanley, 1988: 425), adequate samples of cases and controls drawn, and analyzed with modern multivari-

ate statistics (such a logistic regression or path analysis techniques). *Finally*, it is immensely helpful in the analysis of suicidal developmental models to specify both direct and indirect causal paths to suicide. (28–29)

Other suicidologists have also recommended that the core suicidological concepts be considered in the context of one's entire *lifespan* or *life cycle*. For example, Vaillant and Blumenthal (1990: 2) argue that similar risk factors (male sex, depressive illness, hopelessness, alcoholism, lethal methods, cognitive rigidity, impulsiveness, aging, etc.) appear to operate at various stages of the lifespan of suicides but that their contributory weights (e.g., beta weights in a regression models or path coefficients in a path model) differ. In studying primary psychiatric diagnoses of suicides, Rich, Young, and Fowler (1986b) also found a life-cycle effect. For example, they contended that under age 30, the primary psychiatric diagnosis of suicides was antisocial personality and substance abuse, from ages 20 to 30 schizophrenias and bipolar disorders predominated, from ages 30 to 50 affective disorders were central, and over age 50 (particularly with geriatric patients) psychotic affective disorders and organic brain damage were the key diagnoses.

Case 2.1 sketches the suicidal career of feminist poet Sylvia Plath (note that poet Anne Sexton had a similar suicidal career; see Hendin, 1993, and Middlebrook, 1992). Although Plath gassed herself in an oven in her London flat at age 30, she had in fact a lifelong encounter with suicidogenic factors and forces. For example. she had an ambivalent love–hate relationship with her own father (see her poem "Daddy") and, indeed, with most males (Alvarez, 1970, Ch. 1). She suffered from repeated episodes of depressive illness, she had ECT treatments, and she made numerous suicide attempts. Most of her life she was extremely lonely and isolated (thus, she was enclosed within *The Bell Jar*, the title of her novel; although the "bell jar" symbolized other conditions as well—e.g., psychosis and never being born). Although she had psychiatric treatment (including antidepressant medication and ECT), it apparently did not relieve her depression or her obsession with suicide. Plath had multiple marital and sexual problems, was divorced, and had numerous largely unsatisfying sexual affairs. Eventually Plath apparently grew hopeless (see particularly her metaphor of the fig tree in Case 2.1). Finally, at the time of her death she had a concomitant physical illness (influenza). The concept of a "suicidal career" emphasizes that these multiple biopsychosical factors interact over a lifetime and synergistically produce the final suicidal outcome.

Hypotheses

Once suicidologists have defined their terms and listed their basic concepts, their variables need to be stated as *testable propositions* or "hypotheses" (see Figure 2.1, above). Hypotheses about suicidal behaviors allow for falsification or rejection, statistical testing, and replication of results by independent investigators. For an aborning discipline like suicidology these are extremely important scientific properties. No science can hope to accumulate or advance knowledge, if its claims are not stated in a way that allows them to be tested empirically. In fact, one of the most common reasons for rejecting would-be scientific journal articles is the failure of the author to clearly formulate and adequately test a hypothesis (or a model).

Of course, we all think we already know what a hypothesis is. For our purposes a *hypothesis* can be defined as "a statement about a future event, or an event the outcome of which is unknown at the time of prediction, set forth in such a way *that it can be rejected*" (see Blalock, 1979: 114–116 [emphasis added]). In nonparametric statistics it is customary to assume no relationship (the "null hypothesis") between two variables (see

CASE 2.1. Sylvia Plath's Suicidal Career

As many readers already know, *Sylvia Plath* was a bright female poet who suicided at age thirty after a tortured young adulthood. In a slight deviation from our customary practice of presenting cases from among our own study subjects, we have elected instead to consider Ms. Plath to illustrate the concepts of social isolation, negative interaction, and sexual deviance. Along the way we will also comment on Plath's early trauma, subjective inadequacy, rigidity, depression, and hopelessness. We are aware that in presenting "gifted suicides" (Shneidman, 1971) like Plath or Ernest Hemingway, the very fact of their talent and celebration may be thought to contribute to their being unlike more inconspicuous and uncelebrated suicides. However, less-celebrated suicides are not by that fact alone different from celebrated suicides. Moreover, Plath was articulate and not articulate. We know a great deal about Plath from her poetry, her novel (*The Bell Jar*, 1963), Harriet Rosenstein's critical biography of Plath, the initial chapter of A. Alvarez's *The Savage God* (1970), and more recently from friend and biographer Lois Ames, who also knew and wrote about poet-suicide Anne Sexton. Sylvia Plath was raised in Winthrop and Wellesley, Massachusetts, the daughter of a distinguished Boston University biology professor, an expert on bees, and a woman who taught shorthand and typing. Sylvia herself was an excellent student, graduating Phi Beta Kappa and summa cum laude from Smith College in 1955. After her junior year at Smith, Sylvia received a guest editorship award from *Mademoiselle*. This experience seemed to triggers serious suicidal episodes and resulted in mental hospitalization and electroshock treatments. In 1956 Plath received a Fulbright Fellowship to Cambridge University, where she met and married poet Ted Hughes. In 1957 the Hugheses moved to the United States and Sylvia accepted a position as an instructor in English at Smith College. The following year (1958) they moved to Beacon Hill in Boston, where both wrote. In December 1959, they returned to England, where in the spring of 1960 Sylvia met A. Alvarez, poetry editor of *The Observer*. A daughter was born to the Hugheses in April 1960; a son in the summer of 1962. About the time their son was born Sylvia finished *The Bell Jar*. Sylvia suffered repeated illnesses and for reasons that are not entirely clear she and her husband separated in 1962. The children remained with Sylvia. Finally, after a bitterly cold winter in London and a frenzy of writing poems, including some of the *Ariel* poems, Sylvia Plath suicided by gassing herself in her kitchen. She had been depressed, lonely, burdened by the care of two small children, and periodically ill with the flu. But, of course, there is much more to Sylvia Plath's suicidal-career than the superficial account just given.

To back up as far as we can, Sylvia Plath had a significant love–hate relationship with her father. He died of a long and difficult illness when Sylvia was eight years old. She never worked through her feelings about her father and did not mourn his death until she was an adult (Plath, 1963: 135–37). Some of this ambivalence was captured in her well-known poem "Daddy." It seems likely that what psychiatrist Robert Litman calls "ego-splitting" was a fundamental by-product of Sylvia's relationship with her father. Litman (1967) contends that ego-splitting occurs when a hated external object is internalized (cathected, identified with, etc.), then that death wish for the hated external object is turned beck upon the ego. Of course, Freud (1917) and Menninger (1938) argued along much the

CASE 2.1. (*cont.*)

same lines. Menninger called this phenomenon "murder in the one-hundred-and-eightieth degree." Plath also had very negative feelings toward her mother, feelings verging on hatred (1963: 166). Rosenstein (1972) believed that these early traumas later generalized into dislike and contempt for people in general. In describing Esther Greenwood (nee Sylvia Plath), the central character in *The Bell Jar*, Rosenstein observed:

> While Esther is still pursuing the American Dream, is, indeed, its paragon, her great pleasures are hot baths and anchovy paste. But beyond that, what? Does she like anything? Not men, not children, few, if any women. . . . Esther cherishes her inexplicable rage at arrangements–one cannot call them relationships—she herself has acquiesced in, even initiated. (1972: 48).

What Rosenstein failed to notice with sufficient clarity and compassion was Plath's ultimate contempt *for herself* (Plath, 1963: 61–62). Sylvia's early trauma led to a very basic and tenacious subjective inadequacy. All of her achievements, straight-A grades, prizes, fellowships, and awards could not substitute for her loss of early love and noncontingent approval. Respect and love are very different emotions. "Mother love" is freely given, or withheld, without regard to merit; and later achievements, no matter how grand, can never substitute for early noncontingent acceptance.

This inability to accept self and others led almost inexorably to social isolation. Plath became intensely, even painfully, critical, compulsive, perfectionistic, and rigid (Neuringer, 1961). Unlike Doreen, her roommate during the *Mademoiselle* adventure described in the early pages of *The Bell Jar*, Sylvia lacked animal vitality. Often she could not do anything, became virtually paralyzed (Plath, 1963: 85). In one of the more poignant metaphors of *The Bell Jar*, Plath pictured herself as sitting in the crotch of a fig tree starving, but unable to choose which "fig" to pick.

Men were not tolerable once Plath got to know them (1963: 67). Of course, the ultimate isolation and logical conclusion of her rigidity was the closed world of the "bell jar." Plath was shut off and shut herself off from people, new experiences, reality, and finally from life itself. Thus, the symbolism of the bell jar was closure, the closure of the unborn child in the jar of formaldehyde, of a life that had never been fully lived, of psychosis, and finally of death.

Plath's early trauma and rigidity as a child and adolescent led to further negative interaction and sexual problems as a young adult. Rosenstein notes correctly that Plath's sexual repression was closely related to her general difficulty with human relationships: "That sexuality contaminates is merely an extension of Esther's notion of human relatedness. It's not just kisses that stick. It's people. Her horror of male domination, the "freedom" she thinks she's won with her diaphragm—laudable in the abstract—remain tragically only that. Abstractions, little bell jars, shielding Esther from intimacies odious when she is sane, lethal once she is mad"(*Ms*, 1972: 49). Plath entered into a series of doomed, often sadomasochistic, relationships with men. Her high-school sweetheart, Buddy Willard, was safe; he was a relatively nonaggressive, well-mannered Yale

(*cont.*)

CASE 2.1. (*cont.*)

premedical student, a kind of All-American boy who never seemed to have much in common with Plath.

It was clear that Plath believed that Buddy would never understand her. Later on, Plath turned to more sadomasochistic affairs with men. For example, she decided to be "relieved" [*sic*] of her virginity and chose a Harvard math professor (Plath, 1963: 197–198). When the episode went awry Plath blamed the seduced professor and demanded that he pay the hospital emergency-room bill for treatment of her hemorrhaging. Sex and children were conceived of as "experiences" that might make her a better writer rather than as gratifying ends in themselves (Plath, 1963: 99). Even an initially positive, nonsexual therapeutic interaction with a female psychiatrist, Dr. Nolan, turned out negatively. Plath felt betrayed when she was given unanticipated electroshock treatment. Her final involvement with someone who might have saved her life was negative too. Just prior to her death, A. Alvarez confessed that he was unable to help her even though he anticipated her suicide:

> She must have felt I was stupid and insensitive. Which I was. But to have been otherwise would have meant accepting responsibilities I didn't want and couldn't in my own depression, have coped with. When I left about eight o'clock to go to my dinner party, I knew I had let her down in some final and unforgiveable way. And I knew she knew. I never again saw her alive. (1970: 33)

Of course, it would be a disservice to Alvarez and to our own knowledge of Plath's complex suicidal career to even suggest that Alvarez was responsible for Plath's suicide. Still, it is not difficult to imagine countless other human beings who might have been able to help Plath, at least in the short run. Once again Plath had become involved with someone who seemed to contribute to her undoing rather than to her growth and continued well-being.

Plath's early trauma, rigidity, isolation, and lack of positive human interaction (of which sexual problems were just one facet) meant that her life had become unacceptable—not just unsatisfying, but intolerable. It was not long before the depression that had hounded her all her life turned irreversibly into hopelessness. Plath herself wrote in *The Bell Jar* that Esther's case was not curable. (130). Rosenstein comes to essentially the same conclusion in her critical biography of Plath:

> Plath's late poetry is full of mouths, open, demanding, never satisfied. Those of children, of flowers, of animals, of other women, of men, and of her speakers. One's sense always is that the universe is insatiable because the speaker herself is insatiable. No amount of food, real or symbolic, can fill the emptiness within. And every demand from outside threatens to deplete her still further, provocations thus to terror or rage. Her fate—her dissolution—has in this and many other poems the ring of inevitability (*Ms.*, 1972: 99).

Of course, there had been suicide attempts all along. One of the earliest had probably been when Sylvia skied down a mountainside totally unprepared and unskilled, with the clear thought that such risk-taking might

CASE 2.1. (*cont.*)

kill her, she "only" broke her leg. In fact, in thinking about her descent and possible death, Plath openly observed that happiness lay in that direction (1963: 79). As she became more agitated, depressed, and hopeless, the attempts became more lethal. In the grips of a psychotic depression at age twenty, Plath took about fifty barbiturates and then misled potential rescuers into believing that she had gone for a "long walk." She could very easily have died from this attempt. It is worth noting that her description of mourning for her father is followed immediately by the overdose (1963: 137).

As described by Alvarez (1970: 33—41) and Ames (Plath, 1963: 215—216), the final attempt, with gas, had a kind of quiet desperation about it. It was cold, there were two young children to care for, Sylvia had been ill, she was recently separated from her husband and very lonely, and Alvarez had been unable to help. Yet all of Plath's attempts were also acts of ambivalence. Like most suicides, she wanted to die *and* to live. Plath left a note for her *au pair* girl to call her doctor; she even gave the phone number in the note. When the *au pair* girl could not get in, and no neighbors could be roused (the gas had also knocked out Sylvia's neighbor), the *au pair* girl left for a few hours before trying again. By then Plath was already dead. Although Plath's suicidal career is complex, it is clear that she suffered from an impoverishment of supportive human relationships. There are so many relational "ifs." If her father and mother had been different, if Plath had been able to form deeper friendships, if her marriage had been more gratifying, if she had been able to receive and accept better psychiatric care, if someone had just been there when she gassed herself then she might have had a chance. To be fair to those who tried to help Plath, we must admit that there were other nonsocial factors operating and that suicides often reject the very nurturance that might save their lives. Nonetheless, each needless death diminishes us all. We share Rosenstein's tribute to Plath:

> The final notes. First, a profound sense of loss that a woman of genius, capable of such uncanny beauties and such inspired furies that her work has measurably extended the range of English poetry, abandoned her art at 30. *Winter Trees* attests that loss. Its title poem, "Event," "Mystic," "Child," and "The Other," a poem of great complexity and brilliance, are superb works. Second, an overwhelming compassion for the anguish the woman must have experienced at the end of her life. Of those who write vengefully about Plath's lifelong love affair with death, one can only ask whether their hypothesis renders her suicide any the less terrible, her suffering any the less real, or their resources of pity any the less impoverished. Her loss is, simply, a tragedy. (*Ms.* 1972: 99)

Source: Maris (1981: 127–133). Copyright 1981 by Johns Hopkins Press. Reprinted by permission.

Sonnad, 1992), then, if the test statistic (chi-square, *t*, gamma, *r*, etc.) reaches certain levels, the null hypothesis can be rejected with known probabilities of so-called type I (i.e., rejecting a true hypothesis) or type II (i.e., failing to reject a false hypothesis) errors (see Chapter 3).

In epidemiology, observations of differences in the occurrence of a disease (here, for example, in suicide or suicide rates) lead to the formulation of hypotheses (i.e., testable propositions), which are then accepted or rejected after more extensive studies (Mausner & Bahn, 1985). Two of the major approaches to hypothesis testing are *experimental* (in which some factor or factors are under control of the experimenter) and *observational* (in which the factor or factors are not under experimental control).

The suicide theory construction process involves listing hypotheses, including possible alternative explanations (for good examples of hypothesis testing in suicidology, see David Phillips's work). Investigators should list all relevant hypotheses at the beginning of a study, otherwise they run the risk of not collecting appropriate data to test their hypotheses. In short, a hypothesis must be fully elaborated (cf. Schlesselman, 1982: 70–71). Because space is limited, one example of hypothesis construction and elaboration in suicidology is given here—that of Emile Durkheim's major hypothesis. (One consequence of choosing Durkheim is that the following discussion focuses on *sociological* hypotheses.) We could have just as easily picked Freud's hypothesis that suicide is a retroflexed murderous death wish for another person that gets internalized (Litman, 1967: 334), that suicide is a product of low levels of 5-HIAA in the cerebrospinal fluid or brain (what we might call "the serotonin hypothesis"; see Maris, 1991: 327), or any of a host of other hypotheses.

As is now well known, French social philosopher Emile Durkheim (1897/1951) hypothesized that "suicide varies inversely [or negatively] with the degree of social integration of the social group of which the individual forms a part" (209). However, sociologists Gibbs and Martin (1964) objected that Durkheim never operationally defined "social integration" and, thus, his hypothesis was not testable or falsifiable. They proposed instead the concept of "status integration" (mainly consisting of infrequently occupied status sets), which was more rigorously defined and measured. Henry and Short (1954) complained that Durkheim's hypothesis needed to be elaborated to include not only external constraint and suicide rates but also internal restraint and homicide rates. They hypothesized that suicide rates will be high when there is a conjoint or interactive effect effect of low external constraint and high internal restraint (especially superego restraint). Henry and Short felt that Durkheim's hypothesis neglected social–psychological factors, like frustration and its relation to aggression in general—not just to suicide.

Writing from the theoretical perspective of ethnomethodology, Douglas (1967) disagreed with Durkheim's hypothesis on the grounds that the relevant observations were not objective social conditions of completed suicides as reflected in vital statistics but, rather, what he calls the "situated subjective meanings" of suicide as seen in the first-person accounts of nonfatal suicide attempters. Phillips (1974) went on to argue that it was not just social integration that affected suicide rates but (contrary to Durkheim's contention) specifically media coverage (i.e., contagion or suggestion) that was associated with a rise in suicide rates. Finally, Pescosolido and Georgianna (1989) agreed with Durkheim that, yes, social involvement protected an individual against suicide, but they claimed specifically that disintegrating religious network ties weakened both integrative and regulative social supports and thereby increased suicide rates.

We can see from this brief consideration how Durkheim's major hypothesis was elaborated, specified, and refined by subsequent suicidologists (for a more detailed review of the evolution of Durkheim's hypothesis see Maris, 1992a: 2114–2119).

Models

Hypotheses usually concern rather simple bivariate relationships, perhaps at most assessing interaction effects when a third variable is taken into account. But in real life (or, in this case, real death) causal relations are seldom that simple. In actual suicidal outcomes there are multiple independent or predictor variables, they usually have complex interaction effects, the predictor variables affect suicide over time (e.g., over an entire lifespan or "suicidal career" of a suicide), and there are presumably feedback loops in causal relationships—just to mention a few of the problems in theory construction. One common theoretical method for simplifying the complex processes involved in suicidal outcomes is causal modeling.

Heuristically it is useful to think of such models as simplified pictures of the causal relationships among variables (Blalock, 1985). For example, one could graphically depict Durkheim's hypothesis as follows:

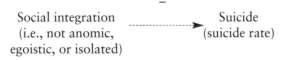

where a broken line and a minus (–) sign indicate a negative (or inverse) relationship and the direction of the arrow indicates the presumed causal order. We could test this simple model by operationally defining "social integration" as Gibbs and Martin's status integration, select a sample, and calculate "r" (Pearson's product–moment correlation; note, causal relationships are customarily measured by regression equations). Given our simple "theory" we would expect on the whole to get negative correlations, and that is exactly what Gibbs has found for the most part (Gibbs & Martin, 1964). We could also state Durkheim's hypothesis positively by saying that social isolation, egoism, and anomie are related positively to the suicide rate.

However, it would not take long for a clinician to realize how relatively useless Durkheim's hypothesis (or simple causal model) is in predicting suicide. Surely a model of suicide ought to have more variables in it, it ought to include psychological, biological, and temporal variables, as well as social variables, and it ought to estimate how the independent or predictor variables interact with each other.

Suppose we tried to construct a more complicated causal model for suicide outcomes with sex (say, where 1 = male and 0 = female) and age as background variables, social isolation, major depressive illness, and substance abuse as intervening variables, and suicide as the dependent or outcome variable. Our model might now be depicted as shown in Figure 2.5. Again, solid lines indicate positive associations and arrows indicate the expected causal relationships. The broken line between sex and depression indicates a negative association (that females are expected to have higher rates of depressive illness than males). The two-headed arrow lines indicate that the model only posits a correlation (a description), not a causal relationship—say, between social isolation and substance abuse. To the extent that such variables are causally related the model is inadequate (poorly specified) and will lead to biased statistical analyses.

Notice how quickly theoretical models become complicated. With only five independent variables (three of them intervening) and one dependent variable, 11 possible relationships have to be estimated. The causal relationships pictured in Figure 2.5 are operationalized by regression equations (see Addy, 1992). With only five independent variables the calculations quickly get cumbersome, especially when we consider interaction effects, feedback loops, indirect effects, and residuals (Pindyck & Rubinfeld, 1981: 47). Without going into details, some of the more common modeling techniques are general linear regression models, logistic regression models, log-linear models, and time-series models (Addy, 1992; Pindyck & Rubinfeld, 1981). Because suicide is a dichotomous (not continuous) dependent variable, logistic regression is usually preferred for suicide research. (For a more recent application of modeling to suicide data see Reed, 1993).

One final caveat: If the reader refers back to Figure 2.1, most of the causal modeling described here is an elaboration of set B. That is, even after modeling of empirical variables there is still a need to deduce the empirical results from a more general set of definitions and theoretical postulates, Although some would disagree, a model is not really a theory. For example, statistical models are not clearly grounded in any one broad theory perspective (such as cognitive, behavioral, psychoanalytic, neurobiological, etc., theory)—except indirectly by the choice of variables for the model.

Research Results

When hypotheses or causal models receive repeated empirical support through significance testing and replication studies (especially when using diverse large random samples and control or comparison groups in different cultural or historical settings), then scientists tend to regard them as verified "research results," or "research findings." Research results are the fundamental empirical regularities of suicidal behaviors and attitudes that our theories strive to explain, to account for, and to be consistent with. That is, theoretically speaking, research results are theorem candidates (see Figure 2.1). More on this later.

Suicidologists have attempted to list these basic suicide research results. For example, Lester published *Why People Kill Themselves: A 1990s Summary of Research Findings on Suicidal Behavior* (1992a). An earlier companion volume was that of McIntosh (1985). However, the specific list of suicide research results chosen as an example here comes from Maris's (1981: 296ff.) compendium of basic research results based on sample surveys of Chicago completed suicides, nonfatal suicide attempters, and natural deaths. Among the most basic findings were the following:

1. There is a positive association between age and the suicide rate.
2. The positive association between age and the suicide rate is strongest for white males.

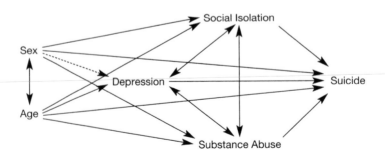

FIGURE 2.5. A simple causal model for suicide.

3. The suicide rate for white females tends to peak between the ages of 45 and 54 and decline slightly thereafter.
4. Suicide completers are more likely to have had suicides in their families of origin than are nonfatal suicide attempters.
5. Birth order is not a predictor of either attempted or completed suicide.
6. Suicide completers are more socially isolated than nonfatal suicide attempters or natural deaths.
7. Socioeconomic status is not a predictor of suicide.
8. Suicide completers have higher unemployment rates at the time of their suicide attempts or deaths than either natural deaths or nonfatal suicide attempters do.
9. About 8–10% of suicide completers are alcoholics.
10. Between 7 and 20% of all alcoholics will eventually suicide.
11. Among patient populations, those with depressive illness have the highest suicide rates, whereas schizophrenics have the greatest absolute prevalence of suicide.
12. Suicide completers tend to make one fatal suicide attempt; this is especially the case for older white males.

A number of questions need to be posed about suicide research results, such as those just listed. *First, is the result really a suicidolological fact?* Research results are notoriously inconsistent, even contradictory. Durkheim wrote, "These being the facts, what is their explanation?" One has to be careful not to explain or account for purported self-destructive behaviors that are in fact eccentric, whimsical, or capricious—not even if they are common suicidological factors. A variant on this problem is that some research results seem more empirical than others. A few so-called research results appear to be mainly theoretical claims.

Second, how many basic suicide research results are there? Of course, there is no simple, straightforward answer to this question; it depends. In Maris's Chicago research (1981) there were 122 main research results, but probably only about 30 were basic. Other suicide researchers have found literally thousands of basic research results.

Third, how are the results weighted? Are some research results more important or more "durable" than others? Probably. For example, suicidologists almost always find an excess of male to female suicides. Suicide is usually more common the older one is. Typically, suicides have one of the affective disorders. Suicides tend to abuse alcohol at a greater rate than nonsuicides. On the other hand, the relative importance of any one predictor can vary widely depending on context, sample, individual, and so on.

Fourth, which disciplinary domain is salient (see Figure 2.2)? Should we pay special attention to psychiatric results, biological results, psychological results, social and economic results, or what and in which situations?

Fifth, how do empirical generalities apply to individual cases? Research results tend to be stated generically. Particular patients, of course, may be the exception to the rule or exhibit complex interactive effects of several different research results. A variant on question 5 is how specific are the research results? Some research findings are limited and have precise operational definitions; others are very general and even vague in their reference.

The final objective of suicide theory construction is to settle on a basic list of suicide research results and then to logically or mathematically deduce these results from a set of definitions and postulates or axioms. After reviewing some of the commonalities and differences of suicides, the chapter concludes with an example of how systematic theory construction in suicidology might proceed. To do so is to skate on thin theoretical ice, as precious few formal theories of suicide have ever been constructed.

COMMONALITIES AND SIMILARITIES

Do all suicides have some traits in common? Are these suicidal commonalities not present among nonsuicides? Edwin Shneidman, one of the founding fathers of suicidology, has answered "yes" to both these questions. Shneidman argues that all suicides tend to share what he calls "the 10 commonalities of suicide," or the common psychological features in human self-destruction (in Shneidman, 1985, 1993). The *10 commonalities* of suicide are:

1. To seek a solution.
2. Cessation of consciousness.
3. Intolerable psychological pain.
4. Frustrated psychological needs.
5. Hopelessness–helplessness.
6. Ambivalence.
7. Constriction.
8. Egression.
9. Communication of intent.
10. Lifelong coping patterns.

Let us elaborate some on these common traits of suicide seriatem, in passing making a few brief asides about their possible implications for suicide prevention.

1. Suicide can be seen as life-problem solving (cf. Shneidman's definition of "suicide" in Table 2.1). Most suicides are in life situations or suicidal careers that seem to demand resolution. Like the chief character in Camus's *Myth of Sisyphus* (1945), suicides' lives are experienced as painful, intolerable, absurd, and meaningless—so much so that suicidal death may seem to be the only way out (Maris, 1982a). Of course, the key response to this commonality is that there usually are other resolutions short of suicide. As Shneidman says, "never buy a patient's syllogism," especially the catabolic conclusion, "Therefore I must die."

2. Shneidman claims that suicides want to interrupt their tortured self-consciousness—to stop the mental pain and anguish. Thus, it is understandable that analogues of suicide—sleep, anesthesia, psychosis, drug abuse, alcoholic stupor, etc.—all involve alteration or cessation of consciousness. Paradoxically, suicide may be a desperate transformation drive (Hillman, 1977; Lifton, 1979), not necessarily a death wish. As the lyrics go in the theme song from the movie *M.A.S.H.*, "Suicide is painless, it brings on many changes . . ." The challenge to suicide prevention here is to facilitate a meaningful change short of death through neurochemistry, psychotherapy, and so on.

3. Lately Shneidman has come to see intolerable psychological pain as the key commonality in all suicides. Shneidman writes (1993):

> Nearing the end of my career in suicidology, I think I can now say what has been on my mind in as few as five words: *suicide is caused by psychache.* . . . . Psychache refers to the hurt, anguish, soreness, aching psychological pain in the psyche, the mind. It is intrinsically psychological—the pain of excessively felt shame. or guilt, or humiliation, or loneliness, or fear, or angst, or dread of growing old, or of dying badly, or whatever. (51)

One absolutely central question for therapists to ask their suicidal patients is, "Tell me where you hurt" (and hope that they know, have insight, are correct, etc.). Often to prevent a suicide one just has to take the edge off the pain, not eliminate the pain.

4. Most suicides have been frustrated in meeting some of their basic psychological needs. These include the 20 to 30 needs originally listed by Harvard psychologist Henry Murray (1938) (e.g., achievement, affiliation, autonomy, nurturance, order, play, succorance, and understanding). They could just as easily refer to the basic psychological and even physical needs cited by Maslow (1963) for security, love, self-esteem, shelter, food, sleep, sexual tension reduction, status, and so on. Often meeting psychological needs entails *resocialization, regression,* and *reparenting.* Although Shneidman would not admit it, it also may involve *rewiring* of one's neurocircuitry through psychopharmacology (Kramer, 1993).

5. Suicides are not just depressed. As Beck (1986) has demonstrated, suicides tend to have become hopeless that their life quality will *ever* improve sufficiently, and they feel helpless to do anything about it. Therapists need to convince the suicidal patient, "You can be helped," or the even more risky, "*I* can help you." As psychiatrist Avery Weisman once commented, "Suicidal patients need at least one significant udder."

6. Suicides both want to die and want to live. It is common for soon-to-be suicides to make appointments (to play golf or tennis, to take part in their child's or grandchild's birthday party or graduation, to take a vacation, to go to their physician or dentist, etc.) for *after* their death. Freud claimed that we all have both life (*eros*) and death (*thanatos*) wishes (see Gay, 1988: 401–402). Readers may recall our earlier remarks about intention: All that is *required* for a suicide is a 51% wish to die at an acute situational crisis (perhaps lower than 50%, if the individual is impulsive). Suicidal treatment and intervention are often justified on the grounds that the therapist is after all just supporting or responding to the life-affirming pole of the would-be suicide's own ambivalence.

7. Shneidman used to ask students in his classes on suicide prevention, "What's the four-letter word in suicidology?" The answer, of course, was *"only"*—as in "it (attempt suicide) was the *only* thing I could do!" One of the salient mental traits of depressed suicidal individuals is the narrowing of their perceived viable alternatives, often to the extreme of dichotomous thinking (Weishaar & Beck, 1992). For example, suicides commonly think to themselves, "I must be either miserable or dead." This pernicious two-valued logic has led some suicidologists (Brandt, 1975) to comment facetiously, "Never kill yourself when you're depressed!" Cognitive therapy, as well as psychopharmacology, is useful in helping the suicidal individual become less perceptually constricted and more able to conceive of viable alternatives to suicide.

8. Recall Ishmael's opening lines in Melville's *Moby Dick* (1851/1988: 2): "Whenever I find myself growing grim about the mouth, whenever it is a damp, drizzly November in my soul . . . , then I account it high time to get to sea as soon as I can." Like Ishmael suicides flee (*fugue*) tormented, painful lives. Most probably just want the pain to stop. Many have tried alternatives short of suicide (e.g., psychotropic medications, various psychotherapies, alcohol and drug abuse, sexual promiscuity, divorce, religious conversion, overinvestment in work and careers, leaving town, sick leave, and leaving jobs) but are now faced with the ultimate egression (i.e., flight from life itself). Sadly, cessation of all experience for many suicidal individuals is seen as preferable to continued existence in this world. The challenge to suicidologists is to stop the egression; to convince the suicidal person (and themselves) that he or she can escape without dying. Sometimes this may mean subverting the lethal means, maybe even saying (careful here!) "give me the gun [or the pills] to hold for you until later on." Sometimes it means hospitalization, involuntary commitment, even seclusion and restraints—whatever it takes, say some. However, this

kind of direct, forceful patriarchal intervention has prompted psychiatrist Thomas Szasz to accuse suicidologists of being part of the police state (Jacobs & Brown, 1989, Ch. 23). It certainly is risky business.

9. A lot of suicides will tell you that they are contemplating suicide, if you listen carefully, are sensitive to indirect behavioral or verbal clues, and generally just pay attention. These may not be clear, dramatic "cries for help" (Farberow & Shneidman, 1961), but they will be at least ambiguous signs. Jobes et al. (1987) have attempted to specify some of the indirect evidence or signs of one's intent to suicide (as we discussed earlier). These may include expressions of hopelessness, preparations for death (like making or revising a will or taking out life insurance), serious depression, partially self-destructive behaviors (especially nonfatal suicide attempts), alcoholism and exacerbation of drinking or drug use/abuse, acquiring the method of suicide (e.g., buying or locating a gun and ammunition), open declarations of suicidal intent or saying farewell (comments like "you'd be better off without me," etc.), being placed in situations of great stress or loss, and isolation and precautions to avoid rescue. Of course, all these presuicidal signs are *ambiguous* and most of the time they identify "false-positive" suicides—that is, people who never in fact kill themselves. Also, clues to suicide are especially clear *after* the fact of suicide, not before, and intervention in false-positive suicides is expensive.

10. Suicides tend to have what we earlier called suicidal careers. They tend to be chronically self-destructive, with a repeated exhaustion of their adaptive repertoire Most suicidal crises are only "crises" because of the long history of partially self-destructive coping and "defective biology" (e.g., neurotransmitter imbalance or postsynaptic receptor "switches" on or off) of the suicidal individual. It would seem to follow that suicide intervention usually cannot just be a "quick fix" of a temporary acute problem in an otherwise healthy, stable person. Later on Shneidman (1987) claimed that his 10 commonalities could be combined into what he called "a theoretical cubic model of suicide." In this model the "suicidal cubelet" or maximum suicide threat condition occurs when psychache (pain), press (stress), and perturbation (agitation) are all at their maximum levels.

DIFFERENCES, TYPES, AND CLASSIFICATIONS

In spite of the fact that suicides tend to share common traits, not all suicides are alike. Most are older, but a considerable number are younger. Most suicides are males, but there are, of course, female suicides. A substantial majority of suicides have a recognizable mental disorder, but by no means all do. Most suicides use highly lethal methods (e.g., guns), but other suicides employ methods of relatively low lethality (e.g., reversible poisons, for which there is an antidote or treatment). In short, the variability in suicides is great. The complexity, variability, or multidimensionality of suicide has some pragmatic consequences for theory construction in suicidology. To be able to understand, predict, or assess suicide or suicidality accurately, we must specify the type of suicide as precisely as possible. Differentiating suicides, typologies, and classifications is a complex undertaking that we have gone into great detail about elsewhere (see Maris, 1992d). Here we can only summarize and highlight our earlier detailed examination.

The crucial question asked in this section is: "Is suicide one thing or many things?" Given this choice, it seems clear that the answer is "many." But how many? In the extreme case a few clinicians might argue that every individual suicide is unique—that no two suicides are alike. If this were true, the predicting and preventing suicide would be virtually impossible. Logically, if all suicidal careers were unique, we could only understand what caused a suicide after it happened, and then it would obviously be too late to intervene in that particular suicide. Fortunately, almost no one believes that all suicides are absolutely unique. What is more plausible to most suicidologists is that suicides share some traits but not others (see, e.g., Figure 1.4, in Chapter 1).

Of course, if there are too many different types of overlapping suicides, the prediction of suicide becomes extremely complex. For example, in the fourth edition of the *Diagnostic and Statistical Manual of Mental Disorders* (DSM-IV; American Psychiatric Association, 1994), there are 18 major types of mental disorders, about 300 subtypes, and a multiaxial system of classification. As readers are well aware, the unreliability and invalidity of specific psychiatric diagnoses are notorious. With this in mind most suicidologists define three or four basic types of completed suicides and two or three subtypes for each basic type. There are good reasons for limiting types of suicide. For one thing, empirically, when a researcher goes beyond (say) 4 to 12 suicide types, he or she runs the risk of having too small a sample to analyze meaningfully. It must be remembered that completed suicide is a rare behavior (i.e., 1 to 3 in 10,000 in the general population). For another thing, theoretically, we could specify a virtually unlimited number of suicide types, but to do so is at some point to create differences that really do not make much of a difference (i.e., specious differences).

We shall review briefly two classical suicide typologies: those of French sociologist Emile Durkheim and Viennese psychiatrist Sigmund Freud (of course, there are many others). Suicide typologies tend to be biased according to the disciplines of their creators. For example, Durkheim focused on broad social types, whereas Freud took a more individualistic, psychiatric approach. *Emile Durkheim* was one of the founders of the scientific study of suicide. Durkheim (1897/1951) argued that there are four basic types of completed suicides (with seven subtypes and six mixed types; see Maris, 1992d: 69–70). The four basic (pure or ideal) types of suicide are (1) egoistic, (2) altruistic, (3) anomic, and (4) fatalistic. Egoistic and altruistic suicides are polar types, as are anomic and fatalistic.

Durkheim hypothesized (as we noted previously) that suicide rates varied inversely or negatively with the degree of social integration of the groups of which the individual formed a part. For example, *egoistic suicide* results from excessive individuation or lack of social integration. As an illustration, other things being equal, Protestants (who tend to advocate a highly individual relationship with God; a "priesthood of all believers") should have higher suicide rates than Catholics or Jews (who tend to be more socially and ritually homogeneous; more bound by traditions, the catechism, the Torah, etc.). On a more individual level, male skid-row social outcasts would be close to the egoistic suicide types. Apathy is thought to characterize egoistic suicides.

Altruistic suicide, on the other hand, results from insufficient individuation and is characterized by energy or activity, rather than apathy. The altruistic suicide type typically finds the basis for existence beyond earthly life. Examples of this type would include religious martyrs (from early Christians in Rome to Jim Jones in Guyana and David Koresh in Waco), soldiers who die for their country (e.g., Japanese kamikaze pilots during World War II), or Indian widows, who until recently were often expected to sacrifice themselves on their husbands' funeral pyres (the custom of suttee).

If egoistic and altruistic suicides are defined by the degree of social participation or involvement, then anomic or fatalistic suicides have to do with social deregulation or hyperregulation. In a sense, egoistic and altruistic suicides operate on the level of social (horizontal) restraint, whereas anomic and fatalistic suicides result from variance in normative (vertical) restraint. *Anomie* literally means "without norms" and *anomic suicide* results from a temporary but abrupt disruption of normative restraint. For example, suicides following stock market crashes and high rates of divorce could be considered anomic. *Fatalistic suicide* (which Durkheim considered only in a footnote) is generated by excessive regulation. Examples might be jail or prison suicides or suicides of very young married couples.

Psychiatric and psychological types of suicide were developed early on by Sigmund Freud and later by his American counterpart, psychiatrist Karl Menninger (1938). As Menninger (and, to a lesser extent, Freud) saw it, all suicides have three fundamental dimensions: hate, depression (melancholia), and guilt. It follows that all suicides are of three interrelated types: (1) *revenge* (a "wish to kill"), (2) *depression/hopelessness* (a "wish to die"), and (3) *guilt* (a "wish to be killed"). The loss of an important love object (such as the death of one's father, as in the case of Sylvia Plath) who has been internalized as part of one's own ego ("introjection") often results in adult melancholia or depression. Freud believed that all suicides involved hostility or a death wish originally directed at an external object (one's father, mother, lover, spouse, etc.). Accordingly, one psychiatric type of suicide is based on anger, rage, hatred, revenge, or a wish to kill (Maltsberger, 1992). Thus, Menninger called suicide "murder in the 180th degree."

Psychologically, trying to kill an introjected object results in ego splitting and regression (Litman, 1967). The suicidal person also feels guilty for harboring murderous wishes toward loved ones. Thus, suicides involve not only a "wish to kill" but also a "wish to be killed" or punished. Finally (of course, we oversimplify immensely here), suicides are depressed, hopeless, and cognitively constricted. As one's ego is destroyed by self-hatred and guilt, a "wish to die" may arise. Freud also thought that the processes of civilization require collective repression of sexuality and aggression, which in turn are channeled into a punitive group superego, fragmenting and otherwise diminishing our egos. In a sense, as Freud saw it, higher suicide rates are one cost of advancing civilization.

At the conclusion of this section we develop a classification of suicidal behaviors that encompasses not only types of completed suicide but also nonfatal suicide attempters, suicide ideators, mixed suicidal types, and indirect self-destructive behaviors. Although space precludes elaboration, most of the subtypes of completed suicides apply *mutatis mutandis* to the other basic forms of self-destructive behaviors and ideas specified in Figure 2.3. For example, there are at least as many different types of *nonfatal suicide attempters* as there are types of suicide completers (i.e., at least four to six basic types and two to three subtypes for each main type). For example (after controlling for age, sex, and race, and keeping it simple by considering only dichotomies), one can readily think of the following differences: psychotic versus nonpsychotic, organic versus nonorganic, interpersonal versus noninterpersonal, self-harm versus harm to others, hopeless versus change motivated, altruistic versus narcissistic, risk taking versus a more genuine wish to die, single versus. multiple attempts, and so on.

Suicidal thoughts or ideas also need to be considered. As we have argued above, many people think about suicide who never attempt or complete suicide. Included here are individuals who plan, obsess, save their pills, consider special circumstances for suicide (e.g., irreversible physical illness and AIDS), make living wills, ruminate, talk about suicide, threaten, fantasize, communicate ideas about suicide, and so forth. Perhaps the largest group of self-destructive behaviors is what Farberow (1980) has labeled ISDB (see Chapter 18). As we saw in Chapter 1, these ISDB include self-mutilation, deliberate self-harm, mismanagment of a physical illness, participation in a risky sport, car accidents, gambling, alcoholism, drug abuse, cigarette smoking, obesity and overeating, anorexia and bulimia, overwork and self-imposed stress, sexual promiscuity, and much more. One final differentiation is that of self-destructive death versus all other deaths. Forensically or pathologically, suicides are often determined by elimination; that is, a suicide is not a natural death, an accident, or a homicide. To make matters even more complicated, manners of death commonly overlap. For example, we may only be able to classify a death as a "suicide/accident/undetermined," "probable suicide," or the like.

Given all the variation in self-destructive behaviors and ideas, the scientific study of suicide (i.e., suicidology) would be advanced immensely by the creation of a single, standardized classification system, similar to DSM-IV or the 10th edition of the *International Classification of Diseases* (ICD-10; World Health Organization, 1992; Cooper, 1994). (It should be noted in passing that there could be *different* [not single] models for classification of suicidal behavior and ideas. For example, there could be a "categorical model" [which defines by criteria of inclusion or exclusion], a "dimensional model" [which relies on factor analytical techniques or derive criteria], or a "prototype model" [which defines correlated features by example]. See Rosenberg et al., 1988.) Theoretically, there is no reason why a diagnostic and statistical manual of suicidal behaviors (and perhaps ideas) could not be developed. One could easily imagine 12 to 18 basic types of suicidal behaviors, each with 6 to 12 subtypes, and even a multiaxial system of classification like that of the American Psychiatric Association's DSM-IV (see Table 2.2).

In effect, the NIMH, Center for the Studies of Suicide Prevention, did just this in 1972–1973. Sixty-two medical and behavioral suicidologists met in Phoenix to consider various aspects of suicide prevention. One of the six committees (chaired by Aaron Beck) developed a classification and nomenclature scheme for suicidal behaviors. Beck still regards this scheme as basically appropriate even today (personal communication, 1999). Essentially, suicidal phenomena are considered either completions, nonfatal suicide attempts, or suicide ideas. Each of these three types is then further specified by (1) certainty of the rater (0–100%), (2) lethality (zero, low, medium, or high), (3) intent to die (zero, low, medium, or high), (4) mitigating circumstances, like confusion or intoxication (zero, low, medium, or high), and (5) methods (one lists the actual method used). Although the Beck committee scheme has the advantage of parsimony, it does not approach the sophistication of classification manuals such as DSM. For example, the Beck committee considers all suicides, nonfatal attempts, and ideas in the same way. Intention is in fact usually not obvious and is difficult to measure. Basic demographic traits are not recorded by Beck and indirect self-destructive behaviors are also left out.

Jobes et al. (1987; and Rosenberg et al., 1988)—plus a committee of scholars from other professional societies—elaborated on the Beck committee's classification scheme, but focused only on completed suicide. They argued that all suicides must be self-inflicted and that the deceased must intend to die. One advantage of the Jobes et al. (1987) classification is that it allows for indirect evidence of intent to die (11 criteria for intent are specified). However, only completed suicide is classified; also, as in the Beck committee scheme, no subtypes are delineated.

Ellis (1988) has explored what he calls the "dimensions" of self-destructive behavior. The Ellis classification does of encompass all major types of self-destruction (including ideation and parasuicide), as well as other descriptive, situational, psychological/behavioral, and teleological concomitants. However, Ellis comes close to confusing classes of suicide with causes of suicide. Definitions should not be explanations.

Although it is far from a finished product and has its own obvious shortcomings, we offer Table 2.2 as a further classification step in the right direction which builds on the seminal work of Beck et al., Jobes et al., and Ellis (as alternative classification approaches, see Rosenberg et al., 1988; O'Carroll et al., 1996; Orbach, 1997). First, on Axis I, the rater has

TABLE 2.2. A Multiaxial Classification of Suicidal Behaviors and Ideation

Suicidal behaviors/ideas	Check (✔)	1. Primary type	2. Certainty	3. Lethal-ity	4. Intent	5. Circum-stances	6. Method	7. Sex	8. Age	9. Race	10. Marital status	11. Occupa-tion
I. Completed suicides												
A. Escape, egotic, alone. no hope												
B. Revenge, hate, aggressive												
C. Altruistic, self-sacrificing. transfiguration												
D. Risk-taking, ordeal, game												
E. Mixed												
II. Nonfatal suicide attempts												
A. Escape, catharsis, tension reduction												
B. Interpersonal, manipulation, revenge												
C. Altruistic												
D. Risk-taking												
E. Mixed												
F. Single vs. multiple												
G. Parasuicide												
III. Suicidal ideation												
A. Escape, etc.												
B. Revenge, interpersonal, etc.												
C. Altruistic, etc.												
D. Risk-taking, etc.												
E. Mixed												
IV. Mixed or uncertain mode												
A. Homicide–suicide												
B. Accident–suicide												
C. Natural–suicide												
D. Undetermined, pending												
E. Other mixed												
V. Indirect, self-destructive behavior (not an exclusive category)												
A. Alcoholism												
B. Other drug abuse												
C. Tobacco abuse												
D. Self-mutilation												
E. Anorexia–bulimia												
F. Over, or underweight												
G. Sexual promiscuity												
H. Health management problem, medications												
I. Risky sports												
J. Stress												
K. Accident-proneness												
L. Other (specify)												

Note. Certainty: Rate 0–100%.
Lethality (medical danger to life): Rate zero, low, medium, high (O, L, M, H).
Intent: Rate zero, low, medium, high.
Mitigating circumstances (psychotic. impulsive, intoxicated, confused): Rate zero, low, medium, high.
Method: firearm (F); poison (solid and liquid) (P); Poison (gas) (PG); hanging (H); cutting or piercing (C); jumping (J); drowning (D); crushing (CR); other (O), none (N).
Sex: Male (M) or female (F).
Age: Record actual age at event.
Race: White (W), black (B), Asian (A), other (O).
Marital Status: Married (M), single (S), divorced (D), widowed (W), other (O).
Occupation Manager, executive, administration (M); professional (P); technical workers (T); sales workers (S); clerical worker (C); worker in precision production (mechanic, repairer, construction worker) (PP); service worker (SW); operator, laborer (OL); worker in farming, forestry, fishing (F); other (O); none (N).
Source: Maris (1992d: 82). Copyright 1992 by The Guilford Press. Reprinted by permission.

to decide whether a suicidal outcome (the focus is on just one outcome at a particular time) is a completion (code I), a nonfatal attempt (code II), an idea (code III), or a mixed or uncertain outcome (code IV). Second, we have assumed from a prior review of the suicide literature, research, and clinical practice that suicidal phenomena are fundamentally either (1) escape, (2) revenge, (3) altruistic, (4) risk taking, or (5) mixed. Each type is elaborated to be as broad as possible and still be relatively homogeneous and yet to be reasonably exclusive with other basic types of suicidal behaviors (see Maris, 1992d: 80–83 for details and examples). Mixed types should be specified (e.g., as 1 and 2). If one type is clearly predominant or primary, it is best not to code the case as mixed. The primary type of suicidal behavior should be checked in column 1.

Like the Beck committee, we recommend that the rater record the certainty of the type (0 to 100% in column 2), the lethality or medical danger to life (column 4), and the mitigating circumstances (column 5). In addition, the method, sex, age, race, marital status, and census occupational category should be coded for each case (columns 6 to 11; see footnotes to Table 2.2). These later variables are not part of the definition, however. Code V records all known indirect self-destructive behaviors (the rater should check all copresent traits in code V, rows A to L in column 1). Code V can be completed for all cases (if the relevant traits are known) and is not an exclusive code. Codes I to IV are mutually exclusive, however. The rate should note that homicide–suicide, uncertain modes of death, pending deaths, and other mixed modes or manners get code IV subcodes.

In effect, suicidal behaviors are being coded in Table 2.2 on three axes: Axis I (primary type; codes I, II, III, or IV), Axis II (secondary characteristics; columns 2–11) and Axis III (ISDBs; code V). For example, the code:

$$IA/75, H,H,M,F,M,55,W,D,P/A,C,H$$

would indicate an escape suicide with a 75% certainty, high lethality and intent, medium mitigating circumstances, and death by a firearm; the individual in this case was a male, 55 years old, white, divorced, and a professional. The code V subcodes (A,C,H) indicate that this man had indirect factors of alcoholism, tobacco abuse, and health management problems. Our scheme is admittedly somewhat incomplete in that it does not rate social or many biological types explicitly.

TOWARD A SYSTEMATIC THEORY
OF SUICIDAL BEHAVIORS

At the beginning of this chapter (in Figure 2.1) we argued that theory construction in suicidology involves taking hypotheses confirmed as research results and converting them into theorems, by deducing them logically or mathematically from sets of general postulates or axioms and definitions. This approach to generating formal or systematic suicidological theory has several advantages. For one, it can ground discrete research results in basic general domain assumptions (e.g., those of cognitive theory, behaviorism, psychoanalysis, psychobiology, or whatever). For another, it integrates diverse theoretical components into a systematic whole. It may also generate novel hypothetical results that can then be tested empirically. Finally, it may force us to specify missing steps or premises (e.g., definitions or provisional assumptions) in our suicide theory in order to complete our inferences.

Systematic theory construction in suicidology is admittedly rare. For whatever reason often our basic assumptions about why people suicide are seldom articulated, let alone systematically interrelated. Early on, Maurice Farber (1968) wrote the ambitious *Theory of Suicide*. But other more recent attempts at constructing formal theories of suicide are hard to think of. Yufit and Bongar (1992) have attempted to state some axiom-like propositions about human development, stress, and suicide outcome. In sociology we see George Homans's work; he attempted to deduce the research results of small group experiments from axioms derived from Skinner's behaviorism and microeconomics (Homans, 1974; cf. Maris, 1970). Peter Blau (1977) made a similar effort to explain structural aspects of human behavior. Of course, one early model similar to that suggested by Figure 2.1 is Euclidean geometry.

In the few pages that remain in Chapter 2 we can only sketch how systematic suicidological theory might be constructed. Given that our sketch will be brief, incomplete, and provisional; it might be best to refer to it as "embryonic theory" or as a suicide "explanation sketch." The focus here is on *form*, not on substance or details. We have considered suicide theory construction in more detail elsewhere (see Maris, 1981: 306–340) and refer readers to that extended consideration.

In our prior suicide theory sketch (Maris, 1981) we stated five axioms or postulates and two provisional assumptions, all derived from broad domain assumptions with psychiatry (and to a lesser degree from existential philosophy; in a research note by Lester, 1994, which compared 15 theories of suicide as to how well they actually described the lives of well-known suicides, the Maris theory sketch virtually tied with Shneidman's theory for second best in prediction behind Beck's top-ranked theory). These "set A" (see Figure 2.1) propositions were formulated in ordinary English and also in Aristotelian logic (using Irving Copi's [1994] notations and rules of inference). They were as follows:

A1. Completed suicide is directly related to the level of one's hopelessness and depression (in managing the human condition) $[(\text{CS} \supset \sim H \cdot D) \text{ or } \text{CS } f(\sim H \cdot D)]$.

A2. Completed suicide is inversely related to satisfaction (with the human condition) $\left[(\text{CS} \supset \sim \text{SA}) \text{ CS} = f\left(\dfrac{1}{\text{SA}}\right)\right]$.

A3. Suicidal hopelessness, depression, and dissatifaction are directly related to the use of lethal methods $\left[(\text{CS}(H \cdot D \cdot \text{SA})\text{LM}) \text{ or CS} = f \dfrac{\text{LM}}{H \cdot \sim D \cdot \text{SA}}\right]$.

A4. Suicidal hopelessness is directly related to depression, repeated life failures, prolonged negative interaction, and social isolation $[(\sim H \supset (D_{1\ldots n} F_{1\ldots n} \text{NI} \cdot \text{SI}_{1\ldots n})$ or $\sim H = f(D_{1\ldots n} \times F_{1\ldots n} \times \text{NI} \cdot \text{SI}_{1\ldots n})]$.

A5. Repeated depression, failure, and negative interaction and social isolation are directly related to early trauma and to a multiproblem family of origin $[(D \cdot F \cdot \text{NI} \cdot \text{SI}) \supset (\text{ET} \cdot \text{MPFO}) \text{ or } (D \cdot F \cdot \text{NI} \cdot \text{SI}) = f(\text{ET} \cdot \text{MPFO})]$.

PA1. Age, male sex, and Protestant religious preference are directly related to completed suicide $[(\text{CS} \supset (A \cdot M \cdot \text{PR}) \text{ or } \text{CS} = f(A \cdot M \cdot \text{PR})]$.

PA2. Age and male sex are directly related to suicidal hopelessnes, lethal methods, work problems, and physical illness and inversely related to satisfaction, repeated depression, negative interaction, sexual deviance, marital problems, drug problems, early trauma, and a multiproblem family of origin $[(A \cdot M) \supset (\sim H \cdot \text{LM} \cdot \text{WP} \cdot \text{PI}) \cdot \sim(\text{SA} \cdot D \cdot \text{NI} \cdot \text{SD} \cdot \text{MP} \cdot \text{DP} \cdot \text{ET} . \text{MPFO}) \text{ or } A \cdot M =$

$$f \frac{\sim H \cdot LM \cdot WP \cdot PI}{SA \cdot D \cdot NI \cdot SD \cdot MP \cdot DP \cdot ET \cdot MPFO}$$

Given these axioms and provisional assumptions, one can now proceed to deduce research results, For example, research result 6 on p. 47 states that completed suicides are socially isolated. We can deduce that result from our set A propositions as follows:

1.	CS ⊃ ~H · D	A1
2.	CS ⊃ ~H	1, simplification
3.	~H ⊃ SI	A4, simplification
4.	/CS ⊃ SI	2,3, hypothetical syllogism

Or again, suppose we wished to deduce that suicide implied physical illness. The argument would be as follows:

1.	CS ⊃ A	PA2, simplification
2.	A ⊃ PI	PA2, simplification
3.	/CS ⊃ PI	1,2, hypothetical syllogism

Finally, what if we wished to conclude that nonfatal suicide attempts implied drug abuse problems. An argument might be constructed as follows:

1.	A ⊃ ~DP	PA2, simplification
2.	DP ⊃ ~A	1, transposition
3.	~A ⊃ DP	2, conversion (by limitation)
4.	AS ⊃ ~A	PA3
5.	/AS ⊃ DP	3,4, hypothetical syllogism

Of course, one can readily find objections to these simple explanation sketches. For example, the inferences seem to work because they are tautologous. That is, the axioms and assumptions contain the outcomes to be inferred. In a sense these theory sketches are substantively trivial and even self-evident. The axioms are not very general, nor do they include all possibly relevant domains . . . and so on. The point here is not to construct useful theory per se but, rather, to indicate how an ambitious suicidologist might go about formal suicide theory construction, as well as what some of the uses of systematic theory in suicidology might be. We only wish to point in a direction, not actually arrive at the theoretical end point. For some of the concepts that would need to be included as axioms, assumptions, and definitions in any sound general theory of suicide, readers are referred to Figure 2.6. (Fuller elaboration of the model in Figure 2.6 is provided in Maris, Berman, & Maltsberger, 1992: 667–669.)

SUMMARY AND CONCLUSIONS

Chapter 2 has described systematic suicidological theory and elaborated its components. We have argued that theory is both a crucial "way of seeing" and a "way of not seeing" (e.g., because of our professional blinders). Theory guides us in what to pay attention to

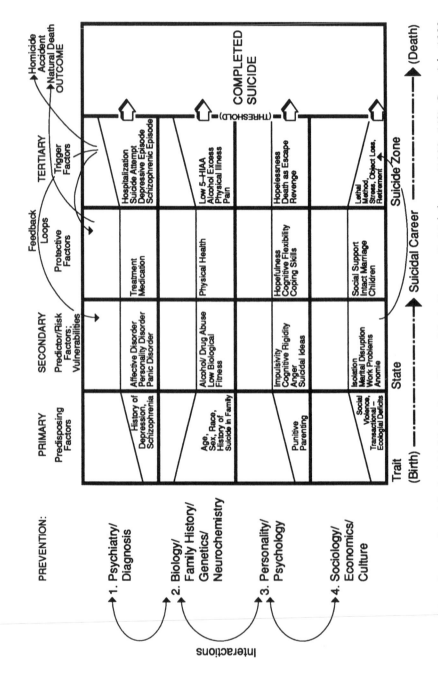

FIGURE 2.6. A general model of suicidal behaviors. *Source:* Maris, Berman, & Maltsberger (1992: 668). Copyright 1992 by The Guilford Press. Reprinted by permission.

clinically as well as in our research. A formal theory can be thought of as sets of laws (law-like propositions, axioms, assumptions, postulates) and definitions that are related logically or mathematically to hypotheses or models confirmed earlier as research results. To deduce research results from broad domain axiomatic propositional assumptions and definitions is to "explain" them, in effect to convert them into theorems. Formal theory has the potential of generating a systematic whole out of isolated, diverse theoretical propositional parts, as well as generating novel propositions for empirical testing.

The building blocks of a systematic theory of suicide include definitions, basic concepts (lethality, motive, intent, suicidal careers, etc.), hypotheses, models, and research results. "Suicide" can be defined as "intentional self-murder." Several implications of this (and other) definitions of "suicide" were discussed. Lethality usually refers to the probability that an action, method, and/or condition will kill you (e.g., the medical certainty of death). Several scales have been designed to measure lethality and a few were presented in this chapter. Lethality can be either acute or chronic. Motives indicate one's presumed reasons for suicide, whereas intent means that the individual understood the consequences of his or her self-destructive act. Suicide-prone biopsychosocial life histories can be thought of as suicidal careers. For example, poet Sylvia Plath's life history was presented as an illustration of a suicidal career.

Hypotheses are usually more focused and limited than are theories. A hypothesis, as a testable proposition, usually implies a systematic test. One important characteristic of hypotheses is their falsifiability. Durkheim's hypothesis that suicide rates vary inversely with the degree of social integration was provided as an example and was operationalized and tested, Models tend to predict interrelationships of several independent variables (as opposed to hypotheses, which are usually bivariate) to an outcome variable (like suicide). Causal models are normally operationalized by regression equations (especially logistic regression for suicide outcomes) but also can include path models, log-linear models, and time-series models.

When hypotheses or causal models receive repeated empirical support in proper research designs in diverse samples and cultures, we tend to regard them as "research results." Research results are the fundamental empirical regularities of suicidal behaviors and ideas that our theories attempt to explain. Chapter 2 listed 12 major research results from Maris's Chicago surveys of suicide as an example and then raised five basic questions about research results in general.

Some concepts are so basic to suicide theories that they can be thought of as "the commonalities of suicide." For example, Shneidman contends that all suicides tend to (1) seek a solution to their life problems, (2) want to cease their consciousness, (3) have intolerable psychological pain ("psychache"), (4) have frustrated psychological needs, (5) be hopeless and helpless, (6) be ambivalent about dying, (7) have constricted, dichotomous thoughts, (8) engage in egression or fugue behaviors, (9) communicate their suicide intentions, and (10) have lifelong self-destructive coping patterns. Taken together with the known predictors of suicide (depression, alcohol abuse, being an older white male, etc.; see Chapter 3) the commonalities of suicide form the core concepts for any potential theory of suicide.

Not only do suicides share common traits, they also are (of course) different, comprise somewhat separate and distinct types, and can be classified by their salient characteristics. Suicide is not one thing but is in fact many different overlapping and yet distinct things. For example, we reviewed Durkheim's four basic types of suicide: (1) anomic, (2) egoistic, (3) altruistic, and (4) fatalistic, as well as Freud/Menninger's three essential psychiatric types (or components): (1) revenge/murder, (2) depression/hopelessness, and (3) guilt.

Our efforts at classification began with a schema by the Beck committee, followed by elaborations and revisions from Jobes et al. (1987) and Ellis (1988), and ending with a proposed classificatory synthesis by Maris. The Maris classification required decisions on three axes: (1) primary type (completed suicide, nonfatal suicide attempt, suicide ideator, or mixed types), (2) secondary characteristics (certainty, lethality, intent, mitigating circumstances, method, age, sex, race, marital status, and occupation), and (3) ISDBs.

Finally, Chapter 2 closed with a few illustrations of how suicide research results might be logically deduced from definitions, axioms, and assumptions to form a systematic theory of suicide. Chapter 3 will in a sense be the "mirror image" of Chapter 2. That is, it focuses on *research and data* issues as opposed to theoretical issues.

FURTHER READING

Copi, I. M. (1994). *Introduction to logic* (9th ed.). New York: Macmillan. A classic introductory logic text divided into sections on language (including informal fallacies and definitions) deduction (with chapters on categorical syllogisms, symbolic logic, rules of inference, proving validity, etc.), and induction. Should help the reader see how valid deductions can be made from definitions and axioms.

Durkheim, E. (1897/1951). *Suicide: A sociological study*. Glencoe, IL: Free Press. One of the seminal works in suicidology. Durkheim argues that suicide rates are explained by external and constraining social facts (such as anomie, egoism, altruism, and fatalism), not by individual psychopathology. Although one of the first empirical studies of suicide death records, the distinguishing trait of suicide is its carefully stated theory and powerful arguments for broad social forces in the variation of suicide rates.

Farber, M. L. (1968). *Theory of suicide*. New York: Funk and Wagnalls. Farber attempts to develop a general psychological theory of suicide based on his empirical research in Scandinavia. Some of his basic postulates are that the less hope, the greater the suicide potential or suicide rate, and that the more acceptable life conditions are threateed and a sense of competence diminished, the less hope and the greater suicide potential. Farber's theory is weak in that it omits biological factors, does not give operational definitions of key terms, and does not systematically interrelate the theory's propositions.

Maris, R. W. (1981). *Pathways to suicide*. Baltimore: Johns Hopkins University Press. This empirical study of completed suicides in Chicago attempts to deduce some 122 major research results from general psychiatric postulates, assumptions, and definitions through the use of Copi's rules of inference (see Chapter 11 of *Pathways*, "Toward a Theory of Suicidal Careers"). Maris also suggests path models to differentiate suicidal careers of suicide versus natural deaths and those of suicide completers versus nonfatal suicide attempters.

Menninger, K. (1938). *Man against himself*. New York: Harcourt, Brace, & World. Although Freud himself had relatively little to say about suicide theory, his American counterpart and founder of the Menninger Clinic in Topeka elaborated Freud's concepts of life-and death-wishes. Menninger claims with Freud that every suicide is a disguised murder (murder in the 180th degree). All suicides have a wish to kill (hate or murder), a wish to be killed (guilt), and a wish to die (hopelessness). Like Freud, Menninger developed a theory of suicide based mainly on psychiatric patients who had attempted suicide, not primarily on suicide completers. A classic study of the various types of suicide and self-destructive behaviors.

Shneidman, E. (1985). *Definition of suicide*. New York: Wiley. Contains a major definition of "suicide" as "a conscious act of self-induced annihilation, best understood as a multidimensional malaise in a needful individual who defines an issue for which suicide is perceived as the best solution" (203). Also elaborates the 10 conceptual commonalities of suicide. Shneidman emphasizes the idiographic (clinical) method and pays homage to Stephen Pepper, James G. Miller, and Henry A. Murray. Contains important chapters on the word "suicide," as well as on classification issues.

3

The Empirical Foundations
of Suicidology

Give me a man's actual findings, so long as he has taken some pains about
his methods of reaching them, and I care not what obviously silly theory he
may have incorporated them into.
—GEORGE CASPAR HOMANS

One of the first heart transplants in the United States was done at the Johns Hopkins Medical School. The donor was a suicide and immediately after receiving his new heart, the recipient became suicidal. One of the professors in the suicidology training program at Johns Hopkins, Edwin Shneidman, remarked facetiously: "Aha, so that's where *it* is!" Since its inception, suicidology has been trying to determine what facts to pay attention to.

"Suicidology" is loosely the *science* of self-destructive behaviors. Surely any "science" worth its salt ought to try to be true to its name and be as objective as it can, make careful measurements, count something. The renowned French founder of the scientific study of suicide, Emile Durkheim, as we observed previously was fond of saying, "These being the facts, what is their explanation?" One needs to as sure as possible that we have our *facts* clear, that something is worth trying to explain, that it is an empirical regularity of a fairly high order.

To be "empirical" means to be guided by practical experience and not just theory, relying on or deriving some facts from systematic observation or experiment. But *what facts* or observations should the suicidologist heed? Is the explanation or cause of suicide found in the mind, the brain, genes, hormones, chromosomes, blood, urine, alcohol, social forces, psychological behavior, neurotransmitters, or where? A corollary of this question is what professional discipline is at the heart of suicidological sciences (psychiatry, psychology, sociology, biology, nursing, social work, physiology, neurochemistry, economics . . .)? Of course, the answer could be "all of the above."

Box 3.1 suggests that suicidal traits may be hidden from easy view. Certainly there are some false negatives in our clinical practices (i.e., people like author William Styron, who manage to conceal their suicidal ideation or plans). Others, who may in fact be more clearly suicidal, may not give us a clue as to how suicidal they are or exactly how or when they plan to suicide. Part of this is inevitable because the sine qua non of suicide is intention, and intention can be shielded in the black box of the mind or the individual him- or herself may

62

BOX 3.1. Are Suicidal Traits Hidden or Observable?

Hidden: Shneidman (1994).

Observable: Stanley and Mann (1988).

Issue Summary:

Hidden: ". . . some desperately suicidal people, like a focused Ahab or a disconsolate Styron, can dissemble and hide their true feelings from the world. If it is true that all the world's a stage, then some players on occasion may wear their masks . . . the key questions . . . are: 'What is going on?' and 'Where do you hurt?' The challenge is to resonate to the other's hidden psychache, to reassemble what the other has dissembled."

Observable: "Because behavioral factors alone have been of limited clinical utility, more recent studies have tried to determine whether there might be biochemical changes associated with suicide and attempted suicide . . . subsequently in the early 1970s clinical studies that examine biogenic amine metabolites in the cerebrospinal fluid (CSF) began to observe a relationship between the serotonin metabolite 5-hydroxyindoleacetic acid (5-HIAA) and suicidal behavior. . . . A review of the neurochemical measures reported in these studies indicates that differences in the concentration of either 5-HT (serotonin) and/or 5-HIAA are the most consistently reported findings."

---

be confused or ambivalent about his suicidal intentions. Yet *suicidology has to have some observables*, otherwise it runs the danger of lapsing into mysticism and alchemy. It does not have to be Stanley and Mann's synaptic cleft or the serotonergic system that we observe and measure, but all science needs to respect *some* facts.

Another factual/observational issue in suicidology is whether the focus should be on the *individual* or on forces *outside the individual*. For example, Freud tended to study individual, neurotic, young, upper-middle-class female suicide ideator outpatients in his private psychoanalytic practice. "Facts" of interest were repressed sexual conflicts, family dynamics, hysteria, characterological (Axis II) personality traits, roots of anxiety and phobia, and so on.

But Durkheim concentrated on completed suicide *rates of groups* and collectivities based on death records (vital statistics). He focused on broad external and constraining social facts such as social integration, abrupt social disruption (e.g., the anomie of divorce), social isolation (egoism), and normative prosuicidal expectations (altruism). Other extraindividual forces related to suicide might include family violence, poverty, unemployment rates, failure of social support networks, and so on.

To be concerned about "facts and observations" implies quantification, numbers, data, counting, measurement, sampling, statistical analysis, methodology, etc. Typical empirical propositions in suicidology have the following form:

- In this large simple random sample of completed suicides 72% were male and the mean age was 47.
- The mean Beck Depression Inventory (BDI) score was 21 and the Hamilton Depression Rating Scale (HAM-D) was 24.
- The 5-HIAA (5-hydroxyindoleacetic) level in CSF was 92.5 nm/liter.
- Age, sex, race, history of major depressive episode, prior suicide attempt, and substance or alcohol abuse explained 65% of the variance (R_2) in suicide outcome.

Science tries to advance and *accumulate knowledge* (see especially Figure 2.1 in Chapter 2). For example, Maris (1981) listed 122 basic research results or empirical generalizations from a 3-year random sample survey of Chicago suicides. Although we have made considerable progess in building the empirical foundations for suicidology, it is embarassing how far we have yet to go. At a recent NIMH meeting on suicide nomenclature in Washington, DC, Patrick O'Carroll of the Centers for Disease Control and Prevention used what he called the "Senate Subcommittee Reality Check" (on just how advanced suicidological knowledge really is; see O'Carroll et al., 1996). The dialogue went something like this:

Senator: How long have y'all been studying suicide?

Suicidologist: About thirty years, sir.

Senator: Well, then, could you tell this committee what suicide is exactly?

Suicidologist: Sorry, sir, we really don't know.

Any bona fide science attempts to be objective, culture free, universal, and impartial and to have valid, reliable, sensitive, and specific propositions. Unfortunately, empirical "realities" are often evasive and chameleonic and change over time, with the country studied or the sample used, and so on. Empirical regularities or "facts," such as those concerning gender and suicide or age and suicide, often show diametrically opposite patterns in different countries or cultures. For example, some countries have virtually a zero suicide rate (Egypt, New Guinea, Antigua, Jamaica, the Philippines), but in other countries the suicide rate is so high as to almost be part of their national character (e.g., Hungary, Germany, Austria, Denmark, Finland, or Japan).

In the remainder of this chapter we examine (1) data sources for the study of suicide; (2) rates of suicide controlling for broad social–demographic and epidemiological variables; (3) empirical predictors of suicide, including some standardized scales; and (4) statistical, methodological, and research design issues in suicidology.

HOW DO WE STUDY SUICIDE (DATA SOURCES)?

Right away, the would-be student of suicide is faced with at least two serious research obstacles. First, suicide is rare, about one to three persons per year per 10,000 in the general population. Thus, much of the time when researchers think they are examining suicide data, they are in fact considering "only" suicide ideation, nonfatal suicide attempts, suicidal gestures, risk-taking behavior, and so on—in short, what epidemiologists call false positives. Second, suicidal respondents cannot respond; they are dead. Most psychological or psychiatric tests or assessments assume living, first-person respondents. If one interviews a spouse, parent, child, or friend (i.e., third-person respondents) in an effort to assess a suicidal decedent's depression, life history, sexual behavior, or whatever, all sorts of unknown errors are incurred. On the other hand, if an investigator attempts a prospective, longitudinal first-person study of high-risk samples who will later go on to suicide, clearly he or she needs huge samples, lots of continuing research funds, and about 35–50 years for the eventual suicides in the sample to die—which raises further ethical and treatment related problems.

Keeping in mind these two research problems, the major data sources for the study of suicide are as follows:

1. Surveys, including epidemiological studies and psychological autopsies.
2. Treatment records, hospital charts, and clinical interviews.

3. Vital statistics, death certificates, and coroner and medical examiner records.
4. Experiments, especially psychopharmacological studies.
5. Diaries, suicide notes, letters, and other first-person accounts.
6. Art, novels, poems, literature, plays, and history.

Items 5 and 6 are the subject of entire chapters later on in this text (Chapters 11 and 4, respectively). However, items 1–4 merit some elaboration here.

Surveys, Epidemiological Studies, and Psychological Autopsies

Surveys of suicides usually start out with a list of names and addresses of all suicides from either a state vital statistics office or the national center for health statistics. Because human subjects are protected and death records are privileged information, it is difficult and time-consuming to get a list of completed suicides, and even then there is no guarantee that the vital statistics are accurate. Because suicide is rare, lists are generally drawn from large cities such as New York, Chicago, Los Angeles, and St. Louis. Because interviews are expensive, the total universe of all suicides is sampled (random, systematic, stratified, proportionate, clustered, with sampling fractions, etc.).

Appropriate comparison and control groups (e.g., of natural deaths, accidents, homicides, nonsuicidal psychiatric patients, and depressed individuals) are usually also sampled (Schlesselman, 1982). The investigator will either use a standardized interview schedule with standard scales or tests, construct a new questionnaire, or mix both types of instruments. Sample sizes are determined conjointly by available money, the statistical power needed to detect significant differences in the experimental and control groups, the number of independent or predictor variables, and the type of statistical analyses to be done.

Typically the informant being surveyed or questioned is the deceased's spouse or other family member. Multiple informants (two or three) per case are the norm, to capture variation and minimize error. Most surveys are retrospective because (as we saw previously) prospective surveys require large samples of living probands, only some of whom will ever suicide, long time frames, sustained research funding, and probably a team of investigators—like the studies of Aaron Beck and his colleagues mentioned earlier. Another issue is how soon after a suicide is committed should the survivors be interviewed. In our own experience the sooner, the better (e.g., a few weeks after the suicide or even as part of the initial death investigation by the medical examiner or coroner).

Analysis includes comparing case or experimental groups with control or comparison groups by percentages, rates, tests of significance, odds ratios, regression and log-linear models, analyses of variance, and so on. Not many large surveys of suicide are being done today given the cutback in federal research funds, such as Maris's (1981) large suicide survey funded by NIMH in Chicago. Two hundred sixty-six suicides were sampled from a total of 1,349 suicides over 3 consecutive years. Comparison groups of 64 nonfatal suicide attempters and 71 natural deaths were also interviewed. The survey took about 10 years from start to finish and cost a few hundred thousand dollars. Today the same survey would cost at least $1 million. The only suicide researchers who have been getting those kind of funds lately are psychologist David Clark and psychiatrist Jan Fawcett of Rush-Presbyterian Hospital in Chicago and epidemiologist Carol Garrison formerly at the University of South Carolina. Aaron Beck (Penn), John Mann (Columbia), and David Shaffer (Columbia) have also had significant suicide funding, but they have tended to do smaller, more experimental studies and not large-scale sample surveys.

A major epidemiological survey is the Epidemiologic Catchment Area (ECA) study (Eaton & Kessler, 1985). This was a five-site survey (New Haven, East Baltimore, St. Louis,

Durham, and Los Angeles) with 3,000 to 5,000 interview cases per site. The Diagnostic Interview Schedule (DIS) and Schedule for Affectives Disorders and Schizophrenia (SADS) were administered and questions were asked about suicide (see Moscicki, O'Carroll, & Regier, 1988; Nisbet, 1996). Epidemiology can be defined broadly as the study of the distribution and determinants of diseases and injuries (here of suicides) in human populations (Mausner & Bahn, 1985). Epidemiologists, among other things, are interested in the "incidence" rate (the number of new cases of a disease divided by the population at risk) and the "prevalence" rate (the number of existing cases of disease divided by the total population at time t). Loosely "primary prevention" concerns reducing incidence, "secondary prevention" reducing prevalence, and "tertiary prevention" reducing the disability of the disease (here, suicide).

A final survey procedure for our purposes is the psychological autopsy. A psychological autopsy can be defined as *a procedure for reconstructing an individual's psychological life after the fact*, particularly the person's lifestyle and those thoughts, feelings, and behaviors manifested during the weeks preceding death, in order to achieve a better understanding of the psychological circumstances contributing to a death (Clark & Horton-Deutsch, 1992: 144). Probably this survey type should be called a biopsychosocial autopsy, because the relevant variables are not restricted just to psychological ones.

In fact the psychological autopsy is not even one standard form but, instead, consists of forms used for diverse purposes. In addition to Maris's (1981) psychological autopsy study, Robins and Murphy did early psychological autopsies in St. Louis (Robins, 1981), as did Rich, Fowler, Young, and Blenkush (1986a) in San Diego and Barraclough and Hughes (1987) in the United Kingdom (West Sussex and Portsmouth). Psychological autopsies often supplement physical autopsies in medical examiners' and coroners' offices and are widely used in death investigations and forensic cases.

Treatment Records, Hospital Charts, Clinical Interviews

Another valuable source of suicide data is treatment records and hospital charts of suicidal individuals. These records are usually of psychiatric inpatients, but they could be of suicidal outpatients compiled by psychologists, social workers, nurses, various mental health counselors, and so on, as well as by psychiatrists. Usually treatment records are "convenience samples," not products of research designs, with proper controls, and so on. Treatment records tend to be of small, biased samples of single individuals (such as in forensic cases). The focus in these documents by definition is treatment (or litigation), usually not research. Finally, treatment records tend to be of nonfatal suicide attempters or living patients with affective disorders, not of completed suicides.

Elsewhere (Maris, Berman, & Maltsberger, 1992: 660–667) we have discussed clinical suicidal data in detail that we cannot go into here. However, a typical medical or psychiatric file on a suicidal patient will include some of the following relevant type of data:

- Admission and discharge summaries
- A social history
- Progress notes by the treatment team
- A mental status examination
- Psychological tests
- Medication records
- Vital signs charts

All these types of data can provide valuable information for the suicide researcher.

The *admission form* contains standard sociodemographic data (address, age, sex, race, occupation, insurance, responsible party, etc.), a provisional diagnosis and DSM code, a list of presenting problems or chief complaints, a physical examination and review of systems (usually within 72 hours), a history and assessment (including medications, medical data, and mental status), other admission notes, and an initial care or treatment plan.

The *discharge summary* has all the admission data plus a history of the present illness and course in hospital, lab studies, and consults (if any), psychological tests, disposition, discharge medications, and prognosis/aftercare. Correct diagnosis is especially important, as treatment turns on accurate diagnosis. Some DSM codes (such as major depressive episode or borderline personality) are more suggestive of suicide than are others. Discrepancies between admission and discharge diagnoses should be noted, as should type, time initiated, and dosages over time of all psychotropic medications. Simple demographic data (like age, sex, and race) often tell us a lot about suicide potential. If the chief complaint involves suicide ideation or suicide attempts, then further assessments and treatment precautions are indicated.

Much of the data needed for a psychological autopsy can be gleaned from a good *social history*. These three to five pages of family and patient history normally will be written by a social worker. Although there is no one standard form, usually topics covered tend to include who the informants were, a family tree highlighting any psychiatric disorders of family members; marital and psychosocial development; education and employment; present and past psychiatric illnesses, hospitalizations, and treatments; history of physical illnesses and injuries; financial status; religious affiliation; family dynamics; military history; legal history; socialization patterns; any substance abuse; a problem list; patient strengths and weaknesses; and assessment and discharge planning. Doing a good social history may include requesting copies of prior psychiatric records.

Social history data can inform the suicidologist about family dynamics (e.g., driving the family member to suicide or, conversely, social support lowering suicide risk), evidence of a "suicidal career" and increasing hopelessness, what medications have worked in the past to reduce depressive disorder, and an explicit record of prior suicide attempts and suicide ideations and the current need for increased suicide precautions.

Hospital *progress notes* provide logged verbatim quotes and comments (particularly by the nursing staff) that can be especially helpful in suggesting suicide intent or specific suicide plans. These notes are in the form of date, time, name of the notemaker, and remarks. They can be almost eerie after the fact of suicide. Following are two examples of progress notes on suicides from our forensic clinical practice; the first by a 69-year-old white male alcoholic suicide who had earlier survived shotgun wounds to his face, and the second by a 38-year-old white depressed mother of four who eventually hung herself.

69-year-old white male

4/18/89	10 P	—Put on close observation for suicide.
4/19/89	1:30 A	—"Let me die soon."
5/16/89	9:30 P	—"My wife don't want me home. I've got no place to go. I'm at the end of the road. I've played a lot of checkers in my life. This is my last move."
5/18/89	8:10 A	—I entered the room. Client found hanging by cotton belt from ceiling (sprinkler) pipe.

38-year-old female

12/17/88	12:30 A	—Remains on 15-minute checks for suicide precautions.
12/18/88	10:40 A	—Spoke of wanting to leave. Expressed hopelessness in the future.

12/22/88	3:10 P	—Interacting very little with the staff.
12/24/88	11:55 P	—Angry affect
12/27/88	7:30 P	—"I don't want to live like this for another 38 years."
1/2/89	10 P	—Patient discovered hanging in shower room. Code blue.

The *mental status examination* checks for confusion, agitation, difficulty concentrating, and disorientation, among other things. It can be considered the psychiatric equivalent of medicine's physical examination and involves a comprehensive examination of a patient's appearance (including grooming and clothes), thinking and speech patterns, and so on. Items evaluated include motor activity, speech, mood, perception, orientation, memory, calculations, reading and writing capacity, attention, visual–spatial ability, abstraction, and insight. Some items are measured by simple observation, others by direct questions, such as those in Figure 3.1's mini-mental status exam. This mental status test for the 69-year-old white male described previously revealed no mental disorientation, confusion, or psychosis (a poignant reminder of how psychological tests can often indicate false negatives)—although the patient did appear tired, depressed, and hopeless to the examiner. Many confused, psychotic schizophrenics or agitated psychotic depressives are by that fact alone at a greater risk for suicide; thus a mental status test can help predict suicide. However, an individual who is able to clearly appraise a situation that is in fact hopeless or extremely difficult and challenging also can elevate his or her suicide potential (e.g., be a "rational suicide").

Maximum Score	Score	
5	(5)	1. Ask the patient to name the year, season, date, day, and month. (1 point each)
5	(5)	2. Ask the patient to give his/her whereabouts: state, county, town, street, floor. (1 point each)
3	(3)	3. Ask the patient to repeat three unrelated objects that you name. Repeat them and continue to repeat them until all three are learned. (1 point each)
5	(5)	4. Ask the patient to subtract 7 from 100, stopping after five subtractions, or to spell the word "world" backwards. (1 point for each correct calculation or letter)
3	(3)	5. Ask the patient to repeat the three objects previously named. (1 point each)
2	(2)	6. Display a wrist watch and ask the patient to name it. Repeat this for a pencil. (1 point each)
1	(1)	7. Ask the patient to repeat this phrase: "No ifs, ands, or buts!" (1 point)
3	(3)	8. Have the patient follow a three-point command such as, "Take a paper in your right hand, fold it in half, and put it on the floor!" (1 point each)
1	(1)	9. On a blank piece of paper write, "Close your eyes!" Ask the patient to read it and do what it says. (1 point)
1	(1)	10. Ask the patient to write a sentence on a blank piece of paper. It must be written spontaneously. Score correctly if it contains a subject and a verb and is sensible. (Correct grammar and punctuation are not necessary.) (1 point)

_____, MD   Patient Plate

Date: _____

Form 270 - 11/87 - MR

FIGURE 3.1. Mini-mental status examination. *Source:* Folstein, Folstein, & McHugh (1975). Copyright 1975 by Elsevier Science. Adapted by permission.

There are a wide variety of *psychological or psychiatric tests* or structured interviews that are used for clinical purposes to aid in psychiatric diagnosis (Andreasen & Black, 1995), personality assessment (Eyman & Eyman, 1992), and even direct suicide potential assessment (Rothberg & Geer-Williams, 1992). Most routine psychiatric inpatient treatment charts will include at least an MMPI (Minnesota Multiphasic Personality Inventory) or the equivalent, usually computer scored and interpreted with an accompanying profile—like that (of our 69-year-old white male) in Figure 3.2.

As the reader can see, this patient had elevated *D* (Depression), *Pt* (Psychasthenia) and *Si* (Social introversion) scale scores. Scores above 70 on the *D* scale indicate patients at increased risk for suicide, especially by hanging (Eyman & Eyman, 1992: 191). Some have argued that an elevated psychasthenia (*Pt*) scale also predicts suicide. "Psychasthenia" indicates indecisive, obsessive–compulsive, overconscientious individuals. Another consistent suicide prediction finding is a high score for males and a low score for females on the *Mf* scale (masculinity–femininity). However, even with a new depression scale on the MMPI-2, no MMPI item, scale, configuration, or profile consistently discriminates suicidal from nonsuicidal patients (Eyman & Eyman, 1992). Psychiatrists are justifiably mistrustful of the suicidal predictive value of most psychological tests.

Other psychological tests (and there are many more not listed here) that may be in a psychiatric patient's file include the following:

- Rorschach (an inkblot projective test)
- TAT (Thematic Apperception Test)
- HAM-D or BDI (Hamilton and Beck Depression inventories)
- SCID (Structured Clinical Interview for DSM-III-R Diagnosis)
- DIS (Diagnostic Interview Schedule)
- SADS (Schedule for Affective Disorders and Schizophrenia)
- SPS (a standardized Suicide Probability Scale; Cull & Gill, 1982)
- SP (Sad Persons checklist for high and low suicide risk; Patterson et al., 1983)
- CIESR (Clinical Instrument to Estimate Suicide Risk, mostly for research; Motto, Heilbron, & Juster, 1985)

The same comment could be made about all of the listed psychological or psychiatric tests that was made about the MMPI; that is, although they may provide useful supplemental data for assessing and predicting suicide, by themselves none provides sensitive, specific, reliable, value, or predictive measures of suicide potential.

Medication records or profiles and doctors' orders provide a useful source of data (which, when, what, how much, when discontinued, increased, reduced, etc.) on psychotropic drugs that were administered. Among the relevant suicide-related questions are the following:

- How soon was medication administered? (Was the patient left unmedicated for too long? Should a patient being watched closely be cleared or purged of prehospitalization medications?)
- Did the medications match the diagnosis?
- Was the dosage appropriate? (Were outpatients given enough antidepressants to overdose on?)
- Was a medication history taken?
- Were the drugs monitored and adjusted carefully?
- Were drug interactions, adverse reactions, and side effects considered and noted (written, e.g., akathisia)?

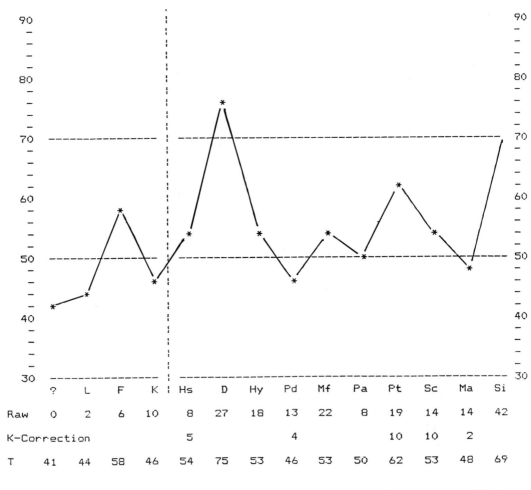

	?	L	F	K	Hs	D	Hy	Pd	Mf	Pa	Pt	Sc	Ma	Si
Raw	0	2	6	10	8	27	18	13	22	8	19	14	14	42
K-Correction					5			4			10	10	2	
T	41	44	58	46	54	75	53	46	53	50	62	53	48	69

F − K (Raw):   −4   Percentage True: 49   Profile Elevation: 55.1
                                                   (Hs,D,Hy,Pd,Pa,Pt,Sc,Ma)
Goldberg Index: 32   Henrichs Rule: Neurotic

Welsh Code: 2'07-13586/84:   F/KL2:

FIGURE 3.2. Minnesota Multiphasic Personality Inventory. Source: Minnesota Multiphasic Personality Inventory. Copyright © by the Regents of the University of Minnesota 1942, 1943 (renewed 1970). Reproduced by permission of the University of Minnesota Press.

- Were drugs given that have possible suicide-related consequences (e.g., Prozac [fluoxetine and the selective serotonin reuptake inhibitors], Halcion [triazolam], the benzodiazepines [e.g., Xanax and Valium] in general, etc.)?

Because some psychiatrists consider treatment and even suicide prevention to be virtually synonymous with psychoactive medication, a patient's drug records are crucial data in suicidology.

Finally, pschiatric nurses keep dated charts of patients' *vital signs*. Samples of such patient care data are as follows:

- Sleep charts
- Eating records
- Weight gain or loss charts
- Bowel and urine movements
- Libido fluctuations
- Pulse, respiration, and temperature
- Personal grooming and hygiene
- Activity therapy notes

One reason we pay special attention to patients' vital signs is that changes in "vegetative symptoms" (sleep, eating, libido, diurnal rhythms, etc., usually as a result of taking antidepressant drugs) often occur *before* a patient's depressed mood lifts. This increased physical energy and arousal level may give the patient a sufficient catalyst or psychic energy to act out a suicide plan. Psychiatric improvement is not uniform on all dimensions. Probably most suicides happen when the patient is getting better physically but lagging behind in mood elevation. Terminal insomnia (insomnia in the last third of the sleep cycle) is also especially predictive of suicide and depressive disorders (Maris, 1981: 222). Clearly weight changes (notably weight loss), depressed libido, restricted activity, and so on, may all be indicative of depressive disorders, which are the subtype of mental disorders most highly associated with a suicidal outcome.

Vital Statistics

All U.S. citizens will have an official certificate of death filled out on them (a disturbing thought!) and filed with a registrar in their state's vital statistics department when they die—such as the one depicted in Figure 3.3 (cf. Despelder & Strickland, 1998: 321, for a California certificate of death). The death certificate is completed primarily by the decedent's "attending" medical doctor, with parts being filled in by the medical examiner or coroner. The death certificate contains sociodemographic information (age, sex, race, marital status, usual occupation, etc.) on the deceased and his or her parents, a section on the death event, its causes (primary, secondary, and tertiary), time of death, autopsy (if any) and physician certification, manner of death (NASH) and injury details, a section on body disposition, and maybe some registration or census tract data. Some jurisdictions have coroner or medical examiner inquests and provide transcriptions of those hearings and jury opinions in addition to the death certicate form, especially if the manner of death is in question and a lot depends on the classification (e.g., insurance money or criminal charges).

This seemingly straightforward document has profound implications for the state and the individual concerning whether or not a crime was committed (such as homicide or assisted suicide), life insurance payoffs, the history of diseases and injuries, pension payments, property rights, social stigma, and much else.

Most of the empirical foundations for state and national suicide rates generated by agencies like the National Center for Health Statistics or the Centers for Disease Control and Prevention are based in the 50 states' death registration system (Garrison, 1992). The empirical investigation of suicide rates based on the official death records has a rich tradition in the social sciences, starting with Durkheim (1897/1951), and continuing with Henry and Short (1954), Gibbs and Martin (1964), Douglas (1967), Maris (1969, 1981), Phillips (1974), Stack (1982), and Pescosolido and Georgianna (1989) (see Maris, 1992: 2115–2117). Pescosolido (1995) has done a major NIMH national coroner and medical examiner suicide study.

Big issues with the U.S. vital statistics are (1) how accurate they are, (2) whether they

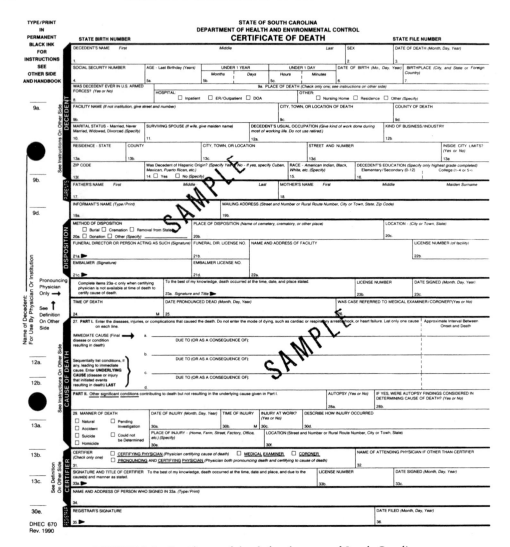

FIGURE 3.3. Certificate of death for the state of South Carolina.

provide a reliable empirical basis for the scientific study of suicide, and (3) whether we need different types of data to understand and control suicide. One of the most outspoken critics of suicide vital statistics has been Jack Douglas (1967). Douglas argues that there may be as many "official statistics" as there are officials. For example, some medical examiners will only certify suicide if a suicide note is left and found, which occurs in only about 15–25% of all suicides (Leenaars, 1988).

The consensus seems to be that the vital statistics undercount suicides (maybe by 10%, even to as much as 50%) and perhaps these errors of omission are greatest in the upper socioeconomic status (SES) groups, as that group is more powerful and effective in avoiding the potential stigma of a suicide classification or losing insurance money. If so, the profiles generated on the basis of death records might be inaccurate.

However, the alternative to vital statistics suggested by enthnomethodologists such as Douglas does not seem much better. Ethnomethodlogists would have us study the first-person accounts (i.e., those of the suicides themselves, not third persons) of serious suicide attempters themselves. Part of his objection is to the types of data death certificates collect (i.e., reducing suicide to dry epidemiological variables) and part is to the presumed error introduced into suicide profiles by interviewing a spouse or family members instead of the suicide him- or herself. Probably suicidology does need data other than death certificates (e.g., those discussed above). However, this author also agrees with Gibbs, Pescosolido, and others that vital statistics may be one of the best objective data sources suicidologists have—a kind of lesser of two "evils." Also, there may not be as much error in the vital statistics as qualitative sociologists such as Douglas suspect.

Experiments

In an experiment, the researcher directly manipulates one or more (independent) variables and then measures the effects on a dependent variable (here, suicide-related outcomes; see Kendall & Hammen, 1995: 144). One does not see many suicide experiments for reasons that should be obvious (however, see Schaefer, 1967). For example, Evans and Farberow's (1988) comprehensive *Encyclopedia of Suicide* has no entry on "experiments."

Usually the experimental design calls for a case or experimental group and a control or comparison group. Both groups experience all the same conditions (are matched) except that the experimental group is exposed to the independent variable, which then presumably causes a different outcome in the dependent variable in the experimental group than in the control group. Subjects are routinely assigned to the experimental or control group randomly and there often is a "double-blind design"; that is, neither the experimenter nor the subjects know until the code is broken whether they are in the experimental or control group(s). Suicide-related experiments are often conducted by drug companies. For example, consider this simple experimental design (many conditions are not specified here to keep it simple):

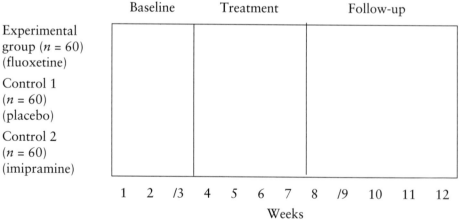

Here 60 subjects each (say, psychiatric patients) are randomly assigned to the experimental or control groups, after a "washout" of all 180 subjects to clear them of other drugs (a risky procedure itself) and doing baseline measurements. Starting with week 3 the experimental group gets 20 mg of fluoxetine per day, control group 1 gets an inert placebo, and control group 2 gets 150 mg/day of the "gold standard" imipramine (Tofranil) for a total of 6 weeks (dosages may vary over the 6 weeks) and then for 4 weeks of follow-up, codes are broken, posttreatment measures (like the HAM-D, the Covi anxiety scale, adverse effects, biological markers, etc.) are taken, and the three groups are tested statistically and then compared for significant differences. One reason we see so few experiments in suicidology is that there are serious ethical and legal issues in withholding treatment that could prevent suicide or in giving a treatment that could induce suicide.

RATES OF SUICIDE

A major component of the empirical foundation of suicidal behaviors is rates and proportions (see Mausner & Bahn, 1985, Ch. 7). A suicide rate is a measure of suicide in relation to the population (general or specific) with some time frame specified. Because suicides are rare, to be able to work with whole numbers (and not fractions) the suicides in the population are multiplied by a constant (usually 100,000). Thus, one common computing formula for suicide rates is simply:

$$\frac{\text{Suicides}}{\text{Population}} \times 100{,}000 = \text{Suicide rate}$$

Suicide rates are normally calculated for each year. For example, a suicide rate of 12 would mean that each year (say, in the United States) for every 100,000 persons in the general population there would be 12 suicides.

Occasionally we see suicide data using bases of a million (e.g., by the World Health Organization). If the behaviors are more frequent (like deaths or births each year), then bases of 1,000 may be used. Rates can be very sophisticated. Instead of a crude suicide rate, we may wish to hold age constant (an "adjusted rate"). But for most of our purposes here simple suicide rates will suffice.

Note that one of the main reasons we use rates instead of frequencies is that frequencies can be easily misinterpreted. For example, reporting that there were 100 suicides per year means something very different in (say) Chicago and a small rural community. Rates standardize for population size.

The discussion of basic suicide rates that follows is somewhat redundant. In a sense we are merely elaborating and updating the suicide incidence and prevalence data section in Chapter 1. Also, Chapters 5, 6, 7, and 9 go into much more detail about age, sex, race, marital status, and suicide rates. Having said this, we now ask, What are some of the fundamental empirical regularities as indicated by rates of suicidal behaviors?

Age

Table 3.1 shows us that suicide rates generally increase with age (especially for white males) until the very oldest age groups (85+), where there usually is a slight dropoff (cf. Table 1.3 for 1950 to 1996 data). Why suicide rates are low in the very young and drop off in the most elderly populations demands an explanation and is the subject of later chapters. Compare the columns of Table 3.2. Suicide rates by age tend to be relatively constant from year to year, especially over short time spans. This raises intriguing questions about optimum, reasonable, lowest, and highest (and so on) suicide rates. Does the constancy of suicide rates suggest they they are about as low as can be expected? Is the optimum suicide rate really zero? Note that a crude death (not suicide) rate of about 8/1,000 in industrialized countries is about as low as we can expect. Observe, too, in the bottom total row that the U.S. suicide rate has stayed at about 12 per 100,000. This has been true since roughly 1900, with slight elevations during economic depressions and slight declines during major wars.

One notable exception to the age constancy of suicide rates in the United States (there are others) is that the adolescent (15–24-year-olds) suicide rate approximately tripled from

TABLE 3.1. Suicide Rates by Age, United States, 1990–1996

Age (years)	1990	1991	1992	1996
5–14	0.8	0.7	0.9	0.8
15–24	13.2	13.1	13.0	12.0
25–34	15.2	15.2	14.5	14.5
35–44	15.3	14.7	15.1	15.5
45–54	14.8	15.5	14.7	14.9
55–64	16.0	15.4	14.8	13.7
65–74	17.9	16.9	16.5	15.0
75–84	24.9	23.5	22.8	20.0
85+	22.2	24.0	21.9	20.2
Total	12.4	12.2	12.0	11.0

Source: National Center for Health Statistics (1996), Advance report of final mortality statistics, 1998. *NCHS Monthly Vital Statistics Report, 46*(1, Suppl.).

1950 until 1980 (actually 1977; see Figure 3.4). This epidemic of teen or adolescent suicide has been so well documented in the media that many laypersons assume wrongly that teen suicide rates are higher than those of the elderly. Easterlin (1987a) argues that the adolescent suicide rate is a mirror image of the proportion of 15–24-year-olds in the U.S. population (a "cohort effect", see Figure 3.4). The cohort effect is such that the more 15–24-year-olds in the population, the higher their suicide rate. Easterlin contends that larger cohorts tend to have more competition for jobs and marriage partners and more stress in general.

Gender and Race

As we see in Table 3.2, suicide is predominantly a male phenomenon. Ratios of male to female suicide rates vary from 2 to 4 for whites and 3 to 5 for nonwhites. Table 3.2 also indicates that about 80% of all suicides are by males. In the next section it will become evident that the higher male suicide rate is explained in part by males' more frequent use of lethal methods (e.g., firearms and hanging), but surely that cannot be the entire explanation. For example, male fetuses have higher *in utero* death rates than do female fetuses. Certainly that differential cannot be the result of stress, occupation, or lifestyle.

About 90% of all U.S. suicides are committed by whites. Specifically, when we rank-order suicide rates by race and gender from highest to lowest, the ranking is (1) white males, (2) nonwhite males, (3) white females, and (4) nonwhite females. Here is an interesting illustration of the point about frequencies. Based on sheer frequencies, whites females (*n* = 5,309) rank ahead of black males (*n* = 1,389). But suicide rates correct for the fact that there are more white females in the U.S. population than black males.

Notice that suicide rates are almost nonexistant among nonwhite females (only 1% of all suicides). Why should that be? It would seem on the surface that black females have much adversity and many of the predictors of suicide (e.g., depression and divorce). The answer apparently lies not so much in their risk factors but, rather, in the counterbalancing protective factors of black females (Nisbet, 1996). For both males and females white suicide rates are about double those of blacks.

Methods of Suicide

Table 3.3 shows that roughly 64% of males and 40% of females commit suicide by firearms. In a real sense, then, much of suicide prevention amounts to gun control. As the

RATE PER 100,000 POPULATION

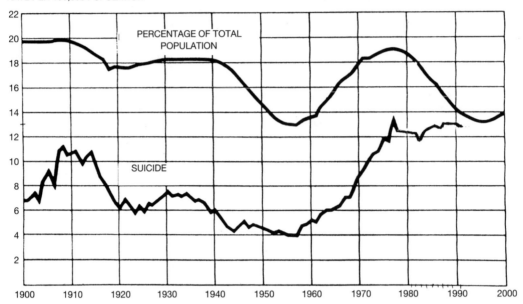

FIGURE 3.4. Percentage of total U.S. population and suicide rate for 15- to 24-year-olds. *Source:* Easterlin (1987a: 104 ff). Suicide rates added from 1978 to 1991. Copyright 1980 by Basic Books, Inc. Adapted by permission.

British studies of coal gas and suicide have shown (Kreitman, 1976), most people do not simply switch methods of suicide if their preferred method is not readily available (i.e., when home coal gas was detoxified in Great Britain, the suicide rate went down and tended to stay down). The second leading method for men is hanging (14%) and for women is drug and medicine poisoning (ca. 25%).

It may be that females have lower suicide rates than males in part because they tend to use methods that are more reversible and allow for higher rescuability (Weisman & Worden, 1974). For both males and females, hanging and asphyxiation are the number one suicide method in hospitals, jails, and prisons. One has to be careful here not to be ethnocen-

TABLE 3.2. Suicide Rates by Race and Gender, United States, 1996

Race/gender	No. of suicides	% of suicides	Rate per 100,000	Rank order
White males	22,547	73.0	20.9	1
White females	5,309	17.1	4.8	3
Black males	(1,389)	(4.5)	(11.4)	—
Black females	(204)	(0.8)	(2.0)	—
Nonwhite males[a]	2,451	8.0	11.3	2
Nonwhite females[a]	596	1.9	2.5	4
Totals	30,903	100.00	11.6	

Source: National Center for Health Statistics (1998), Advance report of final mortality statistics, 1996. *NCHS Monthly Vital Statistics Report, 47*(9).
[a]Includes African Americans, Native Americans, Chinese, Hawaiian, Japanese, Filipino, other Asian or Pacific Islanders, and other.

TABLE 3.3. Methods of Suicide by Age and Sex, United States, 1985–1987

Method	15–24 years No. of suicides	15–24 years % of total	25–44 years No. of suicides	25–44 years % of total	45–64 years No. of suicides	45–64 years % of total	65+ years No. of suicides	65+ years % of total
Males								
All methods	12,652	100.00	27,054	100.00	16,332	100.00	14,973	100.00
Firearms	7,856	62.09	15,562	57.52	10,987	67.27	11,104	74.16
Hanging	2,567	20.29	4,443	16.42	1,856	11.36	1,669	11.15
Solid and liquid poisons	491	3.88	2,158	7.98	963	5.90	460	3.07
Gas poisoning	1,092	8.63	3,064	11.33	1,545	9.46	831	5.55
All other methods	646	5.11	1,827	6.75	981	6.00	909	6.07
Females								
All methods	2,513	100.00	7,459	100.00	5,800	100.00	3,554	100.00
Firearms	1,244	49.50	3,109	41.68	2,203	37.98	1,146	32.25
Hanging	311	12.38	714	9.57	601	10.36	663	18.66
Solid and liquid poisons	482	19.18	2,036	27.30	1,615	27.84	858	24.14
Gas poisoning	306	12.18	968	12.98	772	13.31	355	9.99
All other methods	170	6.76	632	8.47	609	10.50	532	14.97

Source: McIntosh (1992a: 390). Copyright 1992 by The Guilford Press. Reprinted by permission

tric. Methods are often specific to country or culture. For example, hanging is much more common in Europe and firearm suicides are less common.

Carbon monoxide poisoning (the method preferred by Dr. Jack Kevorkian in assisting suicides) is the third leading method of suicide in both men and women. To measure Dr. Kevorkian's and Dr. Humphry's (1996) influence on suicide, one could analyze any increases in the use of carbon monoxide poisoning and/or of plastic bags and drugs. Finally, it should be noted that as men age they tend to be more likely to use firearms to attempt suicide and less likely to use hanging.

Marital Status

Since at least 1897 (Durkheim) we have known that other things being equal, marriage protects against suicide. Durkheim called this empirical regularity the "coefficient of preservation." Table 3.4 reveals that marriage protects men from suicide more than it does women; that is, men have higher coefficients of aggravation (here divorced vs. married). In general, marital status has less influence on the suicide rates for women than for men, although sociobiologists (de Catanzaro, 1992) argue that women with children are more protected against suicide than are those women without children. In general, the highest to lowest suicide rates range in order from the widowed to the divorced, single, and married. Young widowhood is particularly suicidogenic for males.

Country and Gender

As we noted earlier, suicidologists have to be careful not to make ethnocentric errors. Most conspicuously the suicide rates in the United States may not reflect the empirical patterns or regularities in other countries of the world. Table 3.5 indicates that the U.S. suicide rates turn out to be about in the middle of the international rankings. Countries with very *high* suicide rates include Hungary, Finland, Austria, Denmark, France, Japan, and the Falkland

TABLE 3.4. White Suicide Rates by Marital Status, Gender, and Age, United States

Age (years)	Marital status				Coefficient of aggravation (divorced/married)
	Single	Married	Widowed	Divorced	
			Males		
25–29	43.3	15.8	186.6	70.1	4.44
35–39	43.1	15.3	188.2	67.0	4.37
45–49	49.5	17.5	100.5	72.6	4.15
55–59	50.0	19.0	86.3	76.3	4.02
65–69	53.3	25.0	74.6	74.2	2.90
			Females		
25–29	12.2	4.7	26.4	19.5	4.15
35–39	15.8	7.3	17.7	25.6	3.51
45–49	15.1	9.1	23.0	28.1	3.09
55–59	9.9	8.0	15.7	21.4	2.68
65–69	8.6	6.1	11.1	14.4	2.36

Source: Stack (1990b). Copyright 1990 by the National Council on Family Relations. Reprinted by permission.

Islands. Countries with very *low* rates include Egypt, New Guinea, the Philippines, Syria, and Iran. As with very young children it would be interesting to speculate on what protects people who live in low-suicide-rate countries. For example, Catholic and Arabic countries tend to have low suicide rates. But one must also be suspicious of reporting errors in nations that have religion or culture taboos against suicide (e.g., Egypt). Note, too, that almost nowhere in the world is the suicide rate zero.

Table 3.5 also confirms that male suicide rates exceed female suicide rates in almost every country, although the ratio of male to female rates varies considerably. The usual male–female suicide rate is about 3–4:1. In St. Lucia and St. Vincent there are apparently no female suicides. Similarly in the Federal Democratic Republic of Germany presumably the male–female ratio was very high (22:1). However, female suicide rates are nearly equal in Thailand (1.1:1), Hong Kong (1.3:1), and Singapore (1.4:1).

PREDICTION, SCALES, RISK, AND PROTECTIVE FACTORS

In the first chapter of this text we noted that predictions of individual suicides, especially in short time frames, lead to many errors—particularly to false positives (i.e., identifying an individual as a suicide who is in fact not a suicide; cf. Pokorny, 1983, 1993). In Chapter 2 we reviewed Shneidman's commonalities and specific risk and protective factors of suicides (see Figure 2.6). In this chapter we now ask: "Can we identify empirical predictors of individual suicides that are both sensitive and specific ('sensitivity' concerns correctly identifying true positives and 'specificity' concerns correctly identifying true negatives)?"

Psychological tests and suicide scales were discussed in the treatment record section of this chapter. In this section we list and discuss briefly 15 specific single variable predictors of suicide outcome (cf. Tuckman & Youngman, 1968), review a few depression scales (e.g., the Beck and Hamilton scales, as suicide is highly correlated with depressive disorder), note

TABLE 3.5. Suicide Rates (per Million Population) by Country and Gender, World Health Association, 1987

Country	Males	Females	Country	Males	Females
1. Falkland/Maldives	1,000	—	36. Trinidad and Tobago	121	50
2. Hungary	661	259	37. Italy	110	43
3. Suriname	436	128	38. Chile	107	18
4. Finland	430	113	39. Argentina	105	34
5. Austria	421	158	40. Ireland	92	39
6. Sri Lanka	377	197	41. Venezuela	76	20
7. Denmark	351	206	42. Israel	75	35
8. France	331	127	43. Costa Rica	74	15
9. Switzerland	330	132	44. Thailand	60	62
10. Belgium	326	153	45. Spain	68	23
11. Czechoslovakia	292	92	46. Greece	57	25
12. Japan	278	149	47. Ecuador	55	36
13. Federal Republic of Germany	266	12	48. Cape Verde	44	6
14. Sweden	250	115	49. Martinique	44	13
15. Bulgaria	232	94	50. Bahrain	40	6
16. Yugoslavia	228	97	51. Mauritius	40	16
17. Poland	220	44	52. Paraguay	33	15
18. Norway	208	74	53. Dominica	28	—
19. Luxemburg	207	74	54. Mexico	25	7
20. Iceland	206	58	55. Barbados	25	15
21. Canada	205	54	56. Panama	22	5
22. United States	197	54	57. Saint Vincent	20	0
23. Australia	182	51	58. Grenadine	17	—
24. Puerto Rico	176	23	59. Santa Lucia	17	0
25. Scotland	166	60	60. Iran	16	4
26. Uruguay	159	—	61. Belize	13	—
27. New Zealand	157	50	62. Kuwait	12	5
28. El Salvador	148	61	63. Bahamas	10	—
29. Singapore	147	107	64. Guatemala	9	1
30. Netherlands	146	81	65. Philippines	5	4
31. Korea	139	49	66. Syria	2	—
32. Hong Kong	137	107	67. Papua New Guinea	1	2
33. Portugal	136	51	68. Egypt	0	0
34. Northern Ireland	131	39	69. Malta	*a*	6
35. England and Wales	121	57	70. German Democratic Republic	*a*	—
			71. Cuba	*a*	—

Source: Diekstra (1990: 536–537). Copyright 1990 by The Guilford Press. Reprinted by permission.
*a*No data available.

that hopelessness may be a better predictor of suicide than is depression, then examine specific suicide prediction scales. Finally, all these factors and scales are illustrated by a forensic case.

We observed in Chapter 1 that a common type of completed suicide was an older white male who was periodically depressed, alcoholic, and socially isolated and used a gun to commit suicide (like Ernest Hemingway). Table 3.6 elaborates some of these common single variable characteristics of completed suicides. Of course, not all suicides have all these 15 traits, the *common predictors* listed are variously weighted in different individual cases, and there often are interaction effects. We now discuss each of the 15 traits of typical suicides. Note that all these suicidogenic factors are considered in much greater detail in the remaining chapters of this textbook.

1. Almost (but not) all individuals who commit suicide have a *diagnosable mental disorder* (see Chapter 13), usually one of the affective disorders (often major depressive episode [unipolar; DSM-IV code 296.xx and sometimes with psychotic symptoms; cf. Tanney, 1992), although suicide risk is also high among individuals with one of the schizophrenias (especially paranoid schizophrenia) and some personality (Axis II) disorders (including borderline, antisocial, and panic disorders). However, personality disorders are much more common among nonfatal suicide attempters. Bipolar affective disorders are also overrepresented among suicides. It has been estimated that about 15% of hospitalized depressed patients eventually commit suicide and that roughly two-thirds of suicides have a primary depressive disorder (Guze & Robins, 1970). In our own research (using a modified form of the Beck Depression Inventory) several specific items were especially related to a suicide outcome; that is, sleep disturbances (especially terminal insomnia) feelings of hopelessness, dissatisfaction, wanting to die, and loss of interest in other peole (Maris, 1981: 216–224).

2. *Alcoholism* is another major predictor of suicide (see Chapter 15; cf. Murphy, 1992). In a large series of studies of alcoholics, Roy and Linnoila (1986) found that on average, 18% of alcholics eventually commit suicide (although some researchers have found the rate to be much lower [5–15%]; see Murphy, 1992: 236ff.). In Robins's (1981) St. Louis research, 72% of completed suicides were either depressed (45%) or alcoholic (25%). No other single predictor was present in more than 5% of all suicides. Paradoxically, in the short run alcoholism seems to protect against suicide (perhaps by transiently raising low brain serotonin levels), but in the long run (on average over about 25 years) alcoholism is related to higher rates of suicide (over time ethanol lowers brain serotonin levels, disrupts social and economic relationships, lowers impulse control, can destroy the liver and the ability to use alcohol for pleasure; see Styron, 1990). A major factor in alcoholic suicides is disruption of social support and interpersonal relationships. Of course, nonalcoholic drug abuse is also related to suicide, especially among young suicide attempters (Lester, 1992b).

3. Although the relationship of *suicidal ideation* to suicidal action is complex, sometimes the best predictor of suicide is simply to ask those about whom one is concerned

TABLE 3.6. **Common Single Predictors of Suicide**

 1. Major depressive illness, affective disorder
 2. Alcoholism, drug abuse
 3. Suicide ideation, talk, preparation
 4. Prior suicide attempts
 5. Use of lethal methods to attempt suicide (especially guns)
 6. Isolation, living alone, loss of support, rejection
 7. Hopelessness, cognitive rigidity
 8. Being an older, white male
 9. Modeling, history of suicide in the family
10. Work problems, unemployment, occupation
11. Marital and sexual problems, family pathology
12. Stress, negative life events
13. Anger, aggression, low 5-HIAA, impulsivity
14. Physical illness
15. Repetition and "comorbidity" of factors 1–14

Source: Adapted from Maris (1992f: 9). Copyright 1992 by The Guilford Press. Adapted by permission.

whether of not they are thinking about killing themselves (of course, at other times and circumstances asking is an unreliable indicator). In many clinics, hospitals, and jails, asking whether the individual is suicidal in the *only* suicide assessment procedure. If one does ask about suicide, it is also important to inquire: "If you were going to suicide, how exactly would you do it (what methods, specific plans, timing, etc.)"? The suicide literature suggests paying attention to new or altered wills, new or altered life insurance policies (suicidal death within a 2-year period after taking out a policy is usually legal grounds for denying full benefits), giving away previously valued possessions, atypical death or suicide talk, preparations for death, and the like. Suicide notes are not by themselves a reliable indicator of suicide, as only about 10–30% of suicide completers ever leave suicide notes at all, and many people who write suicide notes never suicide (Leenaars, 1988). In our Chicago research (Maris, 1981), 15% of suicides left notes. In random surveys taken in shopping malls about 20% of the general population admit that they have considered suicide at some time in their lives (Linehan & Laffaw, 1982). A skilled clinician can also consider a patient's dreams, use projective tests, and even hypnosis to get at a client's suicidal ideation (although by themselves none of these procedures is valid or reliable).

4. To be sure, before an individual can kill himself, he or she must first make a *suicide attempt* (see Chapter 12). Any person with a history of prior nonfatal suicide attempts is at a much greater risk for eventual suicide than someone who has no history of suicide attempts (Maris, 1992e). Probably about 15% of nonfatal suicide attempters will eventually die by suicide (Maris, 1981a)—of course, that also means that 85% of nonfatal suicide attempters will *never* complete suicide. In the general population the suicide rate is about 12 per 100,000 or .0001 (in the United States). Thus, other things being equal, prior suicide attempts raise the risk of suicide dramatically (.15 v. .0001, or about 1,500 times). However, and this is important, among older white males (the prototypical suicide) who attempt suicide, almost 90% of them die after their *first* attempt (mainly because they shoot themselves in the head and have relatively few protective factors; see Figure 2.6). Nonfatal suicide attempts tend to be more likely among younger persons, especially among females. Even among younger female completers, more than five nonfatal suicide attempts before suicide completion is rare.

5. Since the 1980s in the United States both men and women have preferred *firearms* as the method of choice for suicide. As we saw in Table 3.3, 64% of male completers and 40% of female completers used guns to suicide. The second most common method of suicide for males was hanging (14%) and for females it was drugs and medications (25%)—paradoxically often with the very antidepressant medications given to treat their depression and suicidal ideation. Overall men choose relatively few highly lethal methods to commit suicide, whereas women use a much greater variety of methods, many of which are of relatively low lethality.

Thus, it is no surprise that on average men have suicide rates three to four times higher than those of women, even though women have higher rates of depressive disorder than men by a ratio of about 2 to 1. One interesting question that we must address in this text is *why* women use less lethal methods to attempt suicide than men do. Are they more ambivalent, less familiar with firearms, more concerned about their dependent children, more concerned about disfigurement?

6. Numerous experiments (e.g., with mice and confined human sea travel; Maris, 1981) have demonstrated that prolonged *social isolation* raises levels of irritability, hostility, and aggression (see Chapter 10). As long as social interaction is not negative (e.g., as in one person driving another to suicide), social involvement of all sorts tends to reduce suicide potential and social isolation or living alone tends to increase the risk of suicide. In one

study, 42% of suicidal depressives lived alone as opposed to only 7% of nonsuicidal depressives (Maris, 1981). In Chicago research, 50% of completed suicides had no close friends, compared to only 20% of nonfatal suicide attempters (Maris, 1981). Weisman and Worden's (1974) "risk–rescue ratio scale" takes relative social isolation into account by calculating not only suicide risk but also the probability of rescue or intervention by another person (as a protective factor). Clearly, when one is alone or isolated, the probability of suicidal rescue is diminished.

7. Beck and colleagues (see Weishaar & Beck, 1992) contend that *hopelessness* (see Figure 3.5 and Table 3.7) is a better predictor of suicide, suicidal ideation, and the wish to die than is depressive disorder. Suicidal hopelessness often involves seeing no alternatives to suicide, rigid thinking, or "tunnel vision." At some point in a suicidal career (usually later) repeated episodes of depressive illness may result in a subjective assessment that not only is one's life painful and intolerable but also that it is never going to improve. In one 10-year follow-up study by Beck, Steer, Kovacs, and Garrison (1985), 165 patients were hospitalized with suicidal ideation. Of the 11 patients who eventally suicided, 91% (10 of them) had scores greater than 9 on the Beck hopelessness scale. Only one patient who suicided had a hopelessness score below 10.

8. As we noted earlier, one striking trait of suicide completers is that about 70% of them are *white males* (see Chapter 7; cf. Garrison, 1992). The celebrated rise of adolescent suicide rates in the United States in the late 1960s and early 1970s took place almost exclusively among males. Recent data also indicate significant increases in the suicide rates of older white males (McIntosh, 1992b). Only 22% of all suicides are by white females, and few nonwhite females suicide. In all racial and minority groups in the United States there exists an excess of male to female completed suicide rates by ratios of 3 to 5 to 1 (Earls, Escobar, & Manson, 1990). Some have claimed (de Catanzaro, 1992) that maleness (in the biological, genetic, or chromosomal sense) is related to premature death and to suicide in particular.

9. Suicides and depressive disorder tend to *run in families* (Jamison, 1993). In Chicago research (Maris, 1981), 11% of suicides had at least one other suicide among their first-degree relatives, but none of the natural death comparison group did. This may indicate either *genetic* (Roy, 1992) or *modeling* (Phillips, Lesyna, & Paight, 1992) influences. One study of suicide among the Amish (Egeland & Sussex, 1985) found that both outcomes were gene related (specifically to a narrow portion of chromosome 11). However, a study by Phillips and Carstenson (1986) suggests modeling or imitation as a predictor of suicide (see Chapter 10). Adolescent suicide rates rose by 6.9% above the expected rates 7 to 10 days after New York City adolescent suicide stories were broadcast on television. Adult suicide rates showed only a 0.5% rise in the same circumstances. Still another possiblity is that of *sociobiological* factors, such as having dependent children (which may lower suicide rates, especially among females) or being beyond the years of reproductive fitness (which should raise suicide rates).

10. Although suicide occurs in all census occupational categories (e.g., from professionals to laborers; Wasserman, 1992a) and in all socioeconomic categories (like death, suicide is very "democratic"), it does seem that *work* or productive life activities *protect* one against suicide and, conversely, work problems of all sorts are related to suicidal outcomes (see Chapter 8). In studies (Maris, 1981) about one-third of all suicides were unemployed at the time of their deaths. Suicides typically have erratic work histories. Although suicides occur in all social classes, most studies show higher rates of suicide in the lower socioeconomic classes. A problem in generalizing, however, is that within each broad census occupational category one can find both high and low suicide rates. For example, psychiatrists tend to have high suicide rates, but pediatricians and surgeons usually have low suicide rates—although all are physicians.

11. *Marriage and having a family* are usually associated with lower rates of suicide (see Chapter 9; Stack, 1992). Suicide rates are almost always highest among the divorced and widowed. Suicide completers are also more likely to have never been married (see Durkheim's comments on the unmarried as the "dregs of the country," 1897/1951: 180) than are individuals who die natural deaths. Studies of family development have suggested that certain kinds of family pathology (e.g., early object loss, early separation from one's mother for long periods, physical and emotional abuse by one's father [sometimes by a step-father] or mother [including incest], young adult promiscuity, and frequent moving of one's residence) are all related to subsequent suicide as an adult. One study by Shneidman (1971) found that men's disrupted, hostile, competitive lifestyles and nonsupportive relations as adults with their wives and lovers were especially predictive of suicide.

12. Suicide is sometimes triggered by *undesirable (especially negative) life events or stress* (see Chapter 18; cf. Yufit & Bongar, 1992) over fairly long periods (i.e., "suicidal careers"). These events can include blows to self-esteem, guilt, legal problems, economic strain, interpersonal discord, loss of important social relationships, threat of jail or imprisonment, loss of social status, just being repeatedly overworked, and so forth. Most stress is chronic and accumulates slowly. There can be a few intense, acute "triggering" events preceding a suicide (cf. Figure 2.6), but without a history of stress and other vulnerabilities most of us tolerate time-limited, single, dramatic life events without resorting to suicide. Also, triggering (acute) life events are usually not substantially different from the chronic stressors in one's life. Thus, when the suicide threshold is crossed, friends and relatives of the suicide may not notice anything special going on and often express surprise that the person suicided at all or that they suicided when they did.

13. Because suicide is a violent act, it usually requires some minimal *aggressive* energy (see Chapter 17; cf., Brown, Linnoila, & Goodwin, 1992; van Praag, Plutchik, & Apter, 1990). In addition to being depressed and hopeless, most suicides are also angry, irritated, and dissatisfied. Freud argued that suicides are disguised murders of introjected objects. As Menninger (1938) put it, suicide is "murder in the 180th degree." Murderous revenge is particularly likely among younger suicides, for whom interpersonal factors are more salient. Among older suicides, anger and dissatisfaction may be directed at life itself rather than at specific individuals. One significant repeated biological finding (Brown et al., 1992) is that impulsive, violent suicides are more likely to have lower cerebrospinal fluid levels of 5-HIAA (see Chapter 16). The aggressive component in suicide may also help account for the excess of male to female suicides, in terms of both socialization to be aggressive and violent and hormonal concentrations of testosterone.

14. We know that 30–40% of all suicides have some significant *physical illness* (see Chapter 14; cf. Roy, 1992; de Catanzaro, 1992). Diseases that have been found to be related to suicide include epilepsy, malignant neoplasms, AIDS, gastrointestinal problems, and musculoskeletal disorders (e.g., arthritis and chronic lower back pain), among others. Certainly physical illness in and of itself seldom causes suicide. In Maris (1981) the natural death control group (although they were also older) had far more physical illness than the suicides did. Most physically ill individuals, even terminal cancer patients, do not suicide. Like other single predictors, physical illness has a complex relationship to suicidal outcomes. Because most suicides are older males and that group is more likely to be physically ill, the association between physical illness and suicide is not surprising.

15. Most people bear up under acute insults to their adaptive repertoire. Coping breaks down gradually, usually after about 40 to 50 years of certain kinds of lives. These patterns leading up to suicide can be thought of as *"suicidal careers."* Although the previous 14 single common predictors are present in varying degrees in most suicides and sometimes one or two predictors can be salient and acute, comorbidity (should we

say, "polymorbidity") and interaction of the common suicide predictors over time are the rule.

Of all these 15 individual predictors, some are more predictive of suicide than are others. For example, depressive disorders (see Tanney, 1992) are among the most common and important predictors of suicidal behaviors. Accordingly, systematic scales have been developed to measure depression, hopelessness, and other related suicide risk factors. A *"scale" is a continuum resulting from objective, standardized procedures combining one or more measurements in order to form a single score that is assigned to each individual* (trait, object, etc.; see Selltiz, Wrightman, & Cook, 1976: 403–404). For example, we have already alluded to the depression scale on the MMPI in the treatment section of this chapter.

Two other depression scales commonly used in suicide research and clinical assessment and measurement are the HAM-D (see Hamilton, 1960; Marsella, Hirschfeld, & Katz, 1987: esp., 34ff.) and the BDI (Beck, 1967: 338; Maris, 1981: 216ff.). Both of these scales measure the severity of general depressive symptoms but do not specify a particular DSM diagnostic category. The HAM-D has 17, 21, and 24 item versions. These items measure traits such as depressed mood, guilt, suicide, insomnia, retardation, anxiety, weight changes, and obsessional symptoms. The 17-item HAM-D scores vary from a low of 0 and a high of 50, and the 21-item version from 0 to 62. On the standard 17-item version the following measurements of depression are indicated:

> 25+ = Severe depression
> 18–24 = Moderate depression
> 7–17 = Mild depression
> < 7 = Not depressed or recovered

The BDI is similar to the HAM-D. It has 21 items and scores ranging from a low of 0 to a high of 63, with the following ranges:

> 26+ = Severe depression
> 21–25 = Moderate depression
> 1–20 = Mild depression
> 0 = No depression

The advantages of two such valid and reliable measures of depression that have been used in many situations for a long time are obvious.

In suicidology, such scales allow for comparable, standardized scores on an important variable related to suicide outcome. For example, when Maris (1981: 216–227) gave a modified version (revised from first- to third-person respondents, as suicides cannot respond) of the BDI to suicides and natural deaths (more precisely, to their families), 30% of completed suicides scored 26 or higher on the BDI, compared to only 11% of the natural deaths ($t = -5.6$; $p < .001$). That is, suicides were statistically significantly more depressed than a comparison group sample of natural deaths.

Lately, Beck and his colleagues at the University of Pennsylvania have argued that hopelessness (the seventh predictor in Table 3.6) is a better predictor of suicidal outcome than clinical depression is (Beck, 1986; Beck, Brown, Steer, Dahlsgaard, & Grisham, 1999) and have developed a *hopelessness scale* to test this hypothesis (see Figure 3.5). In a 10-year follow-up study of 165 patients hospitalized with suicidal ideation, of the 11 patients who

True

2. I might as well give up because I can't make things better for myself.
4. I can't imagine what my life would be like in 10 years.
7. My future seems dark to me.
9. I just don't get the breaks, and there's no reason to believe I will in the future.
11. All I can see ahead of me is unpleasantness rather than pleasantness
12. I don't expect to get what I really want.
14. Things just won't work out the way I want them to.
16. I never get what I want so it's foolish to want anything.
17. It is very unlikely that I will get any real satisfaction in the future.
18. The future seems vague and uncertain to me.
20. There's not use in really trying to get something I want because I probably won't get it.

False

1. I look forward to the future with hope and enthusiasm.
3. When things are going badly, I am helped by knowing they can't stay that way forever.
5. I have enough time to accomplish the things I most want to do.
6. In the future, I expect to succeed in what concerns me most.
8. I expect to get more of the good things in life than the average person.
10. My past experiences have prepared me well for my future.
13. When I look ahead to the future, I expect I will be happier than I am now.
15. I have great faith in the future.
19. I can look forward to more good times than bad times.

FIGURE 3.5. Beck et al.'s Hopelessness Scale. *Source:* Beck, Weissman, Lester, & Trexler (1974). Copyright 1974 by the American Psychological Association. Reprinted by permission.

eventually suicided, 10 (91%) has hopelessness scores greater than 9 and only 1 had a hopelessness score below 10 (Beck, 1986). Looking at Table 3.7 we see the following:

- Hopelessness correlates higher with suicidal intent (+.68) than does depression (+.57).
- Hopelessness has a higher negative correlation with wish to live (−.74) than does depression (−.57).
- The relationship between depression and suicide intent is due to a common source of variance (i.e., to hopelessness).

One can also measure suicide potential *directly* (vs. indirectly by scaling depression scores, etc.) with specific *suicide prediction or probability scales* (see, e.g., Rothberg & Geer-Williams, 1992: 202–217). Rothberg and Geer-Williams list 6 first-person scales and 12 third-party scales. We review one of each here. The Western Psychological Services produces a first-person *Suicide Probability Scale* (SPS) (Cull & Gill, 1982; see Figure 3.6). It consists of 36 items, each rated from 1 (low) to 4 (high) by the respondent. In addition to generating an overall suicide probability score, there are four subscales of hopelessness, sui-

TABLE 3.7. Correlations of Beck et al.'s Depression, Hopelessness, Current Suicidal Intent, and Wish to Live Scales

	Hopelessness	Depression	Wish to live
Hopelessness	+.68	—	—
Wish to live	−.74	−.57	—
Current suicidal intent	+.68	+.57	−.76

Source: Kovacs, Beck, & Weissman (1975). Copyright 1975 by The Guilford Press. Adapted by permission.

DIRECTIONS

Listed below are a series of statements that some people might use to describe their feelings and behaviors. Please read each statement and determine how often the statement is true for you. Then circle the letter T in the appropriate box to indicate how often you feel the statement applies to you.

Be sure to rate every item. When you are through, return the completed rating form to the person who gave it to you.

Example:

	None or a little of the time	Some of the time	Good part of the time	Most or all of the time
1. I feel anxious.	T	Ⓣ	T	T

	None or a little of the time	Some of the time	Good part of the time	Most or all of the time
3. I feel I tend to be impulsive.	T	T	T	T
7. In order to punish others I think of suicide.	T	T	T	T
9. I feel isolated from people.	T	T	T	T
17. I think that no one will miss me when I am gone.	T	T	T	T
20. I feel I need to punish myself for things I have done and thought.	T	T	T	T
24. I feel people would be better off if I were dead.	T	T	T	T
25. I feel it would be less painful to die than to keep living the way things are.	T	T	T	T
30. I have thought of how to do myself in.	T	T	T	T
32. I think of suicide.	T	T	T	T
36. I feel I can't be happy no matter where I am.	T	T	T	T

FIGURE 3.6. Selected items from Cull and Gill's Suicide Probability Scale. *Source:* Cull & Gill (1982). Copyright 1982 by Western Psychological Services. Reprinted by permission.

cide ideation, hostility, and negative self-evaluation. Suicide probability scores range as follows:

Probability score (%)	Suicide risk
75–100	Severe
50–74	Moderate
25–49	Mild
0–24	Subclinical

Most suicides have scores of 40–60% or higher. One criticism is that SPS does not rate the lethality of suicide intent well.

A well-known third-person suicide prediction scale is the *Clinical Instrument to Estimate Suicide Risk* (CIESR; Motto et al., 1985; see Table 3.8). The CIESR rates 15 demo-

TABLE 3.8. Motto's Clinical Instrument to Estimate Suicide Risk

RISK FACTOR SCORING TABLE

Item	Response category	Score
1. Age at last birthday	See Age Scoring Table	______
2. Type of occupation	Executive, administrator, or professional	48
	Owner of business	
	Semiskilled worker	48
	Other	
3. Sexual orientation	Bisexual, sexually active	65
	Homosexual, not sexually active	65
	Other	0
4. Financial resources	None or negative (debts exceed resources)	0
	0 or $100	35
	More than $100	70
5. Threat of significant financial loss	Yes	63
	No	0
	Severe	63
	Other	0
6. Special stress: unique to subject's circumstances, *other than* loss of finances or relationship, threat of prosecution, illegitimate pregnancy, substance abuse, or poor health		
7. Hours of sleep per night (approximate nearest whole hour)	0–2	0
	3–5	
	6 or more	
8. Change of weight during present episode of stress (approximate)	Weight gain	
	Less than 10% weight loss	60
	Other	0
9. Ideas of persecution or reference	Moderate or severe	45
	Other	0
10. Intensity of present suicidal impulses	Questionable, moderate, or severe	100
	Other	0
11. If current suicide attempt made, seriousness of intent to die	Unequivocal	88
	Ambivalent, weighted toward suicide	88
	Other or not applicable	0
12. Number of previous psychiatric hospitalizations	None	0
	1	21
	2	43
	3 or more	64
13. Results of previous efforts to obtain help	No previous efforts	0
	Some degree of help	0
	Poor, unsatisfactory, or variable	55
14. Emotional disorder in family history	Depression	45
	Alcoholism	45
	Other	0
15. Interviewer's reaction to the person	Highly positive	0
	Moderately or slightly positive	42
	Neutral or negative	
Total score		____

TABLE OF RISK

Total score	Decile of risk	Relative risk	Approximate 2-year suicide rate
0–271	1	Very low	Less than 1%
272–311	2	Low	1.0%–2.5%
312–-344	3	Low	1.0%–2.5%
345–377	4	Moderate	2.5%–5.0%
378–407	5	Moderate	2.5%–5.0%
408–435	6	Moderate	2.5%–5.0%
436–463	7	Moderate	2.5%–5.0%
466–502	8	High	5.0%–10.0%
503–553	9	High	5.0%-10.0%
554 and over	10	Very high	More than 10.0%

Source: Motto, Heilbron, & Juster (1985: 686). Copyright 1985 by the American Psychiatric Association. Reprinted by permission.

graphic and clinical items and has a maximum score of 1,031. Suicide risk is estimated as follows:

Suicide risk	Level of risk	2-year risk
0–271	Very low	< 1%
272–344	Low	1–2.5%
345–465	Moderate	2.5–5%
466–533	High	5–10%
534+	Very high	10%

A case example from the our clinical practice illustrates the use of many of the scales (see Case 3.1). "VW" was a 45-year-old white male professional who died an equivocal death of carbon monoxide poisoning while washing and waxing his car in an enclosed

CASE 3.1. An Equivocal Suicide: The Case of VW

VW was a 45-year-old white male from a southeastern city who died in July 1990 of carbon monoxide poisoning in his garage at home. He had been washing and waxing his wife's car. VW was a heavy drinker and his CPA business was near bankruptcy. His death was initially listed as an accident by the local medical examiner. But VW's insurance companies were suspicious and refused to pay some of his recent life insurance policies, claiming that VW's death was a suicide. His wife, LW, sued, arguing that her husband's death was indeed an accident. Both sides got their lawyers and experts. At issue was the manner of death of VW. Eventually the wife and the insurance companies settled the case without going to trial.

It had been a hot summer morning when VW washed the car in the driveway. After finishing washing the car, he pulled it into the garage and shut the door, presumably to wax it out of the sun. He left the motor running and the car radio on but had a fan going in the garage. When VW was found by his brother-in-law later that morning, he was sitting in a canvas lawn chair next to the car. There were water buckets, wax, and rags near his feet. One hypothesis was that he had gotten faint or dizzy after washing the car outside and sat down for a minute, intending to shut off the car motor after closing the garage door. Instead he lost consciousness and never recovered. Of course, a more cynical hypothesis is that he was deeply in debt and just staged his own death to look like an accident.

VW had 6 or 7 of the 15 common suicide predictors listed in Table 3.6 (alcohol abuse, hopelessness, being an older white male, work problems, marital problems, stress and negative life events, and anger–irritability). He scored very low (mean of 4) on the Beck Depression Inventory (which was given posthumously to several of his relatives). His overall Cull and Gill SPS (see Figure 3.6) was 15 (the maximum possible is 100), putting his suicide potential in the lowest quartile. On Motto's CIESR scale VW scored 413 (max. = 1031 +), which made him a moderate relative suicide risk. Based on all the empirical indicators VW was still an equivocal suicide.

Other relevant facts were that VW had no suicides in his family and had no prior suicide attempts. VW had been married once and had two sons, the oldest of whom had a history of depression and suicide ideation. After his death VW's debts totaled $7–$10 million. VW had been having an extramarital affair. Just before his death his girlfriend called him at home and his wife found out about the affair. She responded in part by going off to the beach and leaving VW home alone. VW was a very successful CPA (one of his clients was the NFL Atlanta Falcons). VW was in good physical health. He was 6 feet tall and weighed about 215 to 220 pounds. VW had never seen a mental health professional in his life. The week that VW died nothing much unusual happened, other than his girlfriend calling his home and him burning his leg on his car's exhaust pipe.

garage. The issue here was whether VW's death was an accident or a suicide. Natural death and homicide were ruled out as extremely unlikely. Can the various empirical indicators and scales just outlined help us predict VW's manner of death? As the Case 3.1 summary indicates, VW had a maximum of 7 of the 15 individual suicide predictors (47%) and scored very low (did his relatives *lie* on the test?) on the BDI (a mean score of 4).

His Cull and Gill SPS score was 15, which suggested low suicide risk. On Motto's CIESR, VW scored 413 out of a maximum of 1,031, which made him a moderate suicide risk (a 2.5–5% chance of suiciding in the next 2 years). Thus, even considering all single suicide predictors and risk scales, VW was still an equivocal suicide. Accordingly, the family settled this case for less money rather than proceed to trial and risk losing all insurance benefits.

One last caveat: as Figure 2.6 reminds us, when measuring risk factors we also should assess counterbalancing *protective factors*. Protective factors include getting treatment (especially psychtropic medications), being cognitively flexible, having social support, being a younger female, being physically healthy, and being hopeful, among other attributes. There are measurement and scales to assess protective factors, just as we have measured suicide risk factors. In short, a suicidal outcome is not only a joint product of risk, vunerability, and psychiatric disorder but also counterbalanced by protection, competency, and resilience (Silverman & Maris, 1995).

STATISTICS, METHODS, AND RESEARCH DESIGN

Figure 3.7 (from Babbie, 1996: 104) outlines the research process. Clearly, in the few pages we have available here one cannot do justice to the complex subject of research methods and statistics. Fortunately, many of the topics listed in Figure 3.7 have already been discussed in detail. For example, in Chapter 2 we examined issues of *interest, ideas,* and *theory*. One should not forget that research should always start with worthwhile, imaginative ideas. Earlier on in this chapter we also reviewed *concepts*, variables, and *operational definitions* (i.e., measurement), such as using the HAM-D or the BDI to define and measure clinical depression or Beck's Hopelessness Scale to measure the concept of hopelessness. Such standardized instruments allow for accumulation of knowledge, comparability, and replication studies across diverse research projects.

Choice of a *research method* involves selecting a standard procedure for exploring, describing, and explaining a subject or topic of interest (Babbie, 1996: 90). Figure 3.7 lists several basic procedures (e.g., experiments, surveys, field research, content analysis, secondary analysis of existing data, historical research, comparative research, and evaluation) (see Eaton & Kessler, 1985. Most of these research procedures have already been reviewed in this chapter (in the section on data sources), especially *experiments and surveys*, and need not be reiterated here. *Field research* is often conducted by anthropologists and qualitative sociologists (particularly ethnomethodologists). For example, Jack Douglas (1967) urged that suicidologists study the first-person accounts or "situated subjective meanings" of suicide by interviewing actual suicide attempters. *Content analysis* is routinely done on suicide notes (Leenaars, 1988), identifying protocol sentences or recurring themes in the notes. Given the cost and time involved in gathering original data, many suicidologists analyze *existing data sets*. For example, Nisbet (1995) analyzed the ECA data (Eaton & Kessler, 1985) to determine protective factors related to the low suicide rate of black females in the United States.

Kushner (1991) conducted a biopsychosocial historical analysis of U.S. suicide from 1630 to 1988, highlighting the case of explorer Meriwether Lewis—of Lewis and Clark

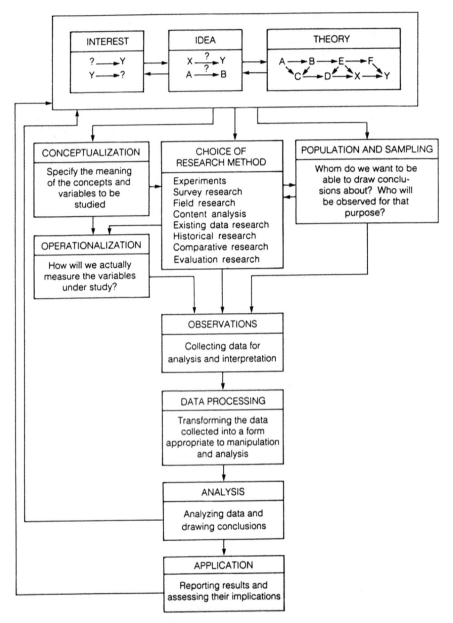

FIGURE 3.7. The research process. *Source:* Babbie (1996: 104). Copyright 1996 by Wadsworth Publishing, a division of Thomson Learning. Reprinted by permission.

fame. Farberow (1975) compared suicides in different countries and cultures, including Israel, Japan, the Netherlands, Austria, Britain, American Indians, Scandanavia, and India. Finally, one could do *evaluation research*. For example, Maris and Connor (1973) conducted an early evaluation of the efficacy of suicide prevention centers (cf. Lester, 1993f).

Next, we have to decide whom we wish to draw conclusions about and whom we wish to *sample* so as to maximize the probability of getting a representative population, being careful to describe the sample fully. Sometimes suicidologists are sloppy and inattentive to sampling, taking so-called convenience samples of their patients or doing nonsystematic hospital chart reviews. Often clinical service or treatment drives the research project, rather than the other way around. Imagine the different conclusions that might be reached, for example, by Freud studying neurotic, upper-middle-class suicide ideators in Vienna at the turn of the century, a medical examiner in Baltimore using suicide autopsy data, or a Los Angeles ER physician doing a chart review of suicide attempters.

Major sampling issues concern whom to sample, the size of the sample (especially as it relates to assumptions of anticipated statistical analyses), methods of subject selection, and the use of comparison or control groups. To begin with, are we interested in ideators, actual suicide attempters, or suicide completers? Next, to whom should our sample be compared: living normals, natural deaths, nonsuicidal psychiatic patients, accident victims, and so on?

Sample size selection (how many subjects should be selected) is a complex process. Sometimes one hears crude rules of thumb, like at least 5 cases expected per cell in a contingency table analysis (e.g., chi square) or *at least* 10 cases per independent variable in a regression equation calculation. Bigger is not necessarily better, if our subjects are not representative (e.g., interviewing 100,000 readers of the magazine *Cosmopolitan* to determine the sexual behavior of the U.S. public).

Generally, our study should be large enough to avoid false positives (type I error) and false negatives (type II error). Statistically, in a case–control design, the probability of making the first type of error is called the "level of signficance" (α), and the probability of making the second type of error is represented by β, where $1 - \beta$ is called the "power" of the study. In a case–control study design (say, of suicides vs. natural deaths), the size of cases is determined by (1) the relative frequency of exposure, Po (say, to depression, alcoholism, or prior suicide attempts), among controls; (2) a hypothesized relative risk, R (say, 2), associated with exposure; (3) the desired level of significance (e.g., $p = .01$); and (4) the desired study power, $1 - \beta$ (see Schlesselman, 1982: 147, where $Po = .3$, $\alpha = .05$, and $\beta = .10$, and the resultant needed sample sizes).

The method of sample selection is usually "simple random sampling," in which the subjects are numbered and selected (by a table of random numbers), until a desired size is reached (correcting for nonresponse, etc.). Samples can also be systematic (such as taking every nth case on a list), stratified (using sampling fractions; see Maris, 1981), or multistage cluster samples (Babbie, 1996: 221). Finally, one needs appropriate comparison or control groups against which to contrast and explain cases. Suppose in the cases of suicide an investigator discovers that 10% of them are alcoholic and 10% have a clinical depression. Is that high? The investigator would have no way of knowing without an appropriate comparison group.

Observations refer to collecting data by, for example, clinical trials of various psychotropic drugs, psychiatric interviews, death records, experiments, surveys, chart reviews, participant observation, and so on. Box 3.2 illustrates some of the controversy in suicidology concerning using death records (here, vital statisics) as observations of suicide.

Data processing usually involves "coding," which is the process of transforming raw data into standard quantitative form (Babbie, 1996: 342). Many data-gathering instruments are precoded. Coding involves specifying and numbering the categories of each variable and may involve constructing an elaborate code book.

Although it need not be, analysis of research data is usually statistical. Statistics are normally divided into simple descriptive statistics, such as rates or percentages, and explanatory statisics (see Johnson, 1992, Ch. 8, or Blalock, 1979: 200). Table 3.9 provides an example of a simple explanatory statistic. Here we ask: Do two different death types differ significantly on depression levels? We assume that there is no difference (the "null hypothesis," or Ho) and then actually test for significant differences, given certain assumptions. If

---

BOX 3.2. Can Official Statistics Be Used to Study Suicide Objectively?

No: Douglas (1967).
Yes: Pescosolido and Mendelsohn (1986).

Issue Summary

No: Douglas claimed that the meanings of suicidal actions are "problematic." Indeed, "suicide" has at least cognitive, moral, and affective meanings. The usual procedure has been to assume that the definitions and meanings of "suicide" are nonproblematic and then to ana-lyze-the official statistics (death certificates, coroners and medical examiners reports, medical records, police files, etc.) as Durkheim and others did. Unfortunately, contended Douglas, there are about as many "official" statistics of suicide as there are officials. It followed, Douglas believed, that official statistics are inadequate for the scientific study of suicide. According to Douglas, the best way to proceed is by "trying to determine the meanings of suicide to the people actually involved; i.e., the meanings to the labeled (viz., the suicide attempters) rather than taking the unknown assumed definitions of public officials" (Maris, 1981: 105).

Yes: "One of the most serious and vexing problems that faces researchers trying to under-stand the factors that underlie suicide lies in the strong criticism that offical state and national data from death certificates are irrevocably flawed. Using several independently collected data sets for county groups in the United States, we find that systematic misreporting does exist. However, misreporting in official statistics has little discernible impact on the effects of vari-ables commonly used to test . . . theories of suicide. . . . To this point no study has demonstrat-ed that the social construction of rates distorts or does not distort the analysis of social corre-lates of suicide."

---

the test statistic (here a *t* test, but others might include χ^2, gamma, alpha, *F*, *Z*, etc.) reaches a certain level (e.g., *p* = .05, .01, .001; the probability of type I error in rejecting Ho), then we reject Ho and assume that there *are* statistically significant differences in depression scores. In Table 3.9, *t* = −5.6, which is significant at the .001 level. Hence, we conclude that natural deaths and completed suicides have different depression levels (eyeballing Table 3.9, we see that suicides are on average *more* depressed than natural deaths.

TABLE 3.9. Beck Depression Inventory Scores for Natural Deaths and Suicide Completers

BDI	Natural deaths (%)	Suicide completers (%)
None (0)	10	2
Mild (1–2)	66	47
Moderate (21–25)	10	17
Severe (26+)	11	30
DK	3	4
	—	—
	100%	100%
	(71)	(266)
$\overline{X}$ BDI score	13	21

Note. t test for significance of means = −5.6, *p* < .001.
Source: Maris (1981: 219). Cf. Johnson (1992, Ch. 8). Copyright 1981 by Johns Hopkins University Press. Reprinted by permission.

More sophisticated statistics involve multivariate analyses and model testing. One could use a general linear model, which measures regression coefficients and an error term on a dependent variable, Y (e.g., some of the predictor variables in Table 3.6, on suicidal outcome) where

$$Y_i = \beta_O + \beta_i X_{1i} + \ldots \beta_p X_{pi} + e_i$$

R^2 is a crude measure of the total variance explained in Y by the predictor (independent) variables (Addy, 1992: 219–223).

However, because suicide is a dichotomous dependent variable (one either suicides or not, 1 or 0), not continuous, logistic regression is generally more appropriate in suicide data analysis. The logistic regression model is:

$$\Pr(Y_i = 1) = \frac{1}{1 + \exp\left[-\beta_O + \beta_i X_{1i} + \beta_2 X_{2i} + \ldots \beta_p X_{pi})\right]}$$

An example of logistic regression estimation for suicide is given in Tables 3.10 and 3.11.

Here Y = the probability of suicide completion and the independent variables are age, prior suicide attempt, and awareness of suicide completion. For example, in this case–control design (see Table 3.11) the odds ratio (OR) of a suicide completer having made a prior suicide attempt compared to the control group would be the exponential of the logistic regression equation, or $\exp(1.4159) = 4.12$. Thus, suicide completers here are four times more likely than controls to have made a prior suicide attempt. Or, if an individual case was (say) 39 years old (i.e., in the third age group), had one prior suicide attempt, and did not know a friend or relative who suicided, his or her predicted probability of committing suicide would be about 20%:

$$0.2075 = \frac{1}{1 + \exp[-(-3.6522 + 0.2987 \times 3 + 1.41590)]}$$

Of course, this is only a brief introduction to the complex topic of statistical testing and inference. Other issues concern measurement of interaction effects, limits to the number of predictor variables that can be estimated in a single model, alternative models, and so on.

TABLE 3.10. Data for Illustration of Logistic Regression Estimation and Prediction of Suicide Completion

Awareness of suicide	Previous attempt	Age groups (years)[a]									
		25–29		30–34		35–39		40–44		45–49	
		Case	Ctl.	Case	Ctl.	Case	Ctl.	Case	Ctl.	Case	Ctl.
None	Yes	6	24	4	16	3	6	4	19	4	9
	No	5	99	5	75	9	80	8	172	6	74
Distant	Yes	18	56	8	23	5	13	5	12	8	4
	No	6	78	14	165	17	164	26	195	37	65
Close	Yes	7	13	18	21	23	19	15	13	9	4
	No	8	59	17	69	20	74	43	134	41	87

Source: Addy (1992: 226). Copyright 1992 by The Guilford Press. Reprinted by permission.
[a]Age is coded as 1, 2, 3, 4, or 5, in logistic model.

TABLE 3.11. Logistic Regression Coefficients for Suicide Completion Data in Table 3.10

Variable	β	Std. error	χ^2	OR
Intercept	−3.6522	0.2302	251.80	
Age	0.2987	0.0472	40.11	1.35
Prior attempt	1.4159	0.1379	105.48	4.12
Awareness of suicide				
Distant	0.7545	0.1737	18.87	2.13
Close	1.4149	0.1700	69.27	4.12

Source: Addy (1992: 227). Copyright 1992 by The Guilford Press. Reprinted by permission.

For a more complete introduction, readers are referred to Addy (1992) and to the Schlesselman and Johnson texts referenced at the conclusion of this chapter.

Finally, research results must be written up and published. In a very real sense if researchers do not publish in the best relevant scientific journals, they did not do the work. In Chapters 21 and 22, we consider implications of suicide research for suicide prevention.

SUMMARY AND CONCLUSIONS

Chapter 3 is the empirical companion for the foregoing theory chapter. Together Chapters 2 and 3 provide a generic overview and introduction to theory and method, thought, and fact in suicidology. To be "empirical" means being guided by practical experience, relying on facts derived from sytematic observation or experiment.

But what data sources are available to the suicidologist to provide a factual basis for the science of suicide? In this chapter we reviewed a panorama of empirical foundation building blocks, including sample surveys, epidemiological case–control studies, psychological autopsies, psychological and psychiatric treatment records and hospital charts, and clinical interviews, ending with formal experiments (especially of psychotropic drugs).

Next we examined the variation in rates of suicide (usually suicides per 100,000 in the general population per year) across standard demographic and epidemiological variables (e.g., age, gender, race, methods, marital status, ethnicity or nationality), as well as some interaction effects. Of course, a detailed examination of suicide rates and other variables continues throughout this text. Especially for white males, suicide rates generally increase with age, until the very oldest ages. Typically rates of suicide are three to four times higher in males than in females. Firearm suicides account for about two-thirds of all male suicides and guns are now the leading suicide method for females as well, although women are much more likely than men to use drugs and medicines for suicidal overdoses. Marriage tends to protect against suicide (especially for men) and widowhood and divorce are factors that aggravate suicide. Suicide rates are high in Hungary, Finland, Austria, Denmark, France, Japan, so high as to almost be part of these countries national character. However, in some other countries suicide rates are so low as to almost approach a zero rate (e.g., Egypt, New Guinea, the Philippines, Syria, and Iran).

Referring back to Figure 2.6, in Chapter 3 we attempted to examine empirical predictors (risk factors) of suicide in concert with protective factors. Although no known set of empirical predictors results in acceptable sensitivity, specificity, or predictive rates, some predictors do identify high suicide risk groups, usually over 1- to 5-year time frames. Among the most important suicide predictors reviewed were depressive disorders, alcohol and substance abuse, suicide ideation, prior suicide attempts, the use of highly lethal method to attempt, hopelessness, being an older white male, a history of suicide in one's family, persistent work and marital problems, negative life events, low brain serotonin levels, and chronic physical illness. We reviewed some depression inventories and suicide scales. Finally, the suicide predictors, various scales, and inventories were applied to a specific suicide case.

Chapter 3 closed with an overview of the generic suicide research process. Issues considered included choice of a research method or design, sampling, data collection, data processing, and statistical analysis. Some elaboration was provided for significance testing and logistic regression analysis.

In the next (and concluding) chapter for Part I, Dutch Professor Anton van Hooff frames our current suicidological knowledge in the contextual sweep of history and art—from the Greek warrior Ajax falling on his sword after defeat in battle (the first known graphic depiction of suicide) to the rape and subsequent suicide of Lucrece (Lucretia); Rubens's Seneca; the suicide of Judas, betrayer of Jesus of Nazareth; the Middle Ages; the 16th to 17th centuries; and Donne's *Biathanatos* and concluding with a review of 19th-century Western Europe, including Emile Durkheim.

FURTHER READING

Babbie, E. (1996). *The practice of social research* (7th ed.). Boston: Wadsworth. A venerable text, now in its seventh edition, on doing social research. Topics include research design, measurement, operational definitions, scaling, sampling. experiments, surveys, field research, analysis of data, and related ethical issues.

Eaton, W. W., & Kessler, L. G. (1985). *Epidemiologic field methods in psychiatry: The NIMH Epidemiologic Catchment Area program*. Orlando, FL: Academic Press. A report on the research methods (sampling, field work, instruments—especially the Diagnostic Interview Schedule, and analysis) utilized in five epdiemiologic research studies in New Haven, Eastern Baltimore, Greater St. Louis, Durham, North Carolina (five counties), and East Los Angeles and Venice, California.

Johnson, R. (1996). *Elementary statistics* (7th ed.). Boston: Wadsworth. A good introductory survey of beginning statistics including, descriptive statistics, probability, inferential statistics (analysis of variance, regresssion analysis, and nonparametric statistics). Useful exercises and technical appendices are provided.

Maris, R. W. (1981). *Pathways to suicide: A survey of self-destructive behavior*. Baltimore: Johns Hopkins University Press. An early example of a major NIMH psychological autopsy survey of suicide in Chicago. Controls included nonfatal suicide attempters and natural deaths. Maris creates an empirically grounded general systematic theory of "suicidal careers." The study has a developmental focus, examining early trauma, social relations, work, substance abuse, depression and hopelessness, and religion—among other predictors. Methods used included path analysis, multiple nominal scale analysis, and an automatic interaction dedection program.

Mausner, J. S., & Bahn, A. K. (1985). *Epidemiology: An introductory text*. Philadelphia: Saunders. A classic introductory textbook in epidemiology. Gives operational definitions of basic terms and methods in epidemiology including rates, risk factors, prevention levels, cohorts, incidence and prevalence, causal relations, morbidity and mortality, vital statistics, life tables, demography, sensitivity, specificity, prediction, infectious disease, odds ratios, and so on.

Schlesselman, J. J. (1982). *Case–control studies: Design, conduct, analysis*. Reviews basic methods for comparing patients (cases) with groups of controls who are disease free. Focus is on discovering factors that differ in the two groups, that may explain the occurrence of the disease in the patients. Examines assessment of risk, procedures for planning a case–control study, matching, bias, determing sample size and power, and analysis (especially logistic regression).

4

A Historical Perspective on Suicide

Anton J. L. van Hooff

> History is bunk.
> —HENRY FORD

At first sight Henry Ford's notorious dictum—"History is bunk"—seems particularly appropriate for the subject of suicide in the past. Tracing the history of self-killing looks like an example of an abstruse topic without any practical significance whatsoever, only suited for experts with a morbid mind. What relevance does it have to a suicidologist who has to deal with present-day people?

In fact, all the human beings a suicidologist meets in his or her clinical practice or research carry parts of the past in their minds. Not only does personal history consist of events that have happened during one's own lifetime, but, to a great degree, it is the result of collective human experience. Each individual bears the marks—some would say the scars—of the value system under which he or she has been brought up. By their nature, moral codes are the product of a slow process in which new rules are piled on existing ones. These moral "layers," which often represent conflicting codes, account for the inward struggles of many a present-day suicide; for example, is killing oneself an act of cowardice, weakness, irresponsibility, escapism, sinfulness, independence, heroism, or some combination of these? All these diverse and often contradictory perspectives have grown during the evolution of mankind. Having a global idea of the variety of attitudes in their development may give the student of suicide a deeper insight into the many conflicting values inside the same human being.

The significance of having an idea of the complexity and the development of the value system with respect to self-killing is particularly relevant in the multicultural society our world has become. Acts of suicidal behavior that a first sight seem puzzling often can be understood as representing another stage in history. Instead of using the word "primitive," one should rather call such behavior "fundamental" or "primary."

Moreover, the student of suicide him- or herself is the product of the past. Being aware of one's own historicity helps to understand as well as brings into question the models that the expert handles as eternal truths. Why does modern science explain self-killing in psychological and sociological terms, whereas people in the past saw it as the most abominable sin (as fundamental Christians still do)? The word "suicide'" itself conveys the concept of man-slaying (cf. "homicide"). But the word "suicide," which looks like a neat Latin word (*suicida/suicidium*) and as such seems a proper scientific euphemism, did not exist among the Romans. There were good linguistic as well as conceptual reasons why the ancients could do without such a term. Already knowing the history of the word that forms the root of "suicidology" is beneficial for the understanding of basic insights.

THE SUICIDAL ANIMAL (BEFORE CIVILIZATION)

Many definitions have been tried to distinguish man's position in relation to other living beings: Does he distinguish himself by walking on his two hind legs, by the refined instruments of his fingers, or by his three-dimensional sight, or is the human species superior because of the use and moreover the fabrication of tools? Is man special by his social organization, cemented by articulate speech, a sexual appetite independent of season, and the rich language of facial expressions? However, man is not only a laughing animal, he is also an *animal suicidale*. The behavior of whales drifting ashore, sparrows flying themselves to death against electrical power lines, and lemmings drowning themselves trying to cross rivers in search of new territories all point to disorientation and defaults of animal instinct rather than *willful* attempts to put an end to their own lives. The closest animals come to self-destructive action is refusing food, a behavior that is sometimes observed when animals are pining away. This "natural" form of euthanasia is also seen among the sick and elderly, regularly in primitive cultures, but also in modern society (see Box 4.1).

In its proper sense suicide presupposes a level of consciousness about existence that is lacking in other animals; human beings have to come to terms with the frightening prospect of having to die one day. Man has to live with death. Many a toddler, shocked with the death of a relative or pet, confronts a parent with the question: "Am I to die too?" The young *homo sapiens* has attained the level of awareness mankind reached tens of thousand of years ago, when it started to give special care to the dead—not simply removing a corpse by way of an hygienic measure but by burying it, adding paint to the flesh and furnishing the deceased with some instruments that might be useful in the hereafter.

There is no way to find out whether there are suicides among the buried of the stone age and whether makers of stone tools ever directed their products against themselves, so we have to resort to anthropological evidence that proves the occurrence of self-killing in all cultures from times immemorial. Refusing food and throwing oneself from a height are basic methods that do not need preparation. The most common way out in all primitive cultures, self-hanging, requires an instrument. The halter has been available since the later stone age, which began some 10,000 years ago, when the techniques of weaving and plaiting were developed. The very brain that made man aware of himself and furnished him with tools also gave him the first ascertained instrument to "lay hands upon oneself." Suicide confronts us with one of the paradoxes of human progress: The ability to produce tools also created means of self-destruction. It is as if an elephant strangles itself with its own trunk or a scorpion poisons itself by its sting.

The noose has all the marks of being the primary instrument of self-killing. "The over-

---

BOX 4.1. A Modern Suicide by Starvation

In 1994 in Holland a teenager was raped and killed by her former boyfriend. Her grandmother was so grief-stricken that she refused to eat. She died in 2 weeks.

whelming method of suicide in Africa is hanging," thus Bohannan (1960: 175) summarized the findings of the collection of papers on self-killing in premodern Africa he edited in 1960. In Bunyoro the halter was used in more than 90% of the cases. One of Bohannan's interviewees used self-hanging and suicide as synonyms.

In all preindustrial societies the rope is by far the most common means. Even nowadays, self-hanging is practiced more in the countryside than in the urban centers. Thus there is good reason to assume that also in the first civilizations self-hanging was the primary method.

A ROMAN DEATH (ANTIQUITY)

Leaving aside non-Western cultures we find in the Greek and Roman world many indications to substantiate the conviction that in real life self-hanging prevailed: Myth, epic, legal texts, sick jokes, and other circumstantial evidence point to self-hanging as the common method. In the cases reported by the literary sources, however, the stress is on the use of weapons. I have gathered more than 1,200 cases (see van Hooff, 1998). In about 40% of these cases swords, daggers, knives and scalpels were used as the tools to bring about voluntary death. This overrepresentation of arms in the official sources is due to the ideal of heroism that dominated the scene. The concept of "Roman death," which has survived antiquity, bears testimony to the significance of the first paradigm of self-killing (see Boxes 4.2, 4.3).

As Figure 4.1 shows, ancient methods were hard and presupposed resoluteness: There was no "gambling with death" by taking a handful of pills. Self-killing was not seen as a cry for help but as an act of will. The most common Greek and Latin terms express this idea: Self-killing is mostly called voluntary death (Greek: *hekousios thanatos*; Latin: *mors voluntaria*). The prototype of ancient suicide is Ajax. In the Trojan war he was unanimously recognized as a hero second only to Achilles. After the death of this champion a controversy arose among the Greek heroes to whom Achilles' armor should be adjudged. Ulysses won the argument by his cunning speech. The fatal blow to his honor made it impossible for Ajax to face his comrades any longer. He thrust himself on his sword. Ajax exemplifies the values of a shame culture in which people mainly see themselves through the eyes of others. Apparently all civilizations go through an epic stage that glorifies the knight who puts his

---

BOX 4.2. The Idea of Roman Death in English Literature

Alexander Pope (1688–1744), *Elegy to the Memory of an Unfortunate Lady* (published 1717), identity of the person—if she was real—unknown:

> What beckoning ghost, along the moonlight shade
> Invites my steps, and points to yonder glade?
> 'Tis she!—but why that bleeding bosom gored,
> Why dimly gleams the visionary sword?
> Oh ever beauteous, ever friendly! tell,
> Is it, in heaven, a crime to love too well?
> To bear too tender, or too firm a heart,
> To act a lover's or a *Roman's part*?

Note. Emphasis added.

BOX 4.3. The Idea of Roman Death in American Literature

Ambrose Bierce, a misanthropic writer (born 1842 in Ohio, disappeared in the chaos of the Mexican revolution in 1913), made, in his story "One Officer, One Man," Captain Graffen-reid stand ready in battle line during an episode of the American Civil War. At his side a man is hit by a rifle bullet. As he has to wait for further development naturally he is very tense. "Suddenly he grew calm. Glancing downwards, his eyes had fallen to his naked sword, as he held it, point to earth. Foreshortened to his view, it resembled somewhat, he thought, the short heavy blade of the *ancient Roman*. The fancy was full of suggestion, malign, hateful, heroic!" Caught by this fascination he throws himself on his sword, thus making the number of losses for the Federal Left Army: one officer, one man.

Note. Emphasis added.

---

fame before everything. The significance of the Ajax model for antiquity is demonstrated not only by his role in epic drama—Sophocles has Ajax kill himself on the stage—and other forms of literature but even more in art. Of about 100 Greek, Etruscan, and Roman representations of suicide, Ajax on his own accounts for more than half of that number. Highly illuminating for his paradigmatic role is the specific use that was made of his suicide: Many a Greek warrior was literally confronted with Ajax's ultimate act of heroism on a bronze plaque that mounted his shield belt (see Figure 4.2).

The perfect female counterpart of a shame suicide was furnished by Lucrece (Latin: *Lucretia*). According to the story, she was forced into sexual intercourse by the son of Tarquinius Superbus, Rome's seventh king. He threatened to kill her as well as a slave and to report to her husband and relatives that he had caught her in the sexual act with the servant. To save her reputation Lucrece gave way, but afterward she called in her people, told what had happened, and stabbed herself to death, thus preserving her honor and lending force to her words (see Figure 4.3). The bewildered witnesses of this heroic act took the

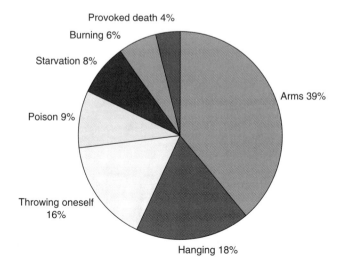

FIGURE 4.1. Methods in ancient self-killing.

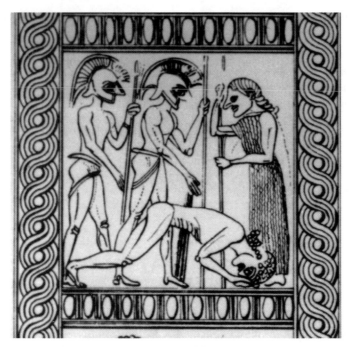

FIGURE 4.2. Many a Greek hoplite (a heavily armed infantry man) had Ajax's heroic self-killing in view, as it was shown on the bronze plaque covering the shield belt.

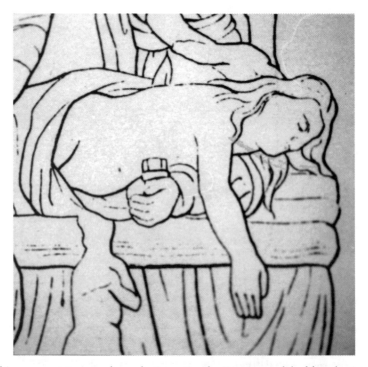

FIGURE 4.3. This woman on a sword may be Lucretia, the Roman model of female virtue who killed herself having been forced into sexual intercourse (detail of an Etruscan urn coffin).

blood-stained dagger and swore on the spot that they would put an end to the rule of kings. Consequently, Rome became a republic and Lucrece became the unchallenged model of female excellence

According to the records many men of quality or noble women modeled their behavior after the two gender paradigms of suicide. In a more complex society into which the Greek city states and the Roman republic developed, the dangers of losing one's reputation could take many forms: politicians not having their way or debtors unable to restore the money paid their tribute to the dominant value of shame. Under the Latin word *pudor*, it comes first in the lists of exculpatory motives for self-killing that were drawn up by Roman legal experts during the Empire and which reflect the common sense of the time (see Figure 4.4).

To put an end to one's life after a defeat was the only means to gain respect. Ancient literature and art paid tribute to the determination shown by enemies who killed themselves having been beaten by the forces of civilization. When King Attalus I of Pergamum defeated the Gauls of Asia Minor, in about 230 B.C., he had a statue erected in his capital showing a group of those barbarians killing themselves.

Three centuries later a similar theme was used for another triumphal monument, Trajan's column in Rome (see Figure 4.5). Like a comic strip, a serpentine in stone winds around the pillar showing the Roman achievements in the Emperor's campaign against the Dacians in present-day Romania. The victory is completed when—on one of the last and highest slabs—King Decebalus cuts his throat just before being overtaken by a Roman horseman, whose name—Valerius Maximus—we happen to know from his epitaph found

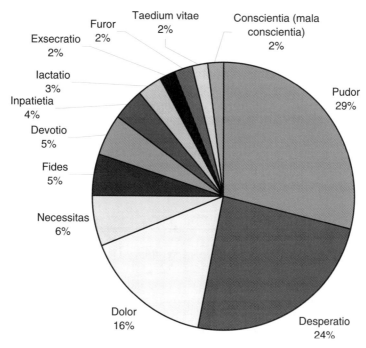

FIGURE 4.4. Motive in ancient self-killing. *Legend* (in alphabetical order): *conscientia* (*mala conscientia*): consciousness of guilt; *desperatio:* despair; *devotio:* sacrificing one's life for the benefit of a community; *dolor:* mourning (over a lost partner); *exsecratio:* bringing a curse over an opponent by a suicide; *fides:* loyalty (shown by a wife or a subordinate); *furor:* fury; *iactatio:* show of (philosophical) contempt of death; *inpatientia* (*doloris*): unbearable bodily suffering; *necessitas:* enforced suicide; *pudor:* shame (in the sense used by anthropologists, as opposed to guilt); *taedium vitae:* being fed up with life.

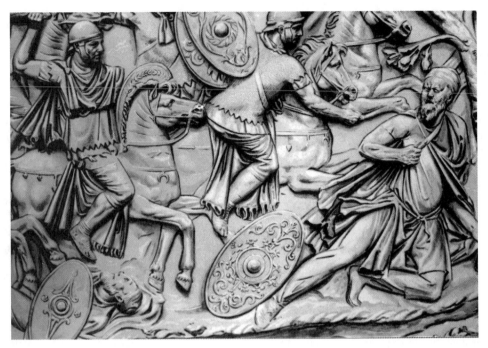

FIGURE 4.5. Decebalus, king of the Dacians (a tribe in Romania), cuts his throat when the Romans are about to capture him. His death made the Roman victory complete. Scene on one of the last slabs of Trajan's column in Rome.

in Romania: He owed his promotion to the fact that he was the one who brought Trajan the head of his formidable enemy.

In times of troubles or during an oppressive regime, in particular by a tyrannical emperor, dying in style was often the only way to save one's honor. When Caesar's bitter adversary Cato had been defeated in North Africa, in 46 B.C., he withdrew in the city of Utica and killed himself, and as "Cato Uticensis" became an icon of honorable suicide (see Box 4.4).

Resoluteness of mind, a philosophical posture, and theatricality made the suicide of a Cato or a Seneca fit for later European drama: Roman death became a common notion. Stoic philosophy, the ancient legitimization of the stiff-upper-lip attitude, gave support to

---

BOX 4.4. Cato's Exemplary Death

Having made arrangements for his comrades to escape and having read Plato's *Phaedo* on the immortality of the soul he retired to bed without rousing any suspicions, behaving and talking just as usual, but secretly took a sword into his bedroom and ran himself through. As he collapsed, still breathing, his doctor and his slaves suspected something and rushed into the room. They began to staunch and tie up his wound, but he ruthlessly pulled it open with his own hands and so deliberately put an end to himself.

—Caesar, *African War* (1955), ch. 88

the established value system that expected every man to do his duty. In principle, Epicure-anism with its stress on the quality of life, was even more permissive with respect to suicide, although its best representatives warned against "frivolous" reasons "to lead oneself out." When could one be absolutely sure that life had irretrievably lost all its meaning? Cynicism was most extreme in exhorting its followers to kill themselves without much ado.

Thus, the world of Greeks and Romans presents itself as a society that permitted and even glorified suicide. As such it has acted as a permanent counterpoint to later Western Christianity. As all learned people of that European society had gone through the school of Latin (and maybe some Greek) they were familiar with that strange world. It made many a literary and philosophical mind question the validity of the existent Christian taboo on sui-cide. As a permanent challenge to Christianity, the pagan world helped moral theologians to refine the Christian doctrine and it furnished critics of alternatives. Therefore, some knowledge of ancient suicide and its impact is indispensable for any expert in the field who is willing to see his or her work in the perspective of Western tradition.

Was suicide really frequent among the ancients as the idea of "Roman death" makes us believe? The impression it was indeed is due to various unforgettable scenes in ancient liter-ature. Above Ajax, Lucrece and Cato have been referred to. Seneca the Stoic, who in his own philosophical writings frequently discusses the theme of suicide, lived up to his own doctrines when Nero ordered him to kill himself in 65 A.D. The detailed description Tacitus gave of his ultimate deed has not failed to move everybody who reads the story in his *Annals* 15: 63 (see Figure 4.6). Among the more than 80 cases of self-killing Tacitus presents in his historical works, it is the most impressive. Stoic champions like Seneca proved to him that the Roman senatorial elite had not completely forfeited its virtue under the tyrannical regime of the emperors. Thus, Seneca as well as Cato could become an example to anybody who wanted to act as a martyr of freedom.

Tacitus and other powerful writers have implanted the impression on Western mind that suicide was frequent among the ancients. However, there is no way to substantiate this idea. The more than 1,200 instances of suicide known from antiquity concern something in the order of 20,000 individuals. This number seems impressive enough, but put against the background of the total population of the ancient world (estimated at 50 million for the Roman Empire) and taking into account the space of time, some 2,000 years, the suicide rate (number of cases per 100,000 per year) is very low: 0.02.

Thus, the idea of Roman death is a myth, albeit it a powerful one. It has to be stressed that the myth is based on highly selective sources and concerns mainly the aristocracy of birth and mind. Below the societal elite we find many traces of ambiguity (e.g., special treat-ment for the corpses of suicides, especially those who hanged themselves). Some philoso-phers expressed doubt about the acceptability of self-killing. Was it not an asocial act that damaged the community (Aristotle)? Was it not a coward's escape?

But there were no laws punishing suicide per se. Only a soldier who "deserted" by try-ing to kill himself was punishable, somewhat inadequately, by death. The prevailing value system never questioned heroic suicide.

Apart from the concept of heroic (Roman) death, antiquity gave shape to romantic sui-cide. Numerous famous lovers were said to have killed themselves (or to have threatened to do so) when their love appeared impossible or when they were deceived in their hopes. Many became part of the Western tradition, like Dido, Carthage's queen forsaken by "pi-ous" Aeneas who obeyed Iove's command to leave North Africa and to set sail for Italy to become the founding father of the Romans. Dido's suicide was to become a popular theme for painting and music (e.g., Henry Purcell's *Dido and Aeneas*).

The Roman poet Ovid (43 B.C.–18 A.D.) gave the tragic couple Pyramus and Thisbe a place in his *Metamorphoses* (see Figure 4.7). As their parents stood in the way of their love,

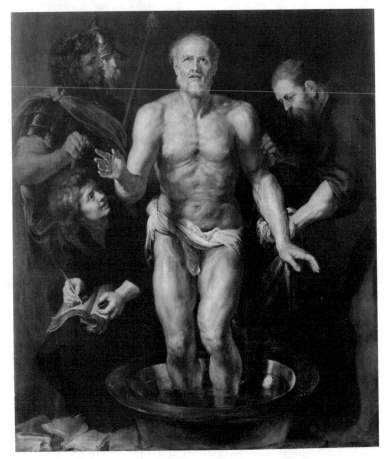

FIGURE 4.6. Tacitus's description of Seneca's suicide inspired many painters from the 16th century onward. Peter Paul Rubens shows the Stoic philosopher dictating his last lessons while his veins are being cut (1611; painting in the Alte Pinakothek, Munich).

the pair arranged a meeting outside the city. Thisbe was the first to arrive, but when a lion turned up she fled in panic, leaving her veil at the spot. When Pyramus arrived somewhat later, he found the veil blood-stained, for the lion had besmeared the cloth with its muzzle, which had the traces of another prey. Assuming that Thisbe had been devoured, Pyramus stabbed himself to death. Dying, he was found by Thisbe, who threw herself on his sword. This tragic pair belongs to the common heritage of Western civilization, and they generated many more tragic love stories, like Romeo and Juliet. The fascination in romantic love as testified by this and other stories signals the growing interest in individuality.

THE MORTAL SIN OF DESPAIR (MIDDLE AGES)

With the fall of the Roman Empire (circa 500 A.D.) came a relapse into barbarism and paganism. Western civilization went through a heroic age, in many ways reminding us of the Homeric world that saw the Ajax type of suicide. Accordingly, epics were composed, glorifying the medieval heroes to whom reputation was their primary concern up to the point of preferring self-chosen death to losing honor. The values of heroism and chivalry occur every

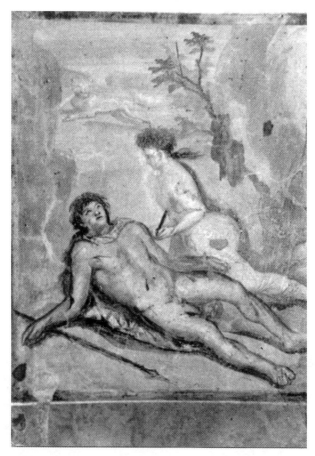

FIGURE 4.7. Thisbe thrusts herself on the sword which her lover Pyramus has used against himself in a tragic misunderstanding (wall painting in Pompeii). Photo: Anton J. L. van Hooff.

time a civilization goes through its first stages. The values are gradually covered over by more sophisticated morals, but they remain a substrate in a developed culture. They persist in certain circles, especially the military, in which self-sacrifice is always admired. Even the capitalist society of our age has some understanding for the self-killing of a politician or someone who went bankrupt and lost face. The heroic values of the early and high Middle Ages (circa 500–1300) got literary praise in the indigenous epics (e.g., *Edda* and *Beowulf*), but the literate men who put them into writing were often familiar with classical stories, so that the extant concepts were easily equated with ancient ideals. Also, the romantic stories of Latin literature found their way into the literary culture of the Middle Ages. Many a tragic couple was clearly modeled if not in name at least in behavior and fate on Pyramus and Thisbe (e.g., *Floire and Blancheflor*, 12th century). Floire is made to believe that his beloved is dead. When even her tomb is shown to him, he is determined to unite with her in the graveyard. He takes the pen that Blancheflor have him as a farewell present, maybe a reminder of Dido's instrument of suicide (i.e., the dagger that Aeneas left her). Just in time Floire's mother wrests the pen from him.

In the Arthurian legend, Queen Guinevere thinks of dying when it is falsely reported to her that "her" knight Lancelot has died in battle. When the false rumor that she has already passed away reaches Lancelot, he tries to strangle himself but is saved by accident. Stories such as these exemplify the courtly love ideal of the Middle Ages, suicide acting as the final proof of devotion.

Often Greco–Roman themes shimmer through these stories. But famous ancient suicides also appear under their own names. The English poet Geoffrey Chaucer (1340?–1400), best known for his *Canterbury Tales*, included Lucrece and Cleopatra in his *The Legend of Good Women*; out of the nine respectable females, five kill themselves. The ability of medieval people to reinterpret the old stories is formidable. Lucrece could be molded into a heroine and martyr of chastity, "a holy pagan," and a prototype of St. Mary. Thus there were extensive domains outside the reach of the Christian Church, which is too readily regarded as the exclusive spiritual force of the Middle Ages.

Even the Bible could be read with a chivalric eye. The Old Testament tells the story of several suicides without misgivings (those of Samson, Saul, and Achitophel, one of the Maccabee brothers and his mother) (see Figure 4.8).

As the main innovation of the Middle Ages is an unqualified condemnation of suicide, special attention must be paid to the origins of new code, which was to be so influential in Western civilization. The roots of this strict taboo on suicide are to be found in classical antiquity. In spite of the general permissiveness undercurrents of doubt and outright rejection had always existed, in particular among those philosophers who held that man consisted of a material body and an eternal soul. This dualistic concept emerged as early as the sixth

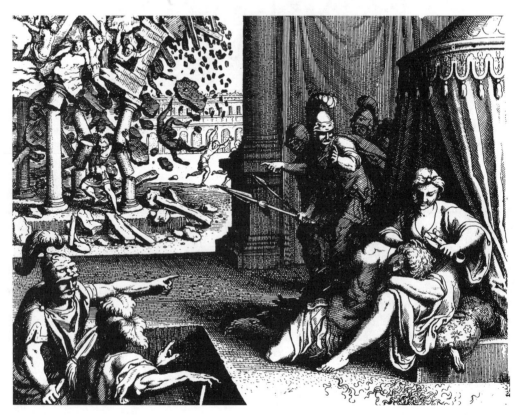

FIGURE 4.8. The Old Testament has some suicides that were a problem for Christians who held to the view that killing oneself was (self)-murder, forbidden by God's commandments. Samson who in a last effort broke the columns to which he was tied and thus killed many enemies, was one of those puzzling self-killers (Plate in a picture bible of 1627).

century B.C. with Pythagoras. In many ways Platonism refined the view that man had no right to force the divine element out of his body's jail. Only God, already seen as the one ruling power, had the command over life and death. Killing oneself was acting like a fugitive slave who steals himself from his master. Only by way of wisdom could the sage try to set free his soul from his body. Platonism in a renewed, highly spiritual form was the school of thinking for all educated people in late antiquity. The Church Fathers who gave a definitive formulation to the Christian doctrine all had undergone the influence of neo-Platonism.

In its early stages the Church had not been very outspoken on self-killing. Christians were exhorted to prevent their brethren from getting so desperate that they killed themselves. Thus the approach was pastoral rather than condemning. Martyrdom, however, roused serious moral and theological problems. The mainstream of Christianity held to the view that nobody should seek death, but in many a case the fervor to become a saint (*sanctus*) caused people to denounce themselves with the pagan authorities. In some cases Christians threw themselves upon the pyres on which their fellow believers were being burned at the stake. Several Christian females are reported to have thrown themselves into the waters to escape the persecutors who threatened to rape them. They were hailed as champions of chastity and Christian counterparts of Lucrece.

In the 4th century, when the Church became dominant, the principled rejection of suicide took shape. Lactantius (ca. 250–ca. 320) put self-killing on par with manslaughter: "For if a homicide is abominable because he is a destructor of man, he falls under the same crime as one who kills himself, for he kills a man" (*Divinae Institutiones* III, 18). Next Lactantius uses the neo-Platonist argument saying that God's revenge will be more severe as a self-killer is encroaching on God's rights over life and death. "So manslayers [Latin: *homicidae*] are all those philosophers and the champion of Roman wisdom himself, Cato."

In a summary of his *Divine Instructions* (Chapter 59) Lactantius is even more explicit: one should neither seek death by provocative words, nor kill or expose a baby nor condemn oneself to voluntary death.

The debate centered in particular on the question whether self-killing was permitted when virginity was at stake. Saint Ambrose in *On Virgins* (III 36ff.) tells the story of Pelagia, her mother, and sisters who were threatened to be caught and raped by "detestable" persecutors. Pelagia ponders: We will die anyway. God is not offended by this solution. Faith wipes out the outrage. And then, having dressed herself as a bride, and going to the water "here," says she, "let us be baptized." Then they entered as in a dance, hand in hand, where the torrent was deepest and most violent. In general St. Ambrose tried to defend the case of some martyrs by suggesting that they had acted on God's instigation.

The definitive doctrine was laid down by St. Augustine (354–430), who has always been the main authority for Christendom in the West. After a prolonged conversion, with much subtlety described in his *Confessions*, he ended his career as the bishop of Hippo in North Africa. There he was confronted with the Donatist Church, a heretic movement that venerated as *sancti* people who had thrown themselves from heights to go to heaven. To fight them effectively on their own ground St. Augustine appealed to their common authority, the Holy Bible. He is the first to explain (in *The City of God*) the commandment "Thou shalt not kill" as meaning "neither another nor oneself." To endorse the biblical argument he refers to the *New Testament* story of Christ being tempted by Satan, who puts Him on the pinnacles of the temple in Jerusalem: If you are God's son, throw yourself. Christ's refusal is seen by St.Augustine and the legion of theologians who were to follow him, as complementary evidence that self-killing is the worst sin imaginable.

It is only in this context that Judas Iscariot gets a new significance. His end is told on two places in the *New Testament*. Matthew (27:5) describes how he tried in vain to return the 30 silver pieces, the premium of his betrayal, to the Jewish priests. "And he cast down the pieces of silver in the temple and departed, and went and hanged himself." The impure money was used by the priest to buy a field to bury the corpses of foreigners. The *Acts of the Apostles* (1:18) tell: "Now this man purchased a field with the reward of iniquity; and falling headlong, he burst asunder in the midst, and all his bowels gushed out." Medieval authors and artists combined both stories having Judas falling with noose and all, his bowels gushing out (e.g. above the porch of Freiburg cathedral, Switzerland).

Judas's suicide was final proof that he completely rejected God's grace, whereas the robber who was crucified next to Christ was redeemed and entered paradise together with the Savior (see Figure 4.9). God's mercy is endless to those who are willing to accept it, but those who reject it, commit the terrible sin of *Desperatio*. Hanging was therefore regarded as the most abominable way out because this type of death left one unable to call for mercy, because one was choked and was unable to express a last-minute repentance (see Figure 4.10).

Thomas Aquinas (ca. 1225–1274), the most influential theologian of the high Middle Ages, says that Judas had a depraved remorse: "Judas indeed had fear and sorrow because he lamented his past sin; but he did not have hope." Self-killing, the theologian argues, "is the most fatal of sins because it cannot be repented of." Moreover it is an offense against self "because everything naturally loves itself, the result being that everything naturally keeps itself in being."

Homicide of oneself is also an offense against society and above these Aristotelian arguments it is a violation of God's sovereignty and ownership of human life. Suicide was seen as the ultimate confession of guilt. Innovative theologians such as St. Augustine had lost the sense of the traditional shame concept. He is only able to understand Lucrece's self-killing as the expression of a guilt. The holy Church Father quite infamously suggested that she had experienced pleasure during the rape by Sextus Tarquinius and that therefore she killed herself. It is a neat example of the opposing value systems of guilt and shame societies.

St. Augustine regards self-killing as the mortal sin of self-murder, without using the

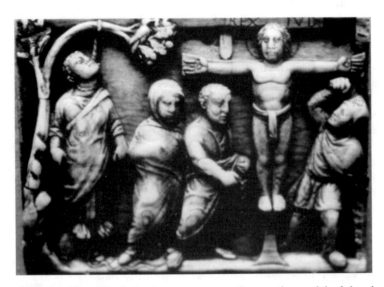

FIGURE 4.9. Judas, who betrayed Christ, became more and more the model of the absolute sinner, who rejects God's mercy even in the moment of death. His shameful death by hanging is a fitting counterpart to Christ the Redeemer on the cross (ivory box for holy objects from about 430 A.D., British Museum). Copyright The British Museum. Reproduced by permission.

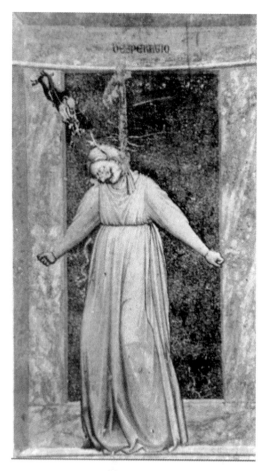

FIGURE 4.10. Having rejected all hope of salvation is the abject sin of "Desperatio." The Italian painter Giotto shows "Desperacio" (a medieval Latin form) on the wall of the Arena Chapel in Padua hanging him- or herself while the devil is fluttering near his or her ear. Photo: Anton J. L. van Hooff.

hateful word *suicida*, which would have been rejected by him as bad Latin, to be compared to English "ownslayer" (see Box 4.5). But medieval writers had less scruples in making up their own Latin. In 1177–1178 a French author, Walter of Saint Victor, attacked those theologians who took ancient philosophers such as Seneca as examples:

> Do you want to know how effeminately he killed himself?[. . .] When that man who was weaker than any woman, was forced to die he took refuge to the baths and there, like a little boy, in perfumed water made lukewarm, as it were in the softest feathers, he buried himself as deep as his neck. Thereupon were the veins of both his arms lightly touched so that he gave up his effeminate soul in the utmost luxury and as it were in his sleep. Thus, with great ingenuity he converted death itself and the pain of death in a great pleasure for himself. That man is not a brother-slayer [*fratricida*], but worse: a self-slayer [*suicida*]; a Stoic by profession, he was an Epicurean in death; do you think that he has been given a place in heaven together with Nero, Socrates and Cato, all self-slayers [*suicidae*]?

Seeing self-killing as the mortal sin par excellence, the Church denied to suicides a decent burial (i.e., in the holy ground of the churchyard). They only got a "dog's burial," their

---

BOX 4.5. On the Word "Suicide" in English

English and other modern languages coined the words "self-murder(er)" and "suicide" only in the 17th century. Suicide first was used by Thomas Browne. In the first edition of his *Religio Medici* (Part I sect. 44, written 1635, but published only 1642) he said of the Stoics: "Yet herein are they extream that can allow a man to be his owne Assassine, and so highly extoll the end of Cato." In the second edition of 1643 he somewhat expanded the passage into the following: "Yet herein are they in extreames, that can allow a man to be his owne Assassine, and so highly extoll the end and suicide of Cato." The neologism "suicide" was accepted in T. Blount, *Glossographia* in 1656. The French accepted the word only in the 18th century.

---

corpses being thrown away like that of other criminals. The secular authorities followed the directives of the Church, seeing ways to profit by confiscating the goods of such outlaws. In the course of the 14th century, English law declared a self-killer a *felo de se* (except in the case of insanity) and automatically liable to the confiscation of property. Until 1961 attempted murder was punishable in English law.

Medieval moralities popularized the Church's doctrine. So the rustic hero called Mankind in the edifying play of that name is prevented from hanging himself by (personified) Mercy. When in those dramas personified Despair appears, she is clutching the dagger that is to stab herself. There were artistic reasons as well to give a role to suicide in plays: A despairing suicide was a highly satisfactory way to get rid of a sinner. Indeed, suicide was often regarded as the most appropriate punishment for a life of sin.

The devil was always looking out for chances. In particular the holy were subject to his temptations. Monks and nuns were considered especially at risk. On their deathbed Satan makes his last assault, fluttering near the ear: "Kill yourself, kill yourself." Woodcuts depict the risks of the last moments thus furnishing a visual lesson in the arts of dying (*Artes moriendi*).

However, at the same time popular story books circulated, for the first time in the vernacular, telling about heroes and knights. This side-by-side existence of the alternative codes of chivalry and Christianity was no problem for a period that is marked by doublethink, as it was to be in later periods of moral offensives.

In this section on the Middle Ages the stress had to be on literature and theology, not only for the sake of the important new concept of suicide that took shape but also simply because concrete data are sparse and selective, mainly concerning cases that came to court. The authorities saw a chance to enrich themselves by confiscating the goods of a suicide. Thus commonly people of some standing were involved. The few cases that are known suggest that self-hanging remained the method most frequently used. In 32 of 54 cases with which a Paris court dealt, the halter was used. Also the sex ratio falls in familiar patterns: 41 males against 13 women (8 hanging themselves).

There is no reason to assume that self-killing indeed was rare in the Middle Ages. It is the Christian taboo that accounts for secrecy. It is highly significant for the prevailing paradigm that no famous *historical* examples of suicide are reported whereas classical antiquity glorified such people as Brutus, Cato Uticensis, and Seneca. Only medieval literature ventured to dream about extraordinary people who did not stick to the Christian doctrine.

MORALE AND MELANCHOLY (EARLY MODERN TIME: 16TH–17TH CENTURIES)

Early modern time, the period of Reformation, Renaissance and Baroque, brought a deeper understanding of human individuality. The revival of classical culture even caused a few to adopt a neopagan attitude and to subscribe to ancient values, glorifying the ancient heroes of suicide without qualification. For most educated people, however, the renewed dialogue with Greeks and Romans resulted in a greater respect for the dignity as well as for the complexity of a human being.

The Reformation and its Roman–Catholic reaction, the Counterreformation, did not question the established doctrine of the Church on suicide. On the contrary, in many ways the religious revival originated a moral offensive, repeating and enforcing the Christian prohibition of suicide. But as individual intention rather than outward behavior counted, both secular and religious thinkers were inclined to qualify or reserve their judgment. Only to God was it to know the last stirrings of the soul.

Thomas More (1477–1535), one of the finest representatives of the Renaissance in Northwestern Europe, revived ancient fantasies on ideal societies. In his "Nowhereland" (Utopia) the members of the ideal state show an exemplary care for the weak (Box 4.6). The Utopians care for incurables by offering them conversation and relief from pain.

More's fantasy reminds us of Plato's totalitarian State (Politeia) and of the ancient stories about communities (e.g., the island of Keos) where the authorities were said to furnish aged people with poison. Thomas More explores the values of a new society marked by responsibility of the individual toward the whole, but also by care of society for those who suffer. However, as a devout Christian, More rejected suicide as an option when he was jailed in the Tower of London. There he wrote his *A Dialog of Confort* in which he adheres to the traditional view that any thought of suicide was inspired by the devil.

The French essayist Michel de Montaigne (1533–1592), who lived among the ancients (in the midst of his books), explicitly chose for man's autonomy. He put his views on suicide as follows: "The most voluntary death is the finest. Life depends upon the pleasure of others, death upon our own. The wise man is one who lives not as long as he can, but as long as he should. Nature has given us only one entry into life, but a hundred thousand ways to leave it. When God reduces us to the state in which it is far worse to live than to die He grants us permission to die."

The Church reformers did not venture to enter into God's rights like Montaigne did. Martin Luther (1483–1546) who, as a former Augustin monk, was steeped in the strict doctrine of the Church Father saw the scheming Satan behind suicide. In a letter to his wife (10 July 1540) he told that the devil was very active in Eisenach. He incited people there to arson and suicide. The German Protestant was adamant in his view that man

---

BOX 4.6. Regulated Self-Killing in Thomas More's *Utopia*

However, those who suffer from incurable diseases that are accompanied by continuous pain are urged by the priests and magistrates not to endure their sufferings any longer. (. . .) But they dishonor a man who takes his own life without the approval of the priests and senate. They consider him unworthy of decent burial and throw his body unburied and disgraced into a ditch.

should care for his health. Who refuses to take medicines, rejects the means supplied by God and risks to become a suicide. So far Luther, whose personality was firmly rooted in rustic society, does not seem to overstep the medieval abhorrence, but he shows himself sensitive to a new approach in refusing to regard a suicide's soul as condemned forever. Nobody but God can know. This kernel of a Lutheran view was developed by pastor Johannes Neser, who in 1617 published an essay on melancholy and its tendency to drive men into suicide. Suicide committed by a sane person leads to damnation. But if melancholy or madness leads men to kill themselves, they are not responsible and are not to be regarded as reprobate.

The exculpating grounds of madness and melancholy played a major role in the public debate of the age. Opponents of Calvinism held that the doctrine of predestination led to melancholy among Calvin's adherents and for that reason to a tendency to kill themselves. The problem of the link between religious belief and suicide was to be tackled by Émile Durkheim (1858–1917) who in his magisterial Le suicide of 1897 laid a sociological link between Protestantism and a predisposition to suicide.

John Calvin (1509–1564) himself did not discuss suicide when dealing with the commandment "Thou shalt not kill," the sixth in the counting of Calvinism and most Protestant churches, the fifth according to Roman Catholics, Lutherans, and Anglicans. Where Calvin refers to the question he stresses the significance of the intentionality. Judas's loss of hope was not real remorse and not an appeal to God's mercy. Therefore his despair constituted "nothing better than a kind of threshold to hell." Generally speaking, Protestant churches present a large variety of opinion (see Box 4.7). Strict views prevailed among the orthodox.

Some pastorally minded Protestant authorities, however, were inclined to accept madness and melancholy eagerly as exceptions to the rule that suicide was the most abominable sin. They exhorted to entrust doubtful cases to the judgment and mercy of God. The exception of mental disturbance was also accepted by the Anglicans and to some degree by Roman Catholic theologians. An example of the latter is Caramuel (1606–1682) (see Box 4.8). For long it was held that he was the first to use the Latin words *suicida* and *suicidium*—(but see p. 109). In the second, much augmented edition of his monumental *Theologia moralis fundamentalis*, which came out in Rome in 1656, he discusses the fifth commandment fully in line with the established doctrine: Under *Fundamentum 55* the moral theologian repeats that any killing of a human being is prohibited by God's order, adding, "You are no more strictly held not to kill yourself than your fellowman" (p. 112). So far there is nothing new, but this section (which significantly also deals with abortion) is followed by a discussion (*Quaestio*) that explores the scope of the commandment. Not only by its subtle judgments the text is of interest. It is illustrated by concrete cases from Caramuel's own experience. They give us glimpses of the reality of the age.

BOX 4.7. On the Continuing Debate among Protestants

In 1994 the mainstream Protestant churches of Holland declared that self-killing could not be called sinful without qualification. A letter to the editor remonstrated against this relaxation: "The sixth commandment of God's Law says: Thou shalt not kill. Is self-killing no killing? Sure it is, so it is sin. God had made us know that His Law will prevail till the Return and therefore cannot be abolished by anyone. What the Church does, is blasphemy. It is not up to man to judge those people, so neither to the Church."

BOX 4.8. Four Cases Discussed by Caramuel

Under the heading "Are all who kill themselves to be called desperate and are they to be regarded as having gone to hell?" the author repeats the doctrine "nobody is allowed to do away with himself." (pp. 115–116) Without suggesting any doubt about this truth Caramuel says that many affected by serious diseases are driven into frenzy (*delirium*); "if those kill themselves, they do not sin." The *first* concrete case concerns a spy, the king's secretary in Brussels. When he was found having hanged himself, the judges ordered the executioner to remove the corpse and to hang it upside down on the gallows outside the city. This harsh treatment was right as an example to others, Caramuel says; as there was no disease, he sinned because of his wickedness.

Caramuel was personally involved in a *second* case. While serving as the deputy to the cardinal–archbishop of Bohemia he had to pass a verdict on the corpse of parish priest, who suffered from a hypochondriac illness. Fits alternated with periods in which he loyally served the Church to full satisfaction. One morning he went to the sheriff, a friend of his, and said: "Oh Sir, how happy I was as long as I had only one head. But already from the day before yesterday I suffer from the burden and would like to remove two to be relieved." A doctor called in was unable to talk the priest out of his conviction that he had three heads. Driven by this fiction the priest went home and hanged himself. Caramuel leaves no doubt that the man acted from illness and that, while trying to remove two of the imaginary heads, he strangled the real one. He had deserved to be treated with respect, but the superstitious Bohemians made an executioner remove and bury the corpse in a field, although in Caramuel's view he could have been buried in sacred soil.

Then there is a *third* case of what we would call religious mania: A lay brother in an unnamed monastery started to get apparitions. He told his friends one Sunday that the Mother of God had given him some relics of her Virginal body. When challenged to produce them he showed two morsels of white wax. That day he persevered in this prejudice. In the following night he strangled himself. The prior had him buried in a secular place. When, after four years, the Inspector of the Order heard the case he ordered the body to be transferred to holy ground, but that was not done. Caramuel sees this case as another instance of delirium so that the victim could have been buried in sacred soil. However, he is willing to respect the prior's motives to act as he did. In his turn the inspector had acted in the right way provided that the corpse could later have been brought to sacred soil without causing scandal and turmoil. Caramuel advised to consecrate the burial site in secret.

His *fourth* case is a priest who strove to be holy, but was a sinner—it is not specified in what way: by masturbation? In consequence he hated himself. Once, when he thought to have been fully reconciled with God, he was afraid to relapse. He confessed all his sins, said mass under many tears, and entered his cell. He opened the Bible and his eyes fell on Job 7:15 "my soul choose hanging." When he was found hanged, his head was shaven to make the tonsure invisible and his face was disfigured. In such a state his corpse was dumped into a river. When he was washed ashore at some distance, the peasants who found him assumed that he was the victim of robbers and gave him a decent burial. Since then the region has been favored by the weather. Caramuel does not know what to make of this miraculous phenomenon. Miracles are expected to edify people. Anyway, the priest had either raved or sinned.

Thinkers like Caramuel were involved in subtly moving Christian morals away from being a rigid system of rules into doing justice to the complexity of human stirrings. Naturally there was a great distance between those pioneers and the people who instructed the masses. Among them the traditional views prevailed, as is proven by a "pictionary" for Latin produced by the Czech pedagogue Comenius (see Figure 4.11) in its first Latin–German edition in 1658. Many generations of kids were educated with this book.

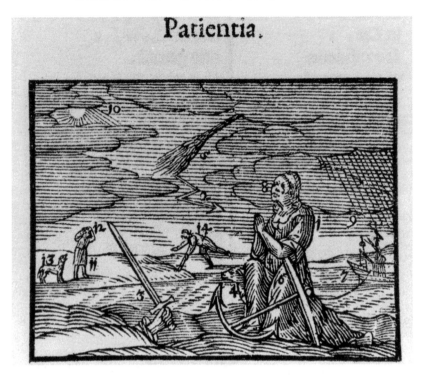

FIGURE 4.11. In his Latin "pictionary," the Czech pedagogue Comenius teaches the sorry consequences of being "impatient" (i.e., not complying with God's ordinances). Such a sinner becomes furi-
ous and throws himself on the sword.

Under the heading of *Patientia*, he tells the sorry consequences of lacking this main
Christian virtue.

In an English edition of 1777 the Latin is rendered as follows: "The impatient Person,
waileth, lamenteth, rageth against himself, grumbleth like a Dog, and yet doth no good; at
the last he despaireth, and becometh his own murtherer." In the Latin text "his own murtherer" is denoted by a Greek word *autochir* (i.e., someone who lays hands upon himself).
The excellent Latinist Comenius refrains from using the word *suicida* (see p. 108). In the
second edition, which came out only 1 year after the first, he added the word *propricida*
(own-killer) in between brackets, betraying his embarrassment.

In early modern times there is much debate about the codes regulating the relation between state and individual. These questions of public and personal morale are the focus of
Samuel Pufendorf's (1623–1694) work *On the Duty of Man and Citizen* (*De officio homin-
is et civis*). In chapter 5, "On duty to oneself," he agrees to the view that self-love is natural:
"It compels man to have a careful concern for himself [. . .] Yet from another point a man
surely does have certain obligations to himself. For man is not born for himself alone; the
end for which he has be endowed by his Creator with such excellent gifts is that he may be
a fit member of human society." Here we have, in a revised form, the ancient Platonic argument that leads to the established Christian view: "No one gave himself life; it must be regarded as a gift of God. Hence it is clear that man certainly does not have power over his
own life to the extent that he may terminate it at his pleasure. He is absolutely bound to
wait until He who assigned him this post commands him to leave." Then Pufendorf argues
that it may be morally correct to shorten one's life by excessive labor as long as it is on be-

half of the common good. On the other hand, the legal rules may order a citizen under threat of the severest penalties not to avoid danger by flight. "He may also take such a risk of his own accord provided that [. . .] there is reason to expect that this action will result in safety for others. [. . .] In general, however, there seems to be no precept of nature that one should prefer another's life to one's own, but things being equal, each may put himself first. Nevertheless, whoever terminates or throws away his life of his own accord must be regarded without fail as violating natural law. . . ." Pufendorf is visibly struggling trying to reconcile the rights of the state and the individual.

Early modern times is also the period that saw the origins of classic European drama. The drama of Shakespeare and his contemporaries exploited suicide because it provided them with inexhaustible opportunities to generate different kinds of ethical complications and emotional effects. These reasons are up to today valid for literature as a means to explore the human situation: An author cannot be made accountable for the extreme things his or her persons do. Literature that has a message has little chance to be more than ephemeral. There is a highly complex interaction between an author and his or her addressees, the audience expecting to have a good time, to be comforted, but also to be challenged albeit not offended. Thus only with much qualification it can be said that Shakespearean drama "reflects" the values of the period.

> To be, or not to be,—that is the question:—
> Whether 'tis nobler in the mind to suffer
> The slings and arrows of outrageous fortune,
> Or to take arms against a sea of troubles. . . .
> (*Hamlet* Act III, Scene I, 83ff.)

Here despair has acquired a widened meaning: Hamlet does not clutch a rope and a dagger as he thinks of suicide. The promptings to self-murder come from within him, not from an evil angel of a personified Despair. The language of his soliloquies is free from the conventional phrases associated with religious despair. He is recognizable to modern man as a complex of drives and anxieties.

As argued earlier, there are intrinsic reasons why drama has a taste for suicide (e.g., deaths being needed to put a radical end to the plot). As to the suicide in Shakespeare's plays, there is a noticeable distinction between good and evil characters. These last (e.g., Lady Macbeth) frequently kill themselves offstage, the most effective way to strip them of either redemptive or heroic connotations. To a dramatist, suicide was a useful way of disposing of female criminals, who could not so readily be killed in battle or single combat. However, the noble suicides of Othello, Brutus, Antony, Cleopatra, and Romeo and Juliet are staged.

By Shakespeare's time suicide had become one of the ways of defining Roman mores and Roman character in the theater. The heroic Stoicism of Cato represented the ideal of Roman death. Macbeth clearly falls short of this model, explicitly saying: "Why should I play the Roman fool?" (V, iii, 1).

A Roman death would have heroic, "manly" qualities that Shakespeare did not attribute to Macbeth. A sinful suicide from despair, on the other hand, would suggest the workings of a conscience, but Macbeth is represented as having gone beyond good and evil. He has surpassed even Judas.

Shakespearean genius shows itself in the Brutus's suicide, which has a tragic complexity. It is not simply nobility but despairing failure; the failure of a man divided against himself. That is why he appears the most tragic Roman of them all and not a cardboard figure. The intense interest in Roman suicides is part of the dialogue and often conflict between the Renaissance and Christianity, classical antiquity challenging the established values.

BOX 4.9. Venereal Disease Triggering a Suicide

In 1590 a woman from Feering in Essex appeared before the Church court on a charge of "committing fornication with Enoch Greve, who drowned himself, being so burned [i.e. with venereal disease] that he could not abide the pains."

It is clear that Shakespeare's suicides have still much to offer to a modern expert. Romeo and Juliet represent death for love, exemplifying the links between *Thanatos* and *Eros*. When Juliet learns of Romeo's exile, she alludes to the ropes with which Romeo was to have ascended to her bedroom:

> Come, cords; come, nurse. I'll to my wedding bed;
> And death, not Romeo, take my maidenhead! (III, ii, 136/7)

Also for the period discussed in this section no systematic data are available. The records show an increase in cases of suspected self-murder that are treated by the *King's bench* between 1510 and 1580, from an average of six to an average of 94 per annum, but this a clearly due to the rule that made it a highly profitable business to have a death established as self-murder. The coroner was rewarded with the payment of 13 s. 4d. for each "successful" case, whereas the confiscated goods were given to the king's chaplain. No wonder that many cases concerned rich merchants.

For the first time in history people tried to find rational explanations for the intriguing act of suicide (see Box 4.9). Melancholy was put forward as triggering self-killing. As the Greek word expresses, it was regarded as a state of mind resulting from an excess of black bile. Thus Robert Burton (1577–1640) expounded in his *Anatomy of Melancholy* (1621) that the imbalance of the four fluids of the body by an overdose of black bile led to self-destruction. He is one of the many who reserve their judgment on suicides: "Of their bodies we can dispose, but what shall become of their souls, God alone can tell. . . . God is merciful unto us all."

For the time being these considerations had no influence on the practices that had developed to treat the corpse of a suicide as an alien. The body was not carried out via the door but via a window or a hole made to that purpose and closed thereafter. The corpse was ignominiously dragged through the streets—sometimes on a sledge—and hanged on the gallows or a two-pronged trunk. When the body had considerably decayed it was buried outside the churchyard, often in ways that inverted normal practice: face below and in north–south direction instead of west–east, which was regarded as ensuring a smooth resurrection. Also, a pole driven through the body prevented the self-murderer from raising from the grave. (See Figure 4.12)

REASON AND SPLEEN (18TH CENTURY)

Although in time John Donne (1572–1631) falls well before the 18th century, his thinking anticipates the Age of Reason. Moreover, only in the 18th century did his essay *Biathanatos* became influential. The monograph, written as early as 1607, but posthumously published by his son between 1644 and 1647, has a Greekish title, *biathanatos* being a Greek compound of "violence" and "death." In antiquity self-killing was classified and discussed as

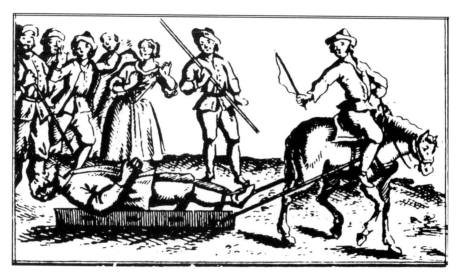

FIGURE 4.12. From the Middle Ages into the 18th century, suicides were being punished posthumously. Their corpses were dragged to the town to the field of the gallows, where it was hung.

just another form of unnatural and immature death, to be compared to death caused by falling stones and other accidents.

Donne, best known as a poet, belonged to a Roman Catholic family, but ended up as a dean of the Anglican St. Paul's Cathedral in London. Both for religious and for economic reasons he had to be cautious. His *Biathanatos* only circulated among trusted friends as the content was explosive. (See Figure 4.13)

On theological grounds, he who in the opening lines of the Preface confesses to have often had that sickly inclination to put an end to his life, argues against a unqualified condemnation of all suicide. To him it is the intention that matters: "to me there appears no other interpretation safe but this, that there is no external act naturally evil, and that the circumstances condition them, and give them their nature." His main argument are the martyrs who sacrificed their lives for an excellent cause: "As therefore Naturally and Customarily men thought it good to dye so and that such a death with charity was acceptable, so is it generally said by Christ, [That the good Shepherd doth give his life for his sheep.] Which is a justifying and approbation of our inclination thereunto. For to say, The good doe it, is to say, They which doe it are good." Conclusive evidence is furnished by the Good Shepherd Himself: Did Christ not sacrifice His life for the best of causes, the redemption of mankind? "And therefore, as He Himself said [No man can take away my soule] And [I have power to lay it down] So without doubt, no man did take it away, not was there any other then his own will, the cause of his dying at that time." So in Donne's highly original arguing Christ is the pure suicide. In Donne we have a sincere Christian trying to reconcile his psychic inclination with Christian doctrine.

Even the most outstanding representative of English Enlightenment David Hume (1711–1776) could not do without religious reasoning. Nowhere in the Bible, he adduced, is suicide explicitly condemned. But for him the biblical argument is only contributory to the main ideas of his essay *On Suicide*. Hume was embarrassed when his text was published without his permission in French in 1770. An English (unauthorized) edition came out 7 years later. The first official version was published in 1783 and as the author had foreseen during his lifetime, it caused much uproar among Christians with strict views, who were

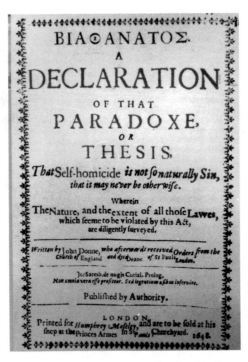

FIGURE 4.13. John Donne, poet as well as priest, argued in his *Biathanatos* that the permissibility of self-killing depended on intention. The Christian martyrs and Christ Himself, who sacrificed themselves for a laudable cause, are Donne's main arguments (title page of *Biathanatos*, only published after the author's death).

sure that it stimulated self-destruction. At that time the Methodist leader John Wesley (1703–1791) urged the British Prime Minister William Pitt Junior to discourage suicide by hanging the corpse in chains for all to witness.

It is no wonder that Hume's strict reasoning shocked people who held to traditional views as he made a frontal attack on the argument that to kill oneself was encroaching on God's established order. Should human beings be absolutely passive in the face of natural occurrences (e.g., the weather) because otherwise they would disturb the natural processes? Is it not allowed to turn one's head aside to avert a falling stone? If it is morally permissible to disturb some operations of nature, then it is morally permissible to avert life itself by diverting blood from its natural course in human vessels. "It would be no crime in me to divert the Nile or Danube from its course [. . .] Where then is the crime of turning a few ounces of blood from their natural channel?" Hume appealed to the individual right of autonomy—"native liberty"—and to the wholesome consequences of some instances of self-caused death. In the end it is up to an individual to decide whether his life is of any value to society. Just as a person can decide to retire from society as a pensioner, whereby no harm is done to the community, an individual has the right to take leave of life, for who is damaged by this action?

Hume's libertine permissiveness was in line with the views expressed by the French *philosophes*. Already Montesquieu (1689–1755) had put into the mouth of a fictitious Persian visiting Europe the argument: Life was given to me as a favor. So I may return it the moment it is not a favor any more. When I commit suicide, I only use the right given to me (*Persian Letters* 76).

As early as 1723 a Dutch publicist, Jacob Weyerman (1677–1747), had already argued for the right of free disposition over one's life. He did so in a weekly magazine, a medium that helped to shape public opinion in the 18th century. He commented on a personal experience some 6 years before in Bristol. There he had made friends with a young merchant who one night suffered from deadly melancholy. His Dutch friend tried as a "sick's comfort" (Dutch: *ziekentroost*) bits of Seneca and Boethius. But even a verse that would have softened a Cato as "molten butter" was of no avail. Finally they went to bed. Next morning the merchant was found to have himself shot with a pistol. This shocking event caused Weyerman to stage a discussion as a process in which the merchant's advocates are the pagan Romans whereas amongst his accusers are the Catholic Romans. The pagan plea sums up all the ancient examples: Cato, Socrates, Cleanthes. The counterargument is summarized as "But man is necessary for the world," immediately refuted by Weyerman's personal view: "Let a bold man not stay so long that de sparrow of death comes and munches the overripe cherries [. . .] Let us live, as long as life pleases us (so the heroic Romans cried, as glorious in their courage as pitiable in their paganism) and not till disease consumes us." For Weyerman as a representative of 18th-century common sense, putting an end to one's life is an act of courage (i.e., a moral virtue). To prolong life is the behavior of a slavish soul, whereas a bold man leaves life as he leaves the table when his appetite is satisfied.

These and similar views that became more and more common encroached on the Church's authority and they paved the way for the principled reassessment of suicide by the French Revolution of 1789.

As for all preindustrial history, we only have filtered facts and anecdotal evidence for the occurrence of suicide. As English society was more open, many cases became known by press publications, even to such a degree that the expression *The English Malady* was coined. It was the title of a work by an alarmed doctor, George Cheyne. In his book, whose full title is *The English Malady, or a Treatise of Nervous Diseases of all Kinds* (1733), he establishes as a fact that England is the country of suicide. The author ascribes the sad record to growing atheism, modern hedonistic philosophy, and the depressing climate.

For the last decades of the 18th century we have an arsenal of cases in Prussia: These concerned 136 instances of drowning, 53 hangings, 42 times use of firearms and 8 throat-cuttings. The material has all the chance to be atypical because about half of the victims were soldiers. Also the preromantic climate is held responsible for the very specific pattern.

Romantic suicide got a major boost from a novel, *Young Werther's Sufferings*, written by the German genius Goethe (1749–1832) in 1774. The work is looked on as the classic example of book causing a wave of suicides among sentimental adolescents who in various ways referred to Werther—by their costume or by having the book as their last reading.

During the Age of Enlightenment there is a marked shift away from condemning to understanding suicide. More than before, a suicide is excused as having been *non compos mentis* (not in his or her right mind). It is no coincidence that the 18th century sees the opening of many an institution for the mentally ill. The old practices of desecrating the corpses of suicides went out of use.

THE MOLOCH OF METROPOLIS (19TH CENTURY)

Abolishing punishment of suicide was only one of the numerous innovations the French Revolution brought to the Western world. As the first modern republic in Europe, France saw itself as ancient Rome reborn. Roman virtues were acclaimed. People called themselves and their children after Roman heroes. In particular, Caesar's murderer Brutus and his principled opponent Cato became popular. When the Revolution devoured its own children, condemning leaders of the first hour, one of its commanders, Pichegru, was found hanged in his cell on April 5, 1804. Next to his corpse was an edition of Seneca opened on the page where the Roman Stoic (and suicide) glorified Cato.

The law codes of the French Revolution had a lasting impact on all the Western nations. Even in England the tradition of burial at the crossroads was ended by statute in 1824, but burial was still done at night and without religious rites Church authorities kept on complaining of slackening moral norms. In 1881 the reverend Isaac Watts said that the Church of England used to rank self-murderers with excommunicated persons and deny them a Christian burial. Civil government backed the Church by ordering that they should be put into earth with utmost contempt, generally in some public cross-way, a stake driven through their dead bodies, which was not to be removed. "It is a pity this practice has been omitted of late years by the too favourable sentence of their neighbours on the jury, who generally pronounce them distracted; and thus they are excused from this public mark of abhorrence."

This protest against slackening morals is but one sign of a radical shift. No longer was a suicide regarded by the public as a sinner but as a sufferer. It was not a pastor who was called in when somebody had attempted suicide but a medical doctor. During the 19th century suicide becoming more and more medicalized, experts looking for clues. At first organic symptoms were diagnosed (e.g., a thick skull bone). Later soul medicine, psychiatry, developed and tried to find mental clues for self-destruction.

A more theoretical, at first rather philosophical, approach was tried by the new branch of psychology that developed hand in hand with sociology—often in hand-to-hand fighting about what approach had the most explanatory power. Modern experts should be aware that they are heir to the 19th century psychosocial tradition. No longer was suicide regarded as an heroic act of free will or as a mortal sin, but as a disease.

The interest in soul and society was the result of the anxious awareness that modern man lived in an unnatural habitat. No longer had he his place in a close network formed by family, village, and church, but he got lost in huge cities. Alienating metropolises like London, Paris, Vienna, and St. Petersburg were notorious for their suicide rates (see Figure 4.14). For, as for the first time mortality was recorded and as suicide emerged as a noticeable death cause in an age whose hygienic offensive dramatically increased life expectancy, suicide fascinated people as the modern urban disease.

Novelists, sensitive to their time, described at length the anxieties that caused young women to drown themselves in the Seine or the Thames River. In the general pattern, these women had come as innocent girls from the countryside trying to find decent jobs in the industrial centers. But they got into evil company and were seduced by arrant villains, most often young gentlemen. The novelists of the great age of the novel proved their genius by varying the theme. Thus, in Dostoyevsky's novel *Demons*, young Kiriloff, who regards himself as being beyond good and evil, is convinced that by committing suicide as an absolutely free act he will become a god, is for the Russian novelist the prototype of the immoral man bred by the world city.

Culturally belonging to the great tradition of the 19th century is the American writer Edith Wharton (1862–1937). In her 1905 novel *The House of Mirth* she describes the decline and fall of the resourceless but beautiful Lily Bart. Lily is in search of a husband who can maintain her in the style she craves in the affluent society of New York City elite. But her chances are annulled when she is rumored to be the mistress of a wealthy man. In several stages she climbs down the social ladder, ending up living in a boarding house: "She put our her hand, and measured the soothing drops into a glass; but as she did so—she remem-

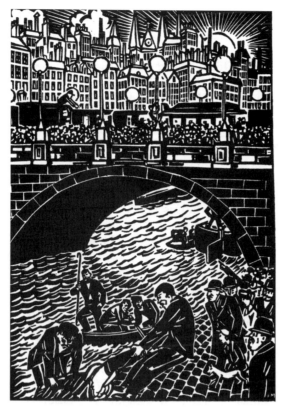

FIGURE 4.14. The big city of the 19th century was assumed to alienate people and drive lonely people into self-killing. Suicides, especially pregnant girls, dragged up from the river were a common phenomenon in the metropolis. (one of the woodcuts in Frans Masereel, *The City*, 1923). Copyright 2000 by Artists Rights Society (ARS), New York/VG Bild-kunst, Bonn. Reprinted by permission.

bered the chemist's warning. If sleep came at all, it might be a sleep without waking. But after all that was but one chance in a hundred: the action of the drug was incalculable, and the addition of a few drops to the regular dose would probably do no more than procure her the rest she so desperately needed. . . ."

This taking a chance—in Lily Bart's case with a fatal outcome—fits well into a new pattern: a suicide attempt as a gamble with death and/or a cry for help. The use of drugs increases considerably according to the statistics that for the first time give a more or less reliable picture.

In Victorian England of 1861 drug use accounted for 7% of all suicides, compared to 48% for hanging. In 1911 it had doubled its share to 14%, whereas hanging had decreased to 29%. New means had entered the scene: using a pistol or throwing oneself in front of a train or from a high construction like the Eiffel Tower or one of the skyscrapers that determined the skyline of cosmopolitan cities.

Modern mass society was believed to make people sick, as was proclaimed by the title of a famous study of the time: *Self-murder as a social mass phenomenon of modern civilization* (*Der Selbstmord als sociale Massenerscheinung der modernen Civilisation*), Vienna 1881. Its author, Thomas Masaryk (1850–1937), would later be the first president of the Czechoslovakia (1918–1935). His book expresses contemporary anxiety, for as Masaryk says "the question of suicide involves the very happiness or unhappiness of mankind." He sees "the relationship between the modern suicidal tendency and widespread nervous afflictions and mental illness" In his study he wishes to identify "the sick, pathological condition of present day." His work is not just a diagnosis, it proposes a therapy as well. The last chapter, "Towards a Remedy for the Modern Suicide Tendency," is a plea for a return to old values: "We need a religion; we need to be religious."

Also Émile Durkheim (1858–1917), the founder of empirical sociology, tries to heal the ailments of fellow men, but he takes into account the new economic and social structures. He is convinced that religion never will be able again to socialize people like it once did. As a return to the old paradise of the village is unthinkable, the workplace is to give man a social framework. Durkheim opts for a political system not based on territorial districts but on corporations of trade and industry.

These rather poor receipts come at the end of a magisterial study that rightly has as its subtitle "A Study of Sociology," for this is what *Le Suicide* (1897) is. Whereas Masaryk and other predecessors mixed all kinds of data (climate, the moon phases) Durkheim consequently sticks to the relation between the social framework and man. Society, he argues, constrains individuals in two ways: by integrating and regulating them. If integration is too strong the individual may be inclined to sacrifice himself in behalf of the whole. This "altruistic" suicide is the perfect opposite to *le suicide égoiste,* which by all accounts is the focus of Durkheim's interest. If the bond with society is too slack and an excessive individualism dominates the individual, he suffers from *disintegration.*

Durkheim pointed to religious differences and divergent family circumstances as the main variables accounting for the large diverse of suicide rates. Catholicism, for instance, demonstrably had a greater integrative power than Protestantism, as nearby Swiss cantons of different denomination proved. Durkheim's *Suicide* looks familiar to the modern suicidologist because of its numerous tables. The figures are sociologically analyzed and show that married people have proportionally lower suicide rates than unmarried people of the same age—one of Durkheim's advisorees is to make marriage less easily dissolvable. Married couples with children have a higher "coefficient of preservation" than do childless ones.

This type of "epidemiological" approach is since Durkheim firmly established. However, not only for his sociological methods Durkheim can be regarded as the founder of suicidology. With his concept of integration versus disintegration he laid down the paradigm that dominates the study of self-killing to our days.

SUMMARY AND CONCLUSIONS: SHAME, SIN, SOCIETY

During our race through history we found that self-killing as an exclusively human behavior has been present since the beginnings of culture. The inarticulate suicide committed by the desperate sick, old, or humiliated, mainly by hanging, always prevailed, but civilization gave birth to the new model of the *shame* suicide requiring the sophisticated means of a weapon.

Growing internalization created the concept of guilt. Suicide became the mortal sin of self-murder in Christian doctrine. This paradigm was challenged by renaissance thinking and refined by Christian reformers, to be fundamentally rejected by the Enlightenment.

Increasing awareness of the complexity of the human soul and the cosmopolitan society originated the extant paradigm of suicide as the problem of disintegration, studied and treated by experts. When such an expert is doing epidemiological research or trying to help an individual, his or her work sometimes looks like the work of an archaeologist, peeling off from the human soul the various skins that history has laid upon it.

FURTHER READING

Much fascinating material on suicide in history, albeit presented in a rather anecdotal way, is to be found in Georges Minois, *History of Suicide: Voluntary Death in Western Culture*, Baltimore, MD: Johns Hopkins University Press, 1999 (translation of *Histoire du suicide: la societé occidentale face à la mort volontaire*, 1995).

For an insight into suicide in primitive society nothing has yet replaced the collection of studies edited by P. Bohannan, *African Homicide and Suicide*, Princeton, NJ: Princeton University Press, 1960.

Suicide among the Greeks and Romans, the data as well as the discourse, is the subject of the monograph by the author of this chapter: Anton J. L. van Hooff, *From Autothanasia to Suicide: Self-Killing in Classical Antiquity*, London/New York: Routledge, 1990.

M. MacDonald and T. Murphy, *Sleepless Souls. Suicide in Early Modern England*, Oxford, UK: Oxford University Press, 1990, is especially valuable as it deals with concrete cases, whereas most studies concern the literary sources (e.g., Rowland Wymer, *Suicide and Despair in the Jacobean Drama*, 1986).

Highly recommended for the historical background of the modern psychological and sociological approach is Olive Anderson, *Suicide in Victorian and Edwardian England*, Oxford, UK: Oxford University Press, 1987.

PART II

SOCIODEMOGRAPHIC AND EPIDEMIOLOGIC ISSUES

5

Age and the Lifespan

with Paul A. Nisbet

> What does a man care about? Staying healthy. Working good. Eating and
> drinking with his friends. Enjoying himself in bed. I haven't any of them.
> —ERNEST HEMINGWAY

As we age, of course, the nearer we are to death. It should not surprise us that the likelihood of suicide grows with age for some groups. The Hemingway quote suggests that not only does our life tend to run out (like sand in the "hourglass" of a lifetime), but also its quality tends to diminish over time. Usually, with age health wanes, depressive disorders increase, there are profound social and interpersonal losses (e.g., through death of a spouse or divorce), alcohol abuse may become "terminal," and, perhaps most crucial, hopelessness may set in.

Although the human life cycle can be subdivided into numerous stages (Erikson, 1950; Levinson, 1978), in this chapter we keep it simple and focus on suicide in just four main life stages: childhood, adolescence and young adulthood, midlife, and the elderly. However, before we examine these four stages, a few introductory general observations on suicide and age are in order.

First, white male suicide rates tend to increase linearly with age, sometimes with a slight drop in rates in the very oldest age groups (Moscicki, 1999, Fig. 2.1). For example, in Table 1.3 the suicide rates of white males ages 55 to 64 were 29.6; from 65 to 74, 46.1; and 85+, 65.4. If we compare these data with those in Chapter 3 (Table 3.1), we see a similar suicide rate increase over age, not controlling for sex or race. Interestingly, black males, white females, and black females all have suicide rates that peak in midlife. Levinson (1978) might suggest to us that suicide rates may increase at life-stage transitions (e.g., adolescence to young adulthood or adulthood to becoming elderly), especially if there is developmental stagnation, acculumation of developmental debits (e.g., failure of marriages or jobs), and abortive life-stage transitions (see Leenaars, 1991).

Second, since about 1950 there has been a striking increase in the suicide rates of 15- to 24-year-olds (see Figure 5.1). In Table 1.3 the increase from 1950 to 1996 is 267%. Garrison (1992: 489) estimates the 15- to 24-year-old suicide rate increase (mostly among young white males) from 1957 to 1987 to be 323%. Maris (1985) calculated the adolescent suicide rate increase from 1960 to 1977 to be 237%. Of course, at a 1950 rate of about 4 per 100,000, the adolescent rate had no place to go but up. Furthermore, even with tripling of

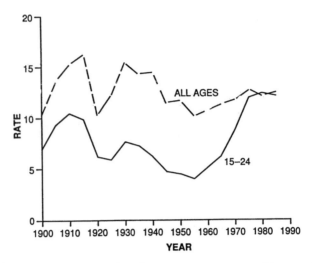

FIGURE 5.1 Suicide rates (per 100,000) for all persons 15–24 years old, United States, 1900–1985, compared to rates for all ages. *Source:* Rosenberg, Smith, Davidson, & Conn (1987: 420). Copyright 1987 by Annual Reviews Inc. Reprinted by permission.

their rates, adolescent suicide rates seldom exceeded the average suicide rate not controlling for age of about 11–12/100,000. Easterlin (1980) and Hendin (1982) tend to see teen suicide rates as a function of a cohort effect (see Figure 3.4). That is, when 15–24-year suicide rates are higher, there are just more 15–24-year olds competing for jobs, spouses, and so on. Suicide clusters tend to occur largely among teenagers (Velting and Gould, 1997: 96).

Third, Table 1.3 indicates that few suicides (there are exceedingly low rates) exist under age 14 in any gender or racial group. In fact, in Maris's study of Chicago suicides, those under age 21 accounted for only 2% of all suicides (Maris, 1981). This striking absence of young suicides could have profound implications for suicide prevention. What is there about being childlike that tends to protect one from suicide?

Fourth, even with the dramatic rise in adolescent suicide rates in recent decades, the highest suicide rates are still found among the elderly. In Table 1.3 white males over age 85 have the highest suicide rates (65.4) of any other gender or racial group (at least in the United States). Those people over 65 in the United States make up about 13% of the population (as of 1996) but commit about 19% of all suicides. Depending on which older age group one looks at (65–74, 75–84, or 85+) from 1950 to 1980 elderly suicide rates tended to decline; however, in 1990, they went back up, only to decrease some in recent years (until 1996). With all the fuss about Dr. Kevorkian, Derek Humphry, and active euthanasia, there is some concern that suicide may increase among the elderly.

Fifth, female suicide rates tend to peak earlier (around ages 45–54) than do male rates and then either decline slightly or hold steady thereafter. Female suicide rates are also about three or four times lower than male rates. Over age 65 white female suicide rates are 5 to 15 times lower than corresponding white male age rates.

Sixth, although the suicide rate has remained essentially constant from 1900 to 2000 (in the United States), from 1970 to 1980 the overall rate dropped from a median age or 47.2 to 39.9 (Buda & Tsuang, 1990). Thus, although the suicide *rates* tend to be the highest in the older age groups, the average age of all suicides falls in midlife, not in old age.

Seventh, black male suicide rates tend to peak earlier than white male suicide rates (i.e., at about ages 25–34), then drop off some in the older age groups. White suicide rates tend

TABLE 5.1. Numbers and Rates of Suicide by Age and Method, United States, 1992

Age Group	All suicides		Poisoning		Strangulation		Firearms		Cutting		Other methods	
	No.	Rate	No.	Rate	No.	Rate	No.	Rate	No.	Rate	No.	Rate
Adjusted rate		11.1		2.0		1.7		6.6		0.1		0.6
Total	30,484	12.0	5,495	2.2	4,678	1.8	18,169	7.1	417	0.2	1,709	0.7
0–4 years	0	0.0	0	0.0	0	0.0	0	0.0	0	0.0	0	0.0
5–9 years	10	0.1	2	0.0	4	0.0	3	0.0	0	0.0	1	0.0
10–14 years	304	1.7	30	0.2	96	0.5	172	1.0	0	0.0	4	0.0
20–24 years	2,846	14.9	302	1.6	547	2.9	1,822	9.6	16	0.1	158	0.8
25–29 years	2,864	14.2	445	2.2	583	2.9	1,639	8.1	30	0.2	167	0.8
30–34 years	3,308	14.9	692	3.1	637	2.9	1,719	7.7	44	0.2	213	1.0
35–39 years	3,177	15.1	800	3.8	510	2.4	1,624	7.7	51	0.2	191	0.9
40–44 years	2,832	15.1	741	3.9	394	2.1	1,455	7.7	46	0.2	192	1.0
45–49 years	2,251	14.7	574	3.7	253	1.7	1,260	8.2	29	0.2	135	0.9
50–54 years	1,767	14.7	393	3.3	224	1.9	1,029	8.5	30	0.3	90	0.8
55–59 years	1,541	14.7	290	2.8	167	1.6	986	9.4	30	0.3	67	0.6
60–64 years	1,564	15.0	283	2.7	188	1.8	974	9.3	25	0.2	93	0.9
65–69 years	1,555	15.6	219	2.2	145	1.5	1,079	10.8	30	0.3	52	0.6
70–74 years	1,483	17.5	176	2.1	139	1.6	1,087	12.8	28	0.3	52	0.6
75–79 years	1,387	21.6	155	2.4	171	2.7	964	15.0	20	0.3	77	1.2
80–84 years	1,021	24.6	112	2.7	154	3.7	679	16.4	16	0.4	60	1.5
85 years and up	714	21.9	86	2.6	129	4.0	424	13.0	16	0.5	59	1.8
Age unknown	13		3		4		2		0		4	

Source: Kachur, Potter, James, & Powell (1995: 31).

to exceed black suicide rates at all ages by a ratio of about 2 to 1. Exceptions to this rule occur in the 15–24 age group (where black and white rates are about the same) and in the 65 and over age group (where white suicide rates far outstrip black rates). Black female suicide rates are *very* low at all ages and peak in the 25-to-34 age group.

Eighth, methods vary by both age and sex (see Chapter 12). There is a greater percentage of firearm methods as one ages among males (see Table 5.1 and cf. Table 3.3).

Finally, suicide rates vary by age and marital status (Table 3.4). Single, married, and divorced people (especially males) have higher suicide rates as they age.

SUICIDE AMONG CHILDREN

Although suicide is extremely rare among children, children do commit suicide (Pfeffer, 1986). In 1970, the first year the National Center for Health Statistics (NCHS) officially reported suicide rates for children ages 5 to 14, the rate was 3 per 100,000. Below age 5, children may lack the conceptual understanding of death as final and, thus, may not be able to intend to die. By 1986, the rate was .8 per 100,000, an increase of 267% (but starting with a small base). Ten years later, in 1996, the rate remained at .8, which is about 302 suicides per year. Less than 1 per 100,000 children and adolescents take their own life (Peters, Kochanek, & Murphy, 1998). As low as this rate is compared to older age groups, it provides little comfort to families that have lost a child to suicide.

Understanding the rationalization behind an older adult taking his or her own life may, perhaps, be easier to understand than the reasons precipitating a youth's suicide. With increasing age we become more susceptible to physical (e.g., cancers, coronary heart disease, hypertension, etc.) and mental (e.g., alcohol dependency, major depressions, anxiety and panic disorders, etc.) illnesses. Once the quality of one's life has long since peaked and is fraught with physical and emotional pain, the wish to end one's own life is somewhat understandable. However, in the prime of life, as a child there is no apparent reason to suicide.

The low rate of suicide among children deserves exploration and could even provide a key to suicide prevention. Several studies indicate that although prepubertal children frequently experience serious suicidal thoughts and impulses (Brent, Kalas, & Edelbrook, 1986; Carlson & Contwell, 1982; Pfeffer, Conte, Plutchik, & Jerrett, 1979, 1980), this age group may be protected against suicide by their cognitive immaturity (Shaffer & Fisher, 1981). Consequently, young children may be unable to plan (and may even lack access to a lethal means, such as a gun) or execute a fatal suicidal act (Brent & Kolko, 1990). Shaffer (1974) found that a greater than expected number of young suicide completers had been shown to have IQs above 130. Shaffer concluded that it is possible, therefore, that intellectual aptitude may override the postulated safeguarding effects of cognitive immaturity. Other factors, such as relatively low incidence of depression and substance abuse and greater familial support, may also protect this age group from completing suicide.

In the United States, the suicide rate is higher among young boys than among young girls (Peters, Kochaneck, & Murphy, 1998). This may be due to males' propensity to resort to impulsive, violent, irreversible methods of suicide, whereas female suicide attempters often use less lethal methods (Brent & Kolko, 1990). In Asian countries, suicide rates are comparable among boys and girls (Kua & Tsoi, 1985). Native American males have the highest child suicide rates in the United States, followed by white males and then black males (Wallace, Calhoun, Powell, O'Neil, & James, 1996).

Although suicide may be rare among children, suicidal behavior or partial self-destruction is not. Pfeffer (1981) reported that 33% of a group of 39 children randomly selected from an outpatient clinic had contemplated, threatened, or attempted suicide, whereas only 10% of a similar group of children in 1960 reported having suicidal ideation (Stillion, McDowell, & May, 1989). Blumenthal (1990) reported that although 12,000 children ages 5 to 14 are admitted to psychiatric hospitals for suicidal behavior annually, no more than 1% of the actual incidence of self-destructive behavior among children is officially reported as "suicidal" each year. Researchers suggest that both rates of suicidal behavior and suicide are underreported in all age groups, but particularly in children. Many families conceal evidence of their children's suicidal behavior because of the associated social stigma. The tendency to deny suicide is especially strong in the case of a child (Stillion et al., 1989).

Factors contributing to suicide among children include demographics (e.g., gender and race), home environment and family, and psychological factors of the individual child. Among children, boys attempt and complete suicide more than girls do (Joffe, Offord, & Boyle, 1983; Pfeffer, 1981). This pattern is not found in persons 15 years and older, where women report more suicide ideation and attempts but men more often complete suicide. However, researchers have not been able to reliably differentiate suicide ideators from attempters and completerers (Goldman & Beardslee, 1999; Kosky, Silburn, & Zubrick, 1990). Thus, the task of identifying and treating those children most at risk is more difficult.

Certain characteristics of the child and the child's family are associated with greater suicidal risk. Children with certain psychiatric disorders (e.g., depression, conduct disorder, specific developmental disorders, and adjustment disorder) are more vulnerable to suicidal behavior. Depression is a major symptom present in suicidal children (Pfeffer, Conte, Plutchik, & Jerret, 1979, 1980). The severity of depression in children has been found to be positively associated with the severity of suicidal tendencies (Carlson & Cantwell, 1982). Evidence shows that a high proportion of child psychiatric patients present serious suicidal ideation or behavior (Brent et al., 1986; Pfeffer, 1982; Pfeffer et al., 1980). The extent of preoccupation with death, recent aggression, and previously stressful experiences (e.g., loss) have also been found to be significantly related to suicide behavior in children (Pfeffer et al., 1986). Suicidal children often report feeling sad, hopeless, and worthless (Pfeffer, 1986).

Suicidal behavior typically occurs in a context of intensely stressful, chaotic, and unpredictable family events. Children who feel incapable of making an impact on these circumstances may use suicide as a desperate, last-ditch effort to affect or coerce those who threaten their well-being (Cohen-Sandler, Berman, & King, 1982a). Self-esteem is considerably diminished in suicidal children (Malmquist, 1983). Children who do suicide have had contact with a friend or relative who has threatened or attempted suicide at a rate of five times greater than a matched control group (Shafii, Carrington, Whittinghill, & Derrick, 1985). Finally, actual or perceived loss of contact in the context of a prevailing sense of loneliness and isolation during the months prior to the suicide can be the proverbial back-breaking straw for these children (Shafii et al., 1985; Mack & Hickler, 1981).

The families of suicidal children often show a high incidence of parental alcoholism and affective disorder (Beardslee, Bemporad, Keller, & Klerman, 1983; Shafii et al., 1985; Famularo, Stone, & Popper, 1985). Affective illness in families extracts a considerable toll from all members, including children. The parents' suicidal children also have a higher rate of marital conflict and seem to model and foster the use of impulsive and ineffective coping strategies in the children (Dugan & Belfer 1989; Shaffer, 1974). Suicidal children have been found to demonstrate a limited ability to find solutions to interpersonal problems. They are less able to consider alternatives and come up with new ideas or solutions to problems (Cohen-Sandler & Berman, 1982; Levenson, 1974). Suicidal, compared to nonsuicidal, children appear less able to generate active cognitive coping strategies (e.g., self-comforting statements and instrumental problem solving) in the face of stressful life events (Weishaar & Beck, 1990).

As Dugan and Belfer (1989) note, the dilemma in preventing child suicide is how to encounter the hopeless, helpless, isolated children and convey a sense of hope and possibility.

SUCIDAL ADOLESCENTS AND YOUNG ADULTS

Before we can hope to understand adolescent suicide and risk taking, we first have to understand *adolescence as a developmental life stage*. Being young in contemporary U.S. urban–industrial society is not easy. We tend to forget that in most preindustrial, agricultural societies, childhood, adolescence, and youth were not recognized life stages (Aries, 1962). Children tended to go directly into adulthood after an initiation ceremony (a *rite de passage* most commonly associated with puberty) marking their assumption of adult responsibility. Even in the first stages of the industrial revolution, marriage tended to be early (certainly by the teenage years), and children went to work in factories and mines.

Only recently, with expanding professionalism and greater demand of skilled and technical labor, have childhood and adolescence emerged as full-blown life stages characterized primarily by dormancy, latency, and prolonged preparation for adulthood (Robertson & McKee, 1980). Adolescence tends to be a time marked by marginality, confusion, and ambiguity. In fact, some have contended that the major problem of adolescence is that adolescents are freed from the responsibilities and rights of adults. As Paul Goodman put long ago in his classic *Growing Up Absurd*, the greatest problem that young people have today is their own *uselessness*.

Adolescents are expected to defer sexual gratification and meaningful employment. Although sexual maturity is reached in late childhood or early adolescence, young people are not expected to act out sexually. Promiscuity, teenage pregnancy, sexual assault, rape, and related erotic problems (whatever else they are) are in part an outgrowth of the lack of routine, regular, acceptable, socially and institutionally approved sexual outlets for adolescents. Unemployment and other economic disenfranchisements (such as subemployment and minimum wages) are particularly acute among teenagers.

Children are expected to remain in school much longer now than at the turn of the century. James Coleman (1961) argues that this prolonged isolation of the young in school has contributed to their developing a counterculture, set against the dominant adult culture. Of course, delayed or blocked work opportunities can also be related to adolescent crime.

Child abuse has also shown dramatic increases (Straus, Gelles, & Steinmetz, 1981). Finally, many believe that substance abuse among the young is related to adolescents being shut out of meaningful participation in society, as well as to the pressures and stresses of being forced to live contingently for prolonged periods of time in an achievement-oriented society.

Little wonder then that young people in our society may have their own special set of social problems, including teen suicide. Adolescence today is a parenthesis that many young people must feel will never end. In this context adolescence can be perceived as a "terminal illness."

Turning specifically to adolescent suicide, Cheryl King (1997) suggests, although "each suicidal adolescent has a unique life story," and, thus "there are no predictive equations with definitive decision-making rules for determining whether a suicidal behavior will occur," the growing body of empirical research focused on adolescent suicidal behavior "provides the backdrop for comprehensive, fine-tuned risk assessments and effective clinical decision making" (61).

As we demonstrated previously, from about 1950 to 1980 suicide frequency among adolescents and young adults increased dramatically. The suicide rate for these groups tripled over a 30-year period dating back to the mid-1950s (Berman & Jobes, 1991; Silverman, 1997). The rate plateaued at approximately 15 per 100,000 and has remained at that rate throughout most of the 1990s.

Approximately 10,200 people ages 15–34 years old kill themselves each year (and about 4,700 from 15 to 24). By 1996, suicide was the third leading cause of death for adolescents and young adults. Important risk factors contributing to suicide among this age group are the decrease in the number of intact homes, increase in family mobility, social isolation, depressive disorders, and the increased availability of alcohol, drugs, and firearms (see Maris, 1985, for distinguishing traits of younger versus older suicides in Chicago).

The suicide rate for adolescents and young adults, ages 15 to 24 years of age, is 12.0 per 100,000 population in the United States (Peters et al., 1998). The rates for completed suicide continue to increase with age (King, 1997). The rate for the 5- to 14-year olds (0.8 per 100,000) is lower than that for the 15- to 24-year-olds, which is lower than that of 25- to 34-year-olds (14.5 per 100,000).

Stressful life events are associated with attempted and completed suicide in adolescence (King, 1997). For example, parent–adolescent arguments as well as difficulties with romantic relationships are common precipitants of suicidal behavior among adolescents (Brent et al., 1988). In a study comparing life stressors and suicide precipitants among suicide victims under and over the age of 30 years, Rich, Young, and Fowler (1986b) found that separation or rejection was a more common precipitant for the younger age group. In the year preceding the suicide, Brent et al. (1993) found that suicide completers were more likely than community-matched controls to have experienced interpersonal conflict, "disruption of a romantic attachment," and "legal or disciplinary problems."

Poor development of coping strategies in childhood may well carry into later years, contributing to legal and disciplinary problems. Lewinsohn, Rohde, and Seeley (1994) found that stressful adolescent life events especially predictive of future suicide attempts are arguments or fights, a relative or friend who had problems with alcohol or drugs, a relative or friend who tried to commit suicide, and the adolescent moving away from or leaving home. Security and comfort in interpersonal relationships seemed to be particulary critical.

King, Naylor, Segal, Evans, and Shain (1993b) documented strong negative associations between perceived social acceptance and depression severity among adolescents in clinical- and community-based samples (King, Akiyama, & Elling, 1996). Past suicide attempts are stronger predictors for future suicidal potential than are stressful life events (Lewinsohn et al., 1994). However, stressful life events may function as proximal risk factors. King (1997) suggests that recent stressors, particularly those that are interpersonal or disciplinary in nature, should be seen as red flags for potentially increased suicide risk among adolescents.

At no time in the human lifespan does the prevalence of alcohol abuse and depression increase at such a rapid rate as during the transition from childhood to adolescents and young adulthood. At no other time in the human lifespan is the ratio of suicide attempts to completions so high (King, 1997).

King (1997) stresses that we must try to understand adolescent suicidal behavior within its social or environmental context and remember that "although variables related to family functioning and psychosocial stress have not always shown specificity to suicidal behavior, they are usually critical aspects of the pathway to suicidal behavior" (88). "At the moment adolescents choose to engage in suicidal behavior, they have crossed their personal threshold for suffering, frustration tolerance, and adaptive coping" (King, 1997: 72).

The risk of suffering a depressive disorder increases across the lifespan. The most dramatic increase is between the ages of 9 and 19. Throughout the lifespan, suicidal behavior is almost always associated with depressive disorders. Indeed, recurrent thoughts of death or suicidal ideation is part of the symptomotology for major depressive episode in the DSM-IV. In a longitudinal study of early-onset depressive disorder, Kovacs, Goldston, and Gatsonis (1993) identified a four- to fivefold increase in suicidal ideation and behavior among youth with major depressive and/or dysthymic disorder, as compared to youth with other psychiatric disorders. Among the youths with depressive disorders, 85% experienced significant suicidal ideation and 32% attempted suicide by the time they had reached their late teens.

However, the high prevalence of depression among this age group limits the specificity of depressive disorders as a predictor of completed suicide. Depression does not have a high specificity as a predictor for completed suicide (King, 1997).

Alcohol abuse impairs judgment, reduces impulse control, and alters moods (Schuckit, 1983). Multiple studies (as reviewed by King, 1997) provide massing evidence for the substantial suicide risk associated with alcohol consumption, documenting a significant connection between the severity of suicidal behaviors, alcohol abuse, and major depression (Pfeffer, Newcorn, Kaplan, Mizrochi, & Plutchik, 1988, King, Hill, Naylor, Evans, & Shain, 1993a; Robbins & Alessi, 1995). Hawton, Fagg, and McKeown (1989) noted that 38% of adolesent suicide attempters had consumed alcohol within 6 hours prior to their attempt. McKenry, Tishler, and Kelley (1982) found that 43% of the 46 adolescent suicide attempters they studied had a history of alcohol and/or substance abuse.

Findings from psychological autopsy studies suggest that more than half the youths who complete suicide had a history of significant alcohol use problems (Abel & Zeidenberg, 1985; Shafii et al., 1985; Rich et al., 1986b). Of course, alcohol or substance abuse with comorbid depressive illness represents an especially high-risk profile for suicidal behavior, repetitive suicidal behavior, and completed suicide among youths (Kovacs et al., 1993; Brent et al., 1993; Rich et al., 1986b). For instance, Shafii, Steltz-Lenarsky, and Derrick (1988) found that 62% of suicide victims had alcohol or substance use disorders, 76% had major depression or dysthymia, and 38% had comorbid alcohol/substance use and depressive disorders.

The majority of psychological autopsy studies on youth suicide to date are generally limited by small sample sizes and/or the absence of appropriate controls. Gould, Shaffer, Fisher, Kleinman, and Morishima (1992) conducted a psychological autopsy study on 119 persons under the age of 20 who had completed suicide. Their analyses revealed that approximately one-third of the victims had made a previous suicide attempt, with more girls (48%) than boys (27%) having had a history of previous attempts. In addition, symptoms of any affective disorder, alone or in conjuction with antisocial behavior and/or substance abuse, were found in nearly 40% of the sample. One-third of the victims also had a history of aggressive and antisocial behavior, boys moreso than girls (e.g., 40% vs. 16%, respectively). Finally, approximately 40% of the suicide completers had a first- or second-degree relative who had previously attempted or completed suicide.

In the United States, firearms are the most common method of suicide among youth for both sexes. In descending frequency, other common methods include hanging, carbon monoxide poisoning, jumping, and overdose (Shaffer & Fisher, 1981). The rate of youth suicide by firearms has increased faster than suicide by other methods (Boyd & Moscicki, 1986; Brent, Perper, & Allman, 1987a) and appear to be a particularly common method when the victim was intoxicated (Brent et al., 1987). There is evidence that the suicide rate by firearms is correlated with the production, sales, and ownership of guns (Kellerman & Reay, 1986; Markush & Bartolucci, 1984) and inversely correlated with the restrictiveness of gun control laws (Lester, 1983; Lester & Murrell, 1980). Brent et al. (1988) found that after controlling for demographic and diagnostic variables, adolescent suicide victims were 2.5 times more likely to have a gun available to them in their homes than were hospitalized suicidal adolescents.

Whereas the number of investigations into the characteristics of youth who commit suicide slowly increases, our profile of the adolescent suicide at this point is incomplete. What we can review are common precipitants of youth suicide. Shaffer (1974) noted disciplinary crises, interpersonal loss, and interpersonal conflict as precipitants common to adolescent suicides. Other studies have indicated that interpersonal conflict and increased number of stressors seem to play a contibutory role (Brent et al., 1988; Shafii, Steltz-Lenarsky, & Derrick, 1988). Two other key elements in precipitants for adolescent suicide are humiliation (Blumenthal & Kupfer, 1988) and, more recently, shame (Lester, 1997b). Shame may play an important role in increasing the risk of suicidal behavior and other symptoms of emotional disturbance (Lester, 1997b; Dwivedi, Brayne, & Lovett, 1992).

SUICIDE IN MIDLIFE

Almost all prior suicide age and developmental studies have concentrated on either adolescents or the elderly, in spite of the mean age of suicide completers in the United States in recent years being about 40 years old. Baby-boomers born in the post-World War II years are now in their 50s. Virtually no one has anticipated the problem of higher young adult and midlife suicide rates as a result of the prior high suicide rates of baby-boomers as adolescents and the cohort effect (Easterlin, 1980). The higher suicide rates of baby-boomer adolescents are expected to carry over into midlife as the cohort ages (Ahlburg & Shapiro, 1984).

This section of Chapter 5 reviews the "suicidal careers" (Maris, 1981) of midlife suicides. The focus here is on white males. Midlife is usually a time when power peaks. By age

40 most of us are pretty much what we are ever going to be. Erikson claimed that stagnation versus creativity was the main developmental crisis of midlife. According to Levinson (1978) between the ages of 40 to 45 we need to reappraise the past and rid ourselves of our earlier illusions. Often midlife brings changes in our life structure (divorce, job plateauing, children leaving home, diminished physical energy, etc.). In midlife we typically turn more inward and become less concerned with the mastery of the external environment. Four polarities (reminiscent of Jungian psychiatric theory) can be involved in midlife individuation: being (1) young versus old, (2) destructive versus creative, (3) masculine versus feminine, and (4) attached versus separated. Essentially in midlife most males need to become more appropriately old, creative, feminine, and able to be alone. At midlife we need to modify the tyranny of our life dream and realize that success does not entail happiness. As the cap given to Maris upon retiring from being a suicide journal editor read: "Never confuse having a career with having a life."

Of course, more than routine midlife developmental problems occur in the psychsocial histories of suicides (Farrell & Rosenberg, 1981). Suicide can be thought of as the ultimate in developmental stagnation. Some midlifers simply cannot negotiate the midlife transition. For example, they can no longer take pleasure in their work and cannot give up the illusions and tyranny of youth—especially if they have nagging, chronic physical illnesses; recurring depressive disorders; alcohol problems; and low economic, emotional, and spiritual resources. Midlife often means (as Hemingway and Styron found out) that one must continue to live without the help of alcohol, work advances, or sexual acting out. Some midlife men kill themselves in part because they do not believe it is possible to change their young adult lifestyles and become viable middle-age people: their "middlescence" does them in.

Robins, West, and Murphy (1977) claim that the distinctive traits of midlife male suicides include: loss of spouse, years of heavy drinking, reaching the age of high depression risk, personal experience with other suicides or suicides in their families, and facing debilitating old age without psychological compensations. Jarvis and Boldt (1980) add occupation loss and stagnated, downward job mobility as another suicidogenic factor. When Darbonne (1969) and others examined the notes of middle-age suicides, they found them to be "the communications of the vanquished." Middle-age suicide note writers displayed less affect (than did younger note writers) and were the least likely age group to give a reason for their suicides. Midlife suicides seemed to have a Darwinian inability to go on.

Of course, the etiology and treatment of midlife suicides are not just psychosocial. Major biological forces are also at work. One always needs to consider antidepressant drugs and electroconvulsive therapy (ECT). Most midlife major depression goes untreated or undermedicated (Isaacson & Rich, 1997). Alcohol abuse is often a complicating factor in midlife suicides. Waning physical energies, lower sexual activity and drive, and related problems of aging are also often present.

Creativity in the face of suicidal forces involves building a life more apropriate for middle adulthood. As we have seen, one may need to be more appropriately old and feminine, be more flexible and less cognitively rigid, to let our dream go. Resignation (especially humor as a defense in crises) and reorganization are important midlife therapy objectives. In midlife one is no longer in a pattern of ascendancy, even if one once was. A central midlife question is: "Is there any good enough future or am I in a pattern of entrophy until death?"

Isolation can be a special problem of midlife, perhaps coupled with overwhelming work demands. Often midlifers need to find new significant others, new lovers and friends, and, perhaps, a newfound or rediscovered religion. In midlife we discover (as we should have realized earlier) that our work will not save us. As in John Updike's novels, we may be working as hard as we can (like a hamster on a wheel) just to stay even (i.e., not to fall off of our midlife plateau). We may find out (too late?) that our own children are a better source of peace and immortality than are money, jobs, books written, work projects completed, sexual affairs, and so on.

For our purposes, we define "middle age" as the age range between 35 and 54 years (although not many of us will live to be 108). In 1996, approximately 11,578 middle-age persons took their own lives (Peters, Kochanek, & Murphy, 1998). Dividing this group in two (e.g., those ages 35–44 and those 45–54) will allow us to be more specific when discussing rates. For instance, the suicide rate is 15.5 per 100,000 (approximately 6,741 suicides per year) for those persons ages 35–44 and 14.9 for the latter group (4,837 suicides per year). However, other than the rate differences, demographic characteristics between the two groups have little effect on the overall suicide risk of the groups. Thus, other than the rates, when we refer to the "middle age" adults, we are referring to the whole group (i.e., all those ages 35 to 54).

Suicidal behavior among middle-age adults has been shown to be related most commonly to an accumulation of negative (or stressful) life events, an affective disorder (especially depression), and alcoholism (Stillion et al., 1989; Barraclough, Bunch, Nelson, & Sainsbury, 1974; Hirschfeld & Blumenthal, 1986; Roy, 1982; Borg & Stahl, 1982; Conwell et al., 1996).

The negative life events commonly associated with suicide in middle age include declining health, financial losses, reduced career opportunities, and interpersonal losses or death of loved ones (see Table 5.2). Such losses appear to be almost universal during this period of life. The major distinction between the stresses of suicidal and nonsuicidal adults seems to be more quantitative than qualitative (Stillion et al., 1989). Thus, the coping strategies we develop throughout our earlier life course play a significant role in how we deal with such negative events in later life. Also, the suicidal adult is more likely to experience a number of negative events within a relatively brief period. If there is an accel-

TABLE 5.2. Frequencies of Life Events during the Last 3 Months among Suicides by Age

	Age					
	20–59 years (n = 803)		≥60 years (n = 219)		Total (n = 1,022)	
Event	%	N	%	N	%	N
Any event	82.9	(641/773)	73.2	(156/213)[a]	80.8	(797/986)
Somatic illness	15.2	(118/779)	48.4	104/215)[a]	22.3	222/994)
Illness in family	12.3	(98/794)	12.3	27/219)	12.3	(125/1,013)
Death	12.8	(99/771)	12.6	(27/214)	12.8	(126/985)
Separation	16.3	(126/773)	4.2	(9/217)[c]	13.6	(135/990)
Separation due to work	3.7	(28/766)	4.6	(10/216)	3.9	(38/982)
Family discord	26.6	(204/766)	12.0	(26/216)[d]	23.4	(230/982)
Residence change	10.3	(82/797)	5.1	(11/218)[e]	9.2	(93/1,015)
Financial trouble	21.7	(168/774)	3.7	(8/218)[f]	17.7	(176/992)
Job problems	34.1	(258/757)	7.3	(16/218)[g]	28.1	(274/975)
Unemployment	19.2	(152/793)	0.5	(1/218)[h]	15.1	(153/1,011)
Retirement	3.9	(31/798)	2.3	(5/216)	3.5	(36/1,016)
Imprisonment	2.2	(17/790)	0.5	(1/128)	1.8	(18/1,008)
Other adverse events	6.3	(49/781)	3.7	(8/216)	5.7	(57/997)

Note. Differences in proportions by age: The chi-square test with Yates's correction [a]χ^2 = 9.49; df = 1; p = .002. correction [b]χ^2 = 105.3; df = 1; p < .001. [c]χ^2 = 20.23; df = 1; p < .001. [d]χ^2 = 19.2; df = 1; p < .001. [e]χ^2 = 5.04; df = 1; p = .025. [f]χ^2 = 36.68; df = 1; p < .001. [g]χ^2 = 58.59; df = 1; p < .001. [h]χ^2 = 45.16; df = 1; p < .001.
Source: Heikkinen & Lönnqvist (1996: 161). Copyright 1996 by Springer Publishing Company, Inc. Reprinted by permission.

eration of these events, the person may indeed begin feeling overwhelmed with disaster—as if his coping strategies are inadequate and that he has lost control over his own life. Suicidal persons often view the act of suicide as the one final thing they can do to control their downward spiraling life.

Interpersonal loss may be the most frequent type of loss among suicidal adults. More than any other kind of loss, separation or divorce from a, and death of a spouse have been found to differentiate suicidal depressed individuals from nonsuicidal depressed individuals (Slater & Depue, 1981). Middle-age adults who commit suicide are more likely to have experienced the death of a spouse, parent, or child. The losses experienced by suicidal adults are not limited to the time period just prior to their suicidal act. Indeed, many suicidal adults are more likely to have a higher than expected incidence of early parental loss through death, divorce, or separation (Adam, Bouckoms, & Streiner, 1982).

Depression is another major factor related to suicide among middle-age adults. Study after study has revealed major depressive disorder to be the most common psychiatric diagnoses associated with suicide among adults (see Table 5.3). From a thorough review of the literature, Pfeffer (1986) concluded that suicide is 30 times more prevalent among adults diagnosed with affective disorder than among than among adults without such a diagnosis. Because the relationship between mental and personality disorders and suicide is covered elsewhere in this text (see Chapter 13), we will not delve into that topic here. Suffice it to say that few suicides occur in the absence of a depressive disorder.

Alcoholism is the third most commonly related factor to adult suicide. Studies indicate that the risk of suicide among alcoholics is 58 to 85 times higher than that of nonalcoholics. (Roy & Linnoila, 1986; Murphy, 1992). Miles (1977) estimates the suicide rate among alcoholics to be as high as 270 per 100,000 population. The majority of alcoholic suicides are

TABLE 5.3. Principal DSM-III-R Axis I and II Diagnoses among 43 Elderly and 186 Younger Suicides

Diagnosis	Victims age 60 years or over (N = 43)		Victims age under 60 years (N = 186)	
	n	%	n	%
Major depression	19	44[a]	50	27
Depressive disorder not otherwise specified	5	12	15	8
Bipolar disorder	0	0	8	4
Dysthymia	1	2	1	0–1
Alcohol dependence	5	12	33	18
Alcohol abuse	0	0	2	1
Alcohol intoxication	0	0	2	1
Schizophrenia	3	7	13	7
Other psychoses	1	2	7	4
Organic mental disorders	1	2	4	2
Anxiety disorders	0	0	2	1
Adjustment disorders	3	7	5	3
Other Axis I diagnoses	0	0	3	2
Any Axis 11 diagnoses	0	0	20	11[b]
No diagnosis of mental disorder	1	2	3	2
Insufficient information for assessment of principal diagnosis	4	9	13	7

[a]$\chi^2 = 4.18$, $df = 1$, $p < .05$.
[b]Fisher's exact test, $p < .05$.
Source: Henriksson (1996: 148) Copyright 1996 by Springer Publishing Company, Inc. Reprinted by permission.

middle-age white males between the ages of 45 and 55 years old who have been abusing alcohol for as long as 25 years. It has been suggested that the reason alcoholic suicides are often in their mid-40s or older is that alcohol-related life problems tend to emerge after an extended history of abuse (family dissolution and social isolation, employment problems, health problems, etc.). Goodwin (1972) proposes that the reason the incidence of alcoholic suicides decreases in old age is because alcoholism leads to early death. The relationship between alcohol abuse and depression is well documented (see, e.g., Chapter 15). Often people self-medicate with alcohol in an effort to combat depression. Ultimately, of course, this does not prove an efficient remedy. Indeed, as alcohol reduces impulse control, depressed persons with suicidal thoughts are more likely to act on their self-destructive ideation.

ELDERLY SUICIDES

"Suicide rates always have been and remain the highest among the elderly" (McIntosh, 1992: 323). Dating from Otto von Bismarck (1815–1898) in Germany arbitrarily setting the mandatory retirement age at 65, "old" has commonly meant over age 65. Obviously, setting "elderly" at age 65 is whimsical (if not downright inaccurate) and glosses over many important differences in the aging process and the aged population.

For example, in the age data we presented earlier (e.g., Tables 1.3 and 3.1) there were groups of 65–74, 75–84, and 85 +. It might be useful to differentiate these groups of the elderly respectively as (1) the young–old, (2) the old–old, and (3) the oldest–old.

Regardless of how we slice up aging or define it (see Maris, 1988: Ch. 4), two facts are clear: (1) the proportion of the elderly in the U.S. population (see Figure 5.2) is growing steadily, and (2) many of the traits associated with aging can be suicidogenic.

What is old age like? Studies of demographic surveys and census analyses tell us that only a century ago most people did not live to see all their grandchildren. Most life-

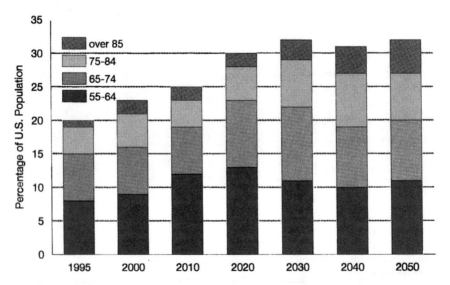

FIGURE 5.2 The graying of America. *Source:* Henslin (1996: 49). Data from *U.S. Statistical Abstract*, various years.

extending technologies (e.g., antibiotics and surgery) did not exist; thus, disease and injury were more often lethal. Only one-third of males born in 1870 lived to be 65. Figure 5.2 shows that all that has changed today.

With longer lives come both opportunities and challenges: for independence, for intimacy (both intra- and intergenerational), and so on. Perhaps in stark contrast to the assumptions of younger generations (e.g., "Old people don't have much to live for"), surveys of older adults have documented that the great majority of our elders maintain personal goals, lead active social lives, and are in regular contact with family members. For example, a recent Gallup poll (1992) of over 800 respondents with a median age of 70 found that almost 9 in 10 enjoyed retirement and 94% agreed or strongly agreed that they looked forward to each day.

However, clearly these findings do not represent the lives of all our elderly citizens. With advancing age also comes multiple losses (e.g., retirement, widowhood, and memory), vulnerabilities, and threats to life—each demanding adaptations and coping responses. For some, the strains of loneliness, financial problems, declining health, and depression may erode both these coping abilities and hope. The longer we survive, the more marginal we tend to become (Kastenbaum, 1992), as age-associated mortality decimates our peers, thus, our reference group, our support system, and our continued sense of viability are also diminished. Anger, despair, and suicidality are all more characteristic of those who have lost their sense of independence due to disability, disease, and social isolation.

Suicide, according to Maris (1981), "results from an inability or refusal to accept the terms of the human condition." Consider the Stoic Seneca's discourse on suicide:

> I will not relinquish old age if it leaves my better part intact. But if it begins to shake my mind, if it destroys its facilities one by one, if it leaves me not life but breath, I will depart from the putrid or tottering edifice . . . if I know that I must suffer without hope of relief, I will depart, not through fear of the pain itself, but because it prevents all for which I would live. (Lecky, 1869, in Osgood, 1985: xix)

Seneca's position on life and death reflects a mixture of individual dynamics (i.e., the refusal to accept . . .) and social pressures (i.e., the burdensomeness of ageism, the devaluation, and agenerativity) that describe most elderly suicides. These themes are represented in most existing theories regarding the elderly suicide's condition.

Briefly, before proceeding to theories of aged suicide, the data on elderly suicides reveal that between 1950 and 1980 suicides ages 65 to 85+ declined (McIntosh, 1992, Fig. 2; Table 3.1). However, in 1990 elderly suicide rates went up some, only to decline again in 1996 (see Leenaars, Maris, McIntosh, & Richman, 1992, Table 2; Pearson & Conwell, 1996: xi; Moscicki, 1996, for international data on aged suicides).

Theories Applicable to Elderly Suicide

Sociological Theory

One of Durkheim's (1897/1951) two major propositions about suicide related (inversely) to an individual's integration into the social group. When social ties and belongingness are weakened (i.e., social integration was low) suicide risk increased. One of Durkheim's four types of suicide, the egoistic, reflects the excessive individuation, social isolation, and constriction of social opportunity (loss of work relationships due to retirement, loss of peer/social relationships due to death, loss of social relationship due to decreased organizational participation, etc.) common to aging.

CASE 5.1. An Isolated Elder

A 78-year-old man was found in his apartment in a decomposed state. Neighbors reported that he had not been seen for three weeks but stated that this was not unusual . . . as he usually "kept to himself." He had no known friends to contact to make the funeral arrangements. The cause of death was a self-inflicted gunshot wound to his head.

Analytic Theory

Carl Jung viewed man teleologically, believing that behavior was conditioned by aims and aspirations, as well as by history. For Freud, from whom Jung broke off relations in 1914, the pursuit of basic instincts largely determined behavior. For Jung, the search for wholeness, completion, and self-actualization guided behavior. According to Jung, when progressive development is thwarted by a frustrating circumstance, the libido makes a regression into the unconscious in an attempt to overcome and proceed (Hall, Lindzey, & Campell, 1997). Thus, in a sense, the self-destructive act is an effort at *rebirth*. For the religious person, this may mean an afterlife or resurrection. For the nonreligious person, death often is seen as life was before birth.

Maltsberger and Buie (1980) describe this illusory belief that the physical or psychological self will survive suicide and find a setting of warmth or peace as magical. The illusion might involve anticipating the grave as a womb with eternal holding by mother earth or a (re)union with a loved object in heaven.

Modern psychodynamic theorists (Buie & Maltsberger, 1989) attempt to describe the psychological vulnerability that predisposes to suicide. These authors describe two threats that underlie suicide vulnerability. First, the loss of psychological self through mental disintegration arises from an intolerably intense experience of aloneness. This aloneness is not equated with the loneliness often seen in later years. Rather, it speaks to the capacity to form introjects, especially internalized memories (of images and feelings) of soothing and holding derived from childhood. Suicidal individuals have few such resources; therefore, they are are more dependent on external resources. Without them they experience aloneness, isolation, hopelessness, and fear. The extremes of aloneness are experienced as impending annihilation, a loss of self. The relationship of such theories to elderly suicide is obvious.

The second threat is that of overwhelming negative self-judgment. When survival is threatened, homicidal rage may animate an individual's response. Suicide may become the

---

CASE 5.2. A Religious Cure?

A 77-year-old widow, known to be despondent over her failing eyesight, jumped to her death from her 10th floor apartment balcony. In her apartment were found a variety of religious items, including a Christian Science Bible with chapters marked relating to sight (e.g., "seeing belongs to God," and "God is all-knowing and all-seeing").

---

psychological equivalent of killing someone else, the unavailable or depriving hated object.

Developmental Theory

Carlista Leonard (1967) proposed that the propensity toward suicide is established within the first years of life, dependent on the relative success of the infant's individuation from mother. For some children who do not accomplish this adaptation well, excessive dependence or a rigid independence results. Leonard described one example of the latter failure to individuate as the unaccepting suicidal type. This person establishes a lifelong pattern of controlling his or her environment in contrast to submitting to the will of another. Often male, this individual is achievement oriented and cannot accept a threatened reduction in self-concept posed by a loss of autonomy due to ill health, retirement, and so on. Suicide allows a way to leave the field "unchanged."

Clark (1993) posits a similar developmental model, based on his psychological autopsy study of elderly suicides. Clark suggests that a fundamental adaptational capacity is missing (and was never developed) in elderly suicidal victims. With the specter of physical decline, limitation, and increased dependency, this character fault leads to a resistance to change. Because of this resistance ordinary life stressors of aging will exceed the individual's tolerance threshold. A suicidal crisis may develop when the individual's defensive denial (the primary coping strategy) collapses and the realities of the aging process flood the individual with intense panic and rage. Suicide, then, provides a means of escaping intolerable anguish, obliterating evidence of decline or dysfunction, punishing the disappointed object (e.g., the failing body), or achieving mastery over that sense of failure through an act of self-control.

The reader will see parallels between these theories and that of Erikson (1950). Erikson described development as proceeding through a series of life stages characterized by distinct psychosocial "crises," or demands to adjust. These crises are turning points, opportunities for progression or regression. The developmental tasks of later adulthood require redirection of energy toward new roles, acceptance of one's life and its accomplishments, and developing a point of view about death (see Maris, 1981: 48). With these accomplished, ego integrity is achieved. If failed, despair and its sequelae may result. One obvious consequence might be suicide.

Sociobiological Theory

Self-preservation is a pervasive function of animal behavior. Suicide is the antithesis of self-preservation. Sociobiological theory asserts that self-preservation may only be favored

---

CASE 5.3. A Failure of Transition

A 72-year-old college professor, described by his colleagues as "driven and achievement-oriented," had recently retired from a tenured university position. He was known to be despondent about his retirement and was terrified of becoming dependent on his wife for life structure and social activity. He was discovered in his bedroom with a self-inflicted gunshot wound to his head.

---

when the individual has some remaining ability to sustain his or her "inclusive fitness" (i.e., one's own welfare and reproductive potential, and those of one's kin). When one's inclusive fitness is seriously impaired, suicide occurs. Thus, the terminally ill, the old and alone, and those with diminished coping capacities are likely to have higher rates of suicide, according to this theory (de Catanzaro, 1992). Again, the reader may note a parallel to Shneidman's concept of "agenerativity," one type of suicidal motive based on a falling out of. . . . Also, Farber's (1968) view of suicide as a disease of hope relates one's suicide risk as inversely proportional to one's degree of personal competence and directly related to one's vulnerability, two themes common to the sociobiological position. Perhaps the simplest model of aging is the most explanatory. With advancing years we generally experience more losses and deficits. From the physical to the social to the cognitive to the financial, these life changes (stressors) may accumulate. They may also overwhelm, depending on the individual's remaining strengths, resources, supports, and coping skills. In a context of decreasing opportunity to contribute and achieve (a further loss of mastery and control), and to be integrated into social groups (Durkheim's "anomic" condition), hopelessness, despair, and depression may ensue. For some, then, suicide may be a consequence of exhaustion—a giving up of the fight; for others, a way to preserve a sense of self rather than having to accept a changed view of self as dependent and increasingly losing control. This fundamental flaw in adaptational capacity may be the most significant distinguishing characteristic of elderly suicides.

Psychological Autopsy Studies of Elderly Suicide

Evidence for this hypothesis may be found in psychological autopsy studies. David Clark (1991) provided detailed information on 72 cases of elderly suicide—age 65 years and older—obtained from a community-based psychological autopsy study in Cook County, Illinois. The sample was predominantly male (4:1) and white (8:1); 53% died by gunshot wounds. At the time of their death, 35% were married and living with their spouses; an equal proportion were widowed. In contrast to expectation, 98% were not socially isolated, defined by at least weekly contact with friends and relatives. Seventy-two percent had forewarned their suicides over the preceding 6 months, yet only 13% were known by informants to have made a prior attempt. A terminal illness was acknowledged in only 13% of these cases and an additional 24% suffered a severe chronic medical illness. Thus, the majority were not severly medically ill. In contrast only one in four cases did not qualify for a psychiatric diagnosis. Most commonly found was a major depression, followed in frequency by alcoholism. Few of these individuals either acknowledged their psychological problems or sought treatment for them.

Although lacking a comparison or control group, Clark (1993) interpreted these findings to suggest that those elderly who suicide do so not because of special stressors but, rather, because a lifelong character fault—a fundamental incapacity to adapt—is unleashed by the forces of aging. He described this as a "narcissistic crisis of aging."

SUMMARY AND CONCLUSIONS

Age is a powerful factor in increased suicide rates, especially among white males. The highest suicide rates in the United States are and always have been found among older white males. For example, we saw that white males over 85 have suicide rates three times higher than 15–24-year-old white males (although, with a slight reversal around 1990, elderly suicide rates have been declining in general). Some of the suicidogenic forces in elderly white male suicides are undiagnosed and untreated depressive disorder, sosial isolation and loss of spouse (through death or divorce), years of alcohol abuse, ready availability of firearms, declining physical health, and coneptual rigidity and failure to adapt to changing life demands. Unlike white males, white females and both male and female African Americans tend to have suicide rates that peak in midlife.

Another major finding of this chapter was the dramatic rise of suicide rates of adolescents and young adults (mainly males), circa 1950 to 1980. Garrison estimated that the rate rise from 1957 to 1987 was over 300%. Although each teen suicide is somewhat unique, adolescent suicides occur in years of rapidly increasing alcohol and substance abuse and depressive illness vulnerability, are often corrlated with the presence of a gun in the home, and are related to social isolation and loss of support, early, sustained negative life events, broken homes, often inadequate parenting, and rising divorce rates.

We saw that children have remarkably low suicide rates (although some children do suicide and many go unreported). In part these low rates are related to the child's conceptual inability to comprehend the concepts of death and suicide early on; and the child's lack of access to lethal means to attempt suicide (e.g., guns); the presence of parents, siblings, friends, and teachers who observe the child (a kind of 24-hour close observation, similar to a suicide watch in psychiatric hospitals), to lower levels of depressive illness in most children, and to shelter from many of life's negative stressors.

Finally, Chapter 5 also examined suicide in midlife (and noted that the average age of most U.S. suicides is about 40 years old), where the loss of a spouse, years of heavy drinking, job stagnation or loss, increased risk of depressive illness, and acculumation of negative life events were all noted as suicidogenic forces.

In Chapter 6 we turn to another major demographic suicide predictor: gender and sex. We ask in Chapter 6, What is there about being a male in the United States that increases one's suicide potential three to four times that of females?

FURTHER READING

Berman, A. L., & Jobes, D. A. (1991). *Adolescent suicide: Assessment and intervention*. Washington, DC: American Psychological Association. One of the basic reference books on adolescent suicide by two of the country's leading youth suicidologists. Has sections on epidemiology, theory, data, risk assessment, treatment, pre- and postvention.

Leenaars, A. A., Maris, R. W., McIntosh, J. L., & Richman, J. (Eds). (1992). *Suicide and the older adult*. New York: Guilford Press. This edited volume has selections from many of the leading gerontological suicidologists (e.g., Robert Kastenbaum, Nancy Osgood, Derek Humphry, John Mann, John McIntosh, Joseph Richman, and others). Topics covered include epidemiology, economics, suicide notes, long-term care, social support, rational suicide, biological factors, and an excellent review of the literature.

Levinson, D. J. (1978). *Seasons of a man's life*. New York: Knopf. A leading Yale developmental psychologist looks at the stages of male development. Companion volume is *Seasons of a woman's life*.

Nuland, S. B. (1994). *How we die: Reflections on life's final chapter*. New York: Knopf. A Yale surgeon talks about the typical types of death (heart disease, cancer, suicide, Alzheimer's, etc.) in great detail, with a focus on physical changes. Gives the reader a sense of what elderly suicides have to cope with before their deaths. Almost "pornographic," as no one has written about the dying process.

Pearson, J. L., & Conwell, Y. (Eds.). (1996). *Suicide and aging: International perspectives.* New York: Springer. Like the title says, the book looks at age patterns in other cultures, nations, and genders. The older male suicide rate excess tends to hold up internationally, but there are some gender and age reversals to the U.S. patterns.

Pfeffer, C. R. (1986). *The suicidal child.* New York: Guilford Press. If there is *one* expert on child suicides, Cynthia Pfeffer is it. She alone has had major NIMH research grants to study youthful suicide. Well written, with ample treatment and clinical asides, indicative of the psychiatrist that she is.

6

Suicide, Gender, and Sexuality

> Women are not imaginative enough and intellectually complex enough to kill themselves.
>
> —EMILE DURKHEIM

Being either male or female is obviously an essential aspect of our biology. But our biology is inadequate for distinguishing differences between males and females. We are born either male or female (with some anomalies). However, we become masculine or feminine. Thus, our identity as either a male or female rests only partly on anatomical differences (Money & Erhardt, 1972). Our awareness of ourselves as "girl" or "boy," as "masculine" or "feminine," is best understood as a consequence of a complex biopsychosocial process, resting on both inner experiences, our sense of being male or female (*gender identity*), and outward expressions, those behavior patterns considered normative and appropriate to our gender (*gender role*).

The complexity of this process needs to be understood if one is to appreciate how gender and sexuality relate to suicide and suicidality. For as males and females differ, so do their suicidal behaviors, the presumed etiologies of these behaviors, and often the contingent reinforcers to these behaviors. In addition, when gender identity and gender role are either confused, dysphoric, or disturbed, there may be sufficient inner conflict or externally imposed stress to predispose a particular vulnerability to suicidal behavior. This vulnerability may be especially relevant to our understanding the relationship between *sexual orientation* (a person's tendency to be attracted to opposite or same sex partners) and suicidality (see "Gender Orientation: Homosexuality," below).

All behaviors, except perhaps those that are reproductive, are found in both males and females. Their expression, or the thresholds for eliciting them, are simply matters of "more" versus "less" in each gender. For example, aggression may have a lower threshold in most males than in most females. Repertoires of aggression as coping behaviors among men are more sanctioned by social acceptance and expectation. Similarly, help seeking is often associated more with females than with males. Some of these differences are determined and governed more by biological (genetic, biochemical; e.g., varying testosterone levels) versus sociocultural (childrearing, reinforcement) factors. Most sexual differences are shaped during childhood but are notably and significantly in evidence with the arrival of hormonal changes at puberty. However, all generalizations have their exceptions.

In many ways males and females appear to have become increasingly similar. This will be evident in our review of historical differences in their suicidal behaviors. Social attitudes, historical trends, and political agendas all influence the relative treatment of males and females, those behaviors considered normative for each gender, and the acceptance or rejection one feels for being this or that gender or for having a minority gender identity.

Consider the following, not-so-tongue-in-cheek description by a family therapist, Dr. Frank Pittman (1992), of how society has shaped gender roles over time:

> Several thousand years ago, while men were off hunting, women made their gathering job more efficient by inventing agriculture. Men, seemingly sterile and eternally awestruck by women's ability to create life, consoled themselves by creating death. Men's part is small and brief in the creation of life, leading to a need for reassurance that their part was big enough. Lacking reassurance, men promptly created an anti-female, anti-sexual male god of war who created man first, delivered woman from man, and encouraged him to be the boss, to fight wars, to kill sons, and to go around naming things after himself.
>
> Men and women back then seem to have struck a deal that men would risk their lives protecting women if women would worship men. At that time, with a world full of saber-toothed tigers, it may have seemed like a fair deal.
>
> Once the tigers were extinct, patriarchy began to collapse. Two hundred years ago, the American and French Revolutions overthrew the divine rights of kings, men's patriarchal power over children, and in time, men's ownership of other men. The world no longer seemed scary enough to warrant all that inefficient fawning over masculine glory. In fact, the growling and stomping of men who didn't feel man enough had become the greater danger.
>
> Patriarchy in Western society, at least, has been shriveling up during the last few decades. Women finally refused to worship men for risking their lives, and let the world know they were fully capable of wrestling any tigers on the prowl. . . . For the past 200 years, each generation of men has had less power, and each generation of women has had more options than the last. Everything a child learns about his or her gender, or about the gender of his or her eventual partner, will be outdated before it can be put into effect. (8)

We are interested in this chapter in exploring how suicidal behavior is gender normative and how exceptions to gender norms affect suicidal behavior. Thus, we present statistical data on how males and females differ in their suicidality and how nonconformity to gender identity or gender role may lead to increased risk for suicidal behavior.

Many questions are raised and answers attempted. For example, are there behavioral differences between the sexes in their suicidal behaviors? Are these differences stable across time and culture? Are any differences noted due to biology, gender roles, or complex interactions between psychological (e.g., needs), biological (e.g., hormones), and cultural (e.g., role expectations) factors?

A brief note about gender differences is appropriate. Although most of us accept a number of gender stereotypes ("Males are . . . /Females are . . ."), research has substantiated only a few, mostly small, disparities between the sexes. Of those relevant to suicidology, even fewer appear germane. In the cognitive domain, females are more verbal than males (Linn & Hyde, 1989). Thus, we might expect to find differences in suicidal communications with females "crying for help" more than males. In the social domain, aggression, both physical and verbal, is more characteristic of males (Eagly, 1987). Thus, we might expect to find more violent behaviors (including suicides) among males. Females are more sensitive than males to nonverbal communications and cues (Hall, 1984). Thus, they are more empathic to the feelings of others and more susceptible to social influence than males (Becker, 1986). Also, there is some suggestive evidence that females are more willing to admit to their fears and anxieties (Hyde, 1985). Thus, we might expect to find more social reactivity and help seeking/help accepting among females.

As modern society demands more androgyny and becomes less patriarchal (i.e., as gender equality becomes more the norm) it becomes less clear what constitutes uniqueness in gender identity. Both males and females may experience more role confusion and display the effects of greater stress in adapting to culturally sanctioned change. One outcome of this leveling effect might be observable in changed suicide rates. As an illustration, Davis (1981) has provided evidence supporting Stack's (1978) hypothesis linking role strain and suicide. Stack (1978) hypothesized that women entering the labor force would reflect increased strain due to increased demands of both outside and household responsibilities. Davis demonstrated that during the 1950s and 1960s, as women increasingly entered and participated in the labor force, their suicide rate did increase. This finding, however, has been contested. Ornstein (1983), using data from British Columbia, for example, found that women in the work force were *less* likely to complete suicide than were either unemployed women or housewives. Moreover, as we shall see, data from more recent decades give evidence for a declining suicide rate among females in general.

As a correlate to these changes, historical differences in gender-specific suicidal behavior may disappear. It may be predicted that as men are increasingly encouraged to shed stereotyped roles of self-control and rationality and to express their fears and anxieties, they, too, will experience less inner tension, be more accepting of help and succorence, and consequently will be less lethal in their suicidality. Interestingly, the data do not appear to substantiate this hypothesis.

For the present, males and females do appear to express psychological distress differently. For example, adult males have higher rates of substance use disorders (alcohol and illicit drug abuse), antisocial behaviors, and gender identity disorders. Adult females have higher rates of anxiety disorders, eating disorders, depression, and prescription drug abuse (Regier et al., 1988). These pathologies (and others that are more age related, such as conduct disorders in adolescent males) are significant risk factors (cf. Chapter 3) for suicidal behaviors.

Similarly, studies comparing homosexual to heterosexual groups have demonstrated higher rates of certain risk factors (such as substance abuse; Fifield, 1975) in the homosexual population, suggesting possible potentiating conditions for more frequent suicidal behavior in this population.

GENDER DIFFERENCES IN HEALTH AND MORTALITY

Generally, males have a greater incidence of serious health problems and a shorter lifespan. Even *in utero* males are less viable (Harrison, 1978). From early childhood through old age, males have higher rates of death than do females for all the leading causes of death. It has been estimated that as much as 75% of the sex difference in life expectancy can be accounted for by gender role behaviors, specifically the greater involvement of men in high-risk health behaviors such as cigarette smoking, alcohol abuse, hazardous activity, and violence (Waldron, 1976). For example, more males than females drink alcohol and considerably more males than females drink alcohol to excess. Consequently, men's rate of death from cirrhosis of the liver is about twice that of women (Eisler & Blalock, 1991). Looking specifically at violent death, males are three times as likely as females to die in motor vehicle accidents and more than four times as likely to die by suicide.

THE EPIDEMIOLOGY OF GENDER DIFFERENCES
IN SUICIDAL BEHAVIOR

Gender

Some of the most consistent findings in suicidology are sexual differences. Males tend to complete suicide more than females and females tend to attempt suicide more than males. However, there are important variants to these generalizations when the data are examined by age groups, race, time, and interactions among these variables.

Temporal Variations in Gender Differences

The ratio of male to female suicide in the United States was 4.4:1 in 1996. That is, the rate of male suicide was more than four times greater than that for females (17.96/100,000 vs. 4.06/100,000). Stated yet another way, in 1996 only 19% of all suicides in the United States were by females. From the 1930s to 1971 (when the suicide sex ratio hit a low of 2.5:1), the ratio of male to female suicide was steady or declined. However, the suicide sex ratio has increased since 1971, due to dramatic increases in younger male suicide and a decline in the female rate (McIntosh & Jewell, 1986).

Cross-Cultural Variations in Gender Differences

Cross-culturally, the ratio of male to female suicide varies markedly, particularly when age is examined. For example, Lester (1991) looked at suicide rates for more than 20 different countries and validated three different patterns to this ratio across the lifespan (i.e., either a linear increase with age, a unimodal peak in middle age, or a bimodal distribution with a minor peak at the younger ages and a major peak in old age).

   The male rate is consistently greater than that for females in almost every culture (Lester, 1984). Exceptions can be found in some subcultures. Rates of suicide among women in the People's Republic of China (PRC) are higher than those of men (Shiang, 1998); similarly, Chinese American women over the age of 45 complete suicide at higher rates than do their male counterparts, yet still well below the suicide rate for white women (Group for the Advancement of Psychiatry, 1989). These older women are generally newer immigrants, having not been allowed to emigrate to the United States until after 1965. As first-generation immigrants they have fewer supports and marketable skills and tend to be more impoverished than Chinese American males (Group for the Advancement of Psychiatry, 1989). In some ethnic subcultures, such as whites living in the East Harlem area of New York City, female rates have been found to be equal to those of white males and two to three times as great as those of Puerto Rican and black females in the same community (Monk & Warshauer, 1974). In the same study, Puerto Rican males living in East Harlem were found to have a suicide rate three times greater than the rate of males living in Puerto Rico.

Age Variations in Gender Differences

In the United States, the greatest suicide rate discrepancy between the sexes is among the older age groups. In 1996, males ages 65–74 were almost six times as likely to complete suicide as same aged females; those ages 75–84 were nine times as likely to complete suicide, and among those age 85 and older the ratio climbed to a staggering 14:1.

   Youth also have a higher ratio of male to female suicide than is observed not controlling for age. Among 15–24-year-olds in 1996, the male–female suicide ratio was 5.9:1. Within the 15–24-year-old age group, some subgroups have been found to have even higher ratios. For example, among Native Americans aged 15–24 who completed suicide in 1980, the male:female suicide ratio was 7:1, more than three times greater than the overall ratio for all Native Americans that year (Group for Advancement of Psychiatry, 1989).

Temporal Variations in Age and Gender Differences

The 15–24-year-old gender ratio, in particular, has shown marked changes over time. For the United States in general in 1911, it was at a low of 0.7:1.0; in 1980 it was 4.7:1.0; in 1990, it had risen to 5.3:1; and in 1996 to 5.9:1. Looked at another way, the discrepancy between male and female youth suicides in 1996 was more than eight times larger than that of 1911. Early in this century (in 1910) the suicide rate for white females ages 15–19 exceeded that for 15–19-year-old white males but then declined thereafter (Dublin, 1963). Table 6.1 depicts a decade-by-decade comparison of male–female suicide rates from 1940 to 1990.

Racial Variations in Gender Differences

White males comprised 73% of all completed suicides in 1996. However, the ratio of male to female suicide is greater among blacks (6:1) than among whites (4.3:1). White females in 1996 had a suicide rate more than twice that of black females. Similarly, white males had a rate almost two-thirds greater than that of nonwhite males.

Temporal Variations in Race and Gender Differences

Between 1970 and 1996 suicide rates have increased for both white and nonwhite males; rates for all females have declined (Table 6.2). The rates of increase among males are most profound in the 15–19-year-old age group, with increases of 103% for white males since 1970 and 144% for nonwhite males. Black females consistently have had the lowest rates of suicide in the United States, accounting for only 1.1% of all suicides in 1996.

As these data are extended in Table 6.3, the ratio of male to female suicide has enlarged by a factor of almost one-third for both whites and nonwhites between the years 1940 and 1996. These ratios have taken a turn in the last 20 years. After declining from 1950 to 1970, they have increased by over 54% for nonwhites and 71% for whites since 1970.

TABLE 6.1. Suicide Rates and Ratios for 15–24-Year-Olds by Sex, United States, 1940–1996

Year	Male Rate	Female Rate	Male:female ratio
1940	8.4	3.8	2.2:1
1950	6.5	2.6	2.5:1
1960	8.2	2.2	3.7:1
1970	13.5	4.2	3.2:1
1980	20.2	4.3	4.7:1
1990	20.9	3.9	5.3:1

Sources: Suicide Surveillance Summary Report, Centers for Disease Control and Prevention, September 13, 1994; National Center for Health Statistics, *Vital Statistics of the United States*, annual volumes.

TABLE 6.2. Suicide Rates by Race and Gender, United States, 1970–1996

Race/gender	1970	1980	1990	1996	% change: 1970–1996
White males	18.2	18.9	22.0	20.9	+ 15%
White females	7.2	5.7	5.3	4.8	−33%
Nonwhite males	10.3	11.3	11.9	11.3	+10%
Nonwhite females	3.3	2.8	2.6	2.5	−24%
All males	17.3	18.0	20.4	19.3	+12%
All females	6.8	5.4	4.8	4.4	−35%

Sources: Suicide Surveillance Summary Report, Centers for Disease Control and Prevention, September 13, 1994; National Center for Health Statistics, Mortality Report, 1996.

Gender Differences in Nonfatal Suicide Attempts

The epidemiology of nonfatal suicide attempts suggests that sex differences may be equally profound here, particularly in the adolescent and young adult age groups. Among children under the age of 14, more boys than girls require hospital treatment for a suicide attempt (see Cohen-Sandler, Berman, & King, 1982). Pfeffer (1986) asserts, however, that there is no difference in the degree of severity of suicidal tendencies (when considering ideation as well as overt behavior) between the sexes at early ages. By their midteens, however, girls outnumber boys as attempters by a ratio of roughly 4:1, although some have estimated this ratio to be as great as 10:1 (Toolan, 1975). The ratio of nonfatal attempts to completions among 15–24-year-old males has been estimated to be 26:1 and among 15–24-year-old females, almost 200:1 (Schuckit & Schuckit, 1989).

This predominance of females as suicide attempters remains consistent through adulthood, although the frequency of attempts peaks among females ages 15–24 (Schuckit & Schuckit, 1989) and is most easily documented by gender differences in histories of *prior* attempts in psychological autopsy studies of completers (see Maris, 1981). In addition, the greater frequency of female attempters can be documented in almost all countries, with the possible exceptions of Poland and India (Weissman, 1974). Case-finding methods may explain some of the observed gender differences in attempted suicide. Weissman (1974) argued that studies relying on hospital admissions will yield a preponderance of women (as more frequent help seekers), whereas cases that include self-injuries in jail and prison settings (which are overwhelmingly male) will reveal a more equal gender ratio. Furthermore, Garfinkel (personal communication, July 1990) asserts that when more rural (vs. urban

TABLE 6.3. Ratio of Male to Female Suicide Rates, United States, 1940–1996

Year	Total	White	Nonwhite
1940	3.22:1	3.22:1	3.43:1
1950	3.45	4.12	3.53
1960	3.37	3.32	3.32
1970	2.55	2.54	2.93
1980	3.38	3.37	4.08
1990	4.21	4.16	4.58
1996	4.38	4.35	4.52
% Increase: 1940–1996	36%	35%	32%

Sources: Suicide Surveillance Summary Report, Centers for Disease Control and Prevention, September 13, 1994; National Center for Health Statistics, Mortality Report, 1996.

hospital emergency room) samples of attempters are studied, the usually observed gender differences wash out.

GENDER AND METHOD

As readers will see in Chapter 12, gender differences have consistently been found in choice of suicide method and may explain part of the gender difference in rates of completed and attempted suicide. Females tend to use a greater variety of methods, many of lower lethality than those of men, particularly drugs (poisons)—which in 1996 accounted for 26% of female suicides, compared to only 6% of male suicides (Table 6.4). Paradoxically, the most frequently used class of drugs in completed suicides is antidepressants.

Ingesting drugs is the preferred method among parasuicides. Tranquilizers and pain relievers are most often used in nonfatal overdoses.

Females, representing both the modal parasuicide and the modal drug ingester, are more likely to survive their attempt. Conversely, males use more lethal methods, particularly firearms and hanging (63% and 17% of all methods, respectively, in 1996), and are more likely to die when they attempt. As a corollary of using more lethal methods, males are more likely to not have as frequent histories of prior attempts before completing suicide (Maris, 1981: Ch. 10).

Some period effects suggest a long-term increasing lethality among female completers who proportionately are using firearms more and poisoning less frequently than in years past (Table 6.4). Since 1980, firearms have been the method of choice for both both males and females, who consequently rarely survive these lethal attempts.

As described in Chapter 12, the reasons for these differences in method choice probably may best be explained by socialization (females are less likely to have experience with or be comfortable with guns), availability (males are more likely to have a gun in their possession and females have greater access to prescription drugs), and association (drugs are painless, easy to use, lack messiness, and do not disfigure the body). These differences also may mark differences in intent, with females being thought to be more ambivalent about dying, wanting to use suicidal behavior more as an instrumental communication (e.g., to coerce change in others and wishing more to be rescued).

TABLE 6.4. Method of Suicide and Gender, United States, 1970–1990

Year/gender	Firearms (%)	Hanging (%)	Drugs (%)	Gas (%)	Other (%)
1970					
Male	58	15	9	11	7
Female	30	12	37	11	10
1980					
Male	63	15	6	8	8
Female	39	11	27	12	12
1990					
Male	66	15	5	7	7
Female	42	12	26	9	7
1996					
Male	63	17	6	6	7
Female	40	17	26	7	11

Source: National Center for Health Statistics, *Mortality Reports,* various years.

HYPOTHESES ABOUT GENDER DIFFERENCES IN SUICIDE

One of the founders of suicidology, Durkheim, was nevertheless the product of his own era and culture. Although his theoretical propositions and empirical findings regarding suicide have stimulated a century of scholars, his view of gender differences, quoted at the beginning of this chapter, was incredibly wrongheaded. There simply is little support relating gender or suicidality to differences in intelligence or creativity. Nor is there much empirical support for differences based on relative strength (e.g., that women are physically weaker), pregnancy, or menstruation (Canetto, 1992; Harry, 1989).

Beginning in the 19th century, explanations for gender differences in suicide were tied to what interpreters believed to be different gender motivations. In men these concerned real or fancied impotence, business embarassments, losses, ungratified ambition, and so on, and in women they included domestic unhappiness, loss of honor or purity (illicit love affairs), disappointed love, and betrayal (Kushner, 1989). Furthermore, women were described as being more protected from suicide by such virtues as being able to cry, having greater religious involvement, and "the relatively less harrassing part she has taken in the struggle for life" (Kushner, 1989: 100).

Twentieth-century hypotheses (outlined in the sections below), as we shall see, may not appear dramatically different from these earlier characterizations, but at least they have been subject to greater empirical testing. Some hypotheses remain colored by the politics of era and culture. Note in particular the following perspective espoused by proponents of the men's movement during the 1980s.

SUICIDE AND GENDER: A MALE PERSPECTIVE

Kammer and Sayles (1987), writing in the magazine *Fast Lane,* which is "For Today's Man," describe the fundamental life problem as a "sort of nutcracker effect," on one side a pressure to succeed and, on the other, an inability to admit weakness and seek help. The social pressure on men, they assert, is "to have it all," from the high-paying job to the European car to the beautiful mate. Failure to achieve this ideal is a given for most men, but their struggle and their pain do not get compassion from others, especially from other men. They may grow hopeless (whereas women are allowed to be helpless) and, if men seek help (which they are not likely to do), they are closer to the edge than a woman would be. Not wanting to be a burden on others, male suicide reflects leaving "like a man."

Warren Farrell, writing in *Why Men Are the Way They Are* (1988), claims that while men feel the pressure to win a woman through performance and material superiority, women continue to reinforce this pressure because (in spite of their increasing liberation and independence) they still cling to the "primary fantasy" of having a man take care of them. So, as women achieve in a traditionally male world, the pressure on men only increases.

Women's increasing independence may also signal changes in their willingness to tolerate problems in men (Hanauer, 1989). Given the message to open up and be more vulnerable with women, a man may become confused and fear abandonment should he express his sense of failure and helplessness to a strong and independent woman he has sought to impress.

In this psychosociobabble there are shreds of truth and a kernel of something very important to understanding both gender differences and their changes over time. And that has to do with differences between males and females in their coping strategies. If overwhelmed, typically women seek help. Females are trained from birth that relationships are to be nurtured and that a dependent position is acceptable. Help seeking is therefore acceptable. A woman's identity is neither compromised nor diminished by turning to others for support.

For males, on the other hand, it simply is not as acceptable to be as openly in need, to self-disclose one's vulnerabilities, or to seek help. Rosenthal (1981) referred to this as a fear of cowardice (fear of social disapproval) among men. Society sanctions self-reliance, toughness, and the avoidance of emotional expression among men, in spite of findings that males do not differ from females in the experience of uncomfortable emotions (Allen & Haccoun, 1976). Indeed, there is evidence to support the notion that others tend to respond to males in suicidal crisis less empathically and with less acceptance (see "Social Acceptability and Suicidality; below).

Moreover, whereas it was predicted that as women increasingly entered the work force (i.e., a traditional male enclave), their suicide rate would increase and ultimately surpass that of males (Neuringer, 1982) under the stress of dual careers (work and family–mothering), as noted earlier this has simply not happened. It would appear that working women have gained from the world of work, in self-esteem, in income, in independence, *and* in the rewards of interacting with other adults on a daily basis. Men, in contrast, have lost some of their dominance and power relative to these shifts in the working culture.

SUICIDE AND GENDER: A FEMALE PERSPECTIVE

For a woman, a decision to kill herself and therefore destroy all relatedness stands in direct opposition to the values most central to her core identity.
—ALEXANDRA KAPLAN AND RONA KLEIN

The importance of relationships and relatedness to others (including childbearing and child care) may provide a core understanding of female suicidal behavior, according to clinical theoreticians at the Stone Center at Wellesley College (Kaplan & Klein, 1989). In their model society is seen as more demanding that women create synergistic interactions with others; that is, a woman's sense of meaning and value (sense of self, self-esteem) is derived from a mutuality of care and responsibility in relationships. A woman's vulnerability to suicide, therefore, increases when her opportunity for growth within relationships is perceived as blocked or distorted.

This model (as opposed to phallocentric developmental models, such as Erikson's, 1982) suggests that women generally strive to preserve relationships, not because of a dependency but because the connection to others maximizes growth opportunities. Suicidal behavior, then, represents a desperate plea for engagement under conditions of threat to that connection. The relatively low suicide rate among women is understandable in this context, as a woman would typically find it more difficult to abandon those perceived as needing her and would be more attuned to and concerned for how others would be affected by her death. Also in this context suicide attempts would be more common among women than men as their primary motivation would be an appeal for connectedness to others (see Lifton, 1983). Box 6.1 offers this motivation as one reason why women ingest drugs more than men do in suicide attempts.

Cumming and Lazar (1981) provide an interesting affirmation of this position through their analysis of Canadian suicide rates. They found that employment appeared to serve a protective function for women, whereas marriage served a protective function for men. For women, work increased opportunities for adult relationship; for men, marriage enabled them to gain a network of affiliations maintained by their wives. It is for this reason, per-

---

BOX 6.1. Do Vanity and Sleeping Beauty Fantasies Influence Female Suicidal Behavior?

Yes: *Various Authors:* Women choose less lethal means to engage suicidal behaviors, particularly drug overdose, because they are more concerned about what might happen to their bodies even after death and do not want to disfigure themselves. The mental image of a violent, mutilating death is, also, associated with suffering and pain. Drug overdoses, moreover, produce both the look of sleep and the opportunity for rescue, akin to the image of Sleeping Beauty being found by her Prince Charming.

No: *Various Authors:* Women simply are not socialized to use firearms the way men are and, in contrast, are prescibed psychotropic medication far more often than are men; therefore, they have drugs readily available for use in overdose. However, increasingly women are turning to firearms when their intent is strong to complete suicide. In 1966, 28% of female suicides were by firearms; in 1996, the proportion was 40%. In contrast, the proportion of female suicides by poisoning decreased from 45% to 26% in this same time period (see Table 6.4). Women who ingest drugs more often wish to alert others to their need for help; males typically are less likely to communicate their need for—or to be willing to accept—help from others.

---

haps, that divorce and separation are more associated with (as precipitants of) male suicides than with female suicides (Maris, 1981).

Social support and social involvement are buffers or protective factors to suicide risk. Studies have consistently shown that women have more close friends, more perceived sources of support, and more interactions in which support is either given or received than do men (Eisler & Blalock, 1991).

SOCIAL ACCEPTABILITY AND SUICIDALITY

Social acceptability may play a significant role in explaining gender differences in suicidal behavior. Linehan (1973) hypothesized that social expectations of suicidal behavior varied as a function of the sex role of the suicidal person. She tested empirically whether social acceptability of suicidal behavior varied by type of suicidal behavior (completed vs. attempted) and sex of the suicidal person. She found that, indeed, completed suicide was considered more "masculine." Similarly, Hammen and Peters (1977) found that males were perceived more negatively for the expression of helplessness, hopelessness, self-depreciation, and passivity and, thus, more positively for acting on versus communicating their suicidality.

Several studies have examined the sex of the observer (i.e., potential helper) as a significant component in the differential labeling and (thus) potential intervention process. Berman (1978) provided stimulus vignettes of stressed or bereaved persons (varying their gender) and asked male and female subjects to rate the severity of their problem, their suicidal risk, their need for intervention, and so on. He found that males (significantly more than females) saw males as more depressed and more pathological than females dealing with identical problems. Similarly, White and Stillion (1988) studied gender-specific responses to suicidal persons. While females (compared to males) were more sympathetic to all troubled people, males were most unsympathetic to suicidal males. Lesham and Lesham (1976) and Wellman and Wellman (1986) also found males to be less sympathetic and more reluctant to respond to suicidal individuals. Thus, cultural norms and social expectations do appear to reinforce the acceptability of suicidal behavior by males, while making completed suicide more gender-inappropriate for females. We note the tautology here. That is, if males indeed do kill themselves more frequently than females, we come to expect that behavior of males more than females.

These findings suggest that contingent reinforcers may shape suicidal behavior in gender-specific ways. As an example, Potts, Burnam, and Wells (1991), studying data on more than 23,000 patients and 500 clinicians, found that depression was generally underdetected in men and overdetected in women. They suggest that in depression screenings, males may be less likely to express their feelings or more likely to deny being depressed. However, it is equally possible that males were not as expected to be depressed or to discuss being depressed and, therefore, were not asked about their symptoms as frequently as women were.

GENDER, MENTAL DISORDERS, AND SUICIDE

The link between diagnosable mental disorders with both completed and attempted suicide is strong (see Chapter 13). Affective disorders, schizophrenias, alcoholism and drug abuse, and comorbid presentation of these disorders with each other and other disorders (e.g., borderline personality disorder, panic disorder, and eating disorder) have especially strong associations with suicide risk (Tanney, 1992).

Overall, women are diagnosed with mental disorders more frequently than men are (Gove, 1979). Some significant gender differences in specific disorders are also evident. Depressive illness (actually several distinct disorders), the disorder most often associated with suicidality, is more common among adult women than among men (Weissman & Klerman, 1977; Nolen-Hoeksema, 1990), presents twice as frequently with a secondary anxiety disorder among women (Ochoa, Beck, & Steer, 1992), and is three times as frequent in chemically dependent female adolescents (Deykin, Buka, & Zeena, 1992). However, no difference in gender has been observed in bipolar disorders (Leutwyler, 1995). Box 6.2 offers two gender-based hypotheses to explain gender differences in depression.

Anorexia is overwhelmingly found (by a 9:1 ratio) among females (Gove, 1979). In contrast, alcoholism and the use of illicit drugs occur four times more frequently among men (Colton & Marsh, 1984). The use of mood modifying prescription drugs, however, is

---

BOX 6.2. Are Gender Differences in Depression Biologically Based or Psychologically Based?

A biological hypothesis: Leutwyler (1995).

Depressive symptoms may be provoked by shifts in hormonal levels in women who are genetically vulnerable to affective disorder or to stress from psychosocial problems. For example, hormonal differences between men and women have been shown to affect sleep cycles and thus mood. Females, also, have been found to produce less melatonin during the summer.

A psychological hypothesis: Neuringer and Lettieri (1982).

Women are more dependent and, thus, are more significantly affected by negative shifts in and loss of relationship (through separation, divorce, etc.). In personality testing they report higher affiliative needs, feelings of helplessness, and/or feelings of inadequacy.

twice as frequent among women as among men (Colton & Marsh, 1984), perhaps explaining their availability for use in nonfatal suicide attempts by women. We should note that there is, in part, an iatrogenic effect here, as physicians prescribe antidepressants (e.g., benzodiazepines) twice as frequently to females.

We need to remember that the preponderance of females in both overall rates of disorder in most of the specific disorders (excluding alcoholism and illicit drug use) is, partly, an artifact of our case-finding methods. Excluding catchment area community surveys, most of our data is derived from emergency room and inpatient admissions. As females are far more likely to seek and accept offers of treatment, they overpopulate these data sites. A good recent example of this concerns the prevalence of schizophrenia, commonly held to affect about equal proportions of men and women. When researchers in Vancouver, British Columbia, concentrated on first episodes of schizophrenia only, as known to a broad sampling of health services and general practitioners (not just ERs and hospitals), they found that more than two-thirds of the sample were men (Iacono & Beiser, 1992).

GENDER, BIOLOGY, AGGRESSION, AND VIOLENCE

Women have essentially the same neurological structures (brains, neurotransmitters, etc.) as men. Thus one cannot argue that there is no physical mechanism for aggression in women (Moir & Jessel, 1991). At the same time, there are clear gender differences in the frequency of observed aggressive acts. There is a great deal of research demonstrating that males have higher levels of aggression than do females.

Learning plays a significant role in the gender-based social acceptability of aggression. Boys are highly encouraged during socialization to use aggressive strategies to cope (Doyle, 1989; Franklin, 1988). Women, on the other hand, as a consequence of many years of training, are generally more inhibited in expressing more direct acts of aggression (Suter, 1976).

In more recent years, our understanding of aggression has benefited from brain biochemistry studies, particularly of the serotonin metabolite CSF 5-HIAA (cerebrospinal fluid levels of 5-hydroxyindoleacetic; see Chapter 16) and its relationship to suicide and especially violent suicide. As most of this research has focused on male suicidal subjects who tend to both have lower CSF 5-HIAA concentrations and account for the majority of violent suicides, it seems reasonable to speculate that gender-based biochemical differences may be significant in explaining differences in observed suicidal behavior. van Praag (1982; cf. Chapter 17) has suggested that depression, hostility, and impulsivity all are traits correlated with disturbed serotonin metabolism and predispose one to both aggression and suicide.

Women have lower concentrations of testosterone than do men (Moore & Gillette, 1992); although there is no known direct relationship between testosterone and suicidal behavior, the link between testosterone and aggression has clearly been made (Hyde, 1990, Ch. 3). Parallel to this, studies have demonstrated that during the course of a woman's menstrual cycle there is a drop in the production of the ovarian hormone estradiol (and other hormones), the consequence of which often are violent and aggressive behavior (Moore & Gillette, 1992). However, as noted earlier in this chapter, there is no consistent research evidence to support an association between stages of the menstrual cycle and suicidal behavior (see Lester, 1988e, for a review of this literature).

It is also important to note that female completed suicide rates peak in midlife (in the United States), particularly in the menopausal years. Whether this observation may be explained by the biological changes inherent in menopause, by life experience losses incurred during these years (e.g., the "empty nest"), or by (more likely) combinations of these or yet other factors cannot be said, as this phenomenon has received no serious research attention.

This age-specific observation may be explained sociobiologically. According to this theory (see de Catanzaro, 1986, 1992), suicide is more likely to occur when our reproductive potential is impeded, that is to say, when our genetic contribution to our species' preservation is either thwarted or no longer present. Thus, suicide would be predicted to be more frequent among the unmarried, the terminally ill, menopausal women, and elderly males. Each of these groups is, indeed, at greater suicide risk.

GENDER DIFFERENCES: SOME RESIDUAL CONSIDERATIONS

Personality differences between males and females have been suggested as explanatory of different patterns of suicidal behavior from the days of Durkheim's observations to the present. Canetto (1992) has reviewed these hypotheses, noting particularly that descriptors of women's character have tended to be pejorative, even if associated with adaptation and survival. For example, women have been described as more passive, suggestible, and malleable than men (Breed & Huffine, 1979) with these characteristics underlying their lower rates of completed suicide. Canetto (1992) argues that women, as a result of their socialization and developmental experiences, may be capable of more complex and flexible coping than men, who have greater need to be in control and, thus, are more rigid. This rigidity, particularly in the cognitive domain, has been thought to characterize the suicidal mind (Neuringer & Lettieri, 1982; Beck, Brown, Steer, Dahlsgaard, & Grisham, 1999). Box 6.3 presents conflicting views on whether cognitive differences can be discerned through analyses of suicide notes. It is reasonable to postulate a gender-based path model that may be central to our understanding of gender differences in suicidal behavior (see Bonner & Rich's [1987] "stress–vulnerability" model). Gender differences in suicidal behavior may reflect a tendency of males to respond with despair and hopelessness (the more rigid position) to stress, conflict, frustration, and so on. Females may have a greater and more socially acceptable response of helplessness and a communicated need for help (a "cry for help" or help seeking) (i.e., a more flexible position). Thus, females tend to maximize their chances for attachment and succorance, while males tend to move more readily to a position of giving up and ending a perceived intolerable state of being.

Studies of utilization of suicide prevention centers confirm the significantly greater tendency for women to seek and benefit from contact with these helping facilities (Miller, Coombs, Leeper, & Barton, 1984). Older males, facing a changing and downward status as a consequence of retirement, physical illness, and loss of peer relationships may need to

---

BOX 6.3. Are Suicide Notes Written by Men and Women Different?

Yes: Black (1989).

Suicide notes written by women have more indications of depression, self-directed hostility, confusion, and despondency over the death of others.

No: Leenaars (1996).

"[There are] no sex differences on intrapsychic and interpersonal aspects [of suicide notes]. There appear to be no sex differences on such issues as 'I love you,' 'I'm in unbearable pain,' 'I'm hopeless and helpless,' 'I cannot cope,' and 'This is the only way out for me.'"

increasingly rely on others for help with everyday activities. However, lacking the same core ability and drive for relatedness and attachments, as females, these older males may too readily move to an isolated and hopeless position, which in turn breeds greater suicide risk.

GENDER ORIENTATION: HOMOSEXUALITY

The preference for a same-sex partner, once considered unto itself to be psychopathological, presents unique stressors to the homosexual. The majority of society is generally homophobic and even hostile. There continues to be a stigma to being gay, promoted by religious conservatives and expressed along a continuum from negative verbal stereotyping and abuse ("faggot") to social isolation to outright physical abuse ("gay bashing"). For those still "in the closet," the recognition and self-identification of one's homosexuality is laden with loneliness, anxiety, and confusion. In their families, many emerging gay youth anticipate rejection as well, prompting an internalization of these negative societal attitudes. The consequence may be one of lowered self-esteem, depression, heightened use of alcohol or drugs, and so on, for the homosexual person. When familial attitudes are rejecting, particularly when the family system is characterized by substance abuse and physical abuse, substantial numbers of emerging gay youth choose to leave home for life on the streets and often a more promiscuous and substance-abusing lifestyle. As if this self-destructive pattern was not enough, now comes the increased risk of HIV infection and the prospect of death from AIDS.

In this matrix of internal conflict and external stressors, we note a number of well-substantiated risk factors for suicidal behaviors—low self-esteem, loneliness, depression, substance abuse, and so on—strongly suggesting that homosexuality (particularly during the anxiety-ridden stage of "coming out") may breed increased suicide risk. Indeed, as we shall see, the few published empirical reports on suicidality among homosexuals do often report high rates of parasuicidal behavior. But where some interpreters declare there to be a clear and consistent relationship (Harry, 1989), others have concluded that to date "virtually nothing is known . . . about the relationship between homosexuality and suicidal behavior" (Clark, 1992: 13).

As is common to all areas of relatively uncharted scientific investigation, the early and few published studies regarding this hypothesized relationship are of relatively poor quality, relying on biased (e.g., recruited) samples and often lacking in control or comparison groups. Although flawed, these approaches do at least call attention to a possible problem and may eventually lead to serious investigations. At present, however, perhaps no area in suicidology is filled with more unsubstantiated and hyperbolic claims, controversy, and political interference in the process of scientific inquiry. Politics and scientific inquiry do not often make good bedfellows. A brief overview of this recent history follows.

Controversy was sparked by the commissioned report on "Gay Male and Lesbian Youth Suicide" (Gibson, 1989) presented to the U.S. Department of Health and Human Service's "Secretary's Task Force on Youth Suicide." In the report's introductory paragraphs, Gibson asserted that "[gay and lesbian youth] may comprise up to 30% of completed youth suicides annually" and that "suicide is the leading cause of death among gay male, lesbian, bisexual, and transsexual youth" (110). While possible, nowhere in his report did Gibson substantiate these claims with empirical data or published studies. In fact, they are not even alluded to again, perhaps because there simply were no supporting data to report. Yet, for some in the gay community, that these assertions appeared in a government-sponsored publication cloaked them with respectability and even validity. Their validity was further affirmed when the report was assailed by some conservative Republican members of Congress who urged the then Secretary of the Department of Health and Human Services, Dr. Louis Sullivan, to repudiate the report (which had recommended greater acceptance of homosexuality) and affirm, in its stead, the traditional roles of family and religious values. Sullivan responded by attempting to distance President Bush's administration from the report and limiting its distribution to the original printing of 2,000 copies (Okie, 1990). These actions served to infuriate the gay community.

To make matters worse, Gibson's assertions have been exaggerated in their retelling. For example, in an article on gay teen suicide in the national gay and lesbian magazine *The Advocate*, Maguen (1991) writes, "Gay and lesbian teenagers are killing themselves in staggering numbers" and "conservatively estimate(s) 1500 young gay and lesbian lives are terminated every year" (40). Later in this article, a director of a gay youth support program is quoted as saying, "National statistics say that gay males are *8 to 9 times* more likely to commit suicide (than straight males)" (47, emphasis added).

In the midst of this political war of words and policy, what can we substantiate about the relationship between homosexuality and suicidality? First, with regard to *completed* suicide, only one study (Rich, Fowler, Young, & Blenkush, 1986a) has appeared to date. Rich et al. reported on a small number of 13 male homosexual decedents (ages 21–42) who were compared to 106 other male decedents in a large psychological autopsy study. No attempt was made to establish the incidence or prevalence of gay suicide. What was of significance in this study was the finding of "few if any differences" between young gay and straight males. Both groups had high rates of prior attempts and prior psychiatric treatment. No significant differences in categories of stressors were found. All the gay male decedents were diagnosable (postmortem) with 12 of the 13 having a history of drug and/or alcohol abuse. The only significant diagnostic difference between groups was a history of schizophrenia among the gays. The other difference of note was in suicide method, with gays being more likely to hang themselves.

With regard to parasuicidal behavior, Clark (1992) has appropriately noted that there have been no truly representative community-based studies comparing suicide rates in homosexual versus heterosexual communities. Clark goes on to recognize the difficulty in ascertaining sexual orientation in epidemiological studies. Underreporting in this culture may be expected due to the stigma attached to openly affirming one's identity.

Data reported in the 1970s were summarized by Harry (1989) and do suggest higher rates of suicide attempt among homosexual versus heterosexual comparison groups. Saghir and Robins (1973) found an attempt rate of 7% among a sample of 89 homosexual males while none of their 35 heterosexual controls reported suicide attempts (the respective proportions for lesbians and heterosexual women were 12% and 5%). Bell and Weinberg (1978) reported a sixfold increase in the prevalence of attempts for gay males (18% vs. 3%) and a much smaller imbalance for lesbians (23% vs. 14%). In a noncontrolled sample of homosexual males, Roesler and Deisher (1972) found 32% admitting to a history of attempt and among a clinical population of psychiatric outpatients reported on by Woodruff, Clayton, and Guze (1972) the proportion of attempters peaked at 50%, four times that of a heterosexual comparison group.

Of research samples of the late 1980s (all studied without comparison to nonhomosexual comparison or control groups), Yates, MacKenzie, and Pennbridge (1988) reported that 53% of gay street youth had attempted suicide, 90% of these attempters having histories of multiple attempts. Among a sample of 108 men drawn from participants in either gay college student organizations or gay community center rap groups, 21% reported a history of prior attempt, with 44% of these having made more than one attempt (Schneider, Farberow, & Kruks, 1989). Ranmefedi, Farrow, and Deiher (1991) sampled 137 gay and bi-

sexual males recruited through newspapers and referrals and found slightly higher proportions: 30% had a history of at least one attempt and slightly less than half had made two or
more attempts. Ramefedi et al. (1991) also found that 85% of attempters reported illicit
drug use, a finding supportive of Rich et al.'s (1986) regarding substance abuse among completers. Of particular interest, Ramefedi et al. (1991) reported that the most frequently stated reason for their subjects' suicide attempts was "family problems" (44%), not "turmoil
with homosexuality" (33%).

Only recently have case–control studies begun to appear. Ramefedi, French, Story,
Resnick, and Blum (1998) studied Minnesota high school youth, finding significantly
more suicidal ideation and attempts self-reported by gay and bisexual males than by
matched heterosexuals. Two Massachusetts studies, based on the Centers for Disease
Control's Youth Risk Behavior Survey, found a greater proportion of active homosexual
and bisexual teens to report suicide attempts in the past year than among heterosexual
teens (Faulkner & Cranston, 1998: 27% vs. 13%) and a greater proportion of teens self-
identifying as gay, lesbian, or bisexual in their orientation to state that they had made a
suicide attempt (35%) than did their heterosexual peers (10%) (Garofalo et al., 1998). A
similar study among Vermont teens (DuRant, Krowchuk, & Sinal, 1998) reported increased rates of self-reported lifetime suicide attempts among male students with multiple
same-sex partners.

Can anything reliably be concluded from these findings? It appears premature to make
definitive conclusions, but perhaps we can venture the following:

1. We have no hard evidence to support higher suicide rates, no less an "epidemic," of
   completed suicide among gay and lesbian teenagers.
2. Among nonclinical samples, the proportion of gay males with a history of suicide
   attempts appears to range from about 20% to 35% and to be about twice that of
   heterosexual males. Roughly one-half of attempters make two or more attempts.
3. Among more disturbed samples (e.g., runaway gay males) perhaps as many as one
   in two have engaged parasuicidal behavior.
4. If validated by better research, these proportions are roughly two to three times
   what would be expected of appropriate comparison samples. (We urge readers to
   consult Moscicki, Muehrer, & Potter, 1995 [see "Further Reading"], for a much
   more sophisticated review of the research needs in this area.)
5. The prevalence of parasuicide among samples of lesbians may be even higher than
   those of gay males. However, given that parasuicidal behavior is much more common among females in general, these proportions may not be significantly greater
   than those of heterosexual female youth. The lesbian population is rarely represented in the published research to date.

It may be hypothesized that the anxiety of declaring their homosexuality to their family or to the wider society is experienced by gay male attempters as the primary stressor precipitating their attempts, more than the internal conflict inherent in coming to terms with
being gay. This may be true particularly in the family in which violence in response to the
gay adolescent's sexual orientation is not uncommon (Prenzlauer, Drescher, & Winchel,
1992). Hendin (1992) supports this notion, providing anecdotal evidence from his studies
of college student suicide. Of those male and female homosexuals among suicide attempters
he studied, Hendin states, "In every case there was a history of early maternal abandonment
which was not present among (non-suicidal homosexual controls). Guilt or shame over being homosexual was not a significant factor in their suicidal behavior (1416)." Harry
(1989) proposes that the older age of the typical lesbian attempter (>20) compared to the

modal gay male attempter (<20) suggests that their attempts may be precipitated by depression consequent to the breakup of a relationship, rather than family conflict.

ACQUIRED IMMUNE DEFICIENCY SYNDROME AND SUICIDAL BEHAVIOR

There is one clear epidemic striking most perniciously in the gay and bisexual community: AIDS. First diagnosed in the United States in 1981, the number of AIDS cases reported worldwide by the end of 1997 was 1,736,958 (World Health Organization, 1999). The cumulative number of reported deaths from AIDS in 1997 worldwide was estimated to be 2.3 million (Osmond, 1998). In the United States, it is estimated that there were 57,000–60,000 new cases diagnosed each year between 1993 and 1996 (Centers for Disease Control and Prevention, 1998).

Although its pathogenesis remains unclear, the disease begins as an acute viral infection (HIV) and proceeds to an asymptomatic stage with as much as a 10-year latency before again becoming symptomatic and developing into full-blown AIDS. The disease is thought to be uniformly terminal, its last stages often involving neurological and wasting syndromes.

Men who have sex with men accounted for 60% of all AIDS cases diagnosed in 1997 (Centers for Disease Control and Prevention, 1997) and continue to be the primary group at risk for contracting the HIV infection through unsafe sexual practices. In spite of widespread preventive education regarding safe sex, disregard appears to be most common among those who who are younger, less well educated, less aware of their HIV serostatus, and intoxicated or use drugs during sexual activity (Valdisserri et al., 1988). The resulting disinhibition, itself a risk factor for suicidal behavior, may mask and potentiate an underlying gamble with death in risking disease transmission. For some, the gamble is more directly suicidal. Flavin, Franklin, and Frances (1986) describe three alcohol-dependent homosexual male patients who consciously and deliberately attempted to contract the disease as a means of committing suicide. All three had depressed mood and suicidal ideation and stated that they either lacked the courage or had found it difficult to directly kill themselves (see also Frances, Wikstrom, & Alcena, 1985).

Depression, psychosis, delerium, and dementia can all be associated with AIDS (Holland & Tross, 1985). Although these syndromes, in addition to the fact of AIDS's universal lethality, all would suggest that persons suffering from this diagnosis would be more at risk for suicide, it was not until 1988 that a definitive epidemiologic survey of known cases of suicide among persons with AIDS was published (Marzuk et al., 1988). This report was a bombshell. Marzuk et al. (1988) conducted a comprehensive case review of medical examiner records and a cross-match of the suicide registry with AIDS surveillance data in New York City for the year 1985. Finding 12 suicides among men ages 20–59 years with the diagnosis of AIDS, they calculated a suicide rate of 681/100,000. This rate was 36 times that of same-age men without the diagnosis and 66 times that of the general population. Persons with AIDS who completed suicide tended to be single, white, homosexual males, with a mean age of 38, who used violent means (jumping [7], hanging [2], firearms [1]) to suicide. Most occurred within 6 months of diagnosis, all within 9 months. All were in relatively early stages of AIDS with minimal evidence upon autopsy of physical or neurological wasting. Clark (1992) recalculated Marzuk et al.'s data to establish a rate specific to males with AIDS, ages 20–59, of 345/100,000, or 18 times that of same-age males.

A more recent national study of 165 suicides by persons with AIDS occuring between 1987 and 1989 was reported by Cote, Bigger, and Dannenberg (1992). This study found a rate of 165/100,000, about seven times greater than among demographically similar men in the general population. In addition, they reported a significant decline in risk from 1987 to 1989.

It is important to note that not all the suicides in the Marzuk et al. study were known to be gay or bisexual (75% were). However, there was no evidence of intravenous drug abuse or history of recent blood transfusion in the remaining cases. Engelman et al. (1988) reported on 13 AIDS-related suicides, all by homosexual males, ages 29–49 (mean age 39), occurring in San Francisco between 1981 and 1986. Although the incidence of AIDS-related suicide was not reported, the proportion of AIDS deaths which were suicides was less than 1%. The methods used were less violent than those of the New York sample (only four died by firearms, hanging, or jumping), and although five of these deaths occurred within the first 6 months of diagnosis (most of these in the first month and one within 5 days), six occurred 13–18 months after diagnosis, suggesting a bimodal distribution of risk. Engelman et al. (1988) also compared the proportion of AIDS-related white male suicides with that of white males with cancer and found a significant difference.

The disease process of AIDS is generally divided into three stages. Thus, the differences found in this San Francisco study (relative to that in New York City) may suggest different stages of risk. It appears clear that those recently diagnosed with AIDS have significant suicide risk. It is at this stage that panic, depression, guilt, and hopelessness may impair one's ability to deal with the diagnosis. The newly diagnosed may lack information about what to expect and may not understand that supportive resources are available. After a midstage (with perhaps a second bout of pneumocystis or advanced Kaposi sarcoma lesions), last-stage issues of pain, dependency, confusion, and loss of bodily functions may inspire new motivations toward suicide (Goldblum & Moulton, 1986).

Until the recent epidemiological studies appeared, nearly all reports of increased suicidality associated with AIDS or HIV had been anecdotal (cf. Pierce, 1987; Frierson & Lippman, 1988). Although these more scientific investigations have begun to inform us of differential suicide risk across the various stages of AIDS (the most severe mainfiestation of HIV infection), they yet fail to signify that risk may be elevated across the entire spectrum of the disease process (i.e., beginning with knowledge of HIV seropositivity). The first published report regarding suicide among those with HIV infections came from Sweden (Rajs & Fugelstad, 1992). In this study, all suicides in Stockholm between 1985 and 1990 where the decedent was found to be HIV positive or to have AIDS were examined. Of the 85 HIV deaths identified (80% male), only one-fourth were homosexual or bisexual males. Twenty-one (25%) of these 85 deaths were suicides, with 12 of these (57%) being homosexual or bisexual males (mean age 37). Five of these 12 gay male suicides had reached the stage of having AIDS. Thus, the majority of these suicides (71%) had asymptomatic HIV infections. In only two cases had the decedent recently learned of his seropositivity. Case 6.1 presents a case of a young man who appeared to seek HIV infection while keeping his sexual orientation secret.

Kessler et al. (1988), in a longitudinal study of gay men, determined that the perception of symptoms ("psychological appraisal") mediated emotional distress in HIV-seropositive subjects more than the biological symptoms themselves. Similarly, Kurdek and Siesky (1990) reported that asymptomatic AIDS patients had significantly more psychological distress than either symptomatic seropositive or seronegative patients. Several studies (Holland & Tross, 1985; Nichols, 1983; Perry & Jacobsen, 1986) have documented a high incidence of depression among HIV-infected patients. One study documented rates of suicide ideation to be highest in the 2 weeks preceeding HIV testing, remaining higher in seropositive subjects in the week after notification of status (Perry, Jacobsberg, & Fishman, 1990). Others (e.g., Zich & Temoshok, 1987) have found less perceived social support to be correlated with measures of depression and hopelessness among HIV-infected individuals

CASE 6.1. The Case of Peter

Peter had spent much of his 22 years attempting to hide and deny his sexual identity. From as early as he could remember he was different. The youngest of four siblings, he was always "the runt of the litter," small, thin, unathletic, uncoordinated, and eccentric in his interests. As a child, he was teased mercilessly by both his brothers and classmates. He learned to hide, to retreat into a fantasy world, and, later, into drugs and alcohol. He acted the part of "the weirdo" in high school, dressing strangely, always staying on the fringe. He never developed many social skills. He probably would have been diagnosed as "schizoid" had he been afforded the opportunity to see a psychotherapist.

At 15 he had his first sexual encounter. He was fellated in the men's room of a department store by an older man. Fellatio and masturbation became compulsive aims over the next several years. By the age of 18, he averaged 25 orgasms a month, mostly by masturbation, about a third through cruising for anonymous sexual encounters in men's rooms. Each of these illicit encounters was described as intense and satisfying. None ever led to a second encounter with the same person.

Relationships and romance were never sought. These were considered by Peter to be unacceptable, for they would solidify his identity as "gay." For that matter, so would anal intercourse, a sexual behavior he neither sought nor allowed. "I can't be gay," he would scream in protest. "If only I could meet the right woman, I would be straight," he would assert. But his interpersonal world centered on his men's room experiences.

Although having dreams of being a movie producer, Peter in fact worked as a secretary in a large hospital. By a trick of fate he was assigned to an AIDS ward and the AIDS ward bathroom became the site of his now not so anonymous trysts. On an unconscious level he may have been seeking the HIV infection, but on a conscious level he knew he would kill himself, if he became HIV positive. That would mean his secret would be out, that he would be exposed and disowned by his family. His identity as gay would be validated. Consequently, he refused to allow himself to be tested. He continues to dodge the bullet he seems to be inviting.

Source: Anonymous.

GENDER DYSPHORIAS

When one's gender identity and role do not conform to the norms considered appropriate for one's anatomical sex, "gender dysphoria" or "gender transposition" occurs (Money & Wiedeking, 1980). These terms encompass transvestism and cross-genderism. In its most extreme form, transsexualism, the individual usually feels from an early age that he or she was born into the wrong body anatomically and that he or she has the personality of, and thus belongs to, the opposite sex. Transsexuals have a persistent preoccupation with being the opposite sex and strongly desire to be transformed surgically and hormonally. Typically associated with this desire is a moderate to severe personality disorder, anxiety, and depression attributed to the inability to live the role of the desired sex (American Psychiatric Association, 1987).

For a few male transsexuals, angry at not being able to obtain or frustrated by the slow pace of getting a surgical transformation to the desired sex, self-surgery in the form of auto-castration (a form of "focal suicide"; Menninger, 1938) sometimes occurs. Krieger, McAnninch, and Weimer (1980) have described three such cases of males literally taking matters into their own hands and removing their testicles. These cases appear different from those genital self-mutilations precipitated by psychotic processes (see Krieger et al., 1980; Pabis, Masood, & Tozman, 1980). However, it appears safe to conclude that these and other forms of severe self-mutilation (e.g., eye enucleation) are certain signs of major psychopathology, such as schizophrenia and mania (Favazza, 1989). With regard to more direct suicidal behaviors, Huxley and Brandon (1961) found that as much as 53% of English transsexuals had a history of suicide attempt. There appears to be only one control group study in the literature. Langevin, Paitich, and Steiner (1977) reported greater frequency of attempt among male transsexuals still living as males compared to those living as females. In turn, these proportions were greater than those of gay patients, gay nonpatients, and straight nonpatients. Without more empirical study of this subgroup, it is difficult to conclude that these findings document significant risk, although these results may be intuitively compelling.

SEXUALITY AND SUICIDE

Maris (1989) has summarized a number of intriguing similarities between sexuality and suicide. Citing Becker's (1973) seminal work, *The Denial of Death*, he notes that promiscuous sexuality attempts to deny the finitude and decay essential to being human. That is, as an ephemeral and temporary pleasure, sex actively attempts to deny death (a "removal activity" involving fleeting ecstasy) and the powerlessness and lack of control we exert over it.

Both sex and parasuicide are drives, "primitive forces that are difficult to deny" (Weisman, 1967), often acted on impulsively and passionately, with intent to decrease tension. As an example, consider the following poem (included in Berman & Jobes, 1991), written by an 18-year-old college sophomore. Try to distinguish the author's meaning. Is his ideation suicidal, is he describing the thrill of excessive risk taking, is this an erotic/masturbatory fantasy, or what?

> My search continues for a blade.
> A razor's edge to skin the fox
> To determine the entrails' configuration
> To ascertain the color of his blood.
>
> My hand jerks down and immortality
> Rises within my soul, with fright
> The dial sweeps from left to right
> Propelling me towards ecstasy again.
>
> My eyes scrutinize the frictionless surface.
> A meticulous search for the final obstacle
> That will jettison my corporeal body
> From reality to hell, via mutilation.
>
> But I will not have existed without fear,
> A surname for insanity, delight.
> In my final wild ride, I change
> Dimensions, entering through a violent,
> Scarlet porthole.

For many individuals both sexual acts and suicidal behavior defend against loneliness and loss of love, serving instrumental and interpersonal goals as attempts to exert control over others, to communicate, to manipulate, and so on. For those driven to sexual acting out, a partial sacrifice of the self in defense of a sagging ego, the consequence of failing to gain control (or love) is a further assault to the ego. Thus suicide risk increases with sexual acting out, which becomes an additional risk factor along the suicidal pathway (see Maris, 1981). Illustrative of this point, Stephens (1987) described one of two types of female adolescents who as adults attempted suicide as fitting a "cheap thrills" pattern of behavior. These girls decribed themselves as "wild" and "unmanageable." They repeatedly ran away from home, used drugs, got into physical confrontations, and had frequent indiscriminant sexual escapades often resulting in pregnancy.

Maris (1981, 1989) states that low-lethality suicide attempts are only partially self-destructive. For some individuals they may even make life possible. In this regard, repetitive suicide attempts represent a sort of "vocation," a way of staying alive through a form of psychic surgery. Maris uses the suicidal career of Sylvia Plath to illustrate this point, describing "a series of doomed, often sadomasochistic, relationships with men" (Maris, 1981: 130) prior to her final and lethal attempt. Similarly, the suicide of the Pulitzer Prize-winning poet Anne Sexton at age 45 culminated an 18-year courtship with suicide, for whom her ultimate death was described by her biographer as an *idée fixe* (Middlebrook, 1991; Hendin, 1993). Sexton's suicidality led to several long-term psychoanalytic treatments, involving intense transferences. To Dr. Martin Orne, her therapist for 8 years, she wrote, "I would like to lie down beside you and go to sleep, and you will never leave me because I am a good girl. . . . My father was a king. The king can have sex with anyone" (Middlebrook, 1991: 403). After her therapy with Orne ended (when he took a position in another city), Sexton had a sexual affair with her next psychiatrist (Hare-Mustin, 1992). One observer described Sexton as a "perverse exhibitionist" (Kaplan, 1992); she was hospitalized 20 times and had made countless suicide attempts before her last and fatal attempt.

Finally, it should be observed that the association between death and sexuality has been personified in the figure of the Harlequin. This double agent of love and death was used by Wold (1971) as a characterization of one distinct type of suicidal person (the "Harlequin syndrome") who contacted the Los Angeles Suicide Prevention Center. The Harlequin syndrome described women who eroticized death. They led a masochistic lifestyle, had a poor self-image covered by a facade of femininity, and were alienated from others. Death, the dark, mysterious lover, is seductive, looked forward to with pleasure. In this regard, readers will perhaps note again Sexton's first line written to her therapist, "I would like to lie down beside you and go to sleep. . . ."

AUTOEROTIC ASPHYXIA

For some, death and self-harm may be courted, played with as in a game of chicken. Like Russian roulette, the intent of the game is not directly suicidal. The aim may even be antisuicidal. Instead of seeking extinction (nonlife), its goal is either that of tension reduction or sensation (arousal) seeking. One form of this behavior, in which sexual behavior and dangerous risk taking are melded, is sexual or "autoerotic" asphyxia.

Autoerotic asphyxia is an arcane, typically private masturbatory behavior involving bondage. Its prevalence is impossible to estimate, but it leads to self-inflicted (usually unintentional) deaths of as many as 1,000 victims annually in the United States (Burgess & Hazelwood, 1983). It is almost exclusively practiced by males, mostly adolescent and young adult. Of 132 deaths investigated by Burgess and Hazelwood (1983), only 5 were female.

Death from this activity results from anoxia caused by constriction of the neck during masturbation. The victim typically ties a rope or ligature around his neck (and sometimes the genitals) to produe constriction of the blood vessels in the neck and, consequently, the blood flow to the brain. The aim of this behavior is to heighten sensation through production of an altered state of consciousness. Protective padding between the skin and ligature and self-rescue mechanisms (slip knots, a knife to cut the rope, etc.) are often used or kept available. However, for some individuals miscalculations, malfunctions, or simply the loss of control associated with ejaculation may carry the anoxia too far, causing the victim to black out and to die.

The typical victim is found nude or partially clothed (about one in five are cross-dressed, typically in female undergarments), in front of a mirror. Pornographic material as a fantasy aid, mechanical aids (e.g., vibrators), or other stimulants are often present. Case 6.2 presents a case of autoerotic asphyxia.

SUICIDE, SELF-INJURIOUS BEHAVIOR, AND SEXUAL ABUSE

By day we were a perfect family. My father, a doctor; successful, well-respected, a giver to those he cared for, those he loved, those in the community less fortunate than we. By day, he was a saint; a man incapable of evil. By night, in my bed, he taught me something different, and he taught me that it never happened. . . . (Anonymous)

Sexual victimization, particularly at the hands of a parent, creates an overwhelming sense of powerlessness, worthlessness, and a felt inability to change or control one's environment. It creates self-loathing, in particular feelings of being dirty, a body loathing. It facilitates internalized feelings of shame, not the guilt of feeling one has done something bad, but a more pervasive sense of being bad. It creates self-blame (Shapiro, 1992).

To be able to survive, I learned to go away. To go away meant some part of me could stay clean, untouched by evil. I learned to exist outside of my body. I refused all awareness of its pain, and paid the price of not knowing its pleasure. I chose to kill a part of my self so I could survive. (Anonymous)

CASE 6.2. A Case of Autoerotic Asphyxiation

The victim, a 27-year-old male, was found nude, hanging in his home bedroom. A cloth was placed between the fatal noose and his neck. Near the body was found a variety of sadomasochistic paraphernalia. A nipple clamp was attached to the decedent's right breast nipple; lubricant cream and several "S&M" magazines were on the bed.

The decedent was an active homosexual with known sadomasochistic and autoerotic behavior. Approximately 1 year prior to his death he had a near fatal autoerotic asphyxiation. After this incident, his brother reported that the decedent had told him he was embarrassed by the rope burns still visible on his neck. Since then, he apparently made it a practice to use a cloth between the rope and his neck.

Source: Anonymous.

Childhood sexual abuse commonly leads to pathological sequelae, most often the development of dissociative states, including multiple personalities, the instability and rage characterized by borderline states, and comorbid unipolar or bipolar depressions. Self-injurious (self-mutilative) attacks on the body (see next section) can be associated with these disorders and with the legacies of early childhood.

While the empirical literature documents a strong relationship between sexual child abuse and subsequent psychiatric problems (cf. Carmen, Rieker, & Mills, 1984), including the development of suicidal ideation and behavior (Briere & Runtz, 1986; Deykin, Alpert, & McNamarra, 1985), it remains unclear whether abuse leaves the child more vulnerable to suicide in particular (Spirito, Stark, Fristad, Hart, & Owens-Stively, 1987). In addition, the severity, duration, and frequency of abuse may be significant codeterminants of subsequent, maladaptive symptoms and behavior.

Shaunesey, Cohen, Plummer, and Berman (1993) investigated the effects of sexual abuse during childhood on later adolescent suicidal behavior. Among a sample of 117 privately hospitalized adolescents (ages 13–18), 36 (30.8%) had a history of sexual abuse. Twenty of these adolescents (56%; 17.1% of the entire sample) had been both sexually and physically abused. Sexually abused patients reported significantly more previous suicide attempts than did those reporting no abuse, irrespective of frequency and duration of that abuse. Females in this study were found to have been significantly more likely than males to have experienced both physical and sexual abuse and were more likely to make suicide attempts. Shaunesey et al. conjecture that the higher frequency of attempts among females may be linked to a history of sexual abuse rather than simply to the fact of being female.

SELF-MUTILATION AND GENDER

As noted previously, some forms of self-mutilation can be quite extreme. Most common are wrist cutting and cigarette burning, typically of the arms. As described by Walsh and Rosen (1988) and Favazza (1989; cf. Favazza, 1996), the most common function and goal of these self-mutilative behaviors is to decrease tension or other intense affect, diminish a sense of alienation, or terminate dissociation (see Case 6.3). Thus, these behaviors are a form of self-stimulation designed to break out of the numbness or deadness otherwise common to these patients' everyday experience—a sort of "I bleed, therefore I am." These patients most often are diagnosed as borderline personality disorders and often present with a comorbid mood or dissociative disorder, and, as noted earlier, often are found in patients with a history of sexual abuse. These patients are more commonly women than men.

SUMMARY AND CONCLUSIONS

Gender plays a complex and important role in suicidal behavior. By early adolescence, males behave more lethally than females and differences in mortality rates continue across the entire lifespan and across cultures. Male suicide appears most significantly tied to an overall greater frequency and level of violence and aggression and the relative lack of social sanction for accepting a helpless-dependent position in a help-giving relationship. On the other hand, the significance of relatedness to others and the importance of social supports appears to serve women most profoundly both as a protection against suicidal urges and as a precipitant for nonfatal suicidal behavior.

With the increased androgyny in U.S. society and entry of great numbers of females into the traditionally male workplace came predictions of male and female suicide rates re-

CASE 6.3. The Case of Suzanne

Berman and Jobes (1991: 81–82) present the case of Suzanne, a 19-year-old female, who presented for outpatient therapy complaining of feeling "locked up" and scared. She had a long history of multiple somatic complaints and had been considerably overweight since puberty. While in an inpatient weight-control program she observed and felt pressured to join promiscuous and perverse group sexual activity among her fellow patients. In response, she began to experience fainting spells accompanied by visual hallucinations of menacing male figures making sexual advances toward her.

By puberty, Suzanne felt conflicted by the doting attention of her father, both wanting his attention and uncomfortable with its Oedipal implications. To complete the Oedipal triad, her mother, a perfectionist, harped on Suzanne's unattractiveness, particularly on her weight and her large breasts. Suzanne incorporated rigid rules for her acceptability (e.g., to be perfect and to not show problems or feelings). When she violated these demands, she began to hear voices urging her to punish herself. She then would have a dissociative episode which ended by the pain inflicted by self-cutting or burning behavior. She chose body sites for these behaviors which were hidden from public view (consistent with her need to not show herself to others) and associated with her unacceptable sexuality (she slashed at her breasts and burned in the area of her uterus, fulfilling her mother's competitive dominance as a female).

gressing toward the mean. However, recent epidemiological trends suggest just the opposite. There is in fact a growing divergence of rates, with male rates increasing and female rates decreasing. At the same time, there is an increasing trend for females to behave like males in their selection of firearms as the modal method of choice to complete suicide. We await further empirical data to assess the relationship of gender identity or gender orientaion on suicide. It appears that our understanding of suicide among homosexuals may be confounded by the significant involvement of substance abuse in these suicides. The impact of AIDS (particularly in the gay community) does appear to be significant as a predisposing condition for depression, decreased social support, increased hopelessness, and thus suicidality. Risk for suicidal behavior, also, must be considered high for serious gender dysphoric conditions such as transsexualism, in which we may expect to find a high frequency of comorbid personality disorders.

Finally, we explored the relationship between sex and suicide, with particular concern for autoeroticism, the impact of childhood sexual abuse, and self-mutilative behaviors. Throughout these discussions winds the binding thread of mental disorder as a predisposing and confounding variable for suicidal behavior (see Chapter 13).

FURTHER READING

Canetto, S. S., & Lester, D. (Eds.). (1995). *Women and suicidal behavior*. New York: Springer. In 19 chapters this excellent edited volume reviews the epidemiology, theories, and research regarding suicidal women. The editors develop hypotheses about suicidal women from a female perspective and emphasize sociocultural factors (social class, social support, gender socialization, etc.) in contrast to psychological determinants of suicidal behavior.

Canetto, S. S., & Silverman, M. M. (Eds.). (1988). Gender, culture, and suicidal behavior [Special issue]. *Suicide and Life-Threatening Behavior, 28*(1). This special issue of this journal consists of 10 articles reporting on interactions between gender and culture on five continents, and their effects on suicidal behaviors, particularly among women.

Maris, R. W. (1971). Deviance as therapy: The paradox of the self-destructive female. *Journal of Health and Social Behavior, 12,* 114–124. Maris contends that nonfatal suicide attempts by females are most appropriately conceived of as partial self-destruction to the end of making life possible, not ending it. In this sense, females attempt suicide as a defense against feelings of worthlessness and inadequacy.

Middlebrook, D. W. (1991). *Anne Sexton: A biography.* Boston: Houghton Mifflin. Middlebrook, a literary teacher and critic, offers us a fascinating look at the life and death of poet Anne Sexton, who completed suicide in 1974. This is biography as psychological autopsy; a character study of a seriously disturbed woman and chronic suicide risk with repetitive, often exhibitionistic attempts, and of a professional patient.

Moscicki, E. K., Muehrer, P., & Potter, L. B. (Eds.). (1995). Research issues in suicide and sexual orientation. *Suicide and Life-Threatening Behavior, 25* (Suppl.). An archive of presentations made to a national conference on this topic, convened by the American Association of Suicidology, the Centers for Disease Control and Prevention, and the National Institute of Mental Health. The focus is on the need for sound empirical research on the topic of gay, bisexual, and lesbian suicide.

Wold, C. (1971). Subgroupings of suicidal people. *Omega, 2,* 19–29. On the basis of a review of many thousands of case files from callers to the Los Angeles Suicide Prevention Center, Wold empirically derives and describes a typology of suicides that is gender specific. Among those more commonly found to be women were the "discarded women," the "I can't live with you," the "I can't live without you," and "malignant masochist" types; in contrast, males are more commonly found among the "down and out, unstable" and "violent" types.

7

Racial, Ethnic, and Cultural
Aspects of Suicide

Throughout a turbulent history of slavery, legal segregation, civil rights
protests, and controversy over affirmative action, African-Americans have
traditionally had low suicide rates compared to White Americans. . . . This
phenomenon has puzzled many social scientists because of the apparent
paradox between the disadvantaged status of African-Americans and their
infrequen use of suicide as a solution to their problems.
                                            —JEWELLE TAYLOR GIBBS

Imagine that you were an anthopology graduate student attempting to do field work on suicide among the Tiv of Nigeria in central Africa. Much to your amazement and chagrin you
discover that suicide is virtually nonexistent among the Tiv. It turns out that suicide rates
vary immensely throughout the world. In some countries, racial groups, or cultures (such as
the Tiv) suicide rates are almost zero, and it is conceivable that the locals may not even
know what you are talking about, whereas in other places (such as Hungary, Germany,
Lithuania, or Finland) and groups suicide rates are so high as to almost be part of the national character (see Chapter 3, Table 3.5).

We know that suicide is rare among the Tiv of Nigeria, Andaman Islanders, and
Australian aborgines (Goldney denies this), and it is relatively infrequent (as the opening
quote by Gibbs indicates) among rural southern black females in the United States (about
2 per 100,000 per year) and Irish Roman Catholics (in spite of their obvious drinking traditions). The *highest* suicide rates in the world are found in Hungary, Lithuania, the
Falkland Islands, the Federal Republic of Germany, Austria (in spite of being a predominantly Catholic country), Scandinavia (especially Sweden, Denmark, and Finland), and
Japan. Some of the *lowest* suicide rates are found in Egypt, Malta, several South
American, Pacific islands, and mainly Catholic countries (note: religion and cults are considered separately, in Chapter 19—including Antigua, Jamaica, New Guinea, the Philippines, Mexico, Italy, and Ireland.

Several times Maris traveled to and lived for months in high-suicide-rate countries in
an effort to partially immerse himself in the culture and daily routine of highly self-destructive places. For example, Maris lived in Vienna, West Berlin, Calgary (Alberta), and Helsinki. Without suggesting any causal associations (yet at the same time suggesting the presence

of a morbid, suicidogenic culture), Maris was struck by the stuffed dead baby animal petting museum on the Ring-Strasse in Vienna and by being chastised by natives to "stay off the grass" in the city parks. In the winter, Helsinki was a land of almost perpetual darkness, Finlandia vodka, and the manufacture of ice-breaker ships. West Berlin had an excessive number of aged widows and widowers and shared the same somber death culture that was experienced in Vienna. Calgary was a boom–bust city with many anomic factors and a macho cowboy/gun mentality.

Of course, readers may become justifiably skeptical and uneasy at these characterizations. Admittedly, race, ethnicity, and culture are major factors in diffentiating human populations, as are age, gender, occupation, mental status, marital status, and so on. But that is the problem: How do we rule out interaction effects? For example, is it the race, the gender, the age, the religion, the family ties, and so on, that produces the low suicide rates of African American females? Again, it could be that suicides and their subcultures in certain countries are suicidal precisely because they are *different* from the prevailing national culture. An important caveat: Always remember that suicide is a multifactorial outcome with many complex interaction effects and individual case qualifers.

Before we proceed with this chapter we need to define key terms. By "race" we mean a division of a species that differs from other divisions by the frequency with which certain inherited physical characteristics (especially skin color, hair, eye and nose shape, and illnesses) appear among its members. A "species" is a population in which any two healthy, sexually mature members of the opposite sex can mate and produce normal, fertile offspring. For our purposes we distinguish four principal races: Caucasoid, Negroid, Mongoloid, and Australoid. Of course, there could be hundreds of races, depending on which traits one chose to specify. In a brief overview of race and suicide we cannot cover all the nuances of racial or ethnic differentiation. Anthropologist Marvin Harris argues that it is impossible to set a limit on the number of races that could be identified.

"Ethnicity," on the other hand, refers to any group that can be set off by race, religion, or national origin. As such, ethnicity is more inclusive than race. It usually connotes national origin. A "culture" is a the total socially acquired lifeway or lifestyle of a particular group of people (Harris, 1971: 136). Language is a particularly important component of culture. Tylor's (1871: 1) classical definition of culture is that complex whole which includes knowledge, belief, art, morals, law, custom, and any other capabilities and habits acquired by man as a member of society.

Finally, a "minority" is any group of people who, because of their physical or cultural characteristics, are singled out for differential and unequal treatment by the majority, and who are, thus, objects of collective discrimination. Of course, it is logically possible that a minority could be a numerical majority (e.g., blacks in South Africa or females in the United States).

In the remainder of this chapter, three major sections are devoted to (1) suicide and race, (2) national character, and (3) cultural variations in suicide. In the section on race, we examine Caucasian, black, and Asian suicides (see Box 7.2, on the novelist/actor Yukio Mishima). More precisely, we review the work of Hendin (1969), Gibbs (1997), and Nisbet (1996) (on young black males and females) and Bohanan (1960) (on Africans), and the research of Headley (1983), Shiang et al. (1997), and Iga (1993) on Asian suicides. We begin our examination of nationality and ethnicity by discussing the World Health Organization's epidemiological study on suicide and attempted suicide in Europe (Schmitke et al., 1994). Special attention is given to Hungary, Germany, Scandinavia, and Austria. Finally, we investigate cultural variations in suicide (usually of Durkheim's altruistic or anomic varieties) among the Yuit Eskimos, Firth's Tikopian islanders, South Americans in Buenos Aires, and native Americans.

RACIAL ASPECTS OF SUICIDE

Suicide among White Populations

In a sense this entire textbook focuses on suicide among older *white* males, with a case such as that of novelist Ernest Hemingway (presented in Chapter 1, Case 1.1) being fairly typical. However, it may not be whiteness that elevates suicide rates. Whiteness may be just a marker for other causal factors, such as higher socioeconomic status, power, relative social isolation, reluctance to seek psychiatric treatment, and so on. Having made these qualifications, it is striking and dramatic that in the United States about 90% of all suicides are by whites (see Figure 7.1; cf. Chapter 3, Table 3.2, for 1996 data). Oversimplifying, suicide in the West is primarily a disease of older white males. Older white males have far and away the highest U.S. suicide rates compared to any other age or gender group (see Figure 7.2).

Of course, we need to control for varying sizes of the races by using *rates*, which is accomplished in Figure 7.2 (cf. Table 3.2). When we do so, the following race/gender suicide ratios (in the United States in 1996) are derived:

> White males (WM):black males (BM) = 1.6
> White males:white females (WF) = 3.9
> White males:black females (BF) = 9.8
> White females:black females = 2.6
> White females:black males = 0.4
> Black males:black females = 6.0

Generally, white U.S. suicide rates exceed black suicide rates by a ratio of roughly two to one (e.g., WM:BM = 1.6 and WF:BF = 2.6). However, white male suicide rates are on average about 10 times (9.8) those of black females. Maleness is a powerful suicidogenic force, such that black male rates exceed those of white females (ratio = 2.4). Black male rates exceed those of black females more (6.0) than those of white males exceed the white female suicide rates (a ratio of 3.9).

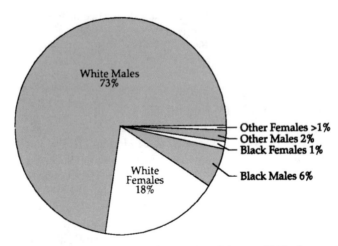

FIGURE 7.1. Distribution of suicides by race and sex, United States, 1992. *Source:* Kachur, Potter, James, & Powell (1995: 9).

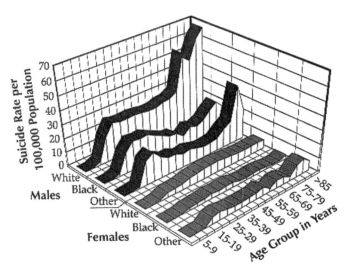

FIGURE 7.2. Age specific suicide rates by race and sex, United States, 1992. *Source:* Kachur, Potter, James, & Powell (1995: 11).

We can also see in Figure 7.2 that the highest suicide rates are to be found among *older* white males: 67.6 at age 85 and higher. The same race/age relationship tends to be true for black (and other) males as well, except that black males do not peak as sharply in the older ages and tend to have high rates in the 25-to-34 age group (Table 7.1). White female suicide rates tend to peak at ages 50–54 and those of black females at ages 30–34, although black females have exceedingly low suicide rates throughout their entire life cycle. When we examine the race/gender ratios of the *highest* suicide rates (e.g., in old age), several of the white male excesses are even more pronounced. Now white male rates exceed black female rates about 18 to 1, white males exceed black males 3 to 1, and white males exceed white females 8 to 1.

Oversimplifying, high suicide rates tend to occur *internationally* among white ethnics (among Hungarians, Finns, Austrian, Danes, the French, Swiss, Czechs, Germans, Swedes, Yugoslavians, etc.; see Table 3.4). When there is a racial high suicide rate exception (e.g., among the Japanese), it is usually argued that the type of suicide varies, too. For example, Japanese suicides tend to be Durkheim's altruistic or anomic types. The assumption is that white suicides tend to be what Durkheim called "egoistic" and depressed types. Hispanics, blacks, and Asians worldwide tend to have low to moderate suicide rates.

Most *explanations* are not of white suicides per se but, rather, of suicides of blacks, Asians, Hispanics, Native Americans, and so on, as contrasted with white suicides (see Henry & Short, 1954; Maris, 1969: 103–107). The argument goes that when white males get into suicidal trouble (e.g., when personal, social, or economic frustration, depressive disorder, or social isolation occurs), whites find it more difficult to blame others than blacks do and, thus, are more likely to aggress against themselves (although, of course, it is more complicated than this). Older white males are less likely to seek and get treatment and have less social support or social constraints than American blacks do. Older white males in the United States tend to have a combination of suicidogenic forces—that is, relatively more power, more social isolation (less social support) and autonomy, more willingness and means to aggress (than females, one should overlook possible hormonal differences as well), more guilt, more perceived responsibility for their own life situations, less willing to seek treatment, fewer alternatives to ventilate accumulated aggression (e.g., less proclivity for homicide or assault), and so on. However, to really test all these hypotheses emprically (and, of course, they are just hypotheses, not facts), one would need to contrast racial rates, controlling for social isolation, depressive disorder, age, gender, alcoholism, culture, presence of a gun, and so on. Until then, the previous ideas are mere speculation. And we all know that speculation is cheap and knowledge is hard to come by.

Suicide among Black (African American) Populations

Typically blacks, especially black females in rural southern United States, have had very low suicide rates. For example, in Table 3.5 there are no black countries (no African countries) with high suicide rates—with the single possible exception of Ceylon/Sri Lanka, an Asian/Indian island of Hindus and Buddhists under British rule. Of course, the term "black" glosses over many racial and cultural subtleties and differences. "Black suicide," in short, is not a homogeneous category. If we had the data to examine, we would probably find as much variation *within* blacks as between nonblacks and blacks.

From the very beginning of Maris's career he has been interested in black suicides. His first book on suicide in Chicago (Maris, 1969) examined possible protective factors in black suicides. For example, Maris found that areas with high populations per household tended to have low suicide rates and areas with low populations per household tended to have high suicide rates. That is, the lower the suicide rate, the more people per household. Specifically, high suicide rate areas in Chicago had on average 2.5 people per household versus 3.7 people in low suicide rate areas ($r = -.72$, $p = .01$). Although one has to be careful of committing the ecological fallacy (i.e., of imputing group characteristics to individuals), the areas with the lowest suicide rates were also predominantly black (52.9%) and the areas with the highest suicide rates had the lowest percentage of blacks (i.e., 8.2%).

As the tease to this chapter suggests, there has always been a paradox about black suicides. Blacks in the United States have more social, economic, and psychological frustration and adversity on average than whites do; yet they have *lower* suicide rates (cf. Henry & Short, 1954; Gibbs's opening quote in this chapter). Why is this? In the United States, black aggression is more likely to be other-directed (e.g., in the form of assault and homicide). It may be that others (not the self) are perceived as the source of black frustration, especially in the United States, with its conspicuous history of slavery and racism (although, like most things, the explanation is not this simple). If this is the case, then ironically blacks tend to assault or kill other blacks. It has been argued that in the United States, suicide and homicide are mutually exclusive choices. For example, in the South (United States), blacks have relatively low suicide rates but high homicide rates (apparently this is not the pattern in Africa, where homicide and suicide rates are often positively related; see Bohannan, 1960).

Transient domestic factors (such as marital conflict) or malfunctions of social interaction (negative interaction, if you will, *not* social isolation) seemed to be crucial factors among Maris's black Chicago suicides. There were also some of what Durkheim would have probably called "fatalistic suicides" among Chicago blacks; that is, suicides in response to hyperregulation (such as conflict with the police or jail and prison suicides; cf. Breed's work in the 1960s on New Orleans suicides, quoted in Hendin, 1969).

Herbert Hendin's early work (1969) and recent work by Jewelle T. Gibbs (1988, 1997) both emphasize the relatively high suicide rates among 20- to 35-year-old urban black males (see Table 7.1). Hendin comments on the murderous rage and self-hatred of young, urban, black males; especially in male homosexuals. Young urban blacks tend to have a

TABLE 7.1. Suicide Rates per 100,000 According to Sex, Race, and Age, 1960–1992

Age (years)	1960	1970	1980	1985	1992
Male					
White					
15–24	8.6	13.9	21.4	22.7	22.5
25–34	14.9	19.9	25.6	25.4	24.7
35–44	21.9	23.3	23.5	23.5	25.2
45–54	33.7	29.5	24.2	25.1	24.0
55–64	40.2	35.0	25.8	28.6	26.0
65–74	42.0	38.7	32.5	35.3	32.0
75–84	55.7	45.5	45.5	57.1	53.0
85–	61.3	50.3	52.8	60.3	67.6
Black					
15–24	4.1	10.5	12.3	13.3	17.3
25–34	12.4	19.2	21.8	19.6	19.2
35–44	12.8	12.6	15.6	14.9	16.9
45–54	10.8	13.8	12.0	13.5	12.4
55–64	16.2	10.6	11.7	11.5	10.1
65–74	11.3	8.7	11.1	15.8	11.8
75–84	6.6	8.9	10.5	15.6	18.5
85–	6.9	10.3	18.8	7.7	17.1
Female					
White					
15–24	2.3	4.2	4.6	4.7	4.1
25–34	5.8	9.0	7.5	6.4	5.0
45–54	10.9	13.5	10.2	9.0	7.9
55–64	10.9	12.3	9.1	8.4	7.2
65–74	8.8	9.6	7.0	7.3	6.3
75–84	9.2	7.2	5.7	7.0	6.6
85–	6.1	6.1	5.8	4.7	6.3
Black					
15–24	1.3	3.8	2.3	2.0	2.1
25–34	3.0	5.7	4.1	3.0	4.3
35–44	3.0	3.7	4.6	3.6	3.3
45–54	3.1	3.7	2.8	3.2	3.0
55–64	3.0	2.0	2.3	2.2	2.0
65–74	2.3	2.9	1.7	2.0	2.0
75–84	1.3	1.7	1.4	4.5	—
85–	—	3.2	—	1.4	3.0

Source: Gibbs (1997: 70). Copyright 1997 by The Guilford Press. Reprinted by permission.

stronger sense of despair and hopelessness (than young whites), both suicidogenic factors. Gibbs emphasizes black suicide risk factors of maleness (See Figure 7.2), substance abuse, depression, family dysfunction, marital conflict, and homosexuality.

At the same time, *black females* (as we observed earlier) in the United States have some of the *lowest* suicide rates of any other racial/gender group. Gibbs hypothesizes that religiosity, older age, southern region, and high social support are all suicide protective factors among black females. Paul Nisbet (1996) explored the issue of suicide protective factors among black females in his master's thesis. Using sophisticated statistical methods (LISREL), Nisbet analyzed data for 2,803 black females gathered from five U.S. sites as part of the NIMH Epidemiologic Catchment Area (ECA) project.

Among other things, he concluded that black females as a consequence of residing in larger households have an increase in the number of supportive familial ties (a network hypothesis). Although black females *attempt* suicide at about the same rate as white females do, having larger familial and friendship support resource systems seems to help keep suicide attempts among black females from becoming fatal (which may explain some of Gibbs's "puzzle" in the opening chapter quote; i.e., black females attempt suicide at about the same rate as other groups, but they are more protected from completing suicide).

White males, who we know tend to have the highest suicide rates, may experience a kind of "iatrogenesis" (illness or disease—here suicide—caused by health care). They seek professional (doctors, psychiatrists, psychologists, etc.) help more and familial support less than do black females, attempt suicide less (i.e., make fewer nonfatal attempts), but complete suicide at higher rates than black females do.

Of course, there may be other protective factors at work, too, for black females, such as religious values that regard suicide as prideful and sinful (see Early, 1992; cf. Davis, 1978), being psychologically "tempered" (like iron is physically tempered; this idea was suggested by George Murphy) by repeated coping with a long history of adversity and having many and intense family ties—especially more children to nurture, more absent husbands (such that suicide of the wife means abandonment and even destruction of her children), and, thus, more likelihood of being heads of single-parent families.

To be complete in our consideration of suicides of black Americans we probably should go back to some of the roots of black violence by citing African studies of suicide. Fortunately for all of us, anthropologist Paul Bohannan (1960) studied homicide and suicide among tribes in Uganda and Nigeria. He and his colleagues provide a wealth of individual case details about this neglected topic. *Un*fortunately, there is not much generic explanation of African suicides in Bohannan's research.

As in the United States, about two-thirds of African suicides were by males, and marital conflict was a major precursor of their suicides. Other common motives included physical distress and fear or shame by the suicide over his or her own prior misdeeds (see Box 7.1). Some African suicides were what Jeffreys (1952) called revenge or "Samsonic suicides" (as in the Old Testament of the Judeo-Christian Bible, where Samson gets even with the Romans by pulling down a coliseum's pillars—thereby killing his enemies and himself as well).

Most African suicides were by hanging. They were often regarded as irrational or as a sure sign that the victim was bewitched (e.g., that someone else wanted him dead). In Africa as in the United States, black homicide was more common (i.e., rates were higher) than black suicide. However, unlike in the United States, it was not uncommon to find tribes in which both the homicide and suicide rates were high. As we have seen, in the United States the argument has been that blacks and whites suffer similar frustrations (with most blacks having somewhat higher levels) but that socioeconomic conditions encourage black homicide and white suicide.

Suicide among Asian Populations

Typically Asians do not have excessively high suicide rates when contrasted internationally with primarily Caucasian countries. For example, of 71 countries in Table 3.5 (above), only Japan is ranked near the top (12th) and even in this case 11 non-Asian countries have higher suicide rates than Japan does. In Table 3.5, Singapore is 29th, Korea is 31st, and Hong Kong is 32nd. In many Asian countries suicide rates parallel the suicide patterns of the West, with suicide rates rising gradually with age and in general being higher

---

BOX 7.1. Suicide among the Gisu (Uganda)

"A person commits suicide if he finds too much trouble" Gisu say. Suicide, in their eyes, is a choice between the alternatives of life and death. Mental illness or insanity is not therefore considered to be a cause of suicide. A mentally unsound person is thought to be incapable of weighing the pros and cons of living and could have no inducement to commit suicide.

However, suicide is not entirely a reasoned decision. It is also a manifestation of *litima*, which is best translated "temper." This is a personal characteristic which, Gisu say, results in the possessor's being liable to fits of anger or violence, or unreasonable jealousy and spite. Gisu believe that traits of character are inherited and therefore a whole lineage or a group of kinsmen may be referred to as bad-tempered, in the sense of possessing *litima*, although they are reluctant to push the argument to its logical conclusion and say that a tendency to commit suicide may be inherited. They are equally reluctant to admit that a member of their own lineage or a close kinsman has committed suicide. Suicide is considered to be evil, for it results from strife, from bad relations between men, or between men and the ancestors.

Suicide is also thought to be contagious in the sense that physical contact with the body or surroundings of a suicide may cause the person who suffered contagion to commit suicide. For this reason the dead body must be removed from the place of death by someone entirely unrelated to the dead man and his kin; the service is repaid by the gift of a bull. A sheep must also be killed to pacify the spirit of the suicide, which is evil. A suicide's hut may be pulled down; it will certainly be smeared with the contents of a sheep's stomach, which is the material used for purification in all cases of ritual defilement. The chyme will be smeared on the agent of death (usually a rope or cord) and thrown round about the spot where the suicide took place. If the suicide hanged himself on a tree, it will be cut down and burnt. Nothing must be left which might cause another suicide by its contagious evil.

Source: Bohannan (1960: 111–112).

---

among males. An important qualification specific to the Orient is that usually Eastern suicide rates do not show as great a male–female difference as in the Occident (For example, see Table 7.2 for comparisons of male–female suicide rate differences in Singapore, Hong Kong, and Japan.)

Asian suicides, like black suicides, are not uniform. Diverse countries would be included in what can loosely be designated "Asian" (e.g., China, Japan, Thailand, Korea, Singapore, Vietnam, Taiwan, the Philippines, Sri Lanka, Burma, Mongolia, Laos, Malaysia, India, and perhaps even some Near Eastern countries such as Pakistan, Iran, and Iraq). (See, e.g., Headley, 1983).

Using Durkheim's typology, Asian suicides are often said to be more *altruistic* (i.e., resulting from insufficient individuation, moral obligations, duty, or self-sacrifice for a higher cause—such as *hara-kiri*, the *kamikaze* in World War II, or India's traditional custom of *suttee*, in which the wife of the deceased was obligated to join her husband on the funeral pyre) or in some cases more *anomic* (resulting from sudden deregulation, rapid social change, economic crisis, intense competition, or high expectations that are rigid and unrealistic—as in some Japanese suicides) (see Iga & Tatai, 1975: 255ff.; Iga, 1993: 301–323; Takahashi, 1997).

In Japan, suicide is permissible or even appropriate in some life circumstances. As a special case of Japanese suicide, consider the exhibitionistic, ritual suicide of Yukio Mishima (see Box 7.2). Mishima was a famous Japanese novelist and playwright who expected to

TABLE 7.2. Suicide Rates per 10,000 Population by Age Group and Sex, Singapore, Hong Kong, and Japan, 1972

Age group	Singapore		Hong Kong		Japan	
	Male	Female	Male	Female	Male	Female
5–14	—	0.7	—	0.6	0.8	0.3
15–24	8.0	7.9	6.8	4.8	18.5	12.4
25–34	10.9	13.3	25.7	13.2	27.0	14.0
35–44	12.6	1.5	19.0	10.7	20.6	11.9
45–54	33.7	9.5	25.7	19.0	23.5	15.0
55–64	58.4	7.4	32.8	17.8	33.1	23.5
65–74	132.1	40.5	52.1	21.1	57.8	49.5
77 and over	83.2	79.9	42.0	75.1	83.4	70.0

Source: Headley (1983: 118). Copyright 1983 by Lee A. Headley. Reprinted by permission.

win the Nobel prize for literature in 1967 or 1968 (it was won in fact by fellow countryman Yasunari Kawabata, for *A Thousand Cranes*). As a child, Mishima was raised primarily by his grandmother, who dressed and treated him as a girl. He was physically frail and led a protected life, mainly indoors. As an adult, Mishima became homosexual and was a fierce bodybuilder a reaction formation?), a champion of Samurai warriors and of Emperor worship. Mishima also became a celebrated movie actor, made millions of dollars, and even created his own private army. Yukio Mishima believed that one should die in the prime of life (his own death was at age 45). On November 11, 1970, Mishima and a few members of his private army captured a Japanese general and forced him to assemble his troops, then Mishima distributed leaflets and lectured the troops on Samurai values, urging them to help overthrow the government. Finally, he committed *hara-kiri* and had himself beheaded by one of his lieutenants.

More recently, Schiang et al. (1997) have studied Asian versus Caucasian suicides in San Francisco, California, and found several interesting differences between the two groups. Among other things Schiang found more female suicides among Asians (a female–male suicide rate ratio of 1 to 2 vs. 1 to 3 among Caucasians; cf. Table 7.3 on Beijing female–male rates) with especially higher suicide rates among very elderly females and a much greater use of hanging as a suicide method (see Figure 7.3). Hanging was a suicide method that was traditionally social and interpersonal in China. It implied great anger and resentment toward one's family or significant others and was seen as one way to get revenge (e.g., ghosts of the dead by hanging were thought to return to haunt the living). There was also much less prominence of alcohol and drugs in the Asian American suicides (8% vs. 31% among the Caucasian suicides). A major factor in the Chinese American suicides was the failure of younger family members of elderly suicides (especially of widowed females) to provide social support for their own aged mothers and fathers.

ETHNICITY, NATIONAL CHARACTER, AND SUICIDE

As we noted earlier in this chapter, ethnic groups are groups that are set apart from others because of their national origin (the Japanese, Germans, Scandinavians, Italians, Irish, Jews, Hispanics, Chinese, etc.) or distinctive cultural patterns (e.g., in the case of *hara-kiri*, *kamikaze, suttee,* or the Heaven's Gate ritual more recently; cf. Schaefer, 1998: 7). Ethnic minority groups are differentiated from the dominant group on the basis of cultural differ-

BOX 7.2. The Suicide of Yukio Mishima

Yukio Mishima, a Japanese novelist, committed suicide in 1970 by disemboweling himself and then having an assistant behead him, the ancient rite of *seppuku*. It may be hard to understand this act of suicide since our culture is so different from the Japanese. Stokes (1974), an Englishman, wrote a biography of Mishima, and we will rely on this to provide information about Mishima's life.

Mishima decided on the romantic image of death as a samurai. He would achieve hero status, and his death would bring together all of the threads in his life. The ideal of the samurai was the pursuit of Literature and the Sword, and Mishima set out to develop both paths.

There are several themes which were portents of Mishima's suicide. For example, in his literary endeavors, he began a long novel in four parts in 1965 that he would finish just prior to his suicide in 1970.

Mishima also became concerned about his physical body. He was a small man, about five foot four and he had loathed his body when he was young. Starting in 1955 he planned a rigorous program of exercise, body building and sun tanning. He specialized in kendo (fencing with a blunt lance), eventually receiving the rank of fifth dan. He developed the idea that it was best to die when your body was still in good shape, rather than as a decayed old man. He came to view his body as beautiful and even had photographs of his body put in a volume about Japanese body builders. However, in 1970, at the age of forty-five, though still in good shape, his body was declining. He was often too stiff for some of the exercises, and he was not able to keep up with younger men.

Mishima was an exhibitionist. He played roles in movies and on the stage. He wrote for all kinds of magazines and newspapers in addition to his serious writings. He delighted in shocking people with his writings and his possessions. He posed for a book of nude photographs in 1963, and in 1966 in the pose of Saint Sebastian.

In 1968, Mishima created his Tatenokai, a group of young men who functioned much like a private army. Using his connections, Mishima obtained permission for his group to train with the Japanese army and to be inspected on ceremonial occasions by military officers. He recruited right-wing students for the group, and the first initiation ceremony is interesting. Mishima and the others cut their fingers and dripped blood into a cup. Each signed their name in blood on a sheet of paper, and then each sipped the blood.

In 1970 he began to plan his *seppuku*. He recruited four students to help, including the leader of his Tatenokai, Morita, probably his lover and who shared his right-wing views. Mishima changed the plan a number of times, but in the end, on November 25th, 1970, the group visited a local military unit, captured General Mashita (the commander of the Eastern Army) and ordered Mashita's officers to gather the troups to hear a speech from Mishima. Mishima tried to get them to rise up and take over the government in the name of the Emperor, but they laughed at him. He went back into the general's room, disemboweled himself, whereupon Morita tried twice to behead him. One of the three assistants, Furu-Roga, took the sword and completed the beheading. Then Morita tried to disembowel himself, but failed, whereupon the Furu-Koga cleanly beheaded him.

Source: Lester (1992: 65, 70, 71). Copyright 1992 by David Lester. Reprinted by permission.

TABLE 7.3. Number of Suicides by Year and Gender, Beijing

Year	Males	Females	Total
1992	237 (42.4%)	322 (57.6%)	559 (100%)
1993	237 (47.0%)	267 (53.0%)	504 (100%)
Total	474 (44-6%)	589 (55.4%)	1,063 (100%)

Source: Jie Zhang (1996: 176). Copyright 1996 by The Guilford Press. Reprinted by permission.

ences; such as language, attitudes toward marriage and parenting, or even food habits. Here we are particulary interested in possible suicidogenic national character. For example, is there something about being German, Finnish, or Austrian that increases one's suicide risk?

The Greek word *ethnos* means people or nation. An ethnic group connoted people who identify with one another on the basis of their ancestry and cultural heritage (Henslin, 1996: 275). Their sense of belonging centers around such cultural factors as their unique customs, foods, physical characteristics, dress, family names, language, music, and religion. It is likely that ethnicity is relevant to suicide outcome.

For example, specific customs regard suicide as being appropriate to avoid shame or atone for defeat in battle (e.g., the suicides of Japanese officers after losing World War II or of Ajax falling on his sword in Chapter 4) or to fulfill a social or economic obligation (e.g., the classical Indian custom of suttee in which the widow of a dead husband was also burned on his funeral pyre) and as religious actions that influence one's spiritual well-being or afterlife (e.g., Muslim terrorists blowing themselves up to kill Jews, and the mass suicides at Jonestown or Heaven's Gate). Elderly, infirm Eskimos ask their families to as-

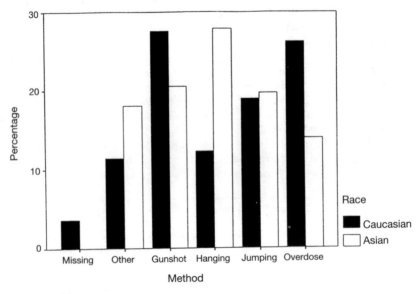

FIGURE 7.3. Percentage of completed suicides by race and method, San Francisco. *Source:* Schiang et al. (1997: 89). Copyright 1997 by The Guilford Press. Reprinted by permission.

sist in their suicide so they will not become a burden on their nomadic hunting and gathering tribe, and even an ethnic character, such as being German, possibly raises suicide risk through traits of rigidity, formality, authoritarianism, and positive attitudes toward death or suicide.

Suicide in Scandanavia

A classical study of the relationship of national character, culture, and suicide propensity was done by psychiatrist Herbert Hendin (1964). In his book, Hendin observes that traditionally the Danes and Swedes have high suicide rates, while Norwegians tend to have somewhat lower (but still elevated) suicide rates (see Figure 7.4; cf. Table 3.5). Hendin attempts to explain these suicide rate differences by alluding to differential ethnic psychosocial characteristics.

For example, in *Denmark* children's discipline tends to be through guilt, there is marked dependency of children on their parents, there is a high level of depressive disorder, suicide is not tabooed, and there is fantasy of reunion with loved ones after death. Hendin argues that these distinctive Danish psychosocial traits are positively related to the Dane's higher suicide rate.

In *Sweden*, males tend to be preoccupied with performance and success, failure to reach overly ambitious goals tends to increase suicide potential, work is inordinantly impor-

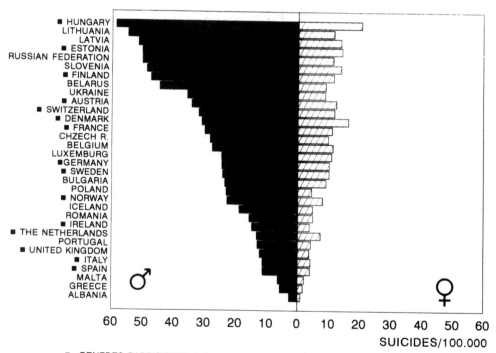

SUICIDE RATES (0–99 YEARS) OF EUROPEAN COUNTRIES
AVERAGE 1989–1993

■=CENTRES PARTICIPATING IN THE WHO/EURO MULTICENTRE STUDY ON PARASUICIDE

FIGURE 7.4. Suicides rates per 100,000 by gender, various countries, 1989–1993. *Source:* Schmidtke (1997: 128). Copyright 1997 by The Guilford Press. Reprinted by permission.

tant, there is early separation from one's mother, female suicides tend to be related to anger over male infidelity and abandonment, there is excessive maternal control of females well into their adulthood, and there is a cultural preoccupation with death (e.g., see the films of Swede Ingmar Bergman).

In *Norway*, females are more involved with their children and less is expected from their husbands, there is more open expression and less internalization of anger, Norwegians are not that competitive, success and achievement are not all that important, and alcoholism (a known suicidogenic factor) is regarded negatively.

It should be noted that Hendin's psychosocial approach has some problems. For one, it assumes that national traits are shared by the suicides of that nation. We do not *know* this without looking at suicidal individuals in the three countries. As, we noted previously, it could be that suicides are suicides partly because they are *not* like their countrymen or do *not* share their country's culture. Furthermore, Hendin tends to emphasize psychoanalytic forces and downplays biodemographic variables. Maybe it is not the parenting but, rather, the age differences that explain the suicide rate differential in Scandinavia?

Suicide in Finland

Achté and Lönnqvist have written an ethnic characterological analysis similar to Hendin's of the high suicide rates in Helsinki, Finland (in Farberow, 1975; cf. *Psychiatria Finnica* by Jouko Lönnqvist, editor, annual volumes which contain several more recent research articles on Finnish suicides). Achté and Lönnqvist note that the Finnish language differs from other Scandinavian languages as well as from Russian language. For the most part, Finland is rural and sparsely populated. Finns tend to believe that the suicide's soul is restless and haunts its survivors. Suicides are mentioned in *Kalevala* (the Finnish national epic). For example, *Aino* is a young female who suicides to avoid an unacceptable marriage. *Kullervo* engages in incest with his sister, in other brutalities, and exhibits much aggression turned on himself. There is also a theme of political suicide in Finnish history (e.g., a Finn who killed himself after assassinating a hated Russian governor).

Achté and Lönnqvist maintain that it "is questionable whether it is legitimate at all to speak of the national character of a people in any scientific sense" (in Farberow, 1975: 104) for some of the same reasons cited previously in discussing Hendin. Having made this caveat, they go on to suggest that Finns tend to be industrious and introverted and given to sulkiness, have violent drinking habits, are prone to depressive disorder, have a masculine ideal of supermen who do not reveal their feelings, have very high violence and violent crime rates, and have unfavorable geographic and climatic conditions (e.g., snow on the ground about half the year and long dark days in the autumn and winter months). Hanging is the number one method of suicide in Finland (about 40% of the total) and suicide is chiefly a problem of the Finnish male.

Suicide in Hungary

As Figure 7.4 indicates, Hungary consistently has the highest suicide rates in the entire world, especially for aged males (in the 60s per 100,000 population; cf. Table 3.5 and Sartorius and Gulbinat, 1994: 42–48). What is there about Hungary or its individuals that results in such a high suicide rate? Much of the recent work on Hungarian suicides has been done by Budapest sociologist Ferenc Moksony (1995, 1996, 1997). In analyzing some 600 Hungarian villages, Moksony argues that it is the lack of social change, the failure to catch up with the rest of society that raises the Hungarian level of self-destruction (but is Moksony's social bias showing?). The presence of a "subculture of suicide" also amplifies the influence of socioeconomic backwardness. For example, the higher the suicide rate for a country, the more permissive the attitudes are toward suicide in the region.

At an international suicide conference in Adelaide (1997) Moksony showed that rural areas with high levels of socioeconomic development tend to have low suicide rates, other things being equal. Moksony argued that Hungarians tend to become vulnerable to suicide because they are stuck in a backward socioeconomic position. Also, people who have sustained a *loss* in social position (e.g., vis-à-vis their parents) are more likely to kill themselves. Moksony (1996) argued that deprivation or backwardness plays a greater role in suicide than does stress or disorganization. In Hungary, Protestants have preserved their elevated vulnerability to suicide.

Suicide in Vienna, Austria, and Germany

As alluded to in the introduction to this chapter, Maris lived in Vienna, Austria in 1979–1980 in order to be immersed in a city, country, and culture with one of the higher suicide rates in the world. A similar research project was undertaken by Farberow (Farberow & Simon, 1975). Austria is somewhat of an anomaly in that it is mainly a Catholic country and yet has the third highest suicide rate (23.1) of the 62 countries considered in Table 3.5 (cf. Figure 7.4) (Germany is ninth highest). The late Professor Erwin Ringel (see Ringel, 1978), argued that in Austria (and elsewhere) there is a presuicidal syndrome, which includes three precursors: (1) constriction of thought, (2) aggression turned on oneself, and (3) suicidal fantasies.

In his research in Vienna, Farberow found that unlike Los Angeles, 38% of the Vienna sample used domestic gas to suicide and far fewer of those in Los Angeles left suicide notes (18% vs. 46% in Vienna). A common Viennese pattern was the suicide of older women, who were basically alone (Maris also found this pattern in West Berlin suicides). Many more of the Austrian suicides were in poor physical health compared to the Americans. In general, the Viennese suicides seemd more socially alienated and isolated than the Los Angeles suicides and were more likely to have poor communication with their spouses, relatives, and friends.

One of the major factors in Berlin suicides was its aged population—especially the preponderance of elderly widows. It was also hypothesized that the German character was involved in Berlin suicides (traits of inflexibility, rigidity, death preoccupation, high alcohol consumption, and depressive tendencies).

Kushner (1989) notes a similar proclivity for suicide among Germans. He comments: "Among immigrants, particularly the Germans, there is a great predisposition toward suicide. One American psychiatry journal reported that in New York City 43 percent of all suicides were by German nationals" (157). Recent research on German suicides has been done by Armin Schmidtke (Schmidtke, Fricke, & Weinacher, 1994). In 1997 Schmidtke noted that "the suicide rates in areas with more 'Germanic' populations is higher than in regions with more Romanic or Slavic populations" (131).

Suicide among Immigrants

Finally, it is well-known that migrants from high-suicide-rate countries tend to maintain their higher suicide rates in their new host countries, at least for a few generations (see Kushner, 1991: 6). Kushner (1991: 150–158) maintains that it is not so much ethnicity, but rather, *migration* that increases the risk of suicide. The census of the United States in 1890 reported that the suicide rate for *any* foreign-born American was almost three times greater than that for native-borns (1989:152). Table 7.4 confirms the higher suicide rates of any

TABLE 7.4. Suicide Rates by Country of Birth, San Francisco, 1938–1942 and 1948–1952

Country	1938–1942	1948–1952
Native-born	25.3	20.7
Foreign-born	48.5	44.0
Germany	65.4	53.3
Italy	37.4	24.9
Russia	59.6	33.2
Ireland	34.9	20.0
England, Wales	36.4	39.3
China	42.2	No data
Canada	32.5	38.2
Denmark	94.2	94.3
Sweden	49.3	45.3
Norway	81.3	91.6
Austria	67.3	34.7
Finland	61.7	90.0
France	20.5	67.4
Poland	32.8	57.8

Source: Kushner (1991: 155). Copyright 1991 by Rutgers University Press. Reprinted by permission.

foreign-born American and that the suicide rates of those in the United States who were born in Denmark, Norway, Finland, Austria, and Germany were especially high (cf. Kushner, 1991: 158).

According to Kushner, immigration itself may be "a strategy of risk-taking" [*sic*]. Because the goal of self-transformation by immigrants is sometimes tied to the repudiation of past "Old Country" values, social or economic failure (if and when it occurs) cannot be diffused by falling back on traditional Old Country values (see Schiang et al., 1997, on Asian American suicides). Furthermore, immigration may also expose the immigrant to more actual loss of kin support in times of crises, as well as reflect the higher suicidogenic character of the country of origin.

CULTURAL FORCES IN SUICIDAL BEHAVIORS

Several important books on suicides have focused on the cultural aspects of self-destruction, from Farberow's *Suicide in Different Cultures* (1975) right up to Leenaars, Maris, and Takahashi's *Suicide: Individual, Cultural, and International Perspectives* (1997). As early as 1971 Anthony Giddens included a major section (III) on the anthropology of suicide in his *The Sociology of Suicide*.

Culture: Definitions and Concepts

As we saw earlier, culture is different from race or ethnicity, because "culture" refers to the total socially acquired life way or lifestyle of a particular group of people (Harris, 1971)—including their self-destructive characteristics, rituals, patterns, language, customs, and so on. Culture is *learned* information and is passed on from person to person and generation to generation (Lenksi, Nolan, & Lenski, 1995: 16). As Harris (1971) puts it, "culture is the learned patterns of thought and behavior characteristic of a population or a society (136)."

Lenski et al. (1995) say much the same thing: "Culture includes a group's total perception reality: its ideas about what is real, true, important, possible, good, beautiful, etc. Because every society has a unique past, every culture is unique" (38)."

Lenski, Nolan, and Lenski (1995) remind us that culture is society's symbol systems and the information they convey (33–35). The most basic symbol systems in any society are its spoken languages.

Languages separate exerience into different units because the experiences of people who create and use languages are so different. For example, Lenski et al. (1995) point out that Eskimos use numerous expression to refer to multifaceted types of "snow," whereas to most of us "snow is snow" (34). In a similar vein, the general public may naively assume that all suicides are basically alike and that one word for suicide will suffice, but expert suicidologists may feel the need to employ many different words to accurately describe the many nuances of different types of self-destructive behaviors (cf. Maris, Berman, Maltsberger, & Yufit, 1992: Chapter 4; O'Carroll, Berman, Maris, Moscicki, Tanney, & Silverman, 1996). As we shall see, there are languages of suicide that reflect the common experiences, traditions, geography, unique experiences, culture, and so on of particular groups of people.

For example, consider the Indian practice of *suttee*. In ancient India widows were expected to throw themselves on their dead husband's burning funeral pyres or to drown themselves in the holy Ganges River. Hindu priests taught that a faithful wife could atone for her deceased husband's sins and thereby open the gates of paradise. Under British rule, *suttee* continued because it was consistent with the British notion that a man's wife was part of his property or estate. It is interesting that even today when Indian families lack the dowry necessary to allow their daughters to get married, some of these young women are found mysteriously burned to death. Suttee was formally outlawed in 1829, but before then in India wives who refused to sacrifice themselves after their husband's death were condemned or even threatened with harsh physical punishment. It might be that *suttee* originated in part from young women suiciding to avoid rape and family dishonor threatened by outside invaders.

Another example of suicide and language would be a related set of words in the Japanese language that reflects their own unique life experiences and culture. We refer to the well-known Japanese words for ritualistic suicides to protect one's honor or atone for shame, epecially for defeat in battle (*hara-kiri* or *seppuku* and the associated concept of *kamikaze*). Originally hara-kiri was an honorable means for a disgraced or defeated Samurai warrior to redeem himself or to prevent capture by disembowelment with his own sword (Evans & Farberow, 1988). Samurais would also commit *seppuku* to show allegiance or respect for a fallen leader, especially to defend or honor their Emperor.

Hara-kiri was an elaborate ritual that sometimes took hours to complete. As with Yukio Mishima (see Box 7.2) the disembowelment was ended by the closest friend of the suicide, beheading the suicide with a sword. Finally, *seppuku* was also a culturally approved way for Japanese nobility condemned to death to avoid the fate of ordinary condemned persons (much like Socrates), who were hung in public squares. In traditional Japanese culture the body was seen merely as a temporary home for the soul (see the Buddhist concept of *muso-kan*) and as such was thought not to be the true self.

A related ritualistic Japanese suicide was *kamikaze*. Literally, *kamikaze* in Japanese means "divine wind" and originally referred to the typhoon that destroyed Kublai Khan's fleet, thus foiling his invasion of Japan in 1281. During World War II more than 1,000 young Japanese pilots were literally welded into the cockpits of their explosive-filled airplanes. The *kamikaze* pilots then crashed and detonated their planes into Allied warships.

Kamikaze suicides were examples of Durkheim's "altruistic suicides"; that is, the lives of the pilots were subjugated to a higher cause, namely, that which placed duty to the Emperor and the welfare of Japan over personal welfare. Because such altruistic suicides were obligatory and expected, of course, not all *kamikaze*'s acted voluntarily.

In traditional Japanese culture, ritualistic suicides to save face, for family honor or loyalty (e.g., of a wife to her husband), to honor and protect the country or prove allegiance to a leader/king were respected and, in a sense, appropriate. However, suicides resulting from personal unhappiness, mental problems, maladjustment, and so on, although not condemned, were met with mixed feelings, short of respect (Hsien Rin & Tua Chen, 1983: 61).

Suicide among the Yuit Eskimos

Many cultural studies of suicide have focused on the basic values and social forces reflected in Durkheim's "altruistic suicide" type (see Maris, 1969: 34). As we know, altruistic suicide is characterized by insufficient individuation. Instead of apathy, we find energy and activity. Whereas Durkheim's "egoistic suicide" no longer finds a basis for existence within this life (no good enough reason to keep on living), the altruistic suicide typically finds the basis for existence beyond this life. The primary attribute of altruistic suicide is duty. Note that in the case of altruistic suicide, even if social integration is high, it cannot protect the individual against suicide because the norms of the society or group themselves are *pro*suicide (as recently in the so-called Heaven's Gate cult; the *kamikaze* pilots are also an excellent illustration of this point).

An anthropological study of predominantly altruistic suicide was done by Leighton and Hughes (1955), who investigated the Yuit Eskimos of St. Lawrence Island. Among the Yuit, suicide is a group activity both in decision and in execution, usually involving relatives and friends. In this nomadic hunting and gathering society, to become old, sick, or infirm might put the group's well-being or even survival at risk.

The custom for a would-be suicide among the Yuit is to ask a family member to help in the suicide. Ordinarily, at first the family member refuses the request. However, if the request is repeated at least three times (i.e., is a persistent wish), relatives must honor the wish of the aspiring suicide. Hunting and killing are part and parcel of everyday life among the Yuit. For hunters killing oneself may not be seen as a dramatic departure from killing animals, given the appropriate circumstances. In certain conditions suicide by the Yuit is even an indication of courage, wisdom, and respect for those in the group on whom the individual is becoming more dependent and whose welfare the individual may be jeopardizing.

Before the suicide the victims dress themselves as if they were already dead; for example, they turn their furs inside out, with the hair of their clothing touching their skin. If possible, the suicidal person walks unassisted to the "destroying place." There the soon-to-be suicide (usually a man) addresses his or her relatives, saying that they (the survivors) are able to take care of themselves, perhaps that they should respect the advice of the elderly, and in general gives the audience a brief statement of their philosophy of life. Then either the wife shoots the husband with a rifle or a number of relatives help hang the victim. The latter means of death is particularly unpleasant, because often it takes up to 30 minutes for the victim to die, during which time the suicide struggles and may defecate and urinate on the hanging site. Clearly, this is an assisted suicide.

Usually a brief period of isolation and purification follows for those who participated in the assisted suicide. A Yuit Eskimo might suicide because of poor health and infirmity or sometimes in an effort to magically save the life of an ill son (almost never to save a daughter). In most cases the suicide's motivation is primarily altruistic. It is motivated by concern for the well-being of other people in the suicide's family and is sanctioned and participated in by the Yuit community.

Risk-Taking Contingencies among Tikopian Suicides

Among the Tikopia, a Polynesian island community in the western Pacific, the suicide rate has always been relatively high (about 50/100,000 per year). But whether risking one's life actually results in a completed suicide or a nonfatal suicide attempt turns on more than just *egoism* (individual isolation) or *anomie* (abrupt social disruption). Firth (1961) argues that there are many *contingencies* in Tikopian risk taking that make a crucial difference in suicidal outcomes.

To begin, suicide does not violate any Tikopian religious prescriptions or basic social norms. The Tikopians' attitude toward suicide is highly related to their attitude toward death in general. Basically they believe that to take one's life is merely to anticipate what will eventually happen anyway. Furthermore, the methods used to suicide reflect the geography and lifestyle of Tikopia. For example, young women swim out to sea and young men put to sea in a canoe (*forau*). Once it is known that someone has put out to sea on a suicidal swim or voyage, the search-and-rescue effort is immediate and enthusiastic—particularly if the suicide attempter is of high social status:

> The Tikopia have a very lively understanding of the whole situation of going off to sea, and a very energetic attitude towards rescue expeditions. As soon as the news of a suicide swim or voyage is known, a searching fleet of organized and hastily paddles out in chase of the fugitive. If the attempt is really serious, the fleet's chances of success are not very high . . . (e.g.,) the escapee goes off at night or in a high wind, which militates against the likelihood of his being spotted and caught in hugh ocean wastes. (Firth, 1961: 213)

Rescuers will not go out beyond sight of land, however. They have to be able to see the top of 1,200-foot Mount Reani. Thus, most serious attempters are not found if they leave secretly and paddle steadfastly out to sea.

However, the are several life-affirming *contingencies* involved in a serious suicide attempt that are often overlooked. *If* the suicide voyager loses sight of land but then returns by himself or *if* he is rescued before losing sight of land, he is completely reinstated within the Tikopean community. All is forgiven by everyone involved. Presumably the suicide attempt atones for both social and personal problems and in the end is paradoxically life affirming. Firth's main point is that among the Tikopia, and presumably among some other sociocultural groups, no one feature of society (social integration, anomie, egoism, etc.) can explain suicide. Other sociocultural and physical *contingencies* that must be considered include a group's attitudes toward death; the social status of the attempter; the seriousness of the attempt; the somewhat whimsical forces of wind, sea, and storms; and the enthusiasm behind the rescue effort.

South American Suicide: The Case of Buenos Aires

Typically Latin American countries have moderate to low suicide rates, owing probably in large part to the relative youth of these countries and to the prophylactic effect of their predominantly Roman Catholic religion. Referring back to Table 3.5, we see that none of the top 25 countries with the highest suicide rates in the world were South American. Of 71 countries, South American suicide rates were ranked as follows:

Rank	Country
26	Uruguay
38	Chile
39	Argentina
41	Venezuela
47	Ecuador
52	Paraguay

Yampey (1975) has provided us with some insight into changes in suicide rate in response to sociocultural forces of one Latin American city: Buenos Aires, Argentina. Buenos Aires, with a population of roughly 3 millon, is the largest city in Latin America. It is a lively port city located on the northeast coast of Argentina, on the right bank of the river *(Rio) de la Plata.* Today Argentina has a suicide rate (not controlling for sex; Argentine male suicides exceed female suicides by a ratio of about 3 to 1) of about 7/100,000. However, at the turn of century its suicide rate stood at about 33/100,000. Why the high suicide rate in Buenos Aires in 1895–1896?

Yampey (1975) claims:

> How should the relationship between the culture of Argentina and the high prevalence of suicide (33) at the turn of the century in Buenos Aires and (then) its gradual decrease (to 7) be interpreted? The factors of massive immigration, quick urbanization and industrialization, and social disorganization must have caused many (suicidal) crises. (55)

In a passage reminiscent of Kushner (1989), Yampey (1975: 52) notes the massive immigration to Bueno Aires in the late 1800s. The adult population in Buenos Aires consisted mainly of foreign-born males. For example, from 1869 to 1914 foreign-born adult males in Buenos Aires outnumbered native-born males by 4 to 1. Other things being equal, being an older foreign-born male immigrant tends to increase the probability of suicide. One detail that is a little puzzling is that about half the Buenos Aires immigrants were Italians and another third were Spanish. We know from Figure 7.4 that Italy and Spain themselves (i.e., the mother countries) both have *low* suicide rates. Perhaps the Italians and Spaniards who migrated to Buenos Aires were nontraditional in some repects (were separated from their families and culture, less likely to married at all, less religious, etc.).

Another suicidogenic force was the rapid growth and urbanization of Buenos Aires as a major trade city. As Buenos Aires moved from an agriculture-based economy to urban industrialism there were no doubt many changes that must have resulted in conflicts, tensions, anomie, and social problems. this rapid socioeconomic transition, Yampey argues, resulted in a loss of prior identity. New cultural forms resulted, which were an amalgam of immigrant heritage and one's new native Argentinian culture. Many of the newcomers to Buenos Aires were uprooted male risk takers. Add to this rapid sociocultural climate of change some preexisting personal vulnerabilities, stress, and untoward, unexpected contingencies and you have a recipe for increased suicide potential.

Finally, Buenos Aires at the turn of the century experienced high levels of social disorganization, especially changes in the family structure. When we discussed the low suicide rates of black females, it was noted that black women, particularly in the rural South, have a large extended kinship social support network and that this tends to protect them against suicide. Yampey (1975:5 4) observes that in Buenos Aires in the late 1890s, the average family size was shrinking rapidly. For example, average family size shrunk from 6.0 in 1869 to 4.3 by 1947. Add to this the influx of foreign-born male immigrants, who were more likely to be unmarried or separated from their families, and you have another major suicidogenic sociocultural factor.

There was also at least one other suicidal force in Buenos Aires around 1900: alcoholism. Argentina has always been a great producer and consumer of wine. About 90% of the Argentine population drinks wine (Yampey, 1975: 64). It is well-known that alcohol use and abuse are highly correlated with violent outcomes, including suicide (see Chapter 15). Yampey (1975: 65) claims that alcoholism became more of a problem in Buenos Aires in the early 1900s. A subculture of alcoholism and drug abuse developed, especially among certain occupational groups (such as harbor stevedores and migrants). Yampey (1975) concludes, in a psychoanalytic interperetation, that "the (migrant) alcoholic reveals great dependence on the mother or upon a subculture that replaces her" (65).

Native American Suicides

As a final example of cultural forces in suicide, consider Native Americans. It is often reported that Native Americans have high suicide rates—up to 10 times higher than those of the overall U.S. population (which, as we know, is about 12/100,000). Factors related to the presumed higher Native American suicide rate are argued to be unemployment, poverty, family stress and disruption, alcoholism and substance abuse, and poor health (see Grossman, Milligan, & Deyo, 1991; Gartrell, Jarvis, & Derkson, 1993). In one study the predicted probability of reported suicide attempts for older adolescent males who smoke, reported heavy alcohol use, had no father in their home, and had a low sense of well-being was 84% (i.e., 84% of native Americans with those traits reported at least on suicide attempt, Gartrell, Jarvis, & Derksen, 1993: 372).

There are at least two major problems with this common view of high Native American suicide rates. First, it is ethnocentric in that it tends to mistakenly view Native American cultures as disturbed forms of European American culture (Webb & Willard, 1975: 17). Second, the early high Native American suicide rate claim was based only on one of the at least six Native American cultural divisions—actually a Shoshone reservation—and was in fact only a Shoshone pattern, not a general Native American suicide pattern. There are at least *six* general cultural divisions of the Native American tribes—the Navajo, the Shoshone, the Papago, the Dakota, the Cheyenne, and the Apache (and more than that depending on your classification criteria)—and they all have discernibly different cultures with discernably different patterns and rates of suicide.

In fact, the *Navajos*, the largest single Native American group, universally *condemn* suicide. Navajos believe that any death that is not the result of old age is unnatural (Webb & Willard, 1975: 27). The rate of suicide among the Navajos is *not* high. In fact, it is *lower* than that of the overall population in the states in which their reservations are located (Arizona and New Mexico). Navajo culture assumes that if a Navajo suicides, the individual will not escape his or her untenable life situation but, rather, will be forced to stay in this bad situation in the altered status of a ghost. So strong was the traditional Navajo's belief in ghosts that nightime reservation activities were curtailed to help them avoid ghosts (Webb & Willard, 1975: 29).

Among other Native Americans there are also cultural variations in self-destructive behaviors. For example, the *Apaches* of the central mountains of Arizona tend to be very aggressive in general and tend to use highly lethal methods to attempt suicide. Almost all males use guns, while a great majority of Apache females used to burn themselves (these cultural patterns have changed some over time with acculturation, education, etc., see Echohawk, 1997). Webb and Willard (1975: 27) contend that Apache suicides are largely the result of expressing unacceptable aggression toward one's spouse or kin (i.e., are often retroflexed anger, assault, or murder).

The *Dakota* and *Cheyenne* used to display a pattern of deliberate headlong rush into death, in which the perpetrator got himself killed—a kind of victim-precipitated homicide. The Dakota and Cheyenne referred to this behavior as "Crazy-Dog-Wishing-to-Die." Finally, the self-destructive behaviors among some (e.g., the *Pueblos*) Native American tribes are largely unstudied and unknown. Given the cultural diversity of the Native Americans, one cannot summarily conclude that there is a uniformly high suicide rate among them.

SUMMARY AND CONCLUSIONS

This chapter opened with the startling contrast of low, virtually absent suicide rates in some countries or populations (as among the Tiv of Nigeria) and extremely high suicide rates in other countries (e.g., Hungary). These vivid differences suggest that suicide rates vary by race, ethnicity, and culture. After defining our key terms, the chapter continued with a consideration of racial aspects of suicide. Of course, the prototypical suicide in the United States and western Europe is an older white male. The suicide rates of older white males are about 10 times higher than those of black females. We examined several hypotheses purporting to explain the high suicide rates of older white men.

Next we discussed the paradox (given their heavy loading on suicidogenic forces such as stress, poverty, absent spouses, and depression) of extremely low suicide rates among black females. We concluded that that black women are protected from suicide by their social support networks, religious values and church ties, and being used to coping with adversity (also, they may make more suicide attempts but fewer suicide completions). The last major racial group the chapter inspected was Asians. It was observed that most Asian countries do not have especially high suicide rates (only Japan is near the top). Suicides in Asian populations tend to be altruistic, as in the ritual self-destruction of *hara-kiri* or *kamikaze* during World War II, although there are some *anomic* Asian suicides related to economic and academic competition and high achievement goals and to rapid social change. As a special instance of Asian suicide, this chapter examined the case of Japanese author Yukio Mishima.

The second major topic in this chapter was ethnicity and national character. We undertook an in-depth review of Herbert Hendin's *Suicide in Scandanavia*. Hendin argued that suicide rates tend to be high among the Danes and Swedes but low among the Norwegians. Danes tend to be guilty and depressed and suicide is not tabooed. Swedes are said to be preoccupied with performance and success. Norwegians are much less competitive, express their anger externally, and usually see alcoholism as negative. Achté and Lönnqvist account for high Finnish suicide rates by their elevated levels of depressive disorder, alcoholism, Finland's inclimatic winter weather, and a male ideal of a "superman," who does not display his feelings.

We then noted that the highest suicide rates in the world are to be found in Hungary. Budapest sociologist Ferenc Moksony claims that Hungarians have a "subculture of suicide," including socioeconomic backwardness, permissive attitudes toward suicide, and loss of relative social position (vis-à-vis other countries). In considering Vienna, Austria and Germany, both of which have high suicide rates, the author discovered aging populations (with an excess of widows), preoccupation with death, character traits of rigidity and inflexibility, high alcohol consumption, and a tendency toward depressive disorder. This section concluded with an observation by historian Howard Kushner that migrants from countries maintain their home country's high suicide rates for a while, and that suicide is further exacerbated by the migration process itself.

The last section of this chapter focused on cultural forces in suicide among the Yuit Eskimos, Tikopian Pacific islanders, Buenos Aires Argentinians, and North American Indians. "Culture" was defined as learned information patterns and behavior (including language, rituals, and customs) passed from person to person and from generation to generation. Examples of the Indian cultural ritual of suttee and the Japanese rituals of *hara-kiri* and *kamikaze* were detailed. Among the Yuit Eskimos it was customary for families to assist suicides—usually older males, who had become infirm, dependent, and sick.

In the Polynesian Pacific island of Tikopia, suicide was essentially risk-taking behavior in which the final outcome depended on several social, behavioral, and natural contingencies. We also considered the high suicide rate in the largest South American city, Buenos Aires, at the turn of the 20th century. Buenos Aires suicides were found to result from large numbers of single male immigrants, rapid socioeconomic change, and high levels of risk taking and alcoholism. This chapter concluded by exposing the myth of a universally high suicide rate among North American Indians. Although poverty, unemployment, family disruption, and substance abuse are correlated with high suicide rates among some Indian tribes (e.g., the Shoshone), in other Indian cultures, such as the Navajos, the Indian suicide rate is actually lower than that of the general non-Indian population in the host states (i.e., in Arizona and New Mexico). There is much diversity in both American Indian culture and suicide rates. In Chapter 8 we explore the crucial role of work (epecially for traditional males), unemployment, and various other economic influences in suicide outcomes.

FURTHER READING

Bohannan, P. (Ed.). (1960). *African homicide and suicide*. Princeton: Princeton University Press. One of the few empirical studies of black African suicides and homicides, by an anthropologist from Princeton and Northwestern. Bohannan and his colleagues collected and analyzed data on the Tiv (Nigeria), the Soga, Gisu, Nyoro, and Alur (Uganda), and the Luyia and Luo (Kenya). Suicide and homicide rates in some areas varied directly, were mainly (two-thirds) by males, were often considered irrational by other black Africans, and were primarily by hanging.

Farberow, N. L. (Ed.). (1975). *Suicides in different cultures*. Baltimore: University Park Press. A collection of studies of suicide patterns around the world (including American Indians, Scandanavians, South Americans, Italians, the Viennese, Bulgarians, Israelites, Indians, Taiwanese, Japanese, Britains, and the Dutch) by one of the founders of the scientific study of suicide in the United States and past president of the International Association for Suicide Prevention. Contains chapters by Achté, Iga, Lönnqvist, Retterstol, Kalish, Reynolds, Rudestam, Speijer, and other well-known international suicidologists. The book opens with an important cultural history of suicide by editor Farberow.

Giddens, A. (Ed.). (1971). *The sociology of suicide: A selection of readings*. London: Frank Cass & Co. In the tradition of French sociologist Emile Durkheim, well-known Cambridge classical sociological theorist Anthony Giddens takes on the suicide liturature. Part III of this anthology has a selection of anthropological studies of suicide—including Firth's risk taking in Tikopia, Leighton and Hughes's article on Eskimo suicides, Jeffrey's paper on revenge suicide in Africa, and Iga and O'Hara on anomic suicides among Japanese adolescents.

Headley, L. A. (Ed.). (1983). *Suicide in Asia and the Near East*. Berkeley: University of California Press. In addition to traditional pieces on fairly well-explored countries (e.g., Japan, India, and Hong Kong), Headley also includes novel chapters on little known counties' suicides (e.g., Iran, Iraq, Egypt, Syria, Pakistan, Kuwait, and Sri Lanka). Because most of our knowledge of suicidal behaviors comes from Western countries, Headley's Eastern and Near Eastern supplement fills many suicidal lacunae. Especially interesting is the preponderance of Near Eastern female suicides.

Hendin, H. (1969). *Black suicide*. New York: Harper & Row. One of the pioneering early social–psychiatric treatises, especially on the higher suicide rates of young adult urban black males and male homosexuals. Hendin anticipates the futility, hopelessness, murderous rage, and self-hatred felt by many contemporary urban black males. Needs to be read in conjunction with Jewelle Gibbs's (1988) book, *Young, Black, and Male in America: An Endangered Species* (Auburn House).

Leenaars, A. A., Maris, R. W., & Takahashi, Y. (Eds.). (1997). *Suicide: Individual, cultural, international perspectives*. New York: Guilford Press. A recent updating of cultural and international perspectives on suicide, with chapters on immigrants, native Americans, African Americans, Asians in San Francisco, and Mexican Americans. There are also chapters on how Canadian suicides differ from U.S. suicides and the latest report from Armin Schmidtke on the World Health Organization/Euro Multicentre project on parasuicide and suicide in Europe.

8

Work and the Economy

Steven Stack

After receiving the Nobel Prize for physics, Harvard's Percy Bridgemen shot himself and left a simple note: "My work is over, why wait?" This note emphasizes the often crucial role work plays in one's sense of well-being, especially among American males. It suggests that occupational problems may be a major factor in the evolution of suicidal careers.
—RONALD W. MARIS

This chapter deals with how aspects of work and the economy can influence suicide risk. The conditions to be discussed are socioeconomic status (SES), unemployment, occupations, business cycles, cohort analysis, work mobility, and executive/professional suicide. Attention is called to how these conditions can affect suicide risk both directly and indirectly.

The influence of the economy on a population's level of suicide risk can be conceptualized in terms of an economist's costs–benefits model. When the terrors of death seem less costly than the terrors of life, suicide risk increases (Hammermesh, 1974). Sociologically, groups faced with relatively high terrors in life include those under economic strain: the poor, unemployed, persons in lower-status occupations, and the large numbers of people who are affected during downturns in the business cycle, and when persons are in a relatively large age or other kind of cohort. This chapter analyzes each of these groups.

Economic strain can also affect suicide risk indirectly. Financial strain, for example, can increase alcohol consumption and marital turmoil, which, in turn, can elevate suicide risk. An unemployed person may migrate to another locality, such as another state, to find a job. The migration process, a result of the strain of unemployment, can increase suicide risk. This is through the intervening process that involves breaking certain suicide-preventing bonds such as those to friends and relatives (Lester, 1992a; Stack, 1982).

The nature of work also influences suicide risk. Excessive work-related strain can contribute to suicide risk; for example, dentists may face hostile patients each day (Stack, 1996a). However, the relationship between work and suicide may decrease or become even insignificant for persons in an occupational category once the covariates of work are controlled. These covariates include age, gender, and race.

Work mobility, the process of changing jobs, can affect suicide risk. Changes, especially if sudden, can result in a sense of disorientation and can elevate suicide risk (Breed,

1963). Such mobility can be horizontal or lateral, upward involving increases in career status, or downward involving losses in one's former prestige.

While the relationship between the status level of broad groups of occupations and suicide risk has been found to be negative in most studies, there is substantial variation within broad occupational groups in the odds of suicide. This chapter also explores this variation within one such occupational group: professionals and executives.

SOCIOECONOMIC STATUS

Some classic works have contended that the poor should have a low suicide rate (Durkheim, 1966: 254; Henry & Short, 1954). The social correlates of poverty have been viewed as offsetting any economic strains. In Durkheim (1966: 254) the poor would be expected to have a low suicide rate because poverty is, in effect, a "school" for doing without, a form of "social restraint." The impoverished would learn to be satisfied with little. They would be less likely to experience anomie in economic downturns as they have little distance to fall through unemployment as compared to rich persons encountering unemployment. More affluent persons would often fall into the trap of wanting more and more, and at some point anomie sets in and aspirations are blocked. Therein suicide potential increases for the "anomic" affluent.

The evidence for Durkheim's (1966) position is not strong. Durkheim had no data on income or occupations, and so he marshaled rather indirect data including those on suicide by sector of employment. The Durkheimian position is often naively said to be supported by high suicide rates among select groups of high-status persons such as physicians and dentists (Lester, 1992a).

According to Henry and Short (1954), the poor have been said to have "strong relational systems" and an obvious "subordinate status." These aspects of poverty enable the poor to blame others and/or society for their financial and other plights. It is assumed that frustration is apt to be vented as aggression against others, not themselves. In short, the poor would be apt to have a high homicide rate and low suicide rate (Henry & Short, 1954). However, Henry and Short measured "subordinate status" not in terms of income or occupation but in terms of social measures, such as race. Although it is true that blacks have a suicide rate lower than that of whites, Henry and Short (1954) did not explore the specific relationships between income or occupation and suicide risk.

Although these classic, works speculated that there was a positive link between poverty and suicide, research based on more direct measures of poverty has tended to find that the opposite is the case. As one goes up the SES ladder, suicide rates tend to fall (e.g. Boxer, Burnett, & Swanson, 1995; Schony & Grausgraber, 1987).

Persons in the lower classes including the poor, tend to have a relatively high suicide rate. Through its association with many suicidogenic conditions, such as family instability, mental troubles such as depression, financial stress, physical illness, alienation from work, alcoholism, and crime victimization, poverty tends to increase (not decrease) suicide risk (Lester, 1992a; Stack, 1982a).

However, it is also true that the poor have an extremely high homicide rate. In fact, they are much more likely to die of homicide, at least in the United States, than of suicide. In this limited sense, Henry and Short (1954) would be correct. Nevertheless, sticking to suicide, their rate is elevated compared to that of persons with a higher SES rating.

Studies at the local and state level have tended to find an inverse association between SES and suicide. In a study of 1,549 suicides in Chicago, Maris reported suicide rates of 33/100,000 for the lower (operatives, service, laborers), 21.9/100,000 for the middle (clerical, sales, craftsmen), and 15.2/100,000 for the upper (professional–technical, managers, and proprietors) SES groups. An analysis of 1,210 suicides in Detroit determined that blue-collar workers had a suicide rate of 44.2 compared to 17.8 for white-collar workers (Stack, 1980). The suicide rate of low-status laborers (87.5/100,000) was 4.6 times as high as that for high-status professional–technical workers (19.1/100,000). For 113 suicides in New Orleans, Breed (1963) also reported an inverse relationship. For example, professionals composed 15% of the population but only 7% of the suicides. Laborers composed only 5% of the population but 13% of the suicides.

In a study of Sacramento County, California, Lampert, Bourque, and Kraus (1984) performed a more refined analysis by including only suicides who were employed at the time of their deaths. This excluded two groups at high risk of suicide: the unemployed and the retired. For the decade of 1965–1974, Lampert et al. (1984) found a ratio of 5 to 1 between the suicide rates of farm laborers (135.1/100,000) and professional–technical workers (26.5/100,000). Large ratios were also found for these two groups in earlier decades (see Table 8.1). In all decades, the rates for male farm laborers and other laborers were more than double the rates for male professional–technical workers. Male clerical workers, a lower-middle-class occupational group, had a suicide rate of 19.7, 26.5, and 31 during each of the three respective decades. These rates were below the average rate of all male workers. Men in sales occupations had suicide rates below the mean as well in all three decades. Managers and administrators also had suicide rates below the male labor force mean.

For the United States as a whole, Stack (1995b) reports that the suicide rate for laborers is 94.4/100,000, a rate eight times the national average. Lalli and Turner (1968) employ national data on suicide rates by broad occupational groups for the year 1950. These data also demonstrate an inverse relationship.

The inverse association between SES and suicide has also been documented in other nations. In a study of 2,536 suicides in Austria, white-collar workers had a suicide rate of 17.9/100,000 compared to rates of 24.2 for unskilled blue-collar workers and 46.8 for skilled blue-collar workers (Schony & Grausgruber, 1987). In the case of Australia, in a

TABLE 8.1. Age-Adjusted Male Suicide Rates (per 100,000 Population) by Occupational Class and Decade of Death, Sacramento County, California, 1945–1974

Occupational class	Decade of death		
	1945–1954	1955–1964	1965–1974
Professional–technical	26.5	20.3	26.5
Farmers–farm managers	2.5*	38.2	29.5
Managerial–administrative	24.4	30.9	45.4
Sales	18.1	28.0	33.4
Clerical	19.7	26.5	31.0
Craftsmen	26.9	37.3	67.7
Operatives	31.9	37.6	81.9
Laborers	68.7	74.8	84.6
Farm laborers	70.6	65.8	135.1
Service	63.1	59.4	61.0
Total number of suicides	253	382	522
Rate all employed	34.2	35.1	48.5

Source: Adapted from Lampert, Bourque, & Kraus (1984). Copyright 1984 by The Guilford Press. Adapted by permission.
*Rate based on one suicide in the 10-year interval.

study of 1,360 suicides, Burnley (1995) found that male manual workers had the highest suicide rate (32.5/100,000). This was compared to a rate of 20.5/100,000 for professional, managerial, and technical workers which was significantly below the average risk of suicide. Male clerical and salesworkers had a rate of 19.4/100,000, also significantly less than average. In the case of Great Britain, an analysis documented an inverse association between SES and suicide risk (Platt 1992: 1199). Kreitman, Carstairs, and Duffy (1991) found that the suicide rate for British and Welch working age males was the highest in the lowest socioeconomic classes.

From epidemiological research, it is not always clear whether economic stress was the actual proximate cause of suicide among the poor. Some individual level analysis has suggested that this is the case. Economic stressors were found to be the second (of eight) most important correlates of suicide in 195 cases of suicide in San Diego. These economic stressors were involved in 24% of suicides. In comparison, conflict–separation–rejection was involved in 31% of the suicides. Medical illness was the next most important stressor, found in 19% of the suicides (Rich, Warsradt, & Nemiroff, 1991).

Some research evidence does not document an inverse association between SES and suicide. In the state of Washington the correlation ($r = .05$, $p > .05$) between the SES score of eight occupational categories and the proportional mortality ratio for suicide was insignificant (Marks, 1980). However, a study also based on eight broad occupational groups found an inverse relationship between standard mortality ratios for suicide and occupational status (Tuckman, Youngman, & Kreizman, 1964). In a similar vein, using national data for the United States for 1950 and a large but select group of occupations, Labovitz and Hagedorn (1971) report no association between occupational prestige scores and suicide. The Labovitz and Hagedorn (1971) study may find no relationship as they give equal weights to suicide rates in small and large occupational categories. Finally, Labovitz and Hagedorn (1971) give no information on how they selected the occupations for analysis; the occupations selected may be a nonrepresentative group.

Caution needs to be exercised in interpreting most findings on SES and suicide because they typically do not factor out the influence of the covariates of lower SES such as divorce. Kposowa, Breault, & Singh (1995) found, for example, that white males with an income of greater than $25,000 had a reduced risk of suicide of 35%. However, when controls were introduced for marital status and six other correlates, this relationship became insignificant (Kposowa et al., 1995). Nevertheless, Burnley (1994) in an analysis of Australia, found that the SES–suicide relationship held up even after controls were included for marital status. In the case of Australia, divorced manual workers had the highest incidence of suicide of any group (Burnley, 1994).

Studies using income as an index of SES tend also to find an inverse relationship. For example, Hasselback, Lee, Yang, Nichol, and Wigle (1991) determined that for 261 Canadian census divisions, a 10% increase in income was associated with a 6.11% decrease in the suicide rate.

Although a majority of studies have documented an inverse relationship between socioeconomic class and suicide risk, there are exceptions. For example, certain high-status occupations are marked by high suicide rates. These include dentists whose odds of suicide are 6.64 times greater than the rest of the working-age population (Stack, 1996a). However, when the suicide rates of these relatively small high-status, high-suicide-risk groups are averaged in with often large, high-status, low-suicide-risk groups such as engineers, the result is a suicide rate that tends to be below average.

There has been a paucity of investigations to determine how efforts at redistributing income to low-status groups affect their suicide potential. One strategy is to explore the influence of welfare spending on suicide. Zimmerman (1987) determined that welfare spending in the 50 states lowered suicide rates. That is, states with relatively high degrees of welfare spending had lower suicide rates. This association was explained in terms of welfare spending being related to lowered divorce rates and increased incomes.

Whereas economic deprivation is related to suicide potential, a neglected concern is whether or not relative deprivation is also so related. That is, is the size of the gap between the deprived and the rich relevant to suicide potential? Persons who are poor in a society in which most people are poor would suffer less, it is assumed, than such persons in a society in which there is a huge gap between the economic conditions of the poor and nonpoor. It is assumed that impoverishment is even more frustrating and suicide potential should increase when there is a large income gap between the poor and the affluent. Income inequality measures have been used in the literature to measure this gap.

Results from investigations on the relationship between income inequality measures and suicide are mixed. In the case of 3,000 U.S. counties, the degree of income inequality was found to be unrelated to suicide in one study (Breault, 1988). However, in another study income inequality was found to be positively related to suicide risk (Kowalski, Faupel, & Starr, 1987). Kowalski et al.'s analysis provides a possible explanation for this discrepancy in findings. If we restrict the analysis to the most urbanized counties there is a strong relationship. This relationship is not found in the least urbanized counties. It is speculated that the urban counties provide better social conduits (e.g., direct encounters with rich persons, direct observation of the lifestyles of rich persons) for the promotion of envy or relative deprivation (Kowalski et al., 1987).

Future research needs to disentangle the effects of SES on suicide from SES's covariates such as divorce. That is, it is still unclear whether or not the impact of SES on suicide is direct. Factors associated with low SES, such as high risk of divorce, may account for part or all of the SES—suicide linkage (e.g., Stack, 1999b).

UNEMPLOYMENT

Unemployment can affect suicide by influencing two groups: the unemployed themselves and their family members. First, unemployment can affect suicide risk of actual unemployed persons in several ways. It can erode the incomes and general economic welfare, reduce self-esteem, increase anxiety, increase a sense of hopelessness, add to marital strain, increase alcoholism, and other suicidogenic factors among the unemployed themselves (e.g., Platt, 1984; Stack & Haas, 1984).

Second, unemployment's effects can reach beyond the unemployed themselves. Unemployment may influence the suicide potential of family members by lowering the standard of living of the family and increasing marital and family-centered strain. In addition, employed persons' suicide potential can increase to the extent that they fear losing their jobs, have been notified of upcoming layoffs, and so forth (Stack & Haas, 1984).

Periods of high unemployment may increase suicide potential for the majority of people in society, both the employed and unemployed. Eras of unemployment are often associated with declines in real wages. For example, most unemployed people find work within a few months, but their new jobs are usually for lower wages. Further, the new jobs of the formerly unemployed are generally lower in skill level. They are, in short, apt to be "underemployed." Such reemployed persons may be high in suicide risk due to relative deprivation (e.g., Stack & Haas, 1984). It is likely that many, if not most, households experience greater economic strain in areas and times of high unemployment.

Perhaps the most common direct test of the unemployment–suicide linkage involves individual-level, cross-sectional studies. This research strategy compares the suicide rate among members of the unemployed to that for employed persons at one point in time. In London, England, for example, the suicide rate for the unemployed was 73.4/100,000 compared to 14.1/100,000 for the general population (Platt, 1984).

Platt (1984) reviewed 17 individual-level, cross-sectional studies on suicide and unemployment. These dated from the 1920s to circa 1980. The studies showed overwhelmingly that unemployed persons have higher suicide rates than their counterparts. However, the studies' results are often difficult to compare as the definition of unemployment (e.g., labor market surveys, union members only surveys) varies among the studies (Lester & Yang, 1997a; Platt, 1984).

The link between unemployment and suicide is sometimes gendered. Women's unemployment was not always related to greater suicide potential (Platt, 1984). According to traditional gender stereotypes, women are not as vulnerable to joblessness as men. Men are still under greater pressure to be breadwinners. Hence, for men, unemployment may carry a greater social stigma than it does for women.

In the 16 years since Platt's (1984) investigation, there have been additional individual-level cross-sectional studies on unemployment and suicide. Summarized in Table 8.2, these have largely shown the same pattern as earlier studies. In Austria, for example, unemployed persons had a suicide rate of 98.3/100,000 compared to 25/100,000 for the general population (Schony & Grausgruber, 1987). In Italy, the unemployed had a suicide rate of 3.2/100,00 compared to 2.1/100,000 for the general population during 1977–1987 (Platt, 1992). For an exception, see Sholders (1981), who found a suicide rate of 13.68 for the unemployed, less than that for the over-16 population (19.3) in Indianapolis.

Some caution should be exercised, however, in interpreting individual level data on unemployment and suicide. It is not clear whether unemployment itself causes suicide among the unemployed. Some authors have tried to gauge the extent to which unemployment plays a role in driving unemployed people to suicide. The few estimates on the issue vary considerably. For example, a study in London suggests that unemployment plays an independent role in 73% of the suicides among the unemployed. A Hong Kong-based study pegged this figure at just 5% (Lester & Yang, 1997a).

As Platt (1984: 95) correctly cautions, the selection process may apply to the association between suicide potential and unemployment. Suicidal people may lose or quit their jobs because their psychological problems prevent them from being productive workers. Hence, psychological problems may be the root cause of job loss and, in turn, eventual suicide. Future work also needs to control for the covariates of unemployment such as marital disruption. Factors related to unemployment may mediate the relationship between unemployment and suicide.

A related, individual-level-based research strategy follows a group of individuals over time to assess their suicide risk. Nearly all of eight studies of this kind found that unemployment increases suicide risk (Platt, 1984). A 25-year follow-up (Hagnell & Rorsman, 1979), for example, found that 50% of the suicides had experienced job problems compared to only 18% of nonsuicides.

TABLE 8.2. Selected Suicide Rates for Unemployed versus Employed Groups

Source	Location	Unemployed	Local population
Platt (1984)	London	73.4/100,000	14.1/100,000
Schony & Grausgruber (1981)	Austria	98.3/100,000	25.0/100,000
Platt (1992)	Italy	3.2/100,000	2.1/100,000
Sholders (1981)	Indianapolis	13.7/100,000	19.2/100,000

A second research strategy used to assess the linkage between unemployment and suicide is based on ecological data. That is, the unemployment rates of populations in ecological areas such as cities, states, or nations are correlated with the suicide rate of such populations. In these ecological or aggregate studies, unemployment and suicide are treated as properties of macrosociological aggregates rather than as properties of individuals. Platt (1984) reviews nine aggregate studies analyzing data at one point in time (cross-sectional). Only one of these studies found a positive association between unemployment and suicide.

At least 14 aggregate cross-sectional studies have been published since Platt's (1984) review. There was at least some evidence in 7 of these 14 that supported a relationship between unemployment and suicide.

The mix in the findings since Platt's (1984) review can be at least partially explained by the level of aggregation (counties, states, nations) that is employed. Research using small units of aggregation is generally considered best because the population in such units is more homogeneous (Platt, 1984: 95). Such research tended to find a link between unemployment and suicide rates. This was true of studies of 3,000 U.S. counties (Breault, 1988; Faupel, Kowalski, & Starr, 1987), and for the largest counties (Kowalski et al., 1987) but not in a less-well-specified model of counties (Breault, 1986). South (1987) documents an association between unemployment and suicide in 292 standard metropolitan statistical areas. However, unemployment was not found to be related to suicide in 294 large cities (Burr, McCall, & Powell-Griner, 1994).

In contrast, almost all work on large units of aggregations (50 U.S. states) found no relationship between suicide and unemployment rates (e.g., Girard, 1988; Breault, 1986; Lester & Yang, 1997a: 103). However, for Canadian provinces, a large unit of aggregation, there was a significant relationship between unemployment and youth suicide rates, especially for those ages 20–29. The latter group is often one of the hardest hit by unemployment given that they lack seniority or experience (Trovato & Vos, 1990). Data from 18 regions in Italy, 25 Swedish counties, and 30 regions in Norway did not support the hypothesis (Platt, 1992; Rossow & Amundsen, 1995; Norstrom, 1995c). Pooled cross-sectional/time series data for the 50 states in the United States, however, gave strong support to the unemployment–suicide linkage (Gruenewald, Ponicki, & Mitchell, 1995).

The weaker findings in aggregated studies may be attributed, at least in part, to unemployed persons moving to areas of low unemployment to try to find work (Platt, 1984: 99). Further, in areas of high unemployment, unemployed people may feel less stress, be less socially stigmatized, and be more socially integrated than are unemployed persons in areas in which unemployment is relatively low (Platt, 1992: 1198).

Individual-level data provide powerful support for a link between unemployment and suicide risk, especially for men. Men, being more tied to work and careers than females, are more subject to stress and suicide risk when faced with unemployment. The research using ecological methods is more problematic. In this area of research, individual-level surveys are still needed to ascertain which groups (unemployed, underemployed, those fearing job loss, etc.) are most affected by high unemployment.

A remaining issue is the extent to which psychiatric morbidity may cause both unemployment and suicide (e.g., Platt, 1992). Shepherd and Barraclough (1980) determined that psychiatric problems affected the ability of people to function at work. This often resulted in job loss, loss of the protective value of belonging to a work force, and suicide. Possibly part of the association between unemployment and suicide is due to preexisting psychiatric problems of the unemployed, whereas part of the association is due to the generation of psychiatric problems among some of the formerly healthy people who are now unemployed.

SPECIFIC OCCUPATIONS

There has been a problem of inconsistent findings in the research evidence on specific occupation and suicide (Bedeian, 1982; Lester, 1992a: 108–112). In 11 of 18 studies of police suicide, for example, a "high" rate was reported; 3 reported an "average" rate, and 4 others concluded that police have a "low" rate (Stack & Kelley, 1994).

Some of these inconsistencies are the result of methodological problems. Such problems include shifts over time in the suicide risk of an occupational group (e.g., Lampert et al., 1984), use of inappropriate reference groups such as the suicide rate of the total population when an occupation is gender segregated, and the use of small numbers of suicides that can bias rates either upward or downward (Stack, 1998b; Stack & Kelley, 1994; Wasserman, 1992a).

A multicausal heuristic model can be used to describe the relationship between occupation and suicide (Stack, 1996a; Wasserman, 1992a). This model is composed of four major factors contributing to occupational suicide risk: demographics, stress associated with work in the occupation, psychiatric morbidity which predates entry into the occupation, and differences in opportunities for suicide. Two or more of these factors can influence the suicide rate of a given occupation at the same time.

Demographics

Occupations have different demographic compositions on such criteria as age, gender, and race. In turn, suicide varies by demographic variables. Whites have a suicide rate twice that of African Americans. Men have a suicide rate four times that of women (Lester, 1992a; Stack, 1982). Further, occupational groups vary in the extent to which their members are divorced, single, and widowed, all risk factors for suicide. Therefore, part of the reason why occupational groups have different suicide rates is simply because they have different demographic compositions (e.g., most physicians are men; most elementary education teachers are women).

In a study of England and Wales, Charlton (1995) analyzed 13,117 suicides and 252,833 natural deaths. In the case of men, only 5 of the 10 occupations with the highest suicide rates continued to have high rates after demographic controls were included in the analysis. In the case of women, only three of such occupations (veterinarian, doctor, and nurse) had significantly higher suicide rates with controls added for demographic variables.

The case of laborers is another illustration of the salience of demographics in generating occupational suicide rates. The suicide rate of laborers is greater than that of the rest of the labor force. When controls for gender, marital status, and other covariates of laborer status are employed, however, the relative odds of suicide for laborers are the same as those for the working-age population. Laborers tend to be men and are more likely to be divorced and single than are the rest of the working-age population (Stack, 1995a, 1995b). An analysis of carpenters found the same pattern (Stack, 1999b).

A majority of studies on police suicide report that the suicide rate of policemen is double or more than that of the general population. It is often argued that this is a result of work stresses such as shift work, the public's antipolice sentiments, and continual danger on the job (Stack & Kelley, 1994). However, the suicide rate for the general population is not an appropriate reference group as most police are men. Men have a suicide rate four times that of women. Using national data, Stack and Kelley (1994) report a suicide rate of 25.6/100,000 for police. This is double the national average of 12/100,000. The suicide rate for age and gender-matched controls (men 15–64) is, however, nearly the same:

23.8/100,000. The difference between these two rates is not statistically significant (Stack & Kelley, 1994). Using data from 26 states, Burnett, Boxer, and Swanson (1992) also report only a marginally elevated suicide rate for police.

Internal Occupational Stress

The nature of an occupation may contribute to stress and the risk of suicide. Client dependence, status integration, and social isolation are aspects of work that can increase the odds of suicide.

Client dependence is essentially the extent to which people in an occupation are dependent on clients for their livelihood. Such occupations include sole business operators and physicians. An exploratory study of 36 occupations found a mean suicide rate of 40.5/100,000 for persons in client-dependent occupations versus a mean of 25.9/100,000 for non-client-dependent occupations (Labovitz & Hagedorn, 1971).

The theory of status integration argues that persons in statistically infrequent role sets (e.g., female laborer) should have higher suicide rates than their counterparts (e.g., female schoolteacher) (Gibbs & Martin, 1964). It is contended that such infrequent role sets are stressful mainly because people have tended to avoid them.

Females in male-dominated occupations can experience additional work stress imposed by a society that does not completely accept females as the equal of their male counterparts (Bedeian, 1982). The category of laborer is a good example of a male-dominated occupation. According to national data, female laborers have higher suicide risk than do females in the rest of the work force (Stack, 1995a, 1995b). The military tends to be dominated by men as well. Females in the air force have a suicide rate 10 times that of other females. In the case of women in the army, the suicide rate of females is three times the general female rate (Bedeian, 1982).

The findings on women's suicide risk in male-dominated occupations are not always consistent. A more general analysis of 623 female suicides in four states found that the suicide rate for women in traditional occupations (33.8/1000,000) was indeed lower than that for women in nontraditional occupations (42.9/100,000) (Alston, 1986). However, women in moderately nontraditional occupations had the highest suicide rate (53.5/100,000). This second finding is at odds with status integration theory.

Social isolation can contribute to suicidal tendencies (Lester, 1992a; Stack, 1982). Occupations characterized by on-the-job isolation may increase suicide risk. Sheepherders are alone for extended periods of time in remote areas. Of 22 occupations studied in the state of Washington, sheepherders were found to have the highest risk of suicide (Wasserman, 1992a).

Psychiatric Morbidity

Occupations differ in the degree to which they recruit personnel at psychiatric risk of suicide. If an occupation attracts personnel with psychiatric problems that put them at risk of suicide, such occupations may be marked by elevated suicide rates. Aspects of such psychiatric morbidity are not necessarily due to occupational stress; they may preexist before entry into an occupation.

It has been postulated that the high suicide rate often reported for psychiatrists is a function of preemployment psychiatric morbidity. Highly educated persons with depressive disorders may tend to select this occupation (Bedeian, 1982; Wasserman, 1992a).

The high suicide rate among artists may also be due to preemployment psychiatric morbidity. Artists have a higher rate of psychiatric morbidity higher than the general population. Andreasen (1987) determined, for example, that 80% of 30 creative writers in her intensive study met the criteria for an affective disorder. Furthermore, 43% met the criteria for a bipolar disorder. For a control group of professional workers, these percentages were only 30% and 10%, respectively. Two of the writers in Andreasen's (1987) study, or 6.7%, had already committed suicide, a figure well above the national average of 1.5%. It is still not clear whether art attracts persons with mental disorders or creates these disorders, or both. Research indicates, however, that mood disorders often facilitate artistic expression. Perhaps both positions are true (Stack, 1996b). Controlling for the covariates of artist status, Stack (1996b) found that artists have a suicide risk 2.25 times higher than for that of the rest of the working-age population.

Opportunity Factors

Opportunities available for access to lethal means of suicide vary among occupations. For example, the availability of lethal drugs in the medical profession (physicians, pharmacists, dentists, nurses) has been linked to corresponding high suicide risk (Burnett et al., 1992; Peipins, Burnett, & Alterman, 1997; Stack, 1996a; Wasserman, 1992a). Therefore, it would be expected that medical and dental assistants would also have high suicide risk, but this is not the case (Wasserman, 1992a).

It would be anticipated that occupations with high gun availability, such as police work and the military, would have above-average opportunities for suicide. These two occupations generally have an average or below-average suicide rate. This is especially true if one controls for the covariates of such work (e.g. gender) (Burnett et al., 1992; Burnley, 1995; Helmkamp, 1996; Milham, 1983; Stack & Kelley, 1994; Wasserman, 1992a).

National Data on Occupation and Suicide

Data on occupation and suicide for a large number of occupations are scarce (Bedeian, 1982; Wasserman, 1992a; Stack, 1996a). Table 8.3 presents national data on suicide risk for 30 occupations (Stack, 1999a). The table presents the odds of suicide or relative risk (RR) of an occupational group relative to the rest of the working-age population for 1990 (Stack, 1999a). Occupations high in suicide risk include dentists, laborers, physicians, and artists. Occupations low in suicide risk include elementary school teachers, clerks, and postal workers. Dentists are 4.45 times more likely to die from suicide, for example, than the working-age population. Elementary school teachers are 46% less likely than the rest of the working-age population to die from suicide. However, most of the RR are not statistically significant. Many occupations simply do not contribute significantly to suicide risk.

Qualitative work needs to be done to sort out occupational stressors from nonoccupational stressors. Interviews with suicide attempters and the significant others of those who complete suicide in an occupation could accomplish this mission. In this fashion we can determine whether an occupation, per se, drives some people toward suicidal behavior as opposed to something associated with the occupation such as psychiatric morbidity.

BUSINESS CYCLES, DEPRESSIONS, AND RECESSIONS

Three theoretical perspectives have guided the research on the business cycle and suicide (Lester & Yang, 1997a). Explanations have contended that (1) suicide increases in both prosperous and recessionary times (Durkheim, 1966), (2) suicide increases only in reces-

TABLE 8.3. Relative Risk Ratios of Suicide for Selected Occupations Relative to the Working-Age Population, 21 States, United States, 1990

Occupation	Relative risk ratio
Managerial/professional	
Executives/Managers	−0.03
Doctors	1.94*
Dentists	4.45*
Lawyers	1.44
Professors	1.13
Accountants	1.17
Engineers	1.21
Mathematicians and scientists	1.85*
Artists	2.12*
Nurses	−0.01
Social workers	1.41
Elementary school teachers	−0.44*
Clerical	
Bookkeepers	−0.28
Clerks	−0.25*
Postal workers	−0.38*
Service	
Police	−0.07
Private security	1.14
Cooks	−0.16
Bartenders	1.25
Agricultural and extractive	
Farmers	0.08
Farm workers	1.13
Miners	1.33*
Skilled manual	
Machinists	1.63*
Auto mechanics	1.41*
Electricians	1.32*
Plumbers	1.63*
Carpenters	2.00*
Semi/unskilled manual	
Welders	1.46*
Laborers	1.31*
Truck drivers (heavy equipment)	1.09

*$p < .05$.

sionary times while it decreases in times of prosperity (Henry & Short, 1954), and (3) suicide increases only in prosperous times and declines in recessions (Ginsberg, 1966). See Figure 8.1 for an illustration of these three views.

Durkheim (1966) argued that suicide rates would increase in times of both economic contraction and expansion. Both represent disturbances of the collective order (Durkheim, 1966: 247). In both cases social regulation and social integration are diminished. In times of prosperity, there is a problem of the unleashing of appetites. Aspirations for material or

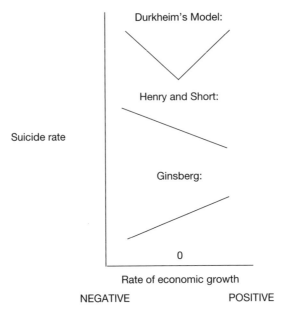

FIGURE 8.1. Three models of the business cycle and suicide. *Source:* Lester & Yang (1997a). Copyright 1997 by Nova Science Publishers. Reprinted by permission.

consumer goods can accelerate faster than the supply, creating a situation of anomie. In addition, a quest after limitless material goods is seen as meaningless. The key to suicide prevention rests in strong social bonds to family, religion, and work. Economic growth and the quest after material goals can detract from maintaining strong social bonds (Durkheim, 1966).

Suicide would also be apt to increase in recessions. In recessions there is a sudden gap between material needs and resources, creating another situation marked by anomie (Durkheim, 1966). Hence, Durkheim's theory of the business cycle and suicide resembles a U-shaped curve. The high points on the curve are the top and bottom of the business cycle. Suicide is in the low range in the transitional period between market highs and lows.

Henry and Short (1954) contended that suicide would increase only in depressions, not in prosperous times. A return to prosperity would reduce suicide. The underlying explanatory mechanism was frustration aggression theory. In economic downturns, frustration increases as an increasing proportion of people cannot realize their financial goals. This frustration can increase aggression, including suicide. In contrast, a trend toward prosperity means that an increasing proportion of people can realize their economic goals. In this case frustration is reduced and suicide should, therefore, decline.

Like Durkheim (1966), Ginsberg (1966) held that suicide increases in economic prosperity. However, unlike both Durkheim and Henry and Short (1954), Ginsberg (1966) argued that suicide should decline in economic recessions. Ginsberg's (1966) perspective has been neglected but was recently restated by Lester and Yang (1997a). Basically, in an argument similar to Durkheim's (1966), during economic expansion, aspirations rise faster than economic growth. This imbalance leads to greater suicide potential. Unlike other theorists, Ginsberg contends that in recessions, economic aspirations decrease faster than declines in economic growth. Thus people expect less than what they receive and suicide potential declines in recessions.

Research on the business cycle and suicide has relied overwhelmingly on unemployment rates as an index of the business cycle (e.g., see the review in Platt, 1984). Other indicators have included the Ayres Index of industrial activity (e.g., Henry & Short, 1954; Pierce, 1967), gross domestic product (GDP) growth rates, change in the stock market index, and the rate of construction of new dwelling units (Lester & Yang, 1997a; Marshall & Hodge, 1981; Pierce, 1967).

Testing the Durkheimian Model

A critical limitation of nearly all of this work is that it tests linear models of the business cycle (Lester & Yang, 1997a, 1997b). That is, no quadratic term is entered into the analysis to test for a curvilinear relationship between the business cycle and suicide. This makes the confirmation or rejection of Durkheim's curvilinear or U-shaped perspective difficult. Ginsberg's procyclical perspective, which posits a largely linear and negative relationship between unemployment and suicide, can be tested with a linear model. The Henry and Short (1954) perspective that argues that suicide rises in depression and falls in prosperity can also be adequately tested with a linear model without a quadratic economic term.

An exception to the lack of rigorous testing of the Durkheimian position with a curvilinear or quadratic model is a study by Lester and Yang (1997b). Lester and Yang (1997b) tested quadratic models for each of 14 nations for the period 1950–1985. Only one of the 14 models had a significant quadratic term. This was for the Netherlands. In 10 cases a significant linear and positive relationship was found between changes in unemployment and changes in suicide rates. The results are largely consistent with the Henry and Short (1954) model.

An alternative to the introduction of a quadratic term in testing the U-shaped Durkheimian hypothesis is to take the absolute value of the differenced data on economic indicators. The Durkheimian (1966) hypothesis argues that it is the rate of economic change, not its direction, that drives suicide rates. Pierce (1967) took the first difference of a variety of economic indicators including unemployment, housing construction, and Ayres Index of industrial activity and then transformed them into absolute values Unfortunately all analyses, except one, of nine indicators were marked by the statistical problem of significant autocorrelation. This condition precludes valid conclusions. Pierce (1967) did find that the absolute value of change in the stock market prices was positively associated with suicide national male suicide rates during 1919–1940. Hence, this confirmed the Durkheimian position that economic change in the business cycle, whether upward or downward, increases suicide risk.

Marshall and Hodge (1981) updated Pierce's (1967) crude correlational analysis with more modern Cochrane Orcutt time-series techniques. In this fashion the problem of autocorrelated error terms, which plagued Pierce's correlational analysis, was remedied. Marshall and Hodge incorporated indicators of both absolute degrees of change (absolute value of stock market prices) as well as directional indicators (first difference of stock market process, and first difference of the unemployment rate). The term representing the absolute value of economic change was insignificant. No support was found for the Durkheimian hypothesis. However, the rate of unemployment emerged as the leading predictor of suicide rates, confirming the Henry and Short (1954) hypothesis.

Lester and Yang (1997a: 39–41) analyzed the suicide rate and the percentage change in the GDP between 1933 and 1986. To the extent that shifts in stock prices may not affect the everyday economic life of most people who do not own appreciable amounts of stock, the percentage change in GDP may be a better index of recession versus prosperity than stock prices. A plot of the percentage change in GDP and change in the suicide rate (suicide rate minus the 5-year moving average) was U-shaped. This indicated support for the

Durkheimian argument. However, this finding is in need of replication. More sophisticated analyses than plots need to be done on the data series.

Testing the Henry and Short Model

The vast majority of studies on the business cycle and suicide were not designed to test Durkheim's (1966) U-shaped hypothesis. The dominant model in research on the business cycle and suicide has used time-series analysis techniques on unemployment as an index of the state of the economy. The unemployment rate of a population, usually a nation, is studied over time, usually a period of 20 or more years. In most of this work, first differences or more advanced differencing techniques are employed so that investigators are actually exploring the relationship between changes in unemployment and changes in suicide rates. Nevertheless, it typically tests the commonsense notion that unemployment trends should be positively related to suicide trends (Henry & Short, 1954). Any work finding the reverse to be the case, that unemployment is negatively related to suicide trends, would be consistent with the Ginsberg (1966) position.

Platt (1984) reviewed 31 such longitudinal, aggregated studies and reported somewhat mixed findings. Of these 31 studies, 21, or two-thirds, supported a significant positive relationship between suicide and unemployment. Basically, the Henry and Short (1954) model was confirmed in this research. However, six studies had mixed findings, and four studies found no relationship between unemployment and suicide. There was no evidence, however, for Ginsberg's (1966) hypothesis.

There have been numerous studies of this type since Platt (1984). Most continue to illustrate a positive link between unemployment trends and suicide trends over time. In some research the relationship is conditional, depending on gender and/or the time period analyzed.

Research documenting a positive relationship between unemployment and suicide trends includes that done with annual U.S. data. The relationship existed for both males and females (Stack, 1987b; Yang & Lester, 1994).

Some U.S.-based research inspects monthly data on trends that might be missed when unemployment and suicide are measured by annual data. Monthly time-series studies on the United States have confirmed the positive link (e.g., Stack, 1987a; Wasserman, 1984).

The relationship between unemployment trends and suicide has also been supported by analyses of other nations. These include analyses of Danish data from 1951–1980 (Stack, 1990a) and data for 1966–1981 in Quebec (Cormier & Klerman, 1985).

Some research illustrates mixed findings in other nations. In the case of Australia, Hassan and Tan's (1989) analysis of data for 80 years dating from 1901–1981 has evidence for males but none for females. Lester's (1992c) results for 20 years dating from 1966–1985 for Australia found no evidence for males. In like manner, Canadian unemployment trends for 1950–1982 were related only to male suicide rates (Trovato, 1986).

Some discrepancies in the work on unemployment and suicide might be resolved if it could be determined that there is a threshold effect; that is, whether or not the unemployment rate has to be at a high level for it to affect the suicide rate. For example, postwar Norwegian unemployment was unrelated to suicide, possibly because full employment policies generally kept it below 2%. This percentage is below a floor where it might affect the national suicide rate (Stack, 1989); however, the relationship holds if the Great Depression era is included (Norstrom, 1995c). In a like manner, evidence for a link in Australia increased by the inclusion of the Great Depression years (Hassan & Tan, 1989; Lester, 1992c).

Historical data indicate that increases in suicide in the Great Depression were often substantial. Sainsbury, Jenkins, and Levey (1980) determined that during the Great Depression, male suicides increased in 15 of 20 nations for men ages 20–39, in 19 of 20 nations for men ages 40–49, and in 15 of 20 for men age 60 and over. In some the increase was very high: 108% for young men in Finland and 96% for young men in Chile. With the Great Depression years left out of an analysis, it would seem plausible that for many nations the link between unemployment and suicide would weaken or even disappear.

Linear (or straight-line) time-series analyses of unemployment and suicide generally support a positive link between suicide risk and unemployment trends. This is true especially for males. The inclusion of periods with high unemployment, such as the Great Depression, also tends to increase the strength of the unemployment–suicide relationship.

Although quadratic models (e.g., such as a U-shaped curve) are not tested in most of this literature, given that linear models tend to fit the data series quite well, it would appear that the U-shaped Durkheimian model might not fit these data series. A test involving time series for each of 14 nations confirmed this point (Lester & Yang, 1997b).

Historical work on monthly suicide trends and the Ayres Index of industrial activity has found mixed results (e.g., Pierce, 1967; Stack, 1988; Wasserman, 1983). For the period 1910–1920, the monthly suicide rate was unrelated to industrial activity. However, industrial activity was negatively related to monthly suicide trends during 1924–1939 (Wasserman, 1983). Wasserman (1983: 717) suggests that the variation in unemployment associated with industrial activity was simply not large enough to influence suicide in the 1910s. However, with the large swings in industrial production and suicide in the 1930s included, one finds such a relationship.

Whereas rigorous tests of the Durkheimian perspective are uncommon, the evidence to date has largely rejected the U-shaped nonlinear relationship suggested by Durkheim. The great bulk of the evidence is consistent with the linear argument of Henry and Short: The greater the prosperity, the lower the suicide rate, or the greater the trend toward recession, the greater the suicide rate. The positive relationship between unemployment and suicide is sometimes marked by a floor effect and often is stronger for men than for women. No evidence has been found for the third position of Ginsberg (1966).

COHORT ANALYSIS

Cohort analysis in suicidology has taken at least three different paths. First, relative cohort size (RCS) models are keyed into the economic strain faced by a relatively large cohort of working-age persons. The suicide risk of the large cohort is measured relative to the size of the cohort with which they are competing on the labor market (e.g., number of 16- to 29-year-olds/number of 30- to 64-year-olds). In this way, measurement errors resulting from shifts in fertility, life expectancy, and the size of the nonworking population are controlled (Easterlin, 1987a). Second, a related model explores the effect of the size of an age group relative to the rest of the entire population, (e.g., groups not in the labor force including the very young and the elderly). This may be, for example, the number of 15- to 24-year-olds/0- to 100+-year-olds (Holinger, Offer, & Ostrove, 1987). A limitation of these models is the measurement error involved in including age groups in the denominator (e.g., 0–15 and 65 and over) with which the target age group (e.g., 15–24) is not competing on the labor market. Finally, there are age-period-cohort models (APC) designed to ascertain whether the high or low suicide rate of a 5-year youthful cohort (e.g., those born between 1933 and 1937) follows them through the life course through the 1980s (e.g., Wasserman, 1989b).

APC models control for the aging process by introducing dummy variables (0,1) for $X - 1$ age categories. For example, Wasserman (1989a) analyzes suicide rates from a table with $X = 13$ age brackets ranging from 15–19 to 75–79. He creates 12 binary variables to measure the aging process with one additional category serving as the benchmark age category. Period effects are generally also measured by introducing binary variables representing 5-year intervals over time. For example, Wasserman (1989a) analyzes 11 time periods, and introduces 11–1 binary variables for such periods between 1933 and 1983 (see Table 8.4). The dependent variable in APC effects are the suicide rates in the cells of the table showing the rates by year and age category. Wasserman's (1989b: 300) table has 11 periods and 13 age brackets; thus there are a total of 143 suicide rates to analyze. In an 11-period × 13-age-bracket suicide rate table there are a total of 16 cohorts, all of which have incomplete data over time. It takes 60 years, or 12 5-year periods, for a cohort to age from 15–24 to 75–79, and there are only 11 5-year periods in the table. Wasserman's (1989b) analysis does not find a cohort effect unless controls are introduced for age and period. Results of APC models need to be taken with caution due to multicollinearity problems and the fact that complete information on suicide rates over the life course is simply unavailable for most cohorts. Hence, developmental paths in suicide are simply not observable for most concrete cohorts. Inferences about cohort effects are largely based on incomplete information (Lester, 1992a). In any event, because none of the APC variables measures economic strain even indirectly, this chapter will not deal with APC models. Further, given the measurement errors in the denominator of cohort variables in the second variety of cohort analyses (e.g., Holinger et al., 1987), this chapter focuses only on the methodologically superior RCS models.

Relative cohort size (RCS) has stimulated a stream of research on suicide risk. This view stresses the negative economic consequences associated with membership in a relatively large cohort (Ahlburg & Schapiro, 1984; Easterlin, 1987a; Pampel & Peters, 1995). Cohort size represents the principal determinant of both income potential and the expected standard of living. The expected standard of living comes from childhood socialization. The baby-boomers, a large cohort, were socialized by a small parental cohort. The relatively high standard of living of a small parental cohort influences the economic expectations of a large birth cohort such as the baby-boomers. When these expectations are not met, the potential for deviant behavior, crime, and suicide increases (Easterlin, 1987a; Pampel & Peters, 1995).

TABLE 8.4. Suicide Rates (per 100,000 Population) among White Males Who Were Born between 1914 and 1918, in the United States, 1933–1983

Age category	Suicide rate (year)
15–19	4.7 (1933)
20–24	14.0 (1938)
25–29	10.6 (1943)
30–34	14.9 (1948)
35–39	17.5 (1953)
40–44	25.6 (1958)
45–49	29.4 (1963)
50–54	30.8 (1968)
55–59	32.1 (1973)
60–64	32.0 (1978)
65–69	29.4 (1983)

Source: Wasserman (1989b). Copyright 1989 by Elsevier Science. Reprinted by permission.

Economic fortunes tend to vary inversely with relative cohort size because large cohorts face problems in three overcrowded institutions. First, crowding in the family reduces the energy and psychological attention that the parent can offer, which results in less than optimal development. Second, crowding in schools deteriorates the quality of education received by a large cohort, as class size increases and the credentials required for teachers, who are in short supply, decline. Such crowding problems reduce the skills that students bring with them to the labor market. Third, the crowded labor market contributes to competition for jobs, underemployment, low wages, a slowing down in the process of promotion, and low income potential (Pampel & Peters, 1995).

Adaptations to such economic strain in a glutted labor market include a transformation of traditional expectations for family life: a lower marriage rate, childlessness in marriage, later age at first marriage, increase in illegitimacy, increase in female labor force participation, lower fertility, and more abortions. With these adaptations, however, men in large cohorts may feel a strain and sense of disappointment to the extent that they have been unable to fulfill traditional male economic roles. The sacrifice of family-oriented goals, in particular, is apt to increase male stress levels. Further, such economic and lifestyle stress can promote family strain, including divorce. In turn, these sources of stress can produce deviant behavior including suicide.

Easterlin (1987b: 3) notes that cohort size will affect the economic and lifestyle outcomes of a large cohort only when other conditions are relatively constant. Certain conditions may offset RCS, or at least reduce its power in shaping behavior.

First, large waves of immigration can offset the importance of RCS in the shaping of suicide risk. The advantages of a small birth cohort can be canceled out by a large influx of immigrants from other nations. Second, female labor force participation can offset the negative economic effects for a large cohort. However, it may also contribute to feelings of failure in traditional men who had expected larger families and traditional family structures such as those in which they were raised as children. Third, RCS arguments may apply more to generating stress among men, to the extent that men are socialized more into the role of breadwinner than are women. Fourth, RCS applies best to developed nations because children are a consumption goal, unlike in undeveloped nations where they are used in agricultural production. Fifth, the influence of RCS can be offset by the extent of the modern welfare state. That is, the state may maintain policies (e.g., full employment and social welfare safety nets for the poor and unemployed) such that they offset the economic stress that would otherwise be faced by a large cohort (Easterlin, 1987b; Pampel, 1993; Pampel & Peters, 1995).

Many of the factors intervening between RCS and suicide can be interpreted from a traditional sociological perspective. For example, by promoting singleness, childlessness, low fertility, and divorce, RCS reduces family integration (Durkheim, 1966).

Ahlburg and Schapiro (1984) performed the first rigorous test of the RCS model as it applies to suicide. RCS was measured as the ratio of the size of the 16- to 29-year-old cohort to that of the 30- to 64-year-old cohort. Using annual data on male suicide for 1948–1976, the authors demonstrated a positive relationship between RCS and the suicide rate of younger male age groups (15–24, 25–34, and 35–44). In turn, RCS was negatively related, as expected, to the suicide rate of the older male groups (45–54 and 55–64) (Ahlburg & Shapiro, 1984: 106). This relationship held up for both men and women for younger cohorts. However, for older cohorts, RCS was unexpectedly positively related to the suicide rates of older women.

Little work is available on how certain contexts mentioned in the theory might offset or multiply the impact of RCS on suicide risk. For example, Pampel and Peters (1995: 168) cautioned that a generous welfare state may be able to cushion or even offset the negative effects of RCS.

Welfare programs for the poor and full employment policies in the Scandinavian nations might act as safety nets for the persons in a relatively large cohort. Further, command economies, such as those in communist and formerly communist nations, might also have welfare policies that reduce the impact of RCS on suicide (Stack, 1997).

Stack (1997) analyzed 12 industrialized nations for the 1950–1980 period. They were classified as capitalist or market economies (e.g., United States and Canada), welfare capitalist (e.g., Scandinavian nations) and command economies (e.g., Czechoslovakia, Hungary, and Poland). Stack (1997) determined that RCS was related to youth suicide rates in market economies (e.g., United States and Canada) and mixed economics (e.g., Sweden). However, it was not so related in command economies. This analysis suggests that the RCS model might be generalizable to most advanced capitalist nations but not to communist nations. The greater degree of state control over the income distribution and employment level in communist nations may have offset the RCS effect.

The available analyses of the RCS suicide model are largely based on data series before the mid-1980s. According to Pampel and Peters (1995), however, the generalized RCS model of social behavior started to break down and not fit previous patterns found for the pre-1980s era. Whether or not this is true for the specific case of suicide is not clear.

WORK MOBILITY

Research on mobility in suicidology has tended to be focused on the relationship between migration from one place to another and suicide. Research has linked such geographic mobility to suicide rates between provinces, states, and nations (e.g., Stack, 1982; Trovato, 1986). Populations marked by high changes in residence tend to have higher suicide rates.

Work mobility involves changes in employment. Conceptually, such changes can take several forms along at least two dimensions. First, work mobility can take on either an intergenerational or an intragenerational form. Intergenerational mobility involves a change in employment status between generations. The son of a bricklayer who becomes a doctor would be an example of upward intergenerational mobility. Downward intergenerational mobility involves a change in work status between generations. The son of a doctor who becomes a bricklayer would be a case in point. Horizontal intergenerational mobility involves a change in occupation between generations that shows no significant change in status. For example, the daughter of a doctor who becomes a corporate lawyer might approximate such horizontal mobility.

Mobility can also refer to intragenerational change in work status when the occupational history of a single individual is compared over time. A bricklayer who goes to night school and ultimately becomes a doctor would be an example of intragenerational upward mobility. If a doctor loses his license and ends up laying bricks to make a living, that is intragenerational downward mobility. If a surgeon goes from working in a hospital in California to a similar one in Connecticut, this would be intragenerational horizontal mobility.

There has been some debate over the nature of the impact of work mobility on suicide risk. Work mobility upward could conceivably lower suicide potential through higher incomes and the many economic lifestyle gains of movement up the ladder. However, some authors suggest that upward mobility should increase suicide risk by breaking down social integration: social bonds to such groups as the extended family and church (Davis, 1980a, 1980b; Porterfield & Gibbs, 1960: 151). Porterfield and Gibbs (1960: 151) also contend that upward work mobility probably increases suicide risk through anxiety over threats to losing status.

Other writers theorize that it is downward work mobility that results in increased suicide risk (Breed, 1963). Downward work mobility is seen as increasing suicide risk through such mechanisms as income loss, disappointment, frustration, decreased approval from peers, and decreased self-respect (Breed, 1963: 184).

Maris (1981: 156) contends that the most meaningful characteristics of suicidal work histories are erratic work histories, unemployment, and developmental stagnation. Erratic work histories characterized by frequent job changes were also noted among suicidal individuals in New Orleans (Breed, 1963). These problems can conceivably take place among both the intergenerational upward and downward groups.

Of the many aspects of economy and suicide, work mobility is perhaps the least studied. Searches through standard databases including MEDLINE, Sociofile, and PsycLIT uncovered less than 60 citations on "mobility" and suicide, from the 1965–1998 period. Moreover, only a few of these dealt with "occupational" mobility. The overwhelmingly majority were on "geographic" mobility. The dearth of current research in this area is reflected in other reviews (Stack, 1982). For example, book-length reviews on suicide do not cover occupational mobility (Lester, 1992a; Maris, Berman, Maltsberger, & Yufit, 1992).

The earliest quantitative study on work mobility and suicide risk was done by Porterfield and Gibbs (1960) in New Zealand. The data all refer to males over 35 years of age. The occupations of 532 suicide victims were compared to those of their fathers. The extent of work mobility from father to son in the suicides was compared to that for a sample of 149 natural deaths. Although Porterfield and Gibbs (1960) concluded that "victims of suicide freely change position between generations on the prestige scale" (150), this view is somewhat contradicted by their own data. The relevant table for assessing the relationship between mobility and suicide risk is absent in their paper but can be readily constructed from their data (Porterfield & Gibbs, 1960: 150). Table 8.5 provides their results on intergenerational work mobility and relative suicide risk. For 28.5% of the completed suicides, the son's work status was lower than that of the father's compared to 16.1% of the controls. Hence, those who completed suicide in New Zealand were nearly twice as likely as those who died natural deaths to have experienced downward mobility in their work careers.

These data from Porterfield and Gibbs (1960) are to be taken with caution because they are not restricted to the working-age population. People who die natural deaths obviously tend to be older than suicide victims. And, as Maris (1981: 156) notes, if one continues to work into retirement, there is a greater chance that one's occupational status will decline in the last years of life. This increases the chances that such persons would be classified as downwardly mobile. Hence, the difference noted in their Table 3 is conservative because the 16.1% downwardly mobile figure for natural deaths is probably exaggerated due to downward changes in occupational status in retirement. As a check on this possibility, an

TABLE 8.5. Intergenerational Work Mobility in Completed Suicides (1946–1951) and Intergenerational Work Mobility among Natural Deaths (1948), Men over 35, New Zealand

	Completed suicides	Natural deaths
Son higher	19.9%	21.5%
Son same	51.6%	62.4%
Son lower	28.5%	16.1%
	100%	100%

Source: Porterfield & Gibbs (1960: 150). Copyright 1960 by University of Chicago Press. Adapted by permission.

analysis of an age-matched control group such as the living working population would have been desirable.

Breed (1963) investigated the work histories of 75 white male suicides who suicided in New Orleans during 1954–1959. The age range, 20–60 years, nearly matched that of the working-age population. This is an important methodological consideration neglected in most other studies that included men in their retirement years. A control group consisting of 169 men drawn from the same neighborhoods as the suicide victims was constructed. Table 8.6 gives the results on the intergenerational work mobility patterns of the suicides and controls. Twenty-five percent of the suicides were sons with a higher status than their fathers (upwardly mobile) This was true of 38% of the controls. Upwardly mobile sons were therefore less likely to die from suicide. At the other extreme, 53% of the sons who died from suicide were downwardly mobile compared to only 31% of the downwardly mobile controls. Downward mobility, then, appears to be associated with increased suicide risk.

In terms of intragenerational mobility, considerable downward mobility or "skidding" was found, and relatively little upward mobility. Using the North Hatt occupational prestige measure developed by North and Hatt Breed (1963) determined that 33% of suicides employed full time at death had been downwardly mobile during their lifetime. This compared to only 5% of the controls. Fifty percent of suicides employed part time at death had experienced downward job mobility in their lifetime. Further, during their own work histories 51% of the suicides had experienced loss of income in the years prior to death compared to only 11% of the controls. Breed's (1963) analysis provides the strongest evidence for a link between downward work mobility and suicide risk.

Shepherd and Barraclough (1980) studied the work histories, including a brief coverage of intragenerational occupational mobility, in a sample of 75 suicides and 150 controls. The suicides showed more unemployment, more job changes, and more absence from work for such reasons as sickness and held their jobs for shorter periods than the controls. Only a limited test of occupational mobility and suicide was performed using just the 2 years preceding death. Only 16 of the 225 persons in the study experienced an observable change in jobs (there were no data available for an unspecified number) for in this time frame. During this 2-year window, movement was downward for five of eight suicides and six of the eight controls who experienced a job change. There was no difference between the suicides and controls in social class mobility during this limited period.

Maris (1981: 149–156) studied the work careers of 160 suicide completers and 49 natural deaths. The suicides were a sample from Cook County, Illinois, during 1966–1968 and the control groups of natural deaths was taken from Baltimore during 1969–1970.

In terms of intergenerational social mobility, Maris's results are in Table 8.7. Fifty-seven percent of the Chicago suicides had been upwardly mobile; they had SES scores higher than those of their fathers. This compared to 41% of the natural deaths. It is also much

TABLE 8.6. Intergenerational Work Mobility in Completed Suicides (1954–1959) and Intergenerational Work Mobility among Natural Deaths, Men between 20 and 60, New Orleans

	Completed suicides	Natural deaths
Son higher	25%	38%
Son same	22%	31%
Son lower	53%	31%
	100%	100%

Source: Breed (1963).

TABLE 8.7. Intergenerational Work Mobility in Completed
Suicides, Chicago (1966–1968), and Intergenerational Work
Mobility among Natural Deaths, Baltimore (1969–1970)

	Completed suicides	Natural deaths
Son higher	57%	41%
Son same	7%	4%
Son lower	36%	55%
	100%	100%

Source: Maris (1981). Copyright 1981 by Johns Hopkins University Press.
Adapted by permission.

higher than the 25% of the suicide completers who were found to be upwardly mobile in New Orleans: 36% of the completers were downwardly mobile compared to 55% of the natural deaths; 7% of the completers and 4% of the natural deaths were horizontally mobile or had the same SES occupational score as their fathers. Hence, suicide risk was associated with upward, not downward, mobility.

The findings of Maris (1981) need to be taken with some caution due to the possible differences in social mobility rates between the cities of Chicago and Baltimore. In addition, the control group of natural deaths were, as Maris (1981: 156) points out, about 20 years older than the suicide completers. For example, 48% of the natural deaths were retired versus 18% of the completers. Given that there has been a tendency for social mobility to increase over time (i.e., there has been an increase in white-collar jobs and a decrease in blue-collar jobs), we would expect to find more intergenerational mobility in a younger age group (suicide completers) than in an older one (e.g., natural deaths). This may minimize the amount of upward mobility found in the control group of natural deaths, thereby inflating the importance of upward mobility in the completed suicide group.

The research findings on work mobility and suicide risk indicate no consistent pattern. Some research finds that suicides are more apt than controls to be downwardly mobile (Breed, 1963; Porterfield & Gibbs, 1960). Other work finds that suicides are more upwardly mobile than are controls (Maris, 1981). Still other work indicates no work mobility difference between suicides and controls (Shepherd & Barraclough, 1980).

Job mobility has been used as a concept in the study of black suicide. There has been a substantial rise in suicide among young blacks. By the late 1970s the suicide rate of young (e.g., less than 40 years old) blacks was essentially the same as that of young whites (Stack, 1982). Davis (1980a, 1980b) contended that this may be due to work mobility. Young, upwardly mobile blacks often reduce or break ties to their extended family and to the church. However, these ties are needed, Davis (1980a) contends, as part of blacks' "survival strategy" against racism.

Historically two institutions accounted for a low suicide rate among blacks: family and church. A key part of this survival strategy was low occupational aspirations. Low occupational aspirations can protect one against failure (due to racism and other problems) in the labor market (Davis, 1980a; Stack & Wasserman, 1995).

As young upwardly mobile blacks reduced their ties to these institutions, their horizontal restraints (Henry & Short, 1954) were reduced. Or, in another vocabulary, their degree of social integration or bonds to family and church was reduced. With horizontal restraints and integration levels lowered, it would be expected that their suicide rate would increase. At the root of these trends, however, is the occupational mobility process (Davis, 1980a). Davis (1980a), however, offered no hard data as evidence for these arguments.

Some work on the related issue of educational mobility offers some indirect support for Davis's (1980a, 1980b) position. Stack (1998a), in an analysis of national data on education and suicide, found that for every year of educational attainment, suicide risk increases 8% for black males. In contrast, one year of educational attainment reduces suicide risk by 2% for white males. Black college graduates are at especially high risk for suicide. Although the data set employed by Stack—the national mortality tapes—has no data on ties to the extended family or church, the notion that highly educated blacks were the most suicidal would mesh well with the notion that blacks with high levels of occupational mobility are the most suicidal. That is, to the extent that education promotes work mobility, this relationship would be anticipated.

La Free, Drass, and O'Day (1992) offer another possible explanation for the rise in black suicide as well as criminality. Although there has been substantial educational mobility among blacks, there has been essentially no change in economic well-being indicators. These economic indicators include the unemployment ratio, mean incomes, and poverty rates between blacks and whites. A gap between educational achievement and job/income aspirations has widened. The resulting gap increases the risk of both suicide and criminal activity (La Free et al., 1992; Stack, 1998a).

The research on work mobility and suicide has been marked by inconsistent findings that are difficult to resolve. In addition, the samples have been relatively small. No national study has been done on occupational mobility and suicide. Further, essentially all the research that exists on the specific problem of occupational mobility and suicide is based on samples that are at least 30 years old. Much more work needs to be done on this issue to have even some consensus on a basic understanding of how work mobility is related to suicide risk.

PROFESSIONAL AND EXECUTIVE SUICIDE

Only a small proportion of the several hundred major occupations have been the subject of empirical research on suicide (Lester, 1992a). Of these, among the most commonly studied are the professions. This section reviews the major findings on the professions and executive/managerial occupations. The professional occupations are broken down into medical and nonmedical categories. The medical category includes physicians, dentists, nurses, and psychiatrists, and veterinarians. Under the nonmedical professional category, studies have been done on occupations such as artists, chemists, engineers and scientists, professors, schoolteachers, and social workers (Boxer et al., 1995; Lester, 1992a).

Physicians

Research on the incidence of suicide among physicians is marked by considerable debate over the extent to which physicians are at risk for suicide (e.g., Bedeian, 1982: 207–210; Brown, 1990; Juel, Mosbech, & Hansen, 1997; Lester, 1992a: 108–110; Revicki & May, 1984; Sonneck & Wagner, 1996; Steffansson & Wicks, 1991; Wasserman, 1992a). Themes in the research include those (1) positing high physician suicide rates, (2) contending that physicians are no more at risk for suicide than are white males, (3) attempting to explain within-group variation or why some physicians suicide and others do not, and (4) focusing on high suicide rates among female physicians.

One body of research reports that physicians are at a high risk of suicide. Early work from the 1960s, which used a questionable methodology based on obituaries in the *Journal of the American Medical Association* (JAMA), is still often cited as evidence for a high physician suicide rate (Brown, 1990). More reliable estimates based on national public health data for 1950 found that physicians were tied for 15th place with civil engineers with a suicide rate of 31.9/100,000. The median rate for the 36 selected occupations was only slightly lower at 27.2/100,000 (Labovitz & Hagedorn, 1971). For the state of Washington between 1950 and 1979 the physician suicide rate was 6th out of 22 occupations surveyed, with sheepherders and dentists having the greatest risk of suicide (Wasserman, 1992a: 533). Data from California indicate a physician suicide rate of 69/100,000 (Brown, 1990: 173; Rose & Rosow, 1973). An analysis of 2,387 physician deaths in Denmark concluded that physicians were at greater risk for suicide than the general population (Juel et al., 1997).

The reasons for this alleged relatively high rate remain unclear. A reported high incidence of alcoholism and greater access to lethal drugs among physicians are often cited as possible explanations (Keeve, 1984; Wasserman, 1992a: 527, 533).

A second body of research reports that physicians are not at high risk for suicide. A key issue is whether or not the rate is compared to the general population or to the population of white males. Because most physicians are white males, and white males have a high suicide rate (about double that of the general population), it is important to control for race and gender effects. Reanalysis of the classic *JAMA* obituary data has found that the suicide rate of physicians (35.7–38.4/100,000) is comparable to that of white males (Brown, 1990; see review in Bedeian, 1982). Further, an analysis of data from North Carolina found no significant difference between the physician and white male suicide rates (Revicki & May, 1984).

Research from other nations also found that male physicians are not at high risk for suicide (Sonneck & Wagner, 1996; Rimpala, Nurminen, Runpala, & Valkonen, 1987). In Sweden, for 1960–1985, male physician suicide was higher than that of the male working-age population only in the period of the 1970s (Stefansson & Wicks, 1991). Arnetz et al. (1987) claim that Swedish male doctors exhibit a high suicide risk relative to other academics but not to the general population.

Stack (1998b) addressed two neglected methodological problems in the second body of research. First, this work has largely overlooked the possible suppressor effect of marital status on physician suicide. Divorce greatly increases the risk of suicide (e.g., Stack, 1990b). However, physicians have a low incidence of divorce. For example, in a study of 1,118 married physicians, after 30 years only 29% of the physicians had been divorced one or more times. In contrast, a majority of married persons in the general population had been divorced (Rollman, Mead, Wang, & Klag, 1997). Without a control for divorce, physician suicide may be underestimated. Second, the past work often fails to control for the working-age population. It uses comparison groups such as "white males over 25" (see reviews in Bedeian, 1982; Brown, 1990). In this fashion, the retired population is included in the analysis. This results in the mixing together of working and nonworking physicians with working and nonworking nonphysicians. The impact of occupation per se on suicide is therefore inaccurately assessed.

Using national data for 1990, Stack (1998a) determined that physicians have a risk of suicide 1.95 times greater than that of the working-age population. However, as anticipated, when divorce and other covariates of physician status were controlled for, this risk factor increased to 2.45 times.

A third body of research explores not whether physicians have a high rate of suicide but why some physicians commit suicide whereas others do not (Brown, 1990; Council on Scientific Affairs, 1987; Lindeman, Luara, & Lönnquist, 1997; see review in Lester, 1992a). For example, a logistic regression model by Brown (1990) of data from the Physician Mortality Project explores nine possible risk factors of physician suicide. Of these nine, only care by a psychiatrist and financial losses (e.g., bankruptcy) discriminated between physicians who died from suicide versus ones who died of other causes.

A fourth stream of research focuses on suicide risk among female physicians. From the standpoint of the status integration theory of suicide, female physicians would be expected to have a high suicide risk given that their role set is statistically infrequent, and, therefore, stressful (Gibbs & Martin, 1964). Female physicians are in a male-dominated occupation, which is associated with a tendency not to be fully accepted by colleagues and/or the general public (Bedeian, 1982). The suicide rate for female physicians is especially high relative to females. The suicide rate for female physicians is four times the national female rate (Bedeian, 1982; Seiden & Gleiser, 1990). See Box 8.1 for a discussion of suicide among dentists.

BOX 8.1. Why Dentists Have a High Suicide Rate

From a basic demographic perspective, one would expect dentists to have an elevated suicide rate because they are mostly white males. In addition, dentists often work beyond age 65. Unless age is controlled, they would be expected to have an elevated suicide rate because elderly white males have a substantially high suicide rate (Stack, 1996a; Wasserman, 1992a).

However, internal occupational stress, psychiatric morbidity, and opportunity factors have been said to play a role in suicide risk among dentists (Hilliard-Lysen & Riemer, 1988; Stack, 1996a; Wasserman, 1992a). Dentists have access to drugs that can provide opportunities for suicide. However, there are also four characteristics of their work life that can promote internal occupational stress.

First, there are problems in the dentist–patient relationship. The nature of much dental work involves pain. Many patients express hostility to the dentist as a result. Second, there are status dilemmas. Some persons believe that dentists are people who were not smart enough to get into medical school. Whereas 90% of physicians are specialists and 10% general practitioners, only 10% of dentists derive prestige associated with being a specialist. Third, dentists have special economic problems not experienced as often by doctors. Insurance covers only 20% of dental patients. This creates more of a problem in collecting fees for work done by dentists. Fourth, dentists are more apt to work alone than are doctors. This creates a higher level of social isolation that can increase suicide risk (Hilliard-Lysen & Reimer, 1988; Stack, 1996a).

Psychiatric morbidity also may play a part in the suicide risk of dentists. The occupational milieu of dentists encourages control of emotional expression in relation to hostile patients. Dentistry is a client-dependent occupation; thus dentists do not have the luxury of offending already hostile patients. Compulsive perfectionism and deferral of gratification also characterize the personality structures of dentists (Bedeian, 1982). Dentistry may attract persons with these traits and/or encourage them after one enters into the profession.

Stack (1996a) notes that there are aspects of dentistry that might be expected to lower suicide risk. These include traditional 9–5 P.M. work hours wherein dentists are far less likely than doctors to be called in after hours on emergencies. Dentists have more potential than physicians for maintaining stable social relationships after work. Also, dentists earn high incomes relative to the general labor force. Relatively high incomes generally lower suicide risk (Stack, 1982).

Seven out of 11 studies that provide information on suicide rates among dentists find elevated suicide risks for dentists (Stack, 1996a). Of the occupations included in various surveys, they had the highest suicide rate in Oregon, third highest rate in California, second highest in Washington, and the third highest of 36 selected occupations in one national study (Stack, 1996a).

Only one study is available that uses national data and controls for the demographic covariates of dentist status. Stack (1996a) determined that even after controls are taken into account, dentists have a suicide rate that is 6.64 times greater than that of the working-age population.

Nurses

Research on U.S. and British nurses has often demonstrated that nurses have an elevated risk of suicide (Boxer et al., 1995; Peipins et al., 1997). The largest study to date on 27 states between 1984 and 1990 found a significant risk of suicide among U.S. nurses (Peipins et al., 1997). From a demographic perspective on suicide risk this is surprising because nursing is a female-dominated profession. Suicide risk may be high for nurses due to opportunity factors (e.g., availability of lethal drugs). In addition, the internal stress associated with this occupation may be responsible for its elevated suicide rate. However, Stack (1999a) did not replicate the finding of a high suicide rate for nurses in 1990.

Pharmacists

Pharmacists might be expected to have an elevated suicide rate due to access to lethal drugs and possible social isolation at work. Using national data for 26 states over 1979–1988, Burnett et al. (1992) found that the suicide risk for pharmacists was more than three times that of the rest of the male labor force.

Veterinarians

Veterinarians might be expected to have a high risk of suicide given their access to lethal drugs. For the state of Washington, Milham (1983) reported that veterinarians were 2.23 times more likely than average to die of suicide. Lester (1992a) reviews four studies indicating high suicide risk among veterinarians in Illinois but not in California. This risk may be restricted or centered on small-animal practice and veterinarian surgeons.

Nonmedical Professionals

Accountants

Accountants were not found to have an elevated suicide rate in a study of 21 states in 1990 (Stack, 1999a).

Artists

Almost all work on suicide among artists focuses on their high level of mental disorders and mentions suicide only in passing (Stack, 1996a). For example, Schildkraut et al., (1994) found that more than 50% of the 15 painters studied had some kind of mental disorder, more than 40% sought treatment, and 20% were hospitalized. Two of the 15 committed suicide. This and other research on mental disorders among artists failed to control for demographics. All of the Schildkraut, Hirshfeld, and Murphy (1994) painters were, for example, men, and men have a high suicide rate. Without controls for demographics, it is difficult to ascertain whether artists have a high suicide rate due to their work or due to their disproportionately being white men (Stack, 1996a).

Stack (1996a), in a study based on 21 states, determined that without demographic controls, artists had a suicide risk of 3.7 times greater than the working-age population. This was reduced to 2.25 times greater with controls. Artists are more than twice as likely to suicide than are other people. However, it is still not clear whether this is due to psychiatric morbidity before or after employment as an artist.

Chemists

Studies report that the suicide rate for female chemists is five times that of the female population (Bedeian, 1982; Seiden & Gleiser, 1990).

Engineers

One might expect engineers to have an elevated suicide risk given that they are disproportionately men. However, mechanical engineers in the state of Washington do not have a suicide risk that is significantly different from the average (Milham, 1983). For 21 states in the United States, Stack (1999a) found that engineers did not have an elevated rate of suicide.

Lawyers

Given male domination of the law profession and an oversupply of lawyers, one might expect an elevated suicide rate. Burnett et al. (1992) found that lawyers had a suicide rate twice that of the rest of the male working-age population.

Mathematicians and Scientists

Stack (1999a) reports that mathematicians and scientists are 1.85 times more likely to die of suicide than are the rest of the working-age population in 1990.

Professors

Professors were not found to have a significantly elevated risk of suicide in a study of 21 states (Stack, 1999a). Arnetz et al. (1987) found that professors had a suicide rate lower than that of the general population.

Psychologists

Burnett et al. (1992) report that male psychologists have a suicide risk that is more than three times that of the rest of the male labor force. Female psychologists have a suicide rate three times the national average (Bedeian, 1982; Seiden & Gleiser, 1990).

Schoolteachers

Given female domination of the teaching profession, we would anticipate a low suicide rate from a demographic perspective. In the United States, the elementary and secondary teaching profession had a rate below the national average (Seiden & Gleiser, 1990; Stack, 1998a). However, British female teachers had a higher than average suicide risk (Roman, Beral, & Inskip, 1985).

Social Workers

In a national study of 21 states, social workers were not found to have an elevated risk of suicide (Stack, 1999a). However, a study of social workers in Rhode Island did find elevated risk of suicide among social workers (Lester, 1992a).

Executives and Businessmen

The literature on suicide risk by occupation has neglected executives. Executives are generally categorized in a larger category of managers. Available information on suicide risk among managers indicates an average or less risk of suicide.

Using national data for the United States for 1990, Stack (1999a) determined that executives and managers had a suicide risk nearly equal to the national average. The suicide rate for businessmen in Hong Kong was not high. Yap (1958) reported that it was lower than that for female domestics, clerks, and shop assistants (Maris, 1967).

Analysis of suicide risk among female managers tends to find an elevated risk. A British study found that female managers were 1 of 11 occupations that had an elevated suicide mortality ratio for females (Roman et al., 1985). Given male domination of this occupational group, this would be expected from the standpoint of status integration theory.

Work on suicide in the professions has been marked by recurrent problems. There are only a few rigorous analyses and these have been restricted largely to a few occupations including physicians, dentists, and artists. Much more descriptive work needs to be done to even determine which professions are or are not at risk for suicide. Further, research exploring the causes of high and low suicide risk in specific professions is even thinner. Much work still needs to be done to determine causality.

SUMMARY AND CONCLUSIONS

Most of the research evidence of the past 30 years has documented an inverse relationship between the general prestige of broad social classes and suicide risk. However, within any social class there is often considerable variation in suicide risk. This can be partially explained by the demographic compositions of occupations, internal occupational stress, preexisting psychiatric morbidity, and differences in opportunities for suicide across occupations. Most detailed work that is available on specific occupations and suicide risk has been done on the professions. Preexisting psychiatric morbidity may play a role in the suicidal careers of artists and psychiatrists. Occupational stress probably plays a key role in producing high suicide risks among dentists. Opportunity factors probably play an important role in the suicides of physicians, dentists, and selected other medical-related occupations. Research evidence to date strongly suggests that females in traditional male occupations are at substantial risk of suicide. These occupations include those in the military, laborers, chemists, and physicians. This is consistent with the status integration theory of suicide.

Of the various economic factors reviewed herein, work mobility is the most thinly researched. Of the four rather limited studies on the subject, two indicate that suicide risk is higher than expected among the downwardly mobile, one finds no difference between controls and suicides on downward or upward mobility but is restricted to the last 2 years of life, and one finds that upward mobility (not downward) puts people at greater risk of suicide but has a control group that is 20 years older, on average, than the suicides. This latter problem probably exaggerates the degree of downward mobility among the controls, making comparisons somewhat problematic. Thus, replication studies are needed in this area before any valid conclusion can be drawn on the issue of work mobility and suicide risk. Such studies need to follow a rigorous research methodology that is competitive with modern standards.

A key predictor of individual-level suicide risk continues to be unemployment. Unemployed persons are generally found to have a suicide rate double or more of that of the working-age population. However, it is not clear to what extent this is due to the pressures of unemployment alone or to preexisting psychiatric morbidity. At most, half of the ecological, cross-sectional work on unemployment rates and suicide rates across cities, states, and nations finds a link at that level. This will continue to present a challenge to researchers on the issue into the next millennium. What is found at the individual level is not generally replicated at the aggregate level. An "individual fallacy" problem may exist under some presently unknown circumstances on this matter. The state of unemployment can predict suicide among individuals much better than it can predict suicide in cities, states, and nations.

The business cycle has proven to be a fairly consistent predictor of suicide trends. This is true of most analyses over time both in the United States and abroad. The nature of this association follows the largely commonsense notion of Henry and Short (1954) that recessions should increase suicide and prosperity should reduce it. Little evidence exists to support alternative interpretations including the U-shaped hypothesis of Durkheim (1966). Although this ecological methodology of aggregated research over time supports individual-level research on unemployment and suicide, the one-shot or cross-sectional ecological work is more problematic, as already noted.

Finally, a relatively new perspective on suicide, the RCS model, was confirmed by research in the United States and most industrial nations. However, replication for periods beyond the 1980s is needed. RCS models of social phenomena other than suicide have found that the RCS model tends not to hold up as well in more recent periods.

The next chapter turns to the role of marital status in the generation of suicidal behavior. That is, how does being single, widowed, divorced, or married relate to the risk of suicide. In addition, Chapter 9 covers gender differences in suicidality.

FURTHER READING

Ahlburg, D., & Schapiro, M. O. (1984). Socio-economic ramifications of changing cohort size: An analysis of U.S. postwar suicide rates by age and sex. *Demography, 21,* 7–105. This is the classic and quite readable overview on why cohort size should be related to suicidality. It analyzes relative cohort size and suicide rates over time using U.S. data.

Boxer, P., Burnett, C., & Swanson, N. (1995). Suicide and occupation: A review of the literature. *Journal of Occupational and Environmental Medicine, 37,* 442–452. This article provides the most comprehensive review of the literature to date on the issue of occupation and suicide.

Lester, D., & Yang, B. (1997a). *The economy and suicide.* Commack, NY: Nova Science. This text provides the most recent book-length treatment of the subject.

Platt, S. (1984). Unemployment and suicidal behavior: A review of the literature. *Social Science and Medicine, 19,* 93–115. This article provides the most rigorous, exhaustive review of the literature on unemployment and suicide through the early 1980s. The author demonstrates that the degree of consistency in the positive relationship between unemployment and suicide varies according to the type of analysis strategy that is employed: cross-sectional individual versus aggregate, and longitudinal individual versus aggregate research.

Stack, S. (1995). Gender and suicide risk among laborers. *Archives of Suicide Research, 1,* 19–26. The research on occupation and suicide has focused largely on high-status occupations such as dentists and physicians. However, many low-status occupations have suicide rates as high or even higher than most high-status occupations. This article analyzes the suicide risk of laborers, an occupational group with one of the highest suicide rates in the labor force.

Wasserman, I. M. (1992). Economy, work, occupation and suicide. In R. W. Maris, A. L. Berman, J. T. Maltsberger, & R. I. Yufit (Eds.), *Assessment and prediction of suicide* (pp. 520–539). New York: Guilford Press. This chapter provides a systematic review of selected issues on the topic of economic conditions and suicide risk.

9

Marriage, Family, Family Therapy, and Suicide

Bruce Bongar, Laura Goldberg,
Karin Cleary, and Kaprice Brown

> The immunity of married persons [to suicide] is due [largely] to the influence not of conjugal society, but of the family society. In itself conjugal society [marriage] is harmful to the woman and aggravates her tendency to suicide.
> —EMILE DURKHEIM

It is well known that marriage and family tend to be protective factors against suicide and are associated with lower suicide rates. Generally speaking (see Figure 9.1), highest to lowest rates in the United States are found in the following order: widowed, divorced, single or never married, married, and married with children. The protective effect against suicide is especially marked among males (cf. Kaplan & Klein, 1989) and whites. In contrast, marriage signals greater risk for suicide among adolescents, as early mariage is more associated with unwanted pregnancy, family conflict, and stress.

Elsewhere in this volume we have considered related aspects to the topic of marriage and family. For example, in Chapter 6 we examined sexuality and gender and in Chapter 10 we look at social relations and isolation. What is there about being married and having a family that tends to protect against suicide?

Is it simply that one is less isolated? Do married people have more to live for? Do the support and comfort of a partner offer succorance and need fulfillment versus deprivation? Could it be that married people simply tend to be physically and mentally healthier and, thus, less likely to suicide? Sociologist Emile Durkheim once commented that the single and never married constitute the "dregs of society."

Whatever the causal relations (multiple factors are likely involved) it is clear that in the United States marriage and family tend to be protective factors and that divorce, widowhood, marital or child problems, death of a spouse, estrangement from a spouse, and so on tend to be risk factors for suicide.

The major focus in this chapter is on treating problems in marriage and family that may be suicidogenic—particularly via family systems and family therapy. Family systems perspectives have changed our view of psychopathology and the context in which it is understood. In contemporary psychological practice, it is no longer unusual to explain symptoms in terms of interaction patterns among intimates. Because suicidal behavior is the most commonly encountered emergency in psychological practice (Bongar, 1991), one might assume that family and marital therapists have studied suicide extensively, but in fact, this is not the case.

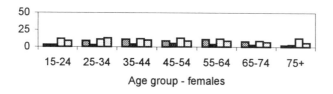

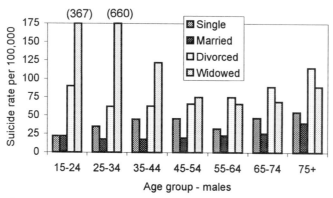

FIGURE 9.1. Suicide rates per 100,000 by marital status and age group, United States, 1996. Data from the National Center for Health Statistics, Vital Statistics of the United States and the U.S. Bureau of the Census, 1998.

Except for Richman's (1986) family work from an object relations perspective, which emphasizes attachment and separation to explain suicidality, and work by (Landau-Stanton & Stanton, 1985), which discusses the treatment of suicidal adolescents and their families, there is little empirical or theoretical literature on family and couple approaches to understanding, managing and preventing suicidal behavior. Wagner (1997) concludes his review of research on family risk factors for child and adolescent suicidal behavior by stating, "Overall, the vast majority of claims regarding family risk factors . . . are not justified by the research designs and empirical findings on which they are based." Pfeffer (1986) and Richman (1986) support this assertion. Turgay (1989) quoted the work of Pfeffer (1986) who stated, "There are no systematic studies evaluating the efficacy of psychotherapy with suicidal patients" (972). She also explained that most of the information from the psychotherapy of suicidal children is obtained from case reports.

If we compare the incidence and costs of suicide in contemporary society, to the amount of consideration given to the topic in the family therapy literature, a large imbalance is apparent. For example, a quick check of two sourcebooks of family therapy information (Piercy, Sprenkle, & Associates, 1986; Simon, Stierlin, & Wynne, 1985) reveals that suicide is not indexed in either one of them. Similarly, *The Family Crucible* (Napier, 1978), which devotes several pages to suicide, does not discuss specific treatment approaches. Thus as a group, structural, strategic, and systemic family therapists have addressed the topic of suicide infrequently (Bongar, 1991).

INTIMACY AND THE SUICIDE SCENARIO

There is consistent evidence indicating an association between suicidal behavior and difficulties in interpersonal relationships. Conflict or loss of a serious, intimate relationship are common precipitants to a suicide attempt (Weissman, 1974). For example, suicidal women were found to have experienced a significantly greater number of arguments with dates, friends, family members (Weissman & Klerman, 1973), and spouses (Paykel, Prusoff, & Myers, 1975), than were nonsuicidal women. For married women, the threat of marital conflict or separation often precedes a suicide attempt. Infidelity, brutality, and battering are also reported by some attempters (Stephens, 1985).

Consider the case of David and Susan, which illustrates that marital strife (coupled with other factors, such as drug therapy) can, indeed, result in suicide (here, a murder–suicide) (see Case 9.1).

Many researchers believe that an individual's suicidal behavior is a multidetermined act in which family tensions, disruptions, and patterns of interaction play a role (Pfeffer, 1981a; Richman, 1979). After studying patterns of communication in suicidal people's fam-

---

CASE 9.1. Controversy: Marital Problems or Drug Reaction?

On the surface, David and Susan had it all. He had recently retired from a successful career in Los Angeles, pocketed a few million from the sale of his business, and built his dream home on the island of Maui in Hawaii. David and Susan had been married for 35 years and had two children, one of whom was an engineer and the other a charter boat captain.

David was about 60 years old when things started to go sour in paradise. He did not adjust well to retirement. He had been an admitted workaholic and began to be irritated with his wife and to argue with her, especially about her newfound fundamentalist Christian religion. He complained about her "God-talk." However, there is no evidence that David ever hit Susan.

As Susan seemed to turn to religion to find comfort that David did not provide her, David separated from Susan. In August 1991, David went to California where he saw a psychiatrist for the first time in his life. David was prescribed Xanax for anxiety and nortriptyline for depression. (For the record, Susan had also been depressed and was given Elavil in 1980 and Prozac in 1987.) Again in July 1992 there was a second marital separation, with David going to live in California again, where his daughter was living.

David and Susan both saw a psychologist during the last 3 months of 1992 and their marriage seemed to improve. They "started over" together in Maui. However, David's anxiety and depression continued into late 1992 and early 1993. He started taking Prozac in February 1993. Two days after being put on Prozac, David felt "200%" better (a "Prozac miracle," said his psychiatrist), but by day 3, David was so anxious (did he have akathisia or "serotonin syndrome"?) that he demanded to be hospitalized.

After being hospitalized for 10 days David was discharged and flown back to Maui to be with his wife and son. The night of March 3, 1993 David stabbed his wife of almost 40 years 15 times and then stabbed himself to death. This was his first act of violence.

The controversy here is: Did the Prozac make David act violently out of character or was it the anger and frustration over continuing marital problems and a growing sense of hopelessness—seeing no other way out?

ilies, Richman (1986) concluded that "suicide is not an individual act, but is part of a collusive communication system that involves an entire family and social network" (147). As we shall see in our discussion of research findings (below), families of a suicidal individual tend to be chaotic and unstable. Pfeffer (1986) stated: "Studies consistently have reported that families of suicidal children are disorganized by parental separations, divorce, and stresses of living in a one-parent family" (125). In support of Richman's (1986) earlier observations, Pfeffer reported that suicidal children were distinguishable from other children by the seriousness of losses as the predominant type of stress and by parental violence, sexual abuse, and psychopathology.

As the *M*A*S*H** theme song goes: "suicide solves many problems," but it certainly creates significant problems for others (see Chapter 22). When a suicide occurs, the self-destructive act has a major impact on friends, families, and health care professionals (Turgay, 1989). Specifically, Eisenberg (1980) noted, "Suicide is the ultimate form of alienation" (319); it "imposes a triple burden on the family: grief at loss, as with any death, rage at desertion, for this was a deliberate death, and guilt at having failed the victim" (315). Some researchers also argue that the suicidal gesture is an ineffective means of promoting change in interpersonal relationships (i.e., in the family) (Kenney & Krajewski, 1980).

Historically, family therapy has certainly not avoided difficult problems. Why then has more attention not been paid to suicide? One possible explanation is that family therapists may consider a suicidal crisis no different than severe psychopathology such as anorexia nervosa or drug addiction (Gurman, 1982). A second possibility may be that the family systems orientation to therapy is a relatively young specialty. As family therapy continues to mature and has less need to defend a systemic orientation against individual orientations (Nichols, 1987), family therapists may find it easier to study suicide and its prevention and treatment.

In the remainder of this chapter, we discuss the personality characteristics of suicidal patients and their families. Second, we summarize the research literature regarding families and suicidal family members. Third, we discuss the treatment of a suicidal individual, followed by a description of desirable therapist characteristics. Finally, we provide a summary of the literature on family therapy treatment of suicidal individuals, including adjunctive and integrative modes of treatment and a brief review of hospital practices. This chapter focuses on families with a suicidal child or adolescent because this family constellation is the most representative in the literature.

SPOUSE/LOVER HOMICIDE–SUICIDES

Case 9.1 descibed a spousal murder–suicide. Although fairly rare (West, 1966, estimates that about 2% of all suicides are murder–suicides; this is consistent with Berman's, 1996, estimate of 400 to 750 "dyadic deaths" per year in the United States), spouse or lover intimacy does occasionally result in murder followed by suicide—as in the case of David (cf. Berman, 1979, 1996; Allen, 1983; Holinger & Kleman, 1982). Paradoxically, here marriage or intimate social involvement does *not* protect one against suicide.

In the majority of murder–suicides men kill women they are romantically involved with or estranged from and then kill themselves (sometimes they also kill their dependent children or their ex-wife's or lover's new lover or spouse). The most typical of these involves partners with a chronic love–hate pattern: They cannot live with each other; they cannot live without each other. The male (typically) batters his partner for affection, as if his life depended on it. When she threatens or manages to sever the relationship, he reacts with jealousy and rage. Her rejection makes him feel shamed, ruined, and rejected, and he reacts further by murdering her and killing himself (Berman, 1996). Berman (1979, 1996) contends that in such cases often the perpetrator's self is enmeshed, sometimes even symbiotically, with the object's (victim's) self. Killing oneself *requires* killing one's spouse and/or family and vice versa. Hemphill and Thornley (1969) referred to these relationshps as "encapsulated units."

A similar explanation has been given for the mass suicide–murders at Jonestown, Guyana (see Chidester, 1991). The argument was that Jim Jones's extended self-concept included his religious cult or "family" (incidentally, many of whom Jones had promiscuous sexual relations with and children by). Thus, when Jones decided to kill "himself," he also needed to persuade 913 others in the Jonestown cult to suicide or else to murder them in order for his own "suicide" to be complete.

Allen (1983) suggests that murder–suicides tend to be older men in despair over relational or interpersonal losses that they cannot tolerate. This reflects a second type of "dyadic death" described by Berman (1996), the dependent–protective type. Here, for example, the perpetrator typically is an older male responsible for the caretaking of his ill or infirm female partner (e.g., wife). When financial or health problems threaten his ability to protect her, the threat to his role and ego becomes suicidogenic. Unwilling to be separated from her or from this protective function, he kills her out of mercy or pity, then takes his own life.

We see similar dynamics in filicide–suicides. Here, the parent (typically, the mother) assumes that the child would suffer in this cruel, harsh world without her protection. As she plots her suicide, the death of her dependent offspring is a necessary and logical extension. After all, the child's ego is but an extension of her own. In Japan, these deaths are called *Oyaku-Shinju*.

Suicides sometimes follow murder out of guilt, hopelessness, or unexpended aggressive energy. Remember that Menninger (1937), following Freud and Steckel, contended that suicides are often retroflexed homicidal energy or rage that is turned back on the homicidal person . . . what Menninger called "murder-in-the 180th-degree."

Allen found that many murder–suicides are by persons with borderline, psychotic, or schizophrenic traits. Often (at least 50% of the murder–suicides studied had been drinking) alcohol abuse is involved (for a more recent consideration of murder–suicide, see Nock & Marzuk, 1999).

Finally (compare Chapters 16 and 17 in this volume), Brown, Linnoila, and Goodwin (1992) contend that aggression may be a more primitive and basic affective response to the environment than depression or suicide is because aggression is found in all species at all ages, but depression and suicide are not.

SUICIDE PACTS AMONG COUPLES

Sometimes a spouse is not killed by her husband but willingly enters into a joint suicide pact. Often such spousal suicide pacts occur among older married couples, when one or both of them are ill. Consider the suicide pact of author Arthur Koestler and his third wife, Cynthia Jeffries, in Case 9.2 (cf. Humphry & Wickett, 1986: 142 ff.; Colt, 1991: 385). Arthur and Cynthia Koestler consummated a suicide pact in March 1983. Arthur was a vice president of the Voluntary Euthanasia Society in London and author of *Darkness at Noon* (an anti-Stalinist novel). He had Parkinson's disease and leukemia. However, his wife, Cynthia, was only 55 and in good health. Both overdosed on barbitu-

CASE 9.2. The Suicide Pact of Arthur Koestler and Cynthia Jeffries

Arthur Koestler was born on September 5, 1905, in Budapest, the only child of Henrik and Adela Koestler. The first trauma for Arthur was an unexpected and unexplained tonsillectomy without anesthesia in 1910. Because of his father's poor business sense and his mother's dislike of Hungary, the family moved to Vienna in 1914 amidst much conflict between his parents.

Shy and insecure, Koestler studied science and engineering, but he became involved in a Zionist dueling fraternity at a polytechnic college in Vienna. The 3 years he spent in this group were very happy and began his involvement in politics. He became a follower of Vladimir Jabotinsky, burned his matriculation papers, and left for Palestine in 1926. After a hard period of adjustment there, he obtained a job as Middle East correspondent for a German publishing company.

In 1929, disillusioned with Palestine, he returned to Europe where he continued to work as a newspaper correspondent. He joined the German Communist Party in 1931 and lost his job as a result. He traveled to Russia to report on events there and returned to Paris to write, though the Communist Party disapproved of many of his articles and books and greatly restricted his freedom. He married Dorothy Asher but separated a few months later. (They were divorced in 1950.)

He made three trips to Spain during the Civil War and was arrested and imprisoned for 3 months by Franco's Nationalists as a spy. He was sentenced to death but freed after British protests. Disillusioned now with Communism, he resigned from the Communist Party. He was detained and imprisoned in both England and France but, after the publication of *Darkness at Noon*, was released and worked for the Ministry of Information in England during the war.

After the war, Zionism again captured his attention, and he traveled to Israel and both reported on events and wrote novels that incorporated his experiences. In 1950 he married Mamaine Paget, but she separated from him in 1951 and died in 1954 soon after their divorce. His third and final marriage was to Cynthia Jeffries in 1965, who had been his secretary since 1950.

He settled in England in 1952 and became a British citizen. He continued to work for and write about political issues. His writings, including both novels, essays, and biographies, always explored the important social issues of the times, and his work has been compared to that of George Orwell's in its impact on the times.

Cynthia Jeffries was 22 when she started working for Koestler. She was from South Africa and had gone to Paris with the aim of working for a writer. There had been stress in her life—her father committed suicide when she was 13 and she had had a brief, unsuccessful marriage. From the time that she joined Koestler, her life was rarely distinct from his.

One of the causes for which Koestler worked was euthanasia. As he grew older, he developed Parkinson's disease and then leukemia. When the effects of these illnesses worsened, he decided to commit suicide, and Cynthia decided that she could not live without him.

(cont.)

CASE 9.2. (*cont.*)

Interestingly, all his wives remained in some way attached to and, for some, devoted to and dependent on him. Dorothy Asher helped free Koestler from prison in Spain. Mamaine Paget, who suffered from his drunken rages, wrote that she would do anything, even leave him, if it were necessary to help him fulfill his destiny.

Cynthia went further. On March 3, 1983, she committed suicide with him in their London home.

Source: Lester, D., 1996, The sexual politics of double suicide, *Proceedings of the Pavese Society, 7,* 21–22.

---

rates. Some commentators have argued that such suicide pacts are often patriarchal (as in the Jonestown case) in that the husband or dominant male coerces the wife to suicide (cf. the Hindu ritual of *suttee,* discussed in Chapter 19). Indeed, in the Koestler–Jeffries case, she had long been dominated by and psychologically abused by him. When he took seriously ill, she became his caretaker. Still interdependent, she appended to his death note, "I cannot face life without Arthur."

A second example of a suicide pacts among older married couples would be that of the parents of Derek Humphry's second wife, Ann Wickett (see her book, *Double Exit,* 1989). In *Double Exit,* Wickett describes the double suicide of her own parents (interestingly, Wickett herself later got breast cancer and suicided alone in a remote area in Oregon, without her husband, Derek Humphry). She tells us that her father (age 92) and mother (78) both suffered from grave illnesses with poor prognoses. It is worth noting that Wickett's uncle (her father's brother) also committed suicide in 1973, after a chronic depressive disorder. To avoid nursing homes and a slow, painful decline, Wickett's mother and father (who were the first two members of the Hemlock society) overdosed on barbiturates and alcohol.

Sometimes suicide pacts are made by younger lovers (such as teenagers whose love is thwarted by their parents or circumstances). Berman (1996) refers to these types as "unrequited love" pacts in which the young lovers fantasize joining in a conjugal grave as both a way to have what has been denied them in life and to punish those (parents) who have opposed their proposed union. A pact to elope to their deaths is preferable to a catastrophic destruction of their relationship. In Japan a love-pact suicide is referred to as *joshi shinju* (see Colt, 1991: 140 ff.) and was a common theme in *Kabuki* and *buraraku* theatre. About one in four dyadic deaths in India are by young lovers who object to forced or parentally arranged intracaste marriages.

A well-known case of love-pact suicide occurs in a short story ("Patriotism") by Yukio Mishima (see Chapter 7, Box 7.2), himself a ritual suicide (cf. Maltsberger & Goldblatt, 1996: 391 ff.). In this story a young officer, a lieutenant, engages in passionate lovemaking, after which he commits *seppuku,* and his wife, Reiko, stabs herself to death. Mishima once wrote: "if you want your beauty to endure, you must commit suicide at the height of your beauty" (Colt, 1991: 141).

Fishbain, D'Achille, Barsky, and Aldrich (1984) found only 20 suicide pacts (involving 40 victims) among 5,895 certified suicides in Dade County, Florida, over a 25-year period. If this sample was representative of the United States as a whole, we would expect to find only about 10 such cases annually.

CHILD SUICIDE IN THE CONTEXT OF THE FAMILY

When the suicidal attempter is a child, it can be thought that the attempt is the symptom of the child's inability to change the disturbing, chaotic, and stressful family environment (Schrut, 1964). As Sabbath (1969) explained: "Suicidal children 'unconsciously respond' to the hostile wishes of the family to get rid of them; the child is 'the expendable child,' one who is not tolerated or needed by the family. The child merely helps to maintain the 'precarious equilibrium within the family structure'" (272–289).

Richman (1971) believed that the factors that help determine suicidal potential are an inability to accept necessary change, an intolerance for separation, a symbiosis without empathy, a fixation on infantile patterns in the primary relationship, and a refusal to mourn past persons or situations. Sometimes a strong symbiotic parent–child relationship exists in a family that prevents the child from developing autonomous functioning. This results in an insufficient establishment of the child's own stable and separate identity (Pfeffer, 1981a). Researchers argue that the child usually experiences a state of extreme helplessness and may fear parental rejection as well (Pfeffer, 1981a).

As a result, the child may experience hostile perceptions of the parents. When turned inward, the child feels as if he or she hates himself or herself, is worthless, or is undesirable. The suicide attempt may be a response to remove these negative self-perceptions that the child has internalized due to the family system (Pfeffer, 1981a, 1989).

CHARACTERISTICS OF THE SUICIDAL FAMILY

Researchers have suggested that certain characteristics are common to the home environment of youthful suicide attempters. Asarnow (1992) indicated that children who attempted suicide or thought about suicide described their families as less cohesive, less expressive, and more conflicted than did nonsuicidal children. Other researchers have found that families tend to be disorganized, unstable, rigid, inflexible, and conflict avoidant with unclear boundaries and roles (Davidson & Linnoila, 1990; Mattson, Seese, & Hawkins, 1969; Mitchell & Rosenthal, 1992; Pfeffer, 1981a).

In addition, Richman (1971) noted that these families tend to possess unbalanced intrafamilial relationships and have role conflicts. Scapegoating, double-binding communications, and communication disturbances are also common occurrences. Richman stated that there is often an excessive secretiveness and prohibition against intimacy that isolates the potentially suicidal person within the family. King (1987) additionally noted that family members tend to interact in a hostile manner when suicide is an issue. As a result, divorce, death, parental separation, family discord, child abuse, parental unemployment, and/or a family history of a psychiatric disorder inclusive of suicidal behavior are common features of families containing a suicide attempter.

Some scholars have presented a generational explanation for families with a suicidal member (cf. Maris, 1997). They argue that parents of a suicidal child may have faulty identifications with their own parents and are, therefore, unable to develop an appropriate capacity to care for their own child (Pfeffer, 1981a). The parent(s) may feel hostility and intense anger that may be openly and indirectly expressed in the family system (Pfeffer, 1981a).

Sometimes the same family has multiple suicides (cf. Jamison, 1993). The loading for suicide and depressive disorder in many of these families far exceeds what we would have expected by chance alone. For example, in the case of author Ernest Hemingway (presented in Chapter 10), Ernest's father, Ed, sister Ursula, brother Leicester, and granddaughter Margaux all committed suicide (i.e., there were five suicides over three generations; see Figure 10.1). Of course, we still have to sort out whether multiple family suicides have a genetic or socialization component, or both. In one study of suicide among Amish families (Egeland & Sussex, 1985), almost three-quarters of 26 suicides clustered in just four family pedigrees (cf. Roy, Rylander, & Sarchiapone, 1997), suggesting that a genetic factor was at work.

Pfeffer (1986, 1989) also noted that severely conflicted couple relationships are a characteristic feature of families containing a suicidal child. The family characteristics described thus far often combine to produce a negative atmosphere that affects the child's personality development and identity.

The atmosphere of fear and terror generated by a suicide attempt can also lead to intense emotions within the family. Family members often feel humiliated; they experience pain and hurt. They also feel that the attempter could not trust them enough to explain his or her current difficulties (Turgay, 1989). Turgay (1989) described the familial recovery process after a suicide attempt. The process occurs in stages yet cannot be clearly separated: "1. Shock and fear, 2. Panic and action, 3. Guilt, 4. Resentment, 5. Reparation, and 6. Partial recovery" (978).

Family members may reach different stages at different times. Often, the family wishes to "punish the suicide attempter or take revenge by threatening to withdraw care and love" (Turgay, 1989: 979). Eisenberg (1980) stated that in a situation in which the distress that led to the suicidal ideas produces a family response that exhibits love and concern, a new opportunity exists for the restoration of psychological equilibrium and personal growth.

FAMILY RISK FACTORS FOR YOUTH SUICIDAL BEHAVIOR: A RESEARCH SUMMARY

Wagner (1997) has reviewed the empirical support, or lack thereof, for five aspects of family dysfunction that have provided a conceptual underpinning to understanding suicide risk and families. These are summarized in this section.

Poor Family Communication and Problem-Solving Skills

It has been alleged that families of suicidal people avoid direct verbal communication, walk out on arguments, have a high degree of secretiveness, feel hostility but discourage its expression to each other, and view transitional events as threats to family stability. In general, Wagner opined, "there is only modest evidence that poor family communication or problem solving is a risk factor" for suicidal behavior. The better-controlled research does suggest that suicidal children and adolescents do experience more negative family and parent–child relationships *and* that much of this may be due to the child's psychopathology, particularly with regard to nonfatal suicidal behavior. In uncontrolled studies, unresolved family problems are the most commonly reported of stressful events in the days prior to both completed and attempted suicide in youths.

Scapegoating

As in Sabbath's (1969) description of the *expendable child*, scapegoating is a family strategy that results in hostile feelings being redirected toward the suicidal child in order to alleviate tension between other family members. A most egregious example of scapegoating involves the physical or sexual abuse of a child. Wagner reports that retrospective reports of abuse are more common among completers than among normal adolescents and that suicide at-tempters are more likely to have been abused than either clinical or normal control groups.

Threatened or Actual Loss of an Attachment Figure

Death or separation, or the threat of separation, have been presented as promoting wishes to reunite (in the grave), guilt and a consequent wish to punish the self for causing the loss, revenge against the lost object, and feelings that one cannot live without the lost object. Sur-prisingly, Wagner reports, there is no evidence that loss of a caregiver to death is a risk fac-tor for suicidal behavior. Similarly, parental separation or divorce, when considered apart from other losses, does not appear to be a significant risk factor for youth suicide. In con-trast, evidence demonstrates that early losses and multiple losses may influence the emer-gence of suicidal symptoms and behavior.

Marital Dysfunction

As noted previously, Pfeffer (1986) described inflexibility, ambivalence, and conflict in the spousal relationship as common among parents of suicidal children. However, Wagner re-ports, there is weak evidence that marital relationships in these families are any less satisfac-tory than in normal controls.

Family Psychopathology

Finally, clinicians have observed that parents of suicidal youth have significant psy-chopathology, ranging from their own depression and suicidality to alcoholism and drug abuse. Pathways, then, might range from genetic (e.g., an inherited predisposition to bipolar disorder) to modeling disturbed behavior as a coping mechanism to negative (e.g., neglect-ful) parenting and its effect on self-esteem and psychopathology in children. Research tends to support this observation in parents of suicidal youth as compared to families of normal controls but not compared to families of clinical controls. Evidence, here, may be strongest with regard to parental substance abuse problems.

FAMILY INVOLVEMENT IN TREATMENT OF SUICIDAL BEHAVIOR

Several researchers have suggested that the family is critical to the effective treatment of a sui-cidal individual. Sokol and Pfeffer (1992) stated "It is essential to establish a working alliance with all family members, and to work closely with them throughout the assessment and treat-ment process. Family members can provide salient information that cannot be obtained from the younger patient" (14). Richman (1992) suggested, "Family therapy is the most effective form of treatment for alleviating a suicidal state" (17). Including the family in the treatment plan is also supported by a number of other authorities (Caine, 1978; Eisenberg, 1980; Motto, Heilbron, & Juster, 1985; Wassenaar, 1987), especially when treating suicidal chil-dren (Pfeffer 1986) and adolescents (Berman & Jobes, 1991). Parents who are guided by in-terventions tend to respond more appropriately to their children (Pfeffer, 1986).

Also, family treatment helps parents to understand their own personal conflicts and en-ables them to provide support for their suicidal child who is trying to both separate from and find a place within the family system. Toolan (1980) supported the idea of involving the par-ents in the therapy of suicidal children because parents were often angry at the child. At times, parents may minimize the seriousness of the child's suicidal ideation due to their anger.

In addition to parents, grandparents, uncles, aunts, siblings, and cousins may be helpful for defining problems and introducing approaches that can achieve resolution of conflicts (Pfeffer, 1986). Some researchers believe that having many people involved in treatment is ideal; however, it is not uncommon for suicidal individuals to be resistant to bringing in the family. Likewise, the family members may feel threatened when the patient enters psychotherapy, afraid of what will be said about them or the "family secrets" the patient will reveal (Richman, 1984). Davidson and Linnoila (1990) proposed that the family and the patient are the most malleable and least resistant and rigid at the time of the suicidal crisis, allowing change to occur.

CHARACTERISTICS OF THE FAMILY THERAPIST AND SUICIDE

When suicide is an issue in treatment, the family therapist can become an indispensable figure in the therapy process and a vital part of the communication network, with a goal of transforming the patient's communications of suicidal despair to communications that are life oriented (Richman, 1986). Richman also believed that the family therapist and family should be open and direct in communication.

To work with suicidal patients in family therapy, some authorities have suggested that therapists must possess special personality qualities and skills. For example, Richman (1984) proposed that when dealing with suicidal adolescents, the family therapist requires special training in addition to a solid background in family therapy. He believes the therapist should possess the characteristics of empathy, sensitivity, self-awareness, and the ability to work through his or her own destructive proclivities.

Also, a family therapist who is well trained, adequately supervised, and well informed and who has worked out his or her own separation/individuation conflicts is able to produce the most positive aspects of the growth process (Richman, 1986).

Golann and Bongar (1987) noted: "The topic of suicide is apparently a difficult one for family therapists. It arouses their personal beliefs, values and epistemologies, and at the same time brings forth questions about accountability and responsibility" (3).

THE FOCUS OF FAMILY THERAPY AND THE SUICIDAL PATIENT

After reviewing the literature, Golann and Bongar (1987: 2) observed, "Explicit discussion of suicide is often surprisingly absent in both theoretical and clinical writings on family therapy."

Some literature, however, does present information on the family system's treatment of a suicidal individual. Landau-Stanton and Stanton (1985) presented strategies and techniques for working with suicidal adolescents in family therapy. They incorporated ideas from many known contemporary models: strategic/structural, experiential, transitional, and contextual. They described guidelines that can be used to treat suicidal cases.

First, it is important to empower the parents and unite them in their behavior toward the patient. Second, family secrets should be exposed in an effort to decrease the adolescent's power. Third, there should be a strong unity in the treatment team, with one member of the team having primary responsibility for the management of the case. The authors also proposed two specialized interventions: (1) the family safety watch, a method of keeping constant watch over the suicidal adolescent 24 hours a day, and (2) resolution of family mourning, the technique of escorting the family through an unresolved mourning or loss within the nuclear or extended family.

Similar to Landau-Stanton and Stanton's ideas, Pfeffer (1981a) also offered guidelines for working with a suicidal young person. First, she believed that therapy should define and offer treatment for the parental conflicts as separate issues from the conflicts of the child. Second, she believed that therapy should provide guidance for parents to respond with better parenting for the child. Finally, she believed that therapy should include a variety of inpatient and outpatient interventions.

Eisenberg (1980) stated: "What is crucial in family therapy is a therapeutic context which permits the rebuilding of hope and the reestablishment of healthy ties among family members" (319). Treatment must convey a sense of caring and restore faith in the possibility of a satisfying future to the patient who feels unloved and unworthy of love.

SPECIFIC METHODS OF FAMILY TREATMENT IN SUICIDE

Richman (1986) proposed that the therapist begin by seeing the entire family, even though the settings, situations, people involved, the seriousness of the suicidal act, and the circumstances surrounding the attempt may be different. He believed that the therapist's contact with the suicidal patient and/or the family can occur anywhere and for any length of time (i.e., one session to several years of sessions). Overall, the timing of the assessment and therapy for both individual and family sessions can be critical (Davidson & Linnoila, 1990).

The family interview is a useful tool for understanding family interactions and can also guide family members toward more positive and helpful types of communication (Pfeffer, 1986; Richman, 1986). During this assessment, the emotions of the family and patient are most likely to be demonstrated. These emotions can include intense anxiety, fear, anger, sadness, and tension.

Turgay (1989) stated that a strong therapeutic relationship with the family members is very helpful. The therapist should also share the risks inherent in repetitive suicidal behavior with the family quite openly and emphasize that decreasing risks and developing new tasks for the family and child are important.

After a family is assessed, additional information can be gathered from the suicidal patient, such as specific details about the crises themselves. This material helps direct the treatment (Richman, 1984). It is the therapist's duty to try to accept the family members as they are without judging them (Richman, 1986).

Richman (1984) also suggested that the therapist see each family member and the suicidal patient individually in order to better understand their individual perceptions of the events that preceded the attempt. After this, the family members are seen together.

At the start of therapy, many family members tend to seek simple answers to the identified patient's suicidal behavior. Turgay (1989) noted: "The therapist should gradually direct their attention to multifactorial etiology and systemic interrelatedness rather than linear thinking during their attempt to solve the problem quickly" (981).

It is also beneficial to the family to participate in an information session with the therapist concerning the suicidal patient's nature, treatment, and possible outcome, thus directing the families attention to the child patient's self-destructive behavior (Turgay, 1989). Family members must be questioned as to whether they feel they have been burdened by the patient, and whether the family believes that the patient's death would be a better solution. From the family members' answers, the conversation continues and tries to "clarify the nature of the stresses within the family and between the family members" (Richman, 1984: 400).

Outbursts may occur during such conversations, but Richman (1984) felt they are beneficial because they clear the air and can have a cathartic effect. Family members should also be asked what they feel can be done to prevent repeated suicidal events in the future. Open and free communication among family members can increase their participation by providing mutual support (Motto et al., 1985).

Richman (1986) noted that the family needs to work at its own pace in therapy, with the major task of facilitating separation at the time and place that are appropriate for the patient, at the same time fostering a proper amount of attachment, which is best for the entire family. The patient and family must heal the splits that occur within the patient and within the family, and the therapist must examine the overall level of ambivalence, as well as disturbed interpersonal and family relationships. Richman (1986) suggested that success can be achieved with direct and honest communication that eliminates double-bind communications or scapegoating.

Motto et al. (1985) described an important treatment task. He believed that the therapist should help the patient understand and accept the family system and teach the family members to accept and understand the patient. Some theorists have also argued that family therapy may be required to restructure the life of the patient so that the parents accept the patient's level of functioning and set their expectations for change accordingly. King (1987) added the value of including efforts to teach the suicidal child better coping skills and attempting to reduce his or her negative self and family outlooks. Interventions must focus on the family in order to increase the child's support.

Finally, Richman (1986) argued that family treatment must work with the family and not in opposition to it. Treatment processes must respect the family's own need to maintain attachments and specific family bonds. Specifically, Sokol and Pfeffer (1992) noted: "The family must always be encouraged to stay involved in the treatment no matter which modality is chosen. Professionals can recommend treatment, but parents ultimately decide what is best for their child" (xx).

Some authorities believe that following a family member's suicide attempt, a healthy change process in the family can occur—unless there is an unhealthy shifting of the balance (Davidson & Linnoila, 1990). If the latter occurs, the family therapist must monitor the process so that suicidal risk is reduced and positive progress is emphasized (Turgay, 1989).

ADJUNCTIVE TREATMENT MODALITIES FOR SUICIDE

When dealing with severe suicidal cases, the therapist may want to include additional treatment modalities: individual psychotherapy, parental–couple counseling, and/or psychopharmacotherapy. These "adjunctive" (Pfeffer, 1986) treatment modalities can improve the patient's intrapsychic functioning and functioning within the family system.

In addition, the parents' ability to appropriately nurture the child can be enhanced (Pfeffer, 1986). Pfeffer (1986) stated "Adjunctive family therapy focuses primarily on reducing family conflict and stress so that the family atmosphere becomes more conducive to the appropriate development of the child; this is essential for the child's successful coping with suicidal proclivities and the underlying conflicts" (262).

This type of family therapy directs the parents toward working together as a unit. They can be taught how to help the child triumph over his or her hopelessness and despair and simultaneously handle their own parental and marital conflicts. When marital problems are resolved, more attention can be directed toward parental responsibilities. Pfeffer (1986) summarized the therapeutic tasks for family adjunctive treatments:

1. Establish empathic relationships between family members.
2. Open avenues for communication between parent and child.

3. Plan alternative ways of dealing with disagreements between parent and child.
4. Develop awareness of feelings, ideas, and needs of others.
5. Achieve a tolerance for change while maintaining a consistently stable family atmosphere.
6. Promote individual autonomous functioning.
7. Decrease tendencies for impulsive and severely aggressive behaviors in both parents and child.
8. Diminish fears of separation between parents and child (262).

AN INTEGRATIVE TREATMENT APPROACH

Turgay (1989) presented another dimension to family therapy: "integrative therapy." Suicidal behavior is considered complex and multifactorial, requiring an integrated response. Various therapeutic strategies and modalities are combined. For example, family therapy or support can be integrated with individual child or adolescent psychotherapy.

Turgay presented three levels of integration. The first integration level is the theoretical orientation. Therapists may use a combination of different schools of family therapy because the needs and characteristics of suicidal patients vary greatly. The second integration level is the "target system for the interventions" (Turgay, 1989: 975). At this level, the therapist may focus on the family as opposed to the child's individual therapy. The third integration level deals with primary, secondary, and tertiary prevention (Maris & Silverman, 1995).

For such prevention, the therapist must also consider genetic and familial aspects of the clinical psychiatric syndromes. Thus, a therapist who is integratively oriented may move from individual outpatient child therapy to pharmacotherapy incorporated in an inpatient milieu, simultaneously providing the family with strong support so that their ability to care for the suicidal patient increases. In integrative therapy, the target intervention systems include the patient, family, friends, school, health care systems, and society (Turgay, 1989).

HOSPITAL INVOLVEMENT AND FAMILY CARE
FOR THE SUICIDAL PATIENT

It is crucial to note that when working with a suicidal patient, hospitalization may be an early and necessary step. However, there are both advantages and disadvantages to using inpatient procedures. One advantage of placing children or adolescents in a hospital setting is that the family may be relieved of anxiety and may gain an understanding of the suicidal behavior as related to the family (Mattson et al., 1969; Berman & Jobes, 1991). Also, family involvement in an inpatient treatment program is usually expected.

Sokol and Pfeffer (1992) suggested that for optimal outcome, a multimodal treatment that coordinates the efforts of family therapist, child psychiatrist, pediatrician, psychologist, social worker, teachers, and family should be used. The case of Mary (Case 9.3), a 16-year-old with a history of suicide attempts and suicidal ideation, illustrates this point.

Hyland (1990) suggested that family involvement is an essential component to short-term and long-term hospital treatment. She proposed a Bowenian family system model in which the focus of treatment is on understanding family "triangles" and the "nuclear family emotional process."

It is also useful to note that some researchers believe that time spent in the hospital

CASE 9.3. The Case of Mary

Mary is a 16-year-old patient whose psychiatrist at the local inpatient emergency psychiatry unit was concerned about her continued wish to die and her impulsive and angry behaviors. Family consultation and evaluation of Mary's suicidality were needed to determine whether Mary could safely go home. The doctors and nurses were concerned about Mary's suicidal ideation, self-mutilation, previous suicide attempts, feelings of lack of self-worth, feelings of hopelessness and helplessness, use of alcohol to reduce her stress, and the intense levels of conflict in her family. The staff felt that Mary might also be suffering from a mild to moderate level of depression.

Mary had been admitted to the emergency unit because of suicidal ideation while intoxicated. Mary, at age 16, already was viewed as an alcoholic with episodic bingeing, blackouts, and delirium tremens. Mary had constant fights with her parents about her boyfriend, who was also a drug abuser. She was sexually active and reported a half dozen boyfriends since age 13. The patient's paternal grandfather had a history of substance abuse and Mary's father had had his own drinking problems in the past. At the age of 11, Mary was raped and sodomized by her uncle. This was reported to the police and Mary testified against her uncle, who was later convicted and imprisoned, in a lengthy court proceeding. Unknown to her family, Mary had previously attempted suicide at age 13 when she tried to hang herself with a belt. Mary had no previous history of psychotherapy except a session or two at the time of the rape with a sexual abuse counselor.

Unlike a number of more straightforward clinical problems, working with suicidal patients and their families is a high-risk, highly individualized endeavor. However, it is essential to involve the family and patient as collaborative risk-management partners. It is often essential to involve the suicidal adolescent and his or her family in the exploration of available options. The therapist must provide pertinent information to both the adolescent and the family over the course of the assessment, and during any subsequent treatment. This not only would allow active collaboration but also would foster close monitoring of the patient's and family's concerns. For Mary, the treatment plan consisted of both individual and family sessions as well as a special group for teenagers who had problems with alcohol abuse.

---

should be kept to a minimum for adolescents, and the family should be actively involved in the decisions regarding the length of the stay and visitation (Kenny & Krajewski, 1980).

Although hospitalization may bring about greater parental involvement in the treatment process, King (1987) warned that such hospitalization does not cure the suicide potential of the patient; rather, it prevents suicide during the time of hospitalization. When the patient leaves the hospital, the risk returns. The decision to hospitalize a patient in place of outpatient therapy can be a difficult one to make. Many factors must be taken into account, including the patient and parent's wishes and the safety of the patient.

Eisenberg (1980) proposed the following:

> If the weight of the risk–rescue ratio is on the rescue side of the fraction and the parents show understanding and concern, counseling on an out-patient basis is feasible. On the other hand, if the parents are indifferent and, worse, if they are angry, show no understanding of the distress represented by the attempt, and are unable to be supportive, then hospitalization will be necessary despite a favorable risk-rescue ratio. Failure of the gesture to bring about an affirmation of genuine concern may serve to confirm the patient's worse fears of being unloved; the parent who belittles the adolescent as a faker may make it necessary for the youngster to try again to save face. (319)

SUMMARY AND CONCLUSIONS

Tables 9.1 and 9.2 summarize the main factors to consider when working with suicidal patients from a family systems point of view. The literature on family therapy and suicide suggests that it is beneficial to involve the family in the treatment process, especially when working with a child or adolescent. The family can provide useful information and insight into the patient's behavior, and the therapist can guide the family to respond in an appropriate and consistent manner to the patient. Often extended family and friends can also be incorporated into the treatment plan. Table 9.2 summarizes the important therapist characteristics and methods of treatment when working with suicidal patients that are reflected in the literature.

Future research needs to more specifically address the role of the family therapist when working with a suicidal patient. Although there are some excellent works on the assessment

TABLE 9.1. Common Characteristics of Suicidal Patients and Their Families

Characteristics of patients

The patient may feel helpless and fear parental rejection.[a]

The patient may feel unloved and worthless.[a]

The individual may be unable to accept change and may have an intolerance for separation.[b]

Nonfatal ideas and actions are common in preadolescents.[c]

The suicidal act may be a cry for help.[c]

Characteristics of the family environment

Disorganized.[a]

Rigid and inflexible.[a]

Unstable.[a]

Conflict avoidant.[a]

Unclear boundaries and roles for family members.[a,b]

Unbalanced intrafamilial relationships.[b]

Excessive secretiveness.[b]

Communication disturbances between members, lack of expressiveness.[b]

Lack of cohesion.[b]

[a]Pfeffer (1981a); [b]Richman (1971); [c]Frances and Pfeffer (1987).

TABLE 9.2. Therapist Characteristics and Treatment Methods When Working with Suicidal Patients

Therapist characteristics

The therapist should be open, honest and direct.[a]

He or she should possess the characteristics of empathy, sensitivity and self awareness.[a]

The therapist should be well trained.[a]

The therapist should accept each family member without being judgmental.

Methods of treatment

The therapist should see the entire family.[a]

A family interview is useful.[a,b]

To better understand the situation, it is helpful to see each family member separately.[a]

The family should work at its own pace.[a]

The therapist should try to clarify the stresses in the family using "open communication."[a]

One goal is to heal the splits that occur within the patient and within the family.[a]

Outbursts that may occur in sessions can be used constructively.[a]

Therapy should define and offer treatment for parental conflicts as separate issues from the conflicts of the individual.[b]

Therapy should provide guidance in parenting.[b]

Therapy should include a variety of inpatient and outpatient interventions.[b]

Adjunctive modalities can be used in addition to individual therapy.[b]

The therapist should form a strong therapeutic relationship with family members.[c]

The therapist should share risks openly with the family.[c]

The therapist should provide insight into the multifactorial etiology of the problem.[c]

Integrative therapy suggests combining various strategies and modalities to treat a suicidal individual.[c]

[a]Richman (1984, 1986); [b]Pfeffer (1981a, 1986); [c]Turgay (1989).

---

of a suicidal individual, too little attention is paid, if any at all, to the context in which suicide occurs, especially the family context (Richman, 1992b).

Chapter 10 continues our examination of the social relations of suicides, but instead of focusing on marriage and family relations we consider more generic issues of social isolation and negative social relations (including stress and contagion).

FURTHER READING

Kaplan, A. G., & Klein, R. B. (1989). Women and suicide. In D. Jacobs & H. Brown (Eds.), *Suicide: Understanding and responding: Harvard Medical School perspectives* (pp. 257–282). Madison, CT: International Universities Press. A psychologist and a physician at the Stone Center at Wellesley College argue that women have a special suicide protective factor (i.e., their nurturing ties to their children [a sociobiological tie] and their interpersonal ties in general). Usually, only when a woman's relational priorities are so blocked or distorted that she perceives no further relational growth possibilities is her suicide vulnerability great.

Maris, R. W. (1997, September). Social and familial risk factors in suicidal behavior. *Psychiatric Clinics of North America: Suicide, 20*, 519–550. Maris begins by discussing the heavy genetic loading for manic-depressive disorder and suicide in the family tree of author Ernest Hemingway (including the suicide of Hemingway as well as that of his father, brother, sister, and granddaughter). Then the history of the sociology of suicide, the role of social isolation to suicide, the contagion of suicide, and stress and negative life events are reviewed.

Pearson, J. L., & Conwell, Y. (Eds.). (1996). *Suicide and aging: International perspectives.* New York: Springer. We tend to assume that the family is youthful or look at only the early stages of married life. Pearson and Conwell remind us that family factors also operate at the other end of the life cycle (i.e., in older or middle ages). See particularly Chapters 5, 9, and 12 on the role of late-life divorce, marital problems, loneliness, and suicide outcome.

Pfeffer, C. R. (1989). *Suicide among youth.* Washington, DC: American Psychiatric Press (especially Chapter 8). Pfeffer has written a great deal on family therapy and family socialization problems among child and youth suicides. The book examines family dynamics in adolescent suicides, depression among baby-boomers, genetics, and biological correlates of suicide among youth.

Richman, J. (1986). *Family therapy for suicidal people.* New York: Springer. Richman has long been a champion of family and social support as major preventive forces in suicidal behaviors. Some of the family characteristics that are seen as suicidogenic are familial role–conflict, scapegoating, and double-bind communications. The book contends that family therapy is the single most effective treatment for alleviating most suicidal states.

Stack, S. (1992). Marriage, family, religion, and suicide. In R. W. Maris, A. L. Berman, J. T. Maltsberger, & R. I. Yufit (Eds.), *Assessment and prediction of suicide* (pp. 540–552). New York: Guilford Press. This chapter notes recurring empirical trends in the United States, such as that for each marital status group by both age and gender, married persons have the lowest suicide rate. Stack presents general data on marriage, family, and suicide (e.g., that divorce rates tend to be a leading predictor of suicide rates).

10

The Social Relations of Suicides

The private experiences usually thought to be the proximate causes of suicide have only the influence borrowed from victim's moral disposition, itself an echo of the moral state of society . . . his sadness comes to him from without.

— EMILE DURKHEIM

Ernest Hemingway, his father, Clarence, brother, Leicester, sister Ursula, and granddaughter Margaux all committed suicide (see Figure 10.1). Ernest's son Gregory had seven "nervous breakdowns" [*sic*], 97 ECT treatments (he was bipolar), and three marriages and divorces (shades of Ernest). Another son, Patrick, also had ECT treatments and a severe head injury from a car accident. Most recently (July 31, 1996) granddaughter Margaux (her father was John, or "Jack") overdosed at age 41 and died, as yet another family suicide, after a history of alcoholism, bulimia, and epilepsy. Margaux described her family as "very, very dysfunctional." Of course, the question we have to answer is how much of the Hemingway family pathology is the result of social relations and how much is from biological or genetic factors—or even psychological forces (cf. Chapter 2, Figure 2.6).

Maris (1969, Ch. 3) has written about social factors in suicide on numerous previous occasions (see also Maris, 1971; Maris, 1981, Ch. 5; Maris, 1992a; Leenaars, Maris, & Takahashi, 1997). The focus in all these works as well as in this chapter is the presence or absence of external and constraining social facts (see Durkheim, 1897, on anomie, egoism, altruism, and fatalism), as reflected in indicators such as the divorce rate, marital status, the number of close friends of the proband, loss of crucial significant others, or sometimes having no one who cares whether the person lives or dies, being shamed or feeling intolerable guilt, sacrificing life for a higher cause or another person, military suicide, and so on.

When we concentrate on the *social* relations of suicides, the implicit contrast is usually with the individual. For example, Durkheim, in the opening quote, draws attention to social facts *outside* the individual and even then examines how social integration and social structure affect group suicide *rates*, not individual cases. The concept of "the Social" involves numbers greater than one *and* some interaction or exchange among the individual or units considered. The Social always has an emergent or even transcendent property to it such that the social sum is not equivalent to its individual parts (e.g., a working clock is more than its disorganized heap of component parts, or water is qualitatively different from two units of hydrogen and one unit of oxygen). Thus, most social suicidologists argue that suicide rates can never be explained by individual cases of suicide. Among the types of "social suicides"

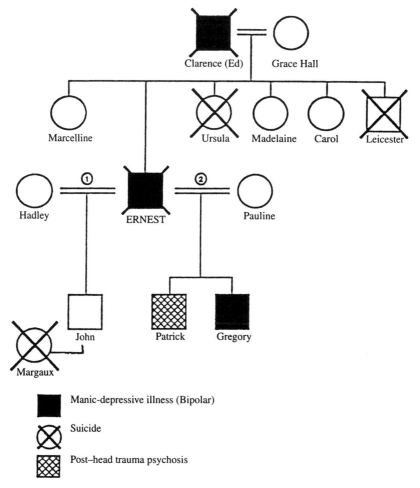

FIGURE 10.1. Psychiatric and suicidal family history of Ernest Hemingway. *Source:* Adapted from Jamison (1993: 229). Copyright 1993 by Kay Redfield Jamison. Adapted by permission.

that suicidologists examine are mass suicides, organizational self-destruction, suicide clusters (including, by extension, suicides in families such as the Hemingways), military suicides and war, murder followed by suicide, suicide pacts, and witnessed suicides among others (cf. Maris, Silverman, & Canetto, 1997).

The social relations of suicides tend to be one of two broad types, either absent or negative. By *"absent" social relations* we refer to social characteristics such as the loss of support (especially in the early socialization years of one's mother), absent parents, disrupted social relations such as anomie, never having been married or being divorced, having few close friends (e.g., Maris, 1981, found that about 50% of Chicago suicides had zero close friends—a statistically significant difference from the natural death control group), having no informant to help fill out a suicide's death certificate, or even no one to identify the body.

"Negative" social relations, or "negative interaction" (Maris, 1981: 116ff.), on the other hand, is *not* being socially isolated but, rather having suicidogenic social relations (e.g., driving an individual to kill himself). Here we refer not to absent parents but to "bad" parenting (e.g., giving a child a parental suicide to model or copy or child abuse). Another

example of negative social relations is suicide cults (e.g., Jonestown, Waco, the Order of the Solar Temple, and Heaven's Gate; see Chapter 19). In such cases one's social relations actually promote, cultivate, or in some cases even "practice" group suicide (e.g., as in Jonestown, Guyana). This type would encompass what Durkheim called altruistic suicides—such as the Japanese *kamikaze* pilots in World War II or the more current Muslim terrorists.

Sociology has a rich tradition in the study of the social relations of suicide (see Maris, 1992), One trend is largely *quantitative* and grows out of the early research of French social scientist Emile Durkheim (1857/1951). Included here would be the work of Henry and Short (1954), Gibbs and Martin (1964), Phillips (1974), Maris (1981), Stack (1982), and Pescosolido and Georgianna (1989).

A second trend is mainly *qualitative* and originated primarily with the "ethnomethodology" of Douglas (1967) and Garfinkel (1967). Among other things, social suicidologists examine *social risk factors* in general models of suicide outcomes, such as those listed in Chapter 2, Figure 2.6 (suicide in one's family, social isolation, marital disruption, stress and life events, loss of social support, etc.) or in Chapter 3, Table 3.6 (suicide predictors such as isolation, living alone, rejection, unemployment, and negative life events).

Other aspects of the social relations of suicides investigated by social scientists include work and the economy (see Chapter 8); sexuality and the family (see Chapters 6 and 9); culture and religion, legal and ethical considerations of euthanasia and death assistance (Chapter 19; imitation; socioeconomic status and suicide; community, organizational, and ecological studies; vital statistics (especially demographic factors such as age, sex, race, marital status, and occupation); temporal variations in suicide rates; mass and cult suicides; military suicides; witnessed suicides (McDowell, Rothberg, & Koshes, 1994); and social analogues of individual suicides, such as industrial pollution as a social overdose.

The remainder of this chapter concentrates on four aspects of the social relations of suicides: (1) a brief history of the sociological study of suicide, (2) social isolation, (3) contagion or imitation, and (4) social stress and negative interaction. We begin with a review of the highlights in the history of social suicidological thought and investigation.

HISTORY OF THE SOCIOLOGY OF SUICIDE

As much of sociology itself, the scientific study of the social relations of suicides began primarily with the work of the eminent French social philosopher Emile Durkheim circa 1897 (see Figure 10.2). In bold defiance of his psychological peer Pierre Janet (for an account of the historical context of Durkheim's *Suicide*, see Maris, 1969: 46–50), Durkheim insisted that suicide, seemingly among the most private and individual of human acts, could only be experienced collectively. Durkheim implored us to think of suicide *rates* (e.g., as in Table 3.4) as external and constraining social facts. Suicide is, thus, a "collective representation" that is admittedly founded in individual suicides, but at the same time transcends them, yet is qualitatively different from individual suicides.

Durkheim (1897/1951) writes:

> Sometimes men who kill themselves have had family sorrow or disappointments to their pride, sometimes they have had to suffer poverty, and sickness, at others they have had some moral fault with which they reproach themselves, etc. But we have seen that these individual peculiarities could not explain the social suicide rate; for the latter varies in considerable proportions, whereas the different combinations of circumstances which constitute the immediate antecedents of individual cases of suicide retain approximately the same frequency. They are therefore not the determining causes of the act which they precede. (297)

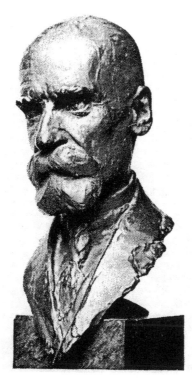

FIGURE 10.2. Emile Durkheim, founder of the social study of suicide.

Durkheim argued that social products such as suicide rates existed on a different explanatory level from the individual suicides that gave rise to the rates. When individuals "associate" or interact, the products of their social interaction (e.g., suicide rates) have an emergent or even transcendent property. It follows that suicide rates can only be explained by broad social conditions such as social integration, *anomie* and egoism. After a detailed empirical examination of the social characteristics (marital status, poverty level, age, mental status, religion, political status, etc.) of the death records from various countries, Durkheim (1897/1951) proceeded inductively to his major hypothesis: "suicide varies inversely with the degree of (social) integration (of the social groups of which the individual forms a part)" (209).

When social integration fails, the suicide rate usually rises (along with other rates, such as crime, divorce, etc.). As readers can see in Table 10.1, social integration can fail in two major ways: through what Durkheim calls anomie (abrupt normative deregulation, such as a sudden rise in the U.S. divorce rate after World War II or the 1929 U.S. stock market crash) or egoism (excessive isolation or being cut off from the support of other human beings, as with homeless skid-row pariahs). Anomie suicide can be thought of as a failure of vertical constraint and egoistic suicide as a failure of horizontal constraint; left to their own, asocial individuals had a greater tendency to self-destruct, because they cannot control themselves, Durkheim reasoned.

There are some anomalies in Durkheim's theory of suicide, as Table 10.1 suggests that social integration does *not always* protect individuals from suicide. With *altruistic* and *fatalistic* suicides, the more social integration, the *higher* (not lower) the suicide rate. Although Durkheim himself never says why these anomalies exist (he just minimizes the importance of the two types; e.g., mentions fatalistic suicide only in a footnote), part of the

TABLE 10.1. Durkheim's Typology of Suicide (Pure and Secondary Types)

	Basic types	Characteristics	Paradigms Secondary Types
A. Egoistic	Excessive individuation, Apathy. Results from man no longer finding a basis for existence in life	Within religions, family domestic society), and politics (wars and revolutions). Protestants vis-à-vis Jews, skid-row pariahs.	A1. Melancholic languor Depressed and inactive. Reflection is egoistic. A2. Epicurean Skeptical, disillusioned matter-of-factness.
B. Altruistic	Insufficient individuation. Energy of passion or will. Activity. Basis for existence appears situated beyond life. Eastern-like asceticism; try to achieve *moksha* or *nirvana*. "Heroic" suicide.	Lower societies, soldiers, religious martyrs, etc. *Hara-kiri, suttee,* the *kami-kaze.*	B1. Obligatory Duty. This is clearest type of altruistic suicide (e.g., North American Indians, Polynesians). B2. Optional Mystical enthusiasm. B3. Acute Renunciation itself is praiseworthy (e.g., India). Note: B2 and B3 derive from B1.
C. Anomic	Literally "deregulation," lack of normative restraint. Irritation, disgust. Anger and weariness. Often violence (nonegoistic) and murder (nonaltruistic). Unregulated emotions. Always accompanied by a morbid desire for the infinite. Lack of power controlling individuals gives rise to anomic suicide. Abrupt social change. Poverty restrains it.	Economic crises, sudden social changes, widowhood, divorce, liberal occupations.	C1. General Violent recriminations against life in general. C2. Particular Violent recriminations against life in particular (e.g., against one specific person—homicide–suicide).
D. Fatalistic	Excessive regulation.	Very young husbands. Childless married women. Slaves and prisoners.	

Source: Maris (1969: 39). Copyright 1969 by Wadsworth Publishing. Reprinted by permission.

explanation could be that *if* social norms are prosuicide (e.g., as in Jonestown, Guyana), social integration has a paradoxical effect. Also, *excessive* social regulation (as in prisons or mental hospitals) may have a paradoxical effect as well (cf. Maris, 1969: 33–42), other things being equal (cf. Pescosolido, 1994: 25, where she claims *moderate* levels of integration and regulation optimally protect against suicide).

It was over 50 years before these issues were again taken up, in Andrew Henry and James Short's *Suicide and Homicide* (1954). *Suicide and Homicide* was primarily an extension of Durkheim's *anomic* type of suicide, because it tested the influence of economic changes on the suicide rate. Henry and Short also expanded Durkheim's concept of external restraint to include a Freudian notion of "internal restraint" (such as a strict or punitive superego) and expanded the possible aggressive outcomes from suicide to homicide rates. Suicide, homicide, internal, and external restraint were all examined interactively, as depicted in Figure 10.3.

If Durkheim's work was sociological *par excellence*, then Henry and Short added im-

	Strong Internalized Restraint	Weak Internalize Restraint
Weak External Restraint	Self-Oriented Aggression (e.g., Suicide)	Unpredictable
Strong External Restraint	Anxiety or Conflict	Other-Oriented Aggression (e.g., homicide)

FIGURE 10.3. Henry and Short's predicted aggressive responses to frustration. *Source:* Henry & Short (1954: 121). Copyright 1954 by The Free Press; copyright renewed 1982 by Mary H. Bloch and James F. Short. Reprinted by permission.

portant dimensions of psychology and economics. The key concepts in *Suicide and Homicide* were (1) Dollard's (Dollard, Doob, Miller, Mowrer, & Sears, 1939) frustration–aggression hypothesis (cf. Berkowitz, 1962), (2) social status, and (3) external and internal restraint. Henry and Short assumed that aggression is often a consequence of frustration, that business cycles produce variation in the differential social status of persons and groups, and that frustrations are generated by interference with the goal response of maintaining a constant or rising position in a status hierarchy.

Henry and Short (1954) claim that reactions of both suicide and homicide rates to the business cycle can be interpreted as aggressive reactions to frustrations generated by the flow of economic forces (see Table 10.1). When external restraints are weak (e.g., because of high social status or social isolation) and internal restraints are *strong* (e.g., having developed an effective superego, taking responsibility for one's own actions, feeling guilt), the self tends to bear responsibility for frustration (i.e., structural circumstances favor *internally* directed aggression). Conversely, when people are subjected to strong external restraint (e.g., by subordinate social status or intense and numerous involvements with other people) and weak internal restraint (e.g., a less punitive superego), it is easier to blame others when frustration occurs and to be assaultive or homicidal (i.e., to aggress *externally*).

Some of the major inadequacies with Henry and Short's theories are that (1) suicide rates in fact often tend to be higher in the lower social classes, (2) there are very high and very low suicide rates in subclasses of both upper- and lower-social-status groups (e.g., high suicide rates for psychiatrists and low suicide rates for surgeons), and (3) status change may be more highly associated with suicide than is status position (Maris, 1981, Ch. 6).

For the last 30 to 35 years, Gibbs has argued that Durkheim's concept of "social integration" was not operationally defined and, thus, was untestable (see Gibbs's most recent statement, Gibbs, 1994). Gibbs has been outspoken, if not outrageous, in his persistent insistence on empiricism in the social study of suicide. In their 1964 book, Gibbs and Martin contend that properly done empirical tests will demonstrate that suicide rates are negatively related to status integration. The heart of status integration theory is that less frequently occupied status sets imply more unstable and disrupted social relationships, more role conflicts, more incompatible statuses, and (thus) higher suicide rates.

"Status integration" is measured in at least three ways: by the simple proportion of individuals occupying a status set (the fewer the occupants, the lower the status integration), by the proportions of status sets squared and summed to give a measure for a more general status set (usually a column is a table), and by the sum of sums of squares, to give a measure for an entire table. For example, Gibbs and Martin (1964: 62) correlate occupational integration measures of race and gender status with their suicide rates and derive a rank-order correlation of −.94. This correlation is both highly significant statistically and is in the direction predicted. Their theory predicts significant negative correlations between various status integration measures and suicide rates.

Table 10.2 provides a more current (1994) example of the relationship of marital status integration to suicide rates. The total measure of marital integration in Table 10.2 would be the average of the ΣP^2 row (i.e., .836 + 1,000 + .250 = .692). Thus, the theory would predict that any marital status set *less* than .692 would have a *higher* suicide rate (here, the set in column 3), and any status set more than .692 would have a *lower* suicide rate (the sets in columns 1 and 2). Status integration theory has been heavily criticized over the years. Clearly, it is only one variable affecting the suicide rate. Also, when one of the statuses is not ascribed or when ascribed statuses are placed in columns (not rows), the Gibbs and Martin results are often not replicated. Note that actual occupancy and role conflict could *both* be low. Finally, the theory is confirmed primarily for occupational, and not other, statuses.

Perhaps the most radical challenge to the Durheimian sociological approach to the study of suicide has come from "ethnomethodology" and Douglas's *The Social Meanings of Suicide* (1967; cf. Douglas, 1970). "Ethnomethodology" concerns uncovering the unstated, implicit, commonsense perceptions held and acted on by participants in a situation (e.g., suicide attempters). Among other things, Douglas and ethnomethodology had fundamental doubts about Durkheim's procedure of founding suicide study on official statistics like death records or death certificates (see quote in Box 10.1 from p. 191). Douglas argued that vital or official statistics (e.g., suicide rates) were unreliable. There could be as many different statistics of suicide as there were officials (see quotes in Box 10.1 from pp. 209, 213).

Coroners and medical examiners use unstated and diverse criteria for certifying a death as a suicide. Thus, "suicide" does not have one meaning. Douglas asks suicidologists to ob-

TABLE 10.2. Gibbs's Measures of Marital Status Integration

Marital status	Occupied state configurations[a]		
	A_3–S_1–E_3 O_4–R_2–O_2 Col. 1	A_4–S_1–E_2 O_3–R_1–P_1 Col. 2	A_5–S_2–E_2 O_1–R_3–P_3 Col. 3
Single	0.912	0.000	0.247
Married	0.063	1.000	0.252
Widowed	0.010	0.000	0.251
Divorced	0.015	0.000	0.250
ΣP[b]	1.000	1.000	1.000
ΣP[c]	0.836	1.000	0.250
W[b]	0.240	0.352	0.408

[a]All possible combinations of occupied statuses in the social unit (a country or a community). In this illustration A signifies age, S sex, E ethnicity–race, O occupation, R religious affiliation, and P parental status. Each number signifies a particular status within a family of statuses (e.g., S_1 would be a male, S_2 a female).
[b]Sum of column proportions.
[c]Measure of marital integration for the status configuration.
[d]Proportion of the social unit's population in the status configuration. The row sum of the W values is 1.000 regardless of the number of columns, but in a real social unit there are likely to be far more than three occupied status configurations.
Source: Gibbs (1994: 46). Copyright 1994 by Charles Press Publications. Reprinted by permission.

BOX 10.1. Excerpts from the Ethnomethodological Critique of Durkheim

- ". . . what Durkheim is doing is assuming his sociologistic theory of suicide to be correct and then explaining away any data that is contrary to it" (p. 177).

- "official statistics cannot be expected to have any significant value in constructing or testing sociological theories of suicide" (p. 191).

- ". . . the more socially integrated an individual is, the more he and his significant others will try to avoid having his death categorized as a suicide, assuming that suicide is judged negatively" (p. 209).

- ". . . the more integrated the deceased individual is into his local community and with the officials, the more the doctors, coroners, and other official responsible for deciding what the cause of death is will be favorably influenced, consciously or subconsciously, by the preferences of the deceased and his significant others" (p. 213).

- "The most important error involved in the use of the official statistics, however, has been the same error as that made in the theories themselves; that is, the assumption that "suidical actions" have a necessary and suficent, unidimensional meaning throughout the Western world" (p. 229).

- ". . . a basic reorientation of sociological work on suicide in the direction of intensive observation, description, and analysis of individual cases of suicide seems to be necessary" (p. 231).

Source: Douglas (1967).

---

serve the "subjective accounts" or "situated meanings" of actual suicidal individuals (i.e., first-person accounts of serious suicide attempters, not third-person accounts of medical examiners). Here, sounding much more like Weber's *verstehen* (1925: 1904–1905) than Durkheim's external and constraining social facts, Douglas urges us to focus on the *subjective meanings* of actual suicidal individuals.

Douglas is making three major claims here: (1) "suicide" has many (not one) different meanings, (2) suicide cannot be explained until we ascertain exactly what it is we are trying to explain (e.g., not simply relying on death certificates, which do not take the meaning of suicide as problematic), and (3) the best way to discover the meanings of suicide is to *observe* the statements and behavior of *individuals* actually engaged in suicidal behaviors—such as suicide attempters (see quote in Box 10.1 from p. 121). Conversely, Douglas argues that it is not possible to predict suicide in abstract collective terms, such as *anomie* or *egoism*.

In spite of Douglas's cogent theoretical critique of Durkheim, over the years social suicidologists have continued to use vital statistics in the study of suicide. In part we use vital statistics because there is no other practical alternative (Gibbs, 1994: 61) and in part because the vital statistics are probably not as inaccurate as Douglas claimed (Pescosolido & Mendelsohn, 1986). Finally, Douglas concentrates mainly on suicide *attempters*, who are a very different self-destructive population than suicide *completers*.

Maris's research (1969, 1981, 1992a, 1997) has combined and extended social suicidology, especially in *Pathways to Suicide* (1981), by (1) adding actual interviews ("psychological autopsies") with a systematic sample of intimate (usually spouses) individual survivors of completed suicides; (2) using a case–control design, with completed suicides as the cases and nonfatal suicide attempters and natural deaths as the control or comparison groups; (3) employing more sophisticated multivariate statistical analyses (i.e., multiple nominal scale analysis and path analysis); (4) developing a biopsychosocial model of suicide outcome (see Chapter 2, Figure 2.2); (5) exploring new data, such as religious attitudes and behavior; and (6) conceiving of suicide developmentally (Maris, 1981: 9–11, claimed that individuals who committed suicide tended to have "suicidal careers" spanning several decades and involving complex interdependent mixes of biological, social, and psychological factors).

In his *early* work, Maris (1969) examined the social structures of Chicago suicides. For example, he investigated the community characteristics of areas in Chicago with high suicide rates (see Figure 10.4) and the relationship of SES and social mobility to suicide rates. In *later* work, Maris (1992f) focused on identifying and specifying 15 major predictors of suicide and then applying them to individual clinical and forensic cases retrospectively. This later work had an emphasis on suicide assessment problems (false positives, false negatives, etc.). Finally, Maris attempted to synthesize prior suicide research by developing a biopsychosocial theoretical model of suicidal careers, as well as to frame the social and cultural contexts of suicide in a more international comparative perspective (Leenaars et al., 1997).

Maris's research was probably more of an approach than an arrival. Suicidology still has not had a truly national sample survey of completed suicide. There are also now more powerful and refined statistical tools available, such as logistic regression, log-linear methods, and event history analysis (see Addy, 1992). The control groups Maris used could also be more systematically drawn, larger, and more diverse.

If Douglas criticized Durkheim methodologically for relying on vital or official statistics, Princeton-trained demographer David Phillips (1974, 1980; Phillips & Cartensen, 1986; Phillips & Lesyna, 1995) took issue with Durkheim's contention that suicides are not suggestable or contagious. In a pioneering article in the *American Sociological Review*, Phillips (1974) demonstrated that front-page *New York Times* newspaper coverage of celebrated suicides (Marilyn Monroe, especially) was associated with a statistically significant rise (an X of about 2–3% and a range of about 1–6%) in the national suicide rate 7 to 10 days after the publicized suicide event (see Table 10.5). The rise in the suicide rate was greater the longer the front-page coverage (a dose–response relationship), greater in the geographic region where the news account ran, and higher if the stimulus suicide and the person presumably copying the suicide were similar (in age, sex or gender, life situation, etc.). The increase due to contagion was less than the separate effects of standard demographic variables such as age, sex, race, or even day of the week (Phillips & Cartensen, 1986). Figure 10.5 illustrates a presumed contagion effect of news publicity, in which Viennese subway suicides declined after curtailment of subway suicide news stories.

In a long series of similar studies (Phillips, Lesyna, & Paight, 1992; Phillips & Lesyna, 1995), Phillips and his colleagues have extended and replicated their first results. For example, the contagion effect appears to be stronger among teenagers than among adults (Phillips & Cartensen, 1986), with teen suicide rates rising about 6.9% after televised news of feature suicide stories. Phillips claims that not only do general suicide rates rise after publicized celebrity suicides but also homicide rates rise after heavyweight championship boxing matches, suicide rates rise after soap opera television suicides, commercial airline crashes rise after publicized murder–suicides, and single-driver vehicle fatalities rise after publicized suicides (although some of these associations seem intuitively far-fetched).

Phillips's ideas about contagion dominated the sociological study of suicide in the 1980s. Work by Stack (1982), Wasserman (1989a), Kessler and Stripp (1984), and others have produced equivocal support for the role of suggestion in suicide (cf. Diekstra, Maris, Platt, Schmidtke, & Sonneck, 1989). Some of the criticisms are that there is no clear evidence that the suicide ever saw the publicized event, that unemployment rates and business

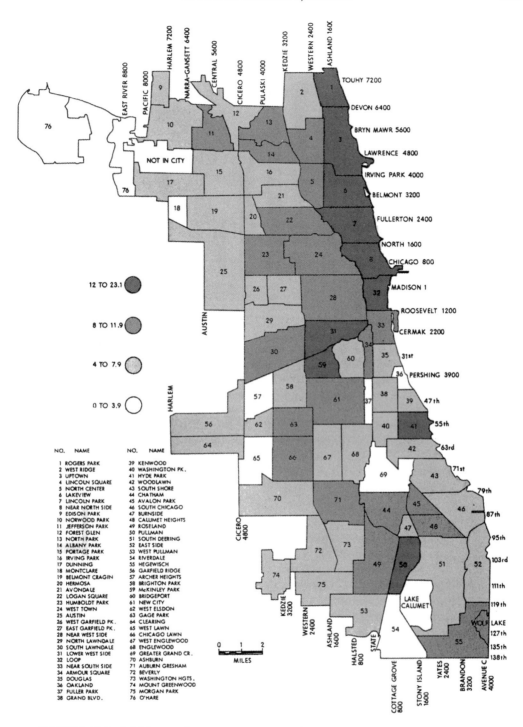

FIGURE 10.4. Suicide rates by community areas of Chicago. *Source:* Maris (1969: 139).

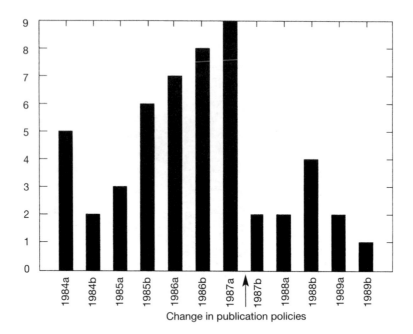

FIGURE 10.5. Number of Viennese subway suicides (in 6-month periods) before and after two major Viennese newspapers curtailed their coverage of subway suicides. *Source:* Phillips (1992: 507). Copyright 1992 by The Guilford Press. Reprinted by permission.

cycles need to be controlled for, and that the *theory* of imitation is underdeveloped. Sometimes one feels that in suggestion studies, precision varies inversely with significance. Finally, because we usually only measure harmful outcomes, we really do not know the beneficial effects of publicized suicide events.

A prolific researcher and publisher who has done work in the same genre as Phillips is Steven Stack. Stack has done a vast number of empirical studies (some with major federal grants) of contagion and suicide and homicide rates and marital status, occupational status, unemployment, religion and family life, and suicide rates. These studies have been published in all the leading sociology journals.

After an early review of 10 years of the literature on suicide, Stack (1982) continued with numerous suicide and contagion studies. For example, he found that suicides rise significantly after both celebrity and noncelebrity suicides and that celebrity suicides and those suiciding afterward tended to have the same characteristics (Stack, 1987a).

In a 1992 review of marriage, family, religion, and suicide, Stack confirmed the low suicide rates of married persons and the high suicide rates among the divorced. He also reminded us that Catholics have lower suicide rates than Protestants and that religiosity and family life are inseparable.

Two recent research pieces have brought Stack nationwide media attention. In 1992, Stack and Gundlach supported the hypothesis that the greater the air time devoted to country music in metropolitan areas, the greater the white suicide rate. A follow-up article (Stack, 1995c) suggests that country music fans are at greater suicide risk, largely because of the indirect effects of greater marital disruption and gun ownership.

Finally, sociologist Bernice Pescosolido is worth noting here because she addresses issues related to Douglas and the reliability of official statistics and also because of her efforts, as she puts it, "to bring Durkheim in the 21st century" by translating and extending his work into network analysis (Pescosolido, 1994: 264). Contrary to Douglas, Pescosolido argues that official statistics of suicide are fairly reliable (Pescosolido & Mendolsohn, 1986; coroners' and medical examiners' study, 1991).

Pescosolido (1994) believes that network theory provides a way to understand how Douglas's level of individual actors and Durkheim's level of *sui generis* social structure are linked by "looking at the network content, [the] structure and cultural context in which social interaction takes place" (268). For example, disintegrating network ties deny suicidal individuals both integrative and regulative protection (Pescosolido & Georgianna, 1989). As a case in point, Roman Catholic and evangelical Protestant (e.g., Southern Baptists) networks protect against suicide, but institutional Protestant networks (e.g., Episcopal or Congregational) do not. Pescosolido (1994: 274; Nisbet, 1996) argues that religious protection comes from their social support communities.

Pescosolido contends that *moderate* levels of both social integration and regulation are optimal in protecting individuals from suicidal impulses. For example, Jonestown, Guyana had *excessive* levels of integration and regulation and, thus, did not protect its members against suicide.

Although linking micro- and macrosocial processes is a crucial task and network theory has much to tell us in social suicidology, *network analysis may not be the answer to bridging the gap between the micro- and macrosocial study of suicide*. Much of formal network analysis in sociology is not interested in any individuals, suicidal or otherwise. Many network sociologists believe that all social behavior must be explained at the *macro*level (Turner, 1998, Chs. 25, 38).

Also, one problem with excessive regulation or integration is that the *norms* of such groups may be prosuicide and their basic group behaviors self-destructive. That is, integration and regulation only protect if the norms and behaviors of the group are *against* suicide.

SOCIAL ISOLATION AND SUICIDE

What, if anything, is suicidogenic about being alone? It has been argued that suicide outcome is enhanced by the loss of necessary social supports; by increases in levels of hostility and aggression accompanied by a corresponding reduction of targets for that aggression other than oneself; by greater impulsivity resulting from lessened social constraints; and by isolation-enhanced depression, sleep disorder, and hopelessness. Durkheim (1897/1951) wrote: "First of all it can be said that, as collective force is one of the obstacles best calculated to restrain suicide, its weakening involves the development of suicide" (209).

In early social–psychological experiments by Solomon Asch (1955: 31–35) it was discovered that individuals tended to go along with group judgments, even when they believed that the group judgment was erroneous. The Asch experiments concerned matching the length of a line from one card with the length of another line on a second card. The second card contained two lines, one of which was obviously the correct match in length. In groups of 10, if 9 confederates gave the wrong answer, the naive subject (who could see easily that all 9 gave a wrong answer) was likely to go along with the false group judgment. But when only one confederate sided with the naive subject, the subject was much less likely to conform to the false judgment. Apparently being isolated was a different situation than was having only one significant other.

In some isolating social situations (e.g., Jews in Nazi concentration camps during World War II; Bettelheim, 1943), aggression seems less prominent than apathy, disorganization, or the simple loss of the will to live. It is worth noting that Bettelheim, himself a survivor of Nazi concentration camps, did not suicide while in the camp but did so later on, on March 14, 1990, at the age of 86, as did author Primo Levi in 1987, after surviving Auschwitz.

When social psychiatrist Peter Sainsbury (1955: 41) studied suicides in London, he found that the suicide rate was significantly ($p < .01$) related to the percentage of persons living alone, of those living alone in just one room, of those living in hotel rooms, and of those divorced. When Maris (1969) did similar work in Chicago, he found that the correlation between population per household and the suicide rate in Cook County's 76 community areas was –.72 (–.60 when age was controlled for). In general, then, the greater the number of people living in a dwelling unit in an area, the lower the suicide rate in that area—although one has to be careful not to imput group traits to suicidal individuals (not to commit the "ecological fallacy").

Nisbet (1996: 325–341), examined protective factors for suicidal black females. He knew that in spite of high rates of family disruption, clinical depression, and economic deprivation, black females have the lowest suicide rates of any race or gender group in the United States—and wondered why. It turned out that black females attempt suicide at about the same rate as white females and at a rate greater than that of all males—but they just are less likely to complete suicide. Nisbet concluded that black females seem to be protected against completed suicide primarily by their social support system (e.g., by a larger average household size and by larger kinship and friendship networks). Finally, black females tended to turn to their family and friends for help, not to doctors or other professionals. This sounds like the old conundrum: "If you're sick, be sure to stay away from doctors and hospitals!"

In one of the few sociological surveys of suicides in a major city (Chicago) Maris (1981: 113–115) found that half the suicides did *not* belong to *any* social organizations. This percentage was lower (without reaching statistical significance) than that for nonfatal suicide attempters (43%) and natural deaths (30%). The relative social isolation of suicides was not a simple consequence of age because the average ages for suicide completers and natural deaths was 51 and 71, respectively.

Also, in the 1981 Chicago suicide survey (Maris, 1981a: 113 ff.) Maris asked, "How many close friends did [the subject] have in the last year; that is, persons [he/she] saw frequently and confided in about highly personal matters?" Table 10.3 reveals that on average, natural deaths had about twice as many close friends as did suicide completers ($p = .001$), even though (as we just saw) they were on average 20 years older than the suicide completers. Suicide completers were much more likely than natural deaths or nonfatal suicide attempters to have *zero* close friends(49%, 33%, and 22%, respectively) and fewer larger groups of friends (e.g., the percentages of natural deaths, attempters, and completers who had "three or more close friends" was 29%, 35%, and 11%, respectively). In general then, in Maris's 1981 Chicago survey, completed suicides tended to be *the most interpersonally isolated* of the three study groups and to experience the highest degree of nonparticipation in organizations and social groups.

We know as well that marriage does tend to protect against suicide (see Chapter 9), especially for white males. Generally, suicide rates are highest among the widowed, followed by those of the divorced, single, and married (usually in that order). Females are much less protected against suicide by marriage; that is, they have what Durkheim called a lower "coefficient of preservation."

A few caveats are in order here. It may be *changes* in the degree of social isolation that is the crucial variable in suicide. For example, witness the high suicide rate of young white males put into solitary confinement, overnight lockups, jails, or even retirement and the increasing marginality of most older white males. Furthermore, not all social relations protect

TABLE 10.3. Number of Close Friends Subject Had in the Last Year before
Suicide, Nonfatal Attempt, or Natural Death

Number of close friends	Natural deaths (%)	Suicide attempters (%)	Suicide completers (%)
0	33	22	49
1	11	11	18
2	13	27	11
3+	29	35	11
DK	14	5	11
Total	100%	100%	100%
	(71)	(64)	(266)
$\overline{X}$ scores*	2.4	2.0	1.0

Source: Maris (1981: 115). Copyright 1981 by Johns Hopkins University Press. Reprinted by permission.

*t tests for significance of means were:

	t	Significance
Natural deaths versus suicide completers	3.8	$p < .001$
Natural deaths versus suicide attempters	0.9	n.s.
Suicide attempters versus suicide completers	4.8	$p < .001$

against suicide. Obviously, if you are a member of the Hemlock Society, were in the Jonestown cult, were a Japanese *kami-kaze* pilot in World War II, or a Muslim terrorist, then social support would *increase* the suicide rate in your group.

In general, when the group norms are prosuicide (see Durkheim's altruistic suicide in Table 10.1), or social relations or interactions are negative (painful, rejecting, deprecating [driving a person to suicide], punitive [jail and prison suicides], revengeful, etc.; see Maris, 1981: 116–121), they tend to *raise* the suicide rate. This anomaly to the social support and suicide hypothesis helps to reconcile contradictions in Durkheim's four types of suicide. That is, anomic and egoistic suicides involve failures of social support, but altruistic and fatalistic suicide do not.

Of course, there are other examples of social suicides—of social involvement being positively (not negatively) associated with the suicide rate—that limited space precludes the development of, such as suicide clusters, mass suicides in religious cults, military suicides, suicide pacts, witnesses suicides, organizational self-destruction, murder–suicides, and so on (see Maris, Silverman, & Canetto, 1997; Leenaars et al., 1997).

CONTAGION, IMITATION, AND SUICIDE CLUSTERS

On the face of it, suicide imitation seems ludicrous or even preposterous. If I suggest, "Why don't you just kill yourself?," would you be likely to reply, "Why didn't I think of that?!," and then summarily do yourself in? Not likely. Common sense (not always a reliable guide) tells us that people who copy other suicides are "peculiar" in some way or otherwise vulnerable and "prepped" to respond.

Yet, don't we often robotically do what our parents or authorities tell us to do (Milgram, 1974)? Furthermore, culture lays the groundwork for the sheer possibility of imitating suicides. Could someone copy a suicide, say, among the Tiv of Nigeria, as their societies virtually have no suicides to copy, and perhaps not even a word for "suicide"? Conversely, in places such as Hungary, Germany, Austria, and Finland, suicide is so common as to almost be part of the national character; thus, contagion would seem much more feasible there.

In the pages that follow we examine the role of contagion, imitation, modeling, suggestion, and so on, in suicidal behaviors. Indeed, much of the contemporary sociology of suicide seems almost obsessed with contagion. This was not the case in the beginning. Durkheim (1897/1951), casually minimized the role of imitation in suicide as follows:

> In short, certain as the contagion of suicide is from individual to individual, imitation never seems to propagate it so as to affect the social suicide *rate*. . . . It is equally inadmissable that a social fact is merely a generalized individual fact. But most untenable of all is the idea that this generalization may be due to some blind contagion. . . . Imitation is not an original factor in suicide. It only exposes a [social] state [like *anomie* or *egoism*] which is the true generating cause of . . . [both] act(s). (140, 142, 141)

The roots of the concept of contagion can be found in epidemiology, public health, behavioral psychology, and behavioral biology. By "*epidemiology*" we mean "the study of the distribution and determinants of diseases and injuries in human populations" (Mausner & Bahn, 1985; cf. Chapter 3). An *epidemic* is "an occurrence in a community or region of a group of illnesses of similar nature (here, of suicides), clearly in excess of normal expectancy (e.g., statistically significantly higher than the average suicide rate for a particular month of the year when the stimulus suicide did not occur)."

Contagion also reminds us of the well-known and voluminous research on stimulus and response (e.g., of classical conditioning in Pavlov's dogs who salivated at the stimulus of a bell originally paired with the presentation of their food, or B. F. Skinner's (1953) instrumental or operant conditioning). When pigeons randomly pecked in a so-called Skinner Box, if they happened to peck a target lever and got rewarded with food (and were hungry), they tended to learn to peck the target (under similar appropriate conditions). In sociology, George Homans (1974) founded his explanation of all small-group behavior in Skinnerian psychology and the classical economics of Adam Smith. Homans argued that of all possible actions, people will tend to do those that are the most rewarded and valuable. Blumer (1969) cautions us that the correct sequence is not simply stimulus–response (S-R), but stimulus–subjective interpretation–response (S-I-R); that is, situations are not defined until those perceiving them add their own subjective meanings or interpretations to the stimuli.

Of course, people do not always respond to a stimulus, especially one that will cost them their lives. Some of the factors in the variation of modeling of a stimulus suicide event are as follows:

1. The copying individual's similarity to the stimulus. For example, thirtish white females would be expected to be more likely to copy Marilyn Monroe's suicide (but always with "other things being equal," or *ceteris paribus*).

2. The dosage or the dose–response relationship. Generally, the greater the stimulus or the longer the exposure to the stimulus, the more likely the copying is. For example, the more days of front-page coverage of a suicide story in a major newspaper, the stronger the copying response (here, the higher the rise in the suicide rate over the normal rate expected for that time and place). One caveat here is that, as Skinner reminds us, often intermittent reinforcement is more effective than constant reinforcement.

3. The praise, glorification, or otherwise rewarding of the original stimulus suicide. For example, after World War II, the suicide of defeated military officers was seen in Japan to be heroic and dignified, as was the use of suicide as a response to shame or as a social

obligation. Under these conditions many others in similar situations probably copied this suicidal resolution to defeat or failure.

4. *Mutatis mutandis.* Teenagers are more likely than adults to imitate stimulus suicides, (Phillips & Cartensen, 1986). Most studies show a 6–7% rise in teen suicides after a teen suicide stimulus is presented, compared to a 2 or 3% rise among adults with an adult suicide stimulus.

As we just saw in the section on the history of the sociology of suicide, the seminal work on contagion and suicide was that of demographer David Phillips. Phillips (1970) initially investigated social forces in death in general in his PhD dissertation (cf. Phillips & Feldman, 1973) at Princeton. Phillips argued that people routinely postpone their deaths, regardless of the manner (even natural deaths are postponed) of death, until just after important social occasions in which they were meaningfully involved—such as their own birthdays, presidential elections, the Apollo moon travel, or *Yom Kippur.*

For example, after constructing a 12 × 12 matrix of birthdays and deathdays for 400 famous Americans, Phillips discovered that there was a statistically significant "death dip" (compared to the normal death rate expected) in the month before their birthdays, while there was a significant rise in deaths (compared to expected frequencies, using a chi-square procedure) in the 4 months consisting of the birth month and the 3 months afterwards. Phillips speculated that persons who are highly integrated into society and involved with its ceremonies tend to die "postmaturely" in order to participate in those important social ceremonies.

Although we have discussed Phillips's (1974) paper, we have not yet presented his data. Table 10.4 shows that the actual incidence of suicide increased significantly (total rise = 1,298.5 suicides) over the expected incidences following front-page coverage of suicides in *The New York Times* (especially after the suicides of Marilyn Monroe and Stephen Ward). Durkheim claimed that suggestion has only a local effect. In the cases of Monroe and Ward the effect was international. Durkheim also contended that suggestion merely precipitates suicides that would have happened later anyway. Phillips stated that if that were the case, we should see a dip in the number of suicides occurring in the months following a front-page story. No such dip was observed. Finally, Phillips thought Durkheim was probably right that the effects of suggestibility are relatively small. For example, in Phillips's *New York Times* data overall, the suicide level increased only about 2.5% after the suicide stories were publicized.

Sociologist Ira Wasserman (1984) criticized Phillips (1974) for relying on a quasi-experimental method. By using a multivariate time-series model, Wasserman argued for refinements and specifications in the original Phillips data. For example, Phillips did not control for unemployment, seasonal effects, or the celebrity status of the stimulus suicide. Phillips found a rise in suicides (179.5 suicides) 1 month after comedian Freddie Prinze suicided (February 1977). However, it may be the economic recession in 1977 followed by a large rise in unemployment in 1978 that explained the rise in suicide after Prinze's suicide.

Second, the smaller the time range used (days vs. months vs. years), the more one is able to specify time effects. This could be important, as Wasserman found seasonal variation in suicide rates (U.S. rates are highest in the months of March, April, and May).

Finally, reexamining Phillips's (1974) data, Wasserman found no overall linkage between front-page *New York Times* suicide stories and subsequent suicide rates. However, he did find a significant relationship between *celebrity* suicides (e.g., that of actor George Sanders) and the subsequent suicide rate.

Steven Stack (1987a) further specified Phillips's and Wasserman's presumed celebrity imitation effects. For example, he discovered that the suicide imitation effect held only for

TABLE 10.4. Rise in the Number of U.S. Suicides after Suicide Stories are Publicized on the Front Page of *The New York Times*, 1948–1967

Name of publicized suicide	Date of suicide story	Observed no. of suicides in mo. after suicide story	Expected no. of suicides in mo. after suicide story	Rise in No. of U.S. suicides after suicide story
Lockridge (author)	Mar. 8, 1948	1,510	1,521.5	–11.5
Landis (film star)	July 6, 1948	1,482	1,457.5	24.5
Brooks (financier)	Aug. 28, 1948	1,250	1,350	–100.0
Holt (betrayed husband)	Mar. 10, 1949	1,583	1,521.5	61.5
Forrestal (ex-secretary of defense)	May 22, 1949	1,549	1,493.5	55.5
Baker (professor)	Apr. 26, 1950	1,600	1,493.5	106.5
Lang (police witness)	Apr. 20, 1951	1,423	1,519.5	–96.5
Soule (professor)	Aug. 4, 1951	1,321	1,342	–21.0
Adamic (writer)	Sept. 5, 1951	1,276	1,258.5	17.5
Stengel (N.J. police chief)	Oct. 7, 1951	1,407	1,296.5	110.5
Feller (U.N. official)	Nov. 14, 1952	1,207	1,229	–22.0
LaFollette (senator)	Feb. 25, 1953	1,435	1,412	23.0
Armstrong (inventor of FM Radio)	Feb. 2, 1954	1,240	1,227	13.0
Hunt (senator)	June 20, 1954	1,458	1,368.5	89.5
Vargas (Brazilian president)	Aug. 25, 1954	1,357	1,321.5	35.5
Norman (Canadian ambassador)	Apr. 5, 1957	1,511	1,649.5	–138.5
Young (financier)	Jan. 26, 1958	1,361	1,352	9.0
Schupler (N.Y.C. councilman)	May 3, 1958	1,672	1,587	85.0
Quiggle (admiral)	July 25, 1958	1,519	1,451	8.0
Zwillman (underworld leader)	Feb. 27, 1959	1,707	1,609	98.0
Bang-Jensen (U.N. diplomat)	Nov. 27, 1959	1,477	1,423	54.0
Smith (police chief)	Mar. 20, 1960	1,669	1,609	60.0
Gedik (Turkish minister)	May 31, 1960	1,568	1,628.5	–60.5
Monroe (film star)	Aug. 6, 1962	1,838	1,640.5	197.5
Graham (publisher)				
Ward (implicated in Profumo Affair)	Aug. 4, 1963	1,801	1,640.5	160.5
Heyde & Tillman (Nazi officials)	Feb. 14, 1964	1,647	1,584.5	62.5
Lord (N.J. party chief)	June 17, 1965	1,801	1,743	58.0
Burros (KKK leader)	Nov. 1, 1965	1,710	1,652	58.0
Morrison (war critic)	Nov. 3, 1965			
Mott (American in Russian jail)	Jan. 22, 1966	1,757	1,717	40.0
Pike (son of Bishop Pike)	Feb. 5, 1966	1,620	1,567.5	52.5
Kravchenko (Russian defector)	Feb. 26, 1966	1,921	1,853	68.0
LoJui-Ching (Chinese army leader)	Jan. 21, 1967	1,821	1,717	104.0
Amer (Egyptian field marshal)	Sept. 16, 1967	1,770	1,733.5	36.5
Total				1,298.5

Source: Phillips (1974: 344).

entertainers and celebrities, not for artists, villains, and the economic elite. The primary rise (statistically significant) in suicide rates comes only after entertainment celebrity suicides (e.g., after the suicides of Carole Landis, Marilyn Monroe, and Freddie Prinze). The rate of suicide increased 1.35 units in the months with a story on an entertainment celebrity.

Stack further speculated that copying a suicide might be related to the similarity in the stimulus and respondent suicides mental or physical health, marital problems, age, gender, or race. He found a significant association with mental, but not physical, health. The suicide of Freddie Prinze was significantly associated with a subsequent rise in *youth* suicide. Prinze's suicide was also significant for subsequent male suicides, but not for female suicides. Finally, none of celebrity suicides was significant in the regression on the nonwhite suicide term, suggesting imitative effects only for whites.

Gould and Shaffer (1986) extended the examination of imitation to *fictional* televised suicides, by examining four made-for-TV movies on teen suicides between October 1984 and February 1985. They then examined suicides and attempted suicides in the Greater New York area by samples age 19 years or younger (this resulted in 31 completed suicides and 220 suicide attempters). Gould and Shaffer inspected rates of attempted and completed suicides 2 weeks before and after the four movie broadcasts of teen suicides.

Broadcast I depicted a male high school student who drove his car off a cliff, broadcast II showed a 17-year-old male high school student who suicides after several interpersonal crises, broadcast III dealt with a male teenager's effort to stop his father's suicide, and broadcast IV concerned a teenage boy and girlfriend who jointly suicided. As Figure 10.6 reveals, there was a statistically significant excess of teen suicide attempts and completions 2 weeks after the broadcast of fictional TV teen suicides. Gould and Shaffer conclude that it seems likely that some of the excess suicidal behavior was prompted by the TV broadcasts. The magnitude of this excess could be considerable, corresponding to about 80 excess deaths nationwide.

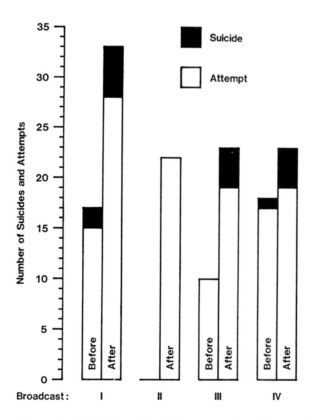

FIGURE 10.6. Number of completed suicides and suicide attempts by adolescents in the Greater New York Area 2 weeks before and after television movies about suicide. *Note.* For Broadcast II, before data and suicide versus suicide attempt data not available. *Source:* Gould & Shaffer (1986). Copyright 1986 by Massachusetts Medical Society. All rights reserved. Reprinted by permission.

Some evidence has accumulated that so-called cluster suicides may be the result of imitative forces. Although the term "cluster suicide" has not been carefully specified, it can be defined as "3 or more linked suicidal events in a series in a common space and usually in a limited, contiguous time frame" (e.g., 7–10 days, 2 weeks, a month, or even longer, just to mention some of the time frames studied; see Berman & Jobes, 1991; Davidson & Gould, 1989). Perhaps about 5% of all adolescent suicides may be clusters (Velting & Gould, 1997). Phillips and Cartensen (1986) suggest that adolescents may be more sensitive than adults to the effects of imitation and, thus, more likely to produce suicide clusters.

On May 4, 1990, in Sheridan, Arkansas, Thomas Smith, age 17, stood up in his American History class, told a girl in his class that he loved her, then pulled a .22 pistol from his pocket and shot himself in the forehead. He died 4 hours later. That evening, between about 10 and 11 P.M., his friend at Sheridan High School, Thomas Chidester, 19, also shot himself in the head (with a .45) and died immediately. The very next day, Jerry McCool, a classmate of Smith and Chidester shot himself at home with a .22. Earlier (March 28 of that year), Ronald Wilkinson had also shot himself.

So, in Sheridan, there were four related suicidal deaths in 2 months, three of them in just 2 days. The teen suicide cluster was reported on the CBS Evening News and on NBC's *Today* show. The town was stunned. Other Sheridan High School students wondered aloud, "Which one of us might be next?"

Answers as to why this had happened were hard to come by. Two of the boys had relatives who had suicided. Two were in ROTC and were known to like and own guns. One of them had a drug problem (Wilkinson) and one had poor grades in school. The nearness in time of the three deaths, especially, suggests copying or imitation. David Phillips, a sociologist quoted in this chapter, has claimed that teenagers are more likely than adults to copy another's suicide or to respond to a similar death stimulus event. Teenagers have suggestability rates for suicide perhaps about twice those of adults.

In an earlier publicized incident (March 1987), four teenagers (two boys and two girls) died in a Bergenfield, New Jersey, garage from carbon monoxide poisoning in a suicide pact. They were Thomas Rizzo, 19, Thomas Olton, 19, and sisters Lisa and Cheryl Burress. All four had signed a suicide note on a paper bag saying they wanted a common wake and a common burial.

The possible clustering effect stemmed from the fact that Rizzo was friends with and witnessed the death of James Majors, 18, who in September of 1986 either fell or jumped to his death off Englewood Cliffs. Furthermore, Majors had been dating Lisa Burress at the time of his death.

All four of the people in the teen suicide pact may have been depressed about the death of their friend, James Majors. It is noteworthy that another friend of the four, Christopher Curley, 21, was run over by a train on June 14, and was killed. At the time, his death was ruled to be alcohol-related and not likely to be suicide.

Note the contiguous nature of these four deaths with other recent deaths of friends, which raises questions of copying or imitative clusters among vulnerable individuals in similar life circumstances.

STRESS, NEGATIVE LIFE EVENTS, AND SUICIDE

As we alluded to in the prologue to this chapter, if isolation is one side of the social–suicidological coin, the other side has to be various aspects of negative social events or negative interpersonal dynamics. Classically suicides are thought of as profoundly alone, low in self-esteem, abjectly depressed, and desperately disconnected from sustaining meaningful social relations. But another important dimension (already touched on in the foregoing section on contagion) is a wealth (not poverty) of social events, relationships, or ties (see Nisbet, 1998) that paradoxically push or drive (Perlin, 1975) the individual toward suicide. In this case, contrary to Durkheim's major conceptual thrust, social relations do *not* protect against suicide.

Often suicidologists refer to negative social events, relationships, or interactions with the terms "*stress*" or "*negative life events.*" House (1986) defines "stress" as when an individual confronts a situation in which his or her usual modes of behaving are insufficient and the consequences of not adapting are serious. Imagine a marginal high school student who has never developed good study habits, has little raw intelligence, and tremendous family pressure to succeed in his first year at a demanding private college. In the past the student had crammed for exams; now this practice no longer works. The student is getting Ds and Fs on examinations, instead of the usual high school Cs. Furthermore, the student's parents have made major financial sacrifices for the student to attend a good private liberal arts college. This freshman who basically finessed high school finds himself in deep trouble and in danger of failing in college, if not in his future career. He is trying his best, but nothing seems to be working. Obviously, this is a stressful situation for the student.

Although such a situation is probably not a life-and-death matter, it nevertheless hints of the anxiety that can be generated with stressful impasses. Typically, suicides experience multiple stressors repeated over long periods. Stress and related problems (especially depression and hopelessness) tend to summate until the only perceived resolution may be to escape *from life itself* by suiciding. Note that stress also indicates a gradual strain on the body and mind associated with measurable physiological changes (Selye, 1982).

One of the classic measurements of stress is Holmes and Rahe's Social Reajustment Rating Scale (see Table 10.5). Holmes and Rahe measure the adjustment time needed for 43 life events. For example, they asked subjects, if getting married took (say) 50 days to adjust to, how many adjustment days would other life events take? Paykel (1992) defines a "recent life event" as a change in the external social environment that can be dated approximately. Table 10.5 presents the results. Basically, subjects were asked to note all 43 events that had happened to them in the last year, then to add up the value of the corresponding life change units in the far right column. Holmes and Rahe defined a "life crisis" as any cluster of life events whose values summed to 150 life change units or more in one year (300 plus = a "major" crisis). Holmes and Rahe's major empirical conclusion was that the greater the summed score of life changes or adaptive requirements, the greater the individual's vulnerability or lowering of resistance to disease (here to suicide attempts or completions) and the more serious the disease that will develop (e.g., the higher your life change score, the more likely a suicide *completion* is). Note that the Holmes and Rahe's stress test includes both positive and negative life events and both socially isolating and socially involving life events.

Closely related to negative life events and stress are the concepts of *early object loss, separation,* and *negative interaction.* Classical Freudian psychoanalytic theory argues that adult depression and adult suicide could be rooted in early object loss, especially of one's mother (or father) in the eventual suicide's first 6 to 12 months of life (Maris, 1981: 70–77). For example, John Bowlby (1973) thought that early attachment to and separation from one's mother (because of her death or prolonged illness of the mother or child) could be followed by pathological anxiety, mourning, and grief and could lead to later depressive disorder, and even suicide of the adult (cf. Melanie Klein, 1948). Rene Spitz (1946) also explored the relationships of early object loss of one's mother, depression, pathological mourning, and premature death of infants. In one study by Spitz of infants separated from their mothers after 2 years, 34 of 91 of the children simply died for no apparent physical reasons, despite acceptable levels of hygiene and asepsis in the hospital. More recently psychiatrist George Murphy (1992) has noticed the crucial importance of object loss among alcoholic suicides. Murphy found that 48% of all alcoholic suicides had experienced an interpersonal loss within 1 year of their suicides; 32% had a loss within 6 *weeks* of their suicides. Howev-

TABLE 10.5. Holmes and Rahe's Social Readjustment Rating Scale

Rank	Life event	Mean value of life change units
1	Death of spouse	100
2	Divorce	73
3	Marital separation	65
4	Jail term	63
5	Death of close family member	63
6	Personal injury or illness	53
7	Marriage	50
8	Fired at work	47
9	Marital reconciliation	45
10	Retirement	45
11	Change in health of family member	44
12	Pregnancy	40
13	Sex difficulties	39
14	Gain of new family member	39
15	Business readjustment	39
16	Change in financial state	38
17	Death of close friend	37
18	Change to different line of work	36
19	Change in number of arguments with spouse	35
20	Mortgage over $10,000[a]	31
21	Foreclosure of mortgage or loan	30
22	Change in responsibilities at work	29
23	Son or daughter leaving home	29
24	Trouble with in-laws	29
25	Outstanding personal achievement	28
26	Wife begin or stop work	26
27	Begin or end school	26
28	Change in living conditions	25
29	Revision of personal habits	24
30	Trouble with boss	23
31	Change in work hours or conditions	20
32	Change in residence	20
33	Change in schools	20
34	Change in recreation	19
35	Change in church activities	19
36	Change in social activities	18
37	Mortgage or loan less than $10,000	17
38	Change in sleeping habits	16
39	Change in number of family get-togethers	15
40	Change in eating habits	15
41	Vacation	13
42	Christmas	12
43	Minor violations of the law	11

Source: Holmes & Rahe (1967: 216). Copyright 1967 by Elsevier Science. Reprinted by permission.
[a]Obviously, this figure should be higher now.

er, Maris (1981) found no significant statistical difference between samples of completed suicides and natural deaths with respect to early object loss or separation.

In one of Maris's (1981: 117 ff.) surveys of Chicago suicides, he decided to test empirically for negative interactions among completed suicides. "Negative interaction" was defined as interpersonal relationships that were painful, unpleasant, rejecting, and/or isolating. Operationally negative interaction included early separation, lack of feeling close to one's mother and/or father, having parents and siblings with major personal problems, having problems as an adult with one's own marriage(s) and/or sex, social isolation, having job and work troubles, having trouble with arrest or with the police, low self-esteem, and conceiving of your death as a way to punish someone else (see Maris, 1981: 122).

There were some negative interaction differences among nonfatal suicide attempters, completers, and natural deaths. For example, attempters and completers were much more likely than natural deaths to conceive of their deaths as a way to get even with others (21% and 47%, respectively, vs. 3%) and to have lost interest in others (57% and 57% vs. 21%). Also, both suicide attempters and completers were much less close to their fathers than the natural deaths were, and were about four times more likely than natural deaths to receive mainly physical discipline as children from their fathers. However, overall the mean negative interaction scores of completed suicides and natural deaths were *not* significantly different. For example, negative interaction scores ranged from a low of 0 to a high of 31+. The mean for natural deaths was 18.5, and for suicide completers it was 20.5. The really striking difference on negative interaction was between natural deaths and nonfatal suicide attempters (18.5 vs. 34.6, $p < .001$).

To understand the relationships for stress and negative events to suicide it is necessary to frame these variables in the context of a *more general model of coping, vulnerability, and problem-solving skills*—such as that presented in Figure 2.6 (cf. Erikson, 1950; Leenaars, 1991; Levinson, 1978). As Yufit and Bongar (1992) write: "Although recent stresses can be important catalytic events in an individual's . . . suicide, these stressful events must be contexualized within a larger overall picture of the individual's personality structure and lifelong charaterological ability to cope with or be vulnerable to stress, failure, and loss" (557). For example, Rich and Bonner (1987) in a stress–vulnerability model discovered that 30% of the variation in suicide ideation was accounted for by negative life events, stress, depression, loneliness, and having few reasons for living.

The reader may wish to flip back to Figure 2.6. Some of the relevant salient factors in this developmental "suicidal careers" model of suicide outcome are early and late stress and negative events (e.g., a history of suicide in one's family, punitive parenting, late object loss—such as of a spouse through death or divorce), depression, hopelessness, protective factors (e.g., Linehan's; see Linehan, Goodson, Neilsen, & Chiles, "reasons for living"), cognitive inflexibility and perfectionism, and so on. It is important to note in any general develpmental model of suicide that stress and negative life events tend to repeat over one's lifetime; that they are usually met with coping adaptations, treatment, medications, hospitalizations, and so on; that most individuals do *not* respond to stress or negative life events with suicide; that those few who do suicide or attempt have various vulnerabilities, are repeatedly threatened; and that everyone has a pain threshold (lower for vulnerable individuals) beyond which he or she cannot tolerate stress, and what Shneidman (1993) calls "psychache," without self-destructive adaptations or suicide (cf. Motto, 1992: 625).

The stress–vulnerability model reminds us that suicidal careers involve complex, multiple stages, divisions, factors, and periods. Some of these aspects of the general model of suicide reflected in Figure 2.5 include *developmental stagnation, abortive life-stage transitions,* and *triggering precursors*. Both Erikson and Levinson argued that early stresses and negative life events such as object losses may result in difficulty for the individual to mature normally and progress easily to subsequent life stages. For example, repeatedly stressed, traumatized individuals may stagnate in their psychosocial development or have abortive life-stage transitions. They may not move readily or smoothly form adolescence to young adulthood, from middle age to retirement, or from being married to being divorced.

One question that often arises is whether life events or stresses just before the suicide "trigger" that suicide. In a survey of suicides in Chicago, Maris compared the immediate (1 week before the event) situational precursors of natural deaths, nonfatal attempters, and completed suicides (see Table 10.6). Although there were differences among the three samples (especially between the natural deaths and the suicidal group), Table 10.6 (when compared with the data for more long-term stresses for the same groups) suggests that suicide attempts are usually *not* triggered, at least in the sense that the immediate precursors are not very different from the long-term causes of suicide attempts. For the most part, the same factors seem to be operating in the week before the attempt (or death) as were mentioned by the subjects as the long-term precursors of the attempt (or death). In short, in suicide, lifelong repetition of problems breaches an adaptive threshold in some vulnerable individuals but not in others.

An issue of *Suicide and Life-Threatening Behavior* (Dean, Range, & Goggin, 1996) provides a summary empirical study for both negative life events and protective factors (here operationalized as "reasons for living"), plus it adds the personality attribute of "perfectionism." "Perfectionism" can be defined as unrealistic high self-expectations and stringent evaluation or censure of self-behavior or needs to attain standards or expectations imposed by significant others.

Some of the relevant empirical associations in Table 10.7 are as follows. Perfectionism and suicide ideation were significantly positively coreelated at .55 ($p < .001$). Negative life events were significantly positively associated with depression (.48), hopelessness (.25), and suicide ideation (.30). Finally, reasons for living were significantly negatively correlated with suicide ideation (−.64). That is, the more reasons for living, the less the suicide ideation.

TABLE 10.6. Immediate (Week before) Precursor Symptoms for Suicide Attempters, Suicide Completers, and Natural Deaths

Immediate situational precursor symptoms[a]	Natural Deaths (%)	Suicide attempters (%)	Suicide completers (%)
Mental problems (depression, hopelessness, anger)	31	88	83
Physical problems (chronic)	75	13	40
Alcoholism	14	14	18
Drug abuse	1	30	6
Loss (including job, divorce, separation, death)	6	14	18
General interpersonal problems	17	78	54
Hospitalization	69	3	7
Financial problems	3	14	17
Total[b]	N = 71	N = 64	N = 266

Source: Maris (1981: 274). Copyright 1981 by Johns Hopkins University Press. Reprinted by permission.
[a]Precursor symptoms could be checked more than once. Interviewers did not ask for the one most common symptom, as they did with causes.
[b]Because respondents could check more than one precursor, columns will not total 100 percent.

TABLE 10.7. Correlation of Life Events, Perfectionism, Depression, Hopelessness, and Reasons for Living with Suicide Ideas

	NLE	PERF	DEP	HOPE	RFL	SI
NLE						
PERF	0.32**					
DEP	0.48**	0.53**				
HOPE	0.25*	0.48**	0.67**			
RFL	−0.15	−0.26*	−0.38**	−0.63		
SI	0.30*	0.55**	0.59**	0.83**	−0.64**	
Mean	12.90	51.45	36.40	2.41	219.88	2.31
SD	10.63	17.52	10.44	3.94	37.63	6.57

Note. NLE, negative life events; PERF, perfectionism; DEP, self-rated depression; HOPE, hopelessness; RFL, reasons for living; SI, suicide ideation.
Source: Dean, Range, & Goggin (1996: 184). Copyright 1996 by The Guilford Press. Reprinted by permission.

SUMMARY AND CONCLUSIONS

Social relations refer to forces that are originally outside and constraining of individuals, usually through interaction with other people. We began the chapter by discussing the extraordinary loading of depressive disorder and suicide in the first-degree relatives of novelist Ernest Hemingway. Of course, one crucial question in cases such as the Hemingways is, How much of the suicide effect is from social modeling and how much is the product of genetics and individual biochemistry (or from some other factor, such as the diseases of depression)?

We provided a brief history of the sociology of suicide. The scientific sociological study of suicide began in late 19th-century France with the quantitative analysis by Emile Durkheim of death records and suicide rates. These empirical regularities were interpreted in a highly biased theory of external and constraining social facts. Sociologists Gibbs, Phillips, Stack, and Pescosolido have all continued largely in the Durkheimian tradition, although they have often criticized Durkheim. Jack Douglas undertook a vastly different approach to the study of the social relations of suicides. Douglas maintained that we should concentrate on the first-person individual accounts of serious suicide attempters, not on the third-person account represented in the vital statistics or on such abstract social concepts as *anomie* and *egoism*. Finally, Henry and Short and Maris have melded and synthesized both individual and social factors in their social theories of self-destructive behaviors.

The social relations of suicide usually are subdivided into two distinct but overlapping areas: (1) absent, or (2) negative relations.

1. It has been well-documented in this chapter that both individuals and groups tend to have higher probabilities or rates of suicide if they are socially isolated. For example, those with absent or deceased parents early in their lives, the never-married and divorced, those with no or few close friends or significant others, and so on—all tend to have a greater individual probability of committing suicide or greater group suicide rates.

2. Negative social relations were discussed in the context of contagion, stress, negative life events, and negative interaction. Social involvement when group norms are prosuicide (e.g., in Jonestown, Guyana, the Hemlock Society, or Heaven's Gate) obviously does not protect one against suicide. We saw that modeling or suicide contagion was more likely if

the stimulus suicide was similar to the potential copier, if the dose or exposure to a suicide event was higher and repeated often, if the stimulus suicide was a celebrity or was otherwise glorified, if the individual copying was vulnerable (e.g., clinically depressed), and if the stimulus and/or responder were younger.

Stress that evacuates in a suicide outcome tends to be multiple and over long suicidal careers. One common suicidal situation is that of a middle-age white male being divorced or separated from his wife or lover. Self-destructive life events need not always be negative. Holmes and Rahe found that the total number of life change units, positive or negative, was related to both the onset of disease and to the seriousness of the disease. Those with higher stress levels were more likely to become ill and were more likely to have serious illnesses.

Chapter 10 concluded with a plea for a contextual model (like Figure 2.6) of coping and vulnerability in which to understand the social relations of suicides. Generally, only the vulnerable respond to stress or pathological social relations with self-destructive behaviors. Older white male perfectionists with clinical depression and alcohol abuse often prove to be especially vulnerable to suicidal outcomes. Social relations also need to be couched in the context of long, developmental, "suicidal careers." Two common developmental traits of suicidal careers are developmental stagnation and abortive life-stage transitions (such as the perceived inability of maturity from adolescence to old age and retirement, or from being married to being divorced). A causal model of suicide like that depicted in Figure 2.6 also reminds us that social relations are clearly not the *only* independent variable producing a suicide. Sometimes the crucial proximate cause of a suicide might be a nonsocial trait or state (such as serotonin disturbance or neurotransmitter imbalance). Social, individual, and biological traits and states usually *interact* in complex time-series equations to produce a suicidal individual or a suicide rate. In the next chapter we explore a specific aspect of social relations: suicide notes.

FURTHER READING

Diekstra, R. F. W., Maris, R. W., Platt, S., Schmidtke, A., & Sonneck, G. (Eds.). (1989). *Suicide and its prevention: The role of attitude and imitation.* Leiden, The Netherlands: E.J. Brill. The World Health Organization sponsored this review of (1) the relationship between suicidal attitudes and behaviors, (2) caregivers' attitudes toward suicidal patients, and (3) the impact of mass media on suicidal behaviors.

Douglas, J. D. (1967). *The social meanings of suicide.* Princeton, NJ: Princeton University Press. A classical first statement of the antithesis of Emile Durkheim's *Le Suicide* by one of the cofounders of ethnomethodology. Douglas argues that instead of basing suicidology on vital statistics, we should focus on the qualitative first-person accounts of actual serious suicide attempters. Like Goffman and Garfinkel, Douglas claims that the emphasis should be on the situated individual meanings of suicides themselves, not on external and constraining social facts such as anomie or egoism.

Giddens, A. (1971). *The sociology of suicide: A selection of readings.* London: Frank Cass & Co. This is a remarkable collection of social science essays by a noted Weber and Marx theory scholar at Cambridge. Although now dated, Giddens reviews (1) the historical context of Durkheim's *Le Suicide*, (2) U.S. sociology of suicide until 1970, (3) major anthropological studies of suicide, (4) community and economic research on suicide, and (5) social–psychiatric correlates of suicide.

Henry, A. F., & Short, J. F., Jr. (1954). *Suicide and homicide: Some economic, sociological, and psychological aspects of aggression.* New York: Free Press. A look by a former President of the American Sociological Association at the interaction of economic, social, and psychological factors as they affect suicide rates. Henry and Short consider the fuller range of the aggression dependent variable.

For example, why a suicide outcome and not homicide, a nonfatal suicide attempt, buglary, robbery, and so on? Adds important examinations of business cycles and of frustration–aggression theory.

Lester, D. (Ed.). (1994). *Emile Durkheim's Le Suicide: One hundred years later*. Philadelphia: Charles Press. Someone had to think of it and Lester got there first (as usual) in his edited homage to Durkheim 100 years after the 1897 publication of *Le Suicide* (Whitney Pope at Indiana also did a review of Durkheim's *Suicide* in 1997). Contains a significant review of the literature by Jack Gibbs, an interesting piece on women's relative immunity to suicide by historian Howard Kushner, and a contemporary network sociological interpretation of suicide by Bernice Pescosolido.

Maris, R. W. (1969). *Social forces in urban suicide*. Homewood, IL: Dorsey Press. An empirical community study reminiscent of Ruth Cavan's Chicago suicides and the University of Chicago's social ecology. Contradicts Durkheim's findings on SES and suicide rates (here they are higher in *lower* social classes), argues for the role of social mobility in causing suicide, looks at variation of social and economic characteristics in Chicago's 76 community areas, and contains an excellent synopsis and critique of Durkheim's theory of suicide.

11

Suicide Notes and Communications

Suicide notes are cryptic maps of ill advised journeys.
—EDWIN S. SHNEIDMAN

Communication implies the exchange of messages (information, emotion, etc.) between sender and receiver. The most commonly studied form of suicide communication, the suicide note, typically intended to convey information to and/or to affect the behavior of the receiver, however, is meant to be one way. The message is given to and for others. But how the receiver will respond has little to do with what the sender expects or wishes. That is determined mostly by the distorted inner logic (*catalogic*; Shneidman & Farberow, 1957a) of the suicidal person's mind.

Suicide notes are communications that also represent the proverbial *last word*. Written typically in the moments just before the fatal suicidal act, they are often the penultimate suicidal behavior. However, the ideations expressed in suicide notes are not limited to this narrow time frame; these final words represent the end products of, perhaps, years of despair in a final frame of hopelessness. In this respect suicide notes have been thought by some observers to be windows to the mind of the deceased (cf. Leenaars, 1992, 1998). Studies of fortuitously surviving attempters who left notes (Beck, Morris, & Lester, 1974; Tuckman & Youngman, 1968), indeed, confirm that the writing of a suicide note is a significant high-risk behavior prognostic of completed suicide. However, as we shall see, these windows are more likely distorting prisms. Equally important to understand is that those most likely to suicide (i.e., elderly white males) are least likely to write suicide notes.

Communications given earlier in the suicidal career of the eventual suicide have more of a signaling function, often directly pleading for a reaction, response, or help. These we call *suicide threats*. The earliest reference to a suicidal threat has been recounted by Hankoff (1979: 27) from a papyrus dated near the end of the third millenium B.C. The narrative tells of a peasant who repeatedly appeals to a nobleman for redress regarding social injustices inflicted upon him. On the ninth appeal, he intimates suicide by stating that he may take his case to the god of the dead. With this, the nobleman properly attends and justice is done.

The word "threat" often connotes manipulation, a pejorative label when applied clinically and a label that does not appropriately describe the majority of verbalized intentions regarding self-harm (see Berman & Jobes, 1991). Yet, the historical example given previously illustrates well that a suicide threat may often produce a desired response (e.g., of attention). In this regard, the suicide threat is a form of *manipulation*, a communication that stresses the possibility of a suicidal act (parasuicide, suicide attempt, or suicide completion) with intent to control or influence the response of others. But threats are typically expressed at times of anguish and desperation, when other attempts to communicate have not accomplished desired ends and when the individual harbors considerable ambivalence about both living and dying. In addition, it typically is given in situations in which prior verbal attempts to connect have failed and when relationship conflict or social isolation interfere with more direct attempts to accomplish better connectedness (empathy, caring, nurturance, etc.). The primary goal of this manipulanda, thus, is captured most aptly by the title of Shneidman and Farberow's classic, *The Cry for Help* (1957b).

Consider the following case example: A 61-year-old single male art curator was known by his coworkers to have been depressed for over a year. A "difficult personality," he at the same time asked others for love and affection while behaving in an offputting manner. During this period, he frequently talked of suicide. When he was informed by the gallery administration that he was to be terminated from his position, he told several coworkers that he was going to take his life. When he failed to show up for work the next day, a coworker called the police. He was found hanging by an electrical cord strung from a basement pipe.

Suicidal behavior, thus, is both a communication itself and a consequence of failures in more adaptive attempts to communicate. It should not surprise us, then, that an estimated four of five suicides (cf. Rudestam, 1971; Brent et al., 1988) have attempted to warn others of their intent through a range of behaviors such as direct verbal statements about suicide, verbalized or written (e.g., diaries and journals) preoccupations with themes of death, statements about joining deceased loved ones, termination behaviors (e.g., inexplicably giving away prized possessions and stating, "I won't be needing this anymore"), and nonfatal suicide attempts. These communications serve as the proverbial *red flags* that call attention to others of the potential risk of more lethal suicidal behavior. At the same time, the vast majority of these communications are not followed by suicidal behavior.

Recipients of these communications often feel anxious and helpless. These feelings, in turn, may be met with defensive reactions such as denial or minimization, thus reducing the likelihood of an empathic connection or active intervention. For some, who have given these suicidal messages over many months or even years, the response may be total disregard, or even anger and contempt. Such a response may become a discriminative stimulus for the suicide's final actions, as in cases in which the recipient directly or symbolically communicates, "So jump already!" For example, a 32-year-old male, depressed over a separation from his common-law wife returned to their apartment to plead for a reconciliation. When she refused, he threatened to kill himself. She answered, "If that's what you have to do, then do it." When she then left the room, he shot himself in the head with a handgun.

Others may unconsciously collude with or not intercede when they know about the suicide's wish to die. Consider the following two examples:

1. A 30-year-old male, depressed over marital problems, killed himself with his shotgun. His outpatient therapist had explicitly told the decedent's wife to hide his weapons, which she did *under their bed*. He killed himself when his wife left for her mother's after an argument.
2. A 52-year-old male died by a self-inflicted gunshot wound to the head. He had a 15-year history of emphysema and was dependent on a portable oxygen system. He told his two sons that he was going to take his life, that he had "nothing left to live for." On the day of his death, he was lying on his living room couch watching television with his wife when he took his gun out from under a pillow. *In front of her* he loaded the weapon and said, "I love you." She left the room, and he shot himself.

CASE 11.1. Adolf Hitler's Suicide Ideation

Hitler spoke of suicide on four occasions, the first time after the failed putsch in November, 1923. In great excitement, he wanted to shoot himself. According to his statement in *Mein Kampf*, he overcame his upset after he resolved to defend his comrades. On 16 September, 1931, he threatened to kill himself after the death of his half-niece, Angela Raubal, Jr. (Geli), with whom he was in love. After one week he recovered sufficiently to continue his election campaign. The third time he expressed suicidal intentions was when the Nationalist Socialist Party threatened to split up in 1932. It seems these threats were cries for help and approval rather than announcements that he would really commit suicide. . . . Hitler realized during the winter of 1941–1942 that he might not win the war . . . , but fought on with determination to be in an advantageous position when the war ended. What mattered to him was retaining his identity as a charasmatic leader, even in the face of major military reversals after 1942. Concomitant with thoughts of survival were thoughts of death. In January, 1942, he severely criticized Field Marshall Paulus for surrendering at Stalingrad rather than committing suicide. After the attempt to assassinate him on 20 July, 1944, Hitler had short bouts of depression. What kept him going was his anger against the allies, the Jews, and his generals, whom he accused of incompetence and treachery. His two somatic illnesses, Parkinson's disease and temporal arteritis . . . , also contributed to his depressed moods. With some self-pity, he made a statement to the effect that a quick death would be a delivery from his suffering. . . .

On April 30, 1945, in a dual suicide, Hitler and his long-time mistress, now wife (they married on the 29th), Eva Braun, died in his chambers. She poisioned herself with potassium cyanide. It is assumed he died by simultaneous ingestion of cyanide and a gunshot wound to the head.

Source: Redlich (1993: 282–283).

Finally, it may be argued that some suicidal communications do not appear to have a dyadic component. Rather, they are intended merely as communicated ideations in a context of depression, stimulated by loss or failure, with no apparent intent to influence a specific other's behavior. However, the very fact that they are given in an interpersonal context ought to make suspect this appearance. Case 11.1, a brief history of Adolf Hitler's suicidality prior to his ultimate suicide on April 30, 1945, illustrates nondyadic suicidality. The central focus of this chapter is end-point communications, that is, suicide notes, the most researched of suicidal communications and ones that appear to offer "an invaluable starting point for comprehending the suicidal act (Leenaars, 1992).

SUICIDE NOTES

The first known example of a suicide note (different from the example of a suicide *threat* given earlier) is probably from Egypt (ca. 1394–1362 B.C.). Allegedly, a seer and adviser to the Pharaoh Amenophis, fearing dire consequences from advice he had given to the Pharaoh, wrote a farewell note and then took his life (Hankoff, 1979: 27).

Like the archaeologist who unearthed this note, Edwin Shneidman by chance discovered in 1949 of a trove of suicide notes in the files of the Los Angeles County Coroner's Office and this initiated the modern era of suicidology. Shneidman believed then that suicide notes presented the best available means of understanding suicidal phenomena: "The golden road to the kingdom of understanding suicide was paved with suicide notes" (Shneidman, 1993: 103).

With this fortuitous beginning, the almost 40 years of research on suicide notes that has followed has branched into essentially five lines of inquiry: (1) the epidemiology and demography of note writing and note writers, (2) distinguishing characteristics of note writers compared to nonwriters and genuine notes compared to simulated notes, (3) how able individuals are to distinguish genuine from faked notes, (4) content analyses of notes (noncomparative studies), and (5) notes as validation of theoretical constructs.

A brief summary of these areas of inquiry follows. No attempt is made here to review the entirety of the empirical research to date on suicide notes, as several excellent reviews already exist in the literature (see Frederick, 1969; Leenaars, 1988, 1992). However, it is noteworthy and instructive to observe that there were two adjustments in the "golden road" Shneidman expected suicide notes to show: (1) a period of reconsideration and disillusionment wherein notes were seen as "flawed guides" (Shneidman, 1973), and (2) the current belief that notes illuminate with meaning only in the context of a detailed life history of the note writer (Shneidman, 1980a). We return at the end of this chapter to explore this last view, after first examining what has been learned about suicide notes and the reasons for Shneidman's midcourse reconsiderations.

Who Leaves a Suicide Note?

The suicide note is left by a minority of those who suicide, although it almost universally indicates that a suicide has indeed occurred. (In at least one city, it has been reported that finding a verifiable, handwritten suicide note was required by the coroner for him to certify a suicidal death; Litman, Curphey, Shneidman, Farberow, & Tabachnick, 1963.) The epidemiological study of suicide notes began with Shneidman and Farberow's (1957c) analyses of an almost complete collection of suicide notes ($N = 721$) written in Los Angeles County in the decade 1944–1953. These notes represented only about 15% of all suicides in the county during these years. Tuckman, Kleiner, and Lavell (1959) reported the prevalence of notes was 24% in the 742 suicides they studied. Cohen and Fiedler (1974), similarly, found notes were written in 21% of the more than 1,000 cases they reviewed. The highest proportion of suicides in which notes were recovered was reported to be 33% by Conway (1960). In an international psychological autopsy study, Farberow and Simon (1975) found notes were left approximately twice as often by suicides in Los Angeles compared to suicides in Vienna, Austria.

With regard to younger-age suicides, Poesner, LaHaye, and Cheifetz (1989) studied all suicides in the age group 10–19 years which occurred in the city of Montreal between the years 1979 and 1982. Of the 136 suicides, only 13 (10%) left notes. Thus, we may conclude that a minority of suicides leave notes, less than one in four among adults and fewer still among teenagers.

However, we should note that these percentages are conservative estimates of the true number of note writers. Family members (or others) who find a suicide note may hide or destroy it. Motives for doing this include attempts to disguise the manner of death in order to protect insurance benefits, feelings of shame and the avoidance of stigma that attends suicidal deaths, a desire to undo any incriminating statements made in the note about the person finding the note, and even a desire to magically undo the suicide itself.

On the other hand, it is possible that a note could have been prepared and left by another person attempting to disguise a homicide. This is the stuff of mystery novels and rarely occurs in everyday life. Simulated note writing, however, has been given research attention (see below).

One working hypothesis about writers of suicide notes is that because they represent a minority of suicides, they must be different from those suicides who do not leave notes. However, studies of demographic differences between those who leave notes and those who do not raise questions about this assumption.

In one comparative study (Tuckman et al., 1959), no differences with respect to age, sex, and marital status were found. Similarly, Shneidman (1980) described note writers as "essentially similar" to nonnote writers. In contrast, Cohen and Fiedler (1974) found that notes were more commonly left by females (26% to 19% for males) who were separated or divorced (40% vs. 31% of single females, 25% of married females, and 16% of widows). In this study, whites were *three times* as likely to leave notes as were nonwhites. Capstick's (1960) study of a Welsh sample of suicide notes found them more commonly left by younger and, again, female suicides. In the Poesner et al. (1989) study of young suicides, however, the male to female ratio was 5.5:1, in stark contrast to the results reported above by Cohen and Fiedler. In this younger sample, again no differences were found between note writers and nonwriters with regard to age or sex; however, there was a slight difference noted in suicide methods; the modal method among note writers in this small sample was shooting (38% compared to 23% of nonwriters).

Yet, in contrast to this finding, Peck's (1986) study of young, predominantly midwestern suicides found that notes were more commonly left by suicides using more passive and lower lethality methods (alcohol and barbiturates, carbon monoxide). Peck opined that less immediate deaths gave time, and thus opportunity, to write a note. This notion is supported by the finding that notes are left more frequently by those who make suicide pacts, typically a planned behavior (Fishbain, D'Achille, Barsky, & Aldrich, 1984) and less frequently by those who die via Russian roulette, typically an impulsive behavior and usually considered to be an accidental death (Fishbain, Fletcher, Aldrich, & Davis, 1987). Finally, no significant differences have been found regarding the socioeconomic status of writers versus nonwriters of suicide notes.

As these reported differences appear minor and sometimes contradictory, it seems reasonable to conclude that writers of suicide notes can tell us a great deal about suicide. On the other hand, at least one suicidologist believes the most significant observation about note writers is simply that they are "good correspondents" (Stengel, 1964).

Genuine versus Faked Notes

A second line of comparative research has explored the question whether suicide note writers are different from those who are not suicidal but who are asked to write a note as if they were suicidal. By analyzing the contents of genuine notes and sytematically comparing these to the contents of simulated (faked) notes, important differences might emerge that could cast light on the cognitive processes that immediately precede suicidal behavior (Lester & Lester, 1971).

The classic experiment of this type (and the prototype) was reported by Shneidman and Farberow (1957d). These researchers matched (by writer demographics) and compared 33 genuine and 33 simulated suicide notes and, then, scored ideas and phrases according to a "discomfort–relief quotient." They found that genuine notes reflected the writer's greater loquaciousness and expressed more discomfort (deeper feelings of hatred, self-blame, and retribution). Also, they were found to be more neutral, that is more often they gave instructions and warnings. Shneidman and Farberow opined that this latter tendency might reflect the suicide's feelings of omnipotence and omniscience.

Genuine notes have been differentiated from simulated notes in both verbal content and style. Osgood and Walker (1959) found genuine notes to be more sterotyped, using fewer words, more phrase repetition, fewer adjectives and adverbs (compared to nouns and verbs), and more absolute (i.e., extreme) words, such as "always" and "never." Furthermore, they reported that genuine notes had more references of farewell; more criticism of spouse; and more references to parents, God, religion, and marital possessions.

Gottschalk and Gleser (1960) reported that genuine notes more often used nouns, pronouns, and references to third persons and places. Similarly, Ogilvie, Stone, and Shneidman (1966) computer-analyzed content differences and found more concrete references (persons and places), more use of the word "love," and less reference to the process of thought and decision in genuine notes. Finally, genuine notes have been found to be less explicit about the suicidal act, mention suicide less frequently, give more instructions, and show greater disorganization (Spiegel & Neuringer, 1963).

Other comparisons between genuine and specific notes have failed to show differences on level of social maturity (Tuckman & Ziegler, 1968), the need for affiliation (Lester, 1971), and temporal perspective, measured by verb tense used in the notes (Lester, 1993d).

These studies, of course, may say as much about the thinking of non-suicidal people attempting to mimic the suicidal experience as they do about the dynamics of suicide. Lester and Leenaars (1988) and Lester (1989b), for example, have demonstrated that writers of simulated notes underestimate the suicide's anger and need to leave instructions. On the other hand, one study that added a third comparative sample of notes written by people who *faked* suicide by claiming (in their notes) to have jumped from the Golden Gate Bridge ("Hoax" notes) found anger to be more frequent in these hoax notes than in both genuine and simulated notes (Lester, Seiden, & Tauber, 1990).

Moreover, as the majority of these studies used the same set of notes (Shneidman and Farberow's original 33 pairs), all generalizations based on them may apply only to white male, native-born, married Protestants (the writers of the original set of genuine notes). Lester (1988c), for example, has shown that there are gender differences in simulated note content written by female versus male undergraduates.

CAN A SUICIDE NOTE'S AUTHENTICITY BE JUDGED?

A parallel line of research has asked the question whether observers/judges are capable of distinguishing in blind analyses genuine from simulated suicide notes. Lester and Lester (1971) assert that this question has important forensic implications (e.g., when a fake suicide has been written by a perpetrator in order to disguise a homicide). This line of research, in general, corroborates that naive judges do no better than chance in identifying genuine notes when presented in paired comparison to simulated notes and that experienced judges (trained professionals) are capable of performing better than chance evaluation. For example, Osgood and Walker (1959) found that graduate students could correctly identify an average of only 16.5 (50%) of Shneidman and Farberow's 33 paired notes.

Frederick (1969) presented 45 sets of notes, 1 original and 3 control notes, rewritten by hand by writers of the same age and sex as that of the true suicide note writer, to three sets of judges: graphologists, detectives, and secretaries. The handwriting experts were able to distinguish the genuine handwriting significantly better than both chance expectation and the control judges, although they were not able to specify discriminative clues in these notes.

Similarly, Arbeit and Blatt (1973) presented Shneidman and Farberow's note sample to four groups at various levels of clinical training. They concluded that the only factor distinguishing these groups in their ability on this task was the rater's clinical sensitivity and skill. The latest of these studies (Lester, 1993d) compared the judgments of college students to those of 20 editors of the journal *Suicide and Life-Threatening Behavior* (this had the potential to be quite embarrassing). As should be, the editors ("experts") performed significantly better than both chance and the college students.

Content Analyses

Noncomparative content analyses of suicide notes have attempted to explore what can be learned of the writer's dynamics, motivations, emotions, cognitions and associated linguistic characteristics. Here, classification schemes and typologies abound. For example, one early investigator (Jacobs, 1967) was able to classify all but 10 of 112 notes into four categories: (1) notes that beg forgiveness, specifying that the suicide's endurance has been exceeded, that death is necessary, and the awareness that the reader will not understand (see Figure 11.1); (2) notes thematically focused on an incurable or painful illness; (3) accusatory notes placing responsibility (thus guilt) for the suicide on the addressee; and (4) instructional notes (impersonal last wills). In support of this last type, Cohen and Fiedler (1974) found the largest proportion (31%) of the almost 200 notes they analyzed to contain advice, instructions, or requests.

Other classifcations of note content have reported on four types based on the logic used by the writer (Shneidman & Farberow, 1957c) and emotional content (Tuckman et al., 1959). Lester and Heim (1992) have compared a small sample of German notes by gender. However, the only true comparative studies of content involve genuine versus simulated notes (see earlier) and studies of older versus younger note writers.

Age Differences

Suicide note writers over age 60 more often than younger note writers give physical illness, pain, and disability as reasons for their suicides (Capstick, 1960; Darbonne, 1969). They

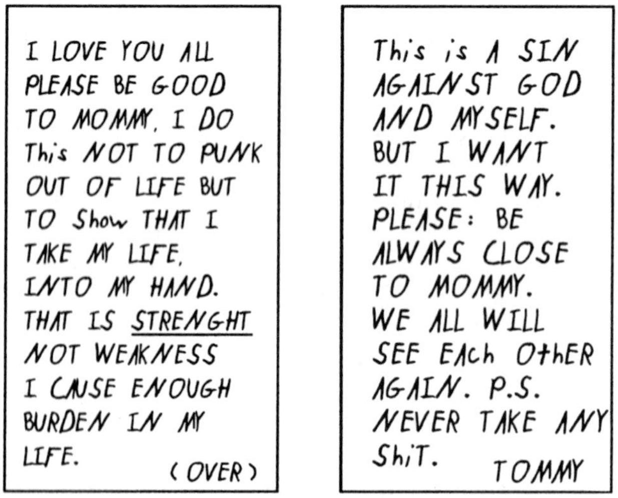

I LOVE YOU ALL
PLEASE BE GOOD
TO MOMMY. I DO
This NOT TO PUNK
OUT OF LIFE BUT
TO Show THAT I
TAKE MY LIFE,
INTO MY HAND.
THAT IS STRENGHT
NOT WEAKNESS
I CAUSE ENOUGH
BURDEN IN MY
LIFE.   (OVER)

This is A SIN
AGAINST GOD
AND MYSELF.
BUT I WANT
IT THIS WAY.
PLEASE: BE
ALWAYS CLOSE
TO MOMMY.
WE ALL WILL
SEE EACh OTHER
AGAIN. P.S.
NEVER TAKE ANY
ShiT.   TOMMY

FIGURE 11.1. An explanatory suicide note.

also show more signs of depression, isolation, loneliness, and general life exhaustion. Consistent with this last finding, Farberow and Shneidman (1957) classified 483 notes according to Menninger's three components of the suicidal act: the wish to kill, the wish to be killed, and the wish to die. They found the wish to die increased with age (with odds ratios ranging from over four to six times its occurrence in middle- and younger-age note writers), whereas both the wish to kill and the wish to be killed decreased with age.

Consider the following two case examples:

1. A 70-year-old male gunshot wound suicide, long ill with emphysema and scheduled for surgery to improve circulation in his legs, wrote: "Were I young and able I would go for the retreads—but this old carcass needs more than legs. Beside physical disability my mind has not functioned normally for more than a year."
2. A 62-year-old male gunshot wound suicide said: "I'm too sick to work and too poor to retire. So what's left?"

Notes as Tests of Theoretical Constructs

As noted previously, psychodynamic and psychoanalytic theory have been applied to the study of suicide notes (cf. Farberow & Shneidman, 1957; Duncan & Edland, 1974; Poesner, LaHaye, & Cheifetz, 1989). In an extensive series of investigations (see Leenaars, 1992), Leenaars and colleagues have translated an array of theories into "protocol sentences" (i.e., theory-derived testable hypotheses) which are then verified as present or absent by judges using suicide notes as objects of analysis. As a result of these studies, clusterings of the 35 protocol sentences, which either described suicide note content or discriminated genuine from simulated notes, were derived to describe suicide. These clusters described unbearable psychological pain, problematic interpersonal relationships, rejection–aggression, inability to adjust, conflict–ambivalence, unmet emotional needs/desire to escape, ego deficit, and cognitive constriction.

MOTIVES OF SUICIDE AS INDICATED IN SUICIDE NOTES

Leenaars's groupings reflect a psychoanalytic understanding of suicide. Themes of ambivalence toward a lost love object and aggression turned against the self may well be expected to appear in notes written to a current or recent love object. From this perspective, suicide notes are "insight documents . . . filled with psychodynamic information, genuinely explaining the human reasons for the act and giving rather clear hints as to the unconscious reasons behind it" (Shneidman, 1993: 98–99). This position is supported by other psychodynamic observers (cf. Posener et al., 1989) who see suicide notes as potentially "most revealing of the motive for suicide" (Hendin, 1982: 150).

However, this position contrasts sharply with Shneidman's "reconsiderations" (Shneidman, 1973), which focused more on the psychic pain, cognitive constriction, and psychodynamic denial that characterize the acutely suicidal state, during which notes typically are written and which, from Shneidman's perspective, preclude the suicidal individual from having true insight. Gottschalk and Gleser (1960) present yet a third position, that sampling bias exists; that is, the psychopathology of the note-writing suicidal person is different from the nonwriter, reminding us of the one significant difference between these two groups—their wish to communicate with others.

Thus considerable question has been raised as to whether or not suicide notes truly reveal the motives of the suicidal individual. Irrespective of whether one or all of these positions is correct (they are by no means mutually exclusive), there is little doubt that individual suicide notes often provide unique and personal glimpses into the final cognitions and cognitive processes of the writer.

From our experience, suicide notes run the gamut from the banal to the insightful. When they do provide thematic insight into the motive and intent of the writer, they often do so with remarkable clarity.

Motivations for suicide range from hostility to guilt, from intrapsychic (e.g., to destroy intolerable impulses within oneself) to interpersonal (e.g., to punish others by inducing guilt or pain), from escape to control. Edland and Duncan (1973) suggested five classifications of motives derived from their study of over 300 notes: (1) retaliatory abandonment, (2) retroflexed murder, (3) reunion, (4) rebirth, and (5) self-punishment. A less theoretical and more varied classification system has been proposed by Bryan L. Tanney (personal communication January 24, 1992; see Table 11.1), providing us with a guide for both understanding suicide motive and applying a template to suicide notes. Examples of these motivations follow, using illustrative excerpts from actual notes (previously unpublished); each is captioned according to Tanney's reasons for suicide and, when applicable, described by other (e.g., theoretical) systems of categorization.

Reunion Suicide

A 51-year-old female, severely depressed since her husband's death, jumped from the 18th floor of a modern, urban hotel after drinking a large quantity of alcohol. Her suicide note, found in her hotel room, stated, "Without my husband, I cannot live. I want to be buried with my husband, if possible." Motivated by grief, this "I can't live without you" type of suicide (Wold, 1971) expresses both her inability to endure the psychic pain and aloneness caused by the loss of relationship and the magical wish to unite with her spouse in a conjugal grave.

Pain avoidance and a wish to be comforted in the arms of already deceased loved ones similarly motivate suicides of those with severe unendurable conditions such as physical and mental illnesses or overwhelming fear. In this sense, the astute reader will note elements of riddance, rebirth, and respite (see Table 11.1), also, in these reunion suicides. In a similar

TABLE 11.1. Reasons for Suicide

Reason	Motivation/intent
Rescue	To appeal to others; to communicate
Reunion	Aloneness; disrupted attachment, retaliatory abandonment, reconciliation
Respite	Pain cessation; relief, management of affect and disappointment
Rigidity	Tunnel vision; constriction; control; power, if helpless; mastery, omnipotence
Gamble	Ambivalence; avoidance
Rebirth	Fantasy; self-completion
Revenge	Rage; aggression
Ridance	Low self-esteem; despair; worthlessness; hopelessness
Reparation	Self-punishment; guilt

Source: Tanney (personal communication, January 24, 1992).

sense, religious persons often write of seeking sanctuary with the all-loving (God, Jesus . . .) such as the following:

1. From a 33-year-old, unemployed male gunshot wound suicide with a history of in-patient treatment for schizophrenia, depression, and alcoholism: "As the years went by the mental illness just got worse. Don't call this a murder. Too much pain in my brain. I'm going to see grandmom and Jesus."

2. From a 51-year-old, married male with bipolar disorder who overdosed with chloral hydrate in his hotel room: "Jesus: I want you. The time has come. Please take me. Please take me with you."

3. From a 22-year-old male found hanging in his prison cell after being gang raped by 10 men in his prison cell; he was fearful of being raped again:

   Dearest Mother:

   I really am sorry I have to pain you this last time. I find it hard to be—live. Pray for me the Lord shows mercy on my soul. Hell is on earth and I hope my brothers learn from this. Join God is the only way to a happy live [*sic*].

Wahl (1957) described suicide as a "magical act, actuated to achieve irrational, delusional, and illusory ends" (23). Suicides motivated by a wish to replace an intolerable life condition with an afterlife of salvation, rescue, protection, resurrection, or spiritual rebirth in the arms of God have this theme, albeit a culturally sanctioned one. Some terminal communications describe these themes not in the form of a direct note but, rather, through indicated passages in the Bible left at the scene or in the residence of the decedent (see Case 11.3, later in this chapter, as one example). The following case explictly illustrates these dynamics: A 71-year-old retired widow jumped to her death from the window of her 10th-floor apartment. She was known to be despondent over her failing eyesight. In her apartment was found a variety of religious items including a Christian Science Bible with chapters and verses marked relating to sight (e.g., "Seeing belongs to God" and "God's mind sees") as well as references in her handwritten notes relating God's ability to be "all-knowing and all-seeing."

Rebirth Suicide

Related to reunion fantasies as a reason for suicide is the concept of rebirth, typically involving fanatasies of passing to a new existence, of transformation. Berman and Jobes (1991: 139) present, for example, the case of a 14-year-old who left a note to his parents to explain his suicide by hanging. After reading the novel, *Watership Down*, about and written from the perspective of a sophisticated culture of rabbits, he wrote that he wanted to die in order to transform himself into a rabbit.

A similar kind of magical thinking is apparent in the notes left by 16-year-old Craig Hunt, who, in the summer of 1983, drove his Porsche to a scenic waterfalls and jumped 320 feet to his death. Hunt was a popular, straight "A" student, captain of his high school soccer team, and class president. His classmates had also voted him "most inspirational student." His surface successes, however, obviously belied his deep inner pain and sense of worthlessness. In his good-bye note to his girlfriend, he wrote, "I'm going down and I know you're going up . . . I hope you will find someone truly worth your love." And in a note to his family, he spoke of the effect of too high expectations and insufficient immediate reward: "I have ended my life of my own free will to satisfy my own selfish desire . . . because the happiness I found in life could no longer overcome my wonder of what would come after it."

Figure 11.2 depicts the remainder of his note to his parents and the inversion of his affect from pain to hope.

Rage–Revenge Suicide

Problematic and conflict-laden interpersonal relationships are common to both suicides and some commonly observed antecedent conditions to suicide, such as alcoholism and bipolar disorders. Concomitant with these are themes of rage, expressed psychodynamically by terms such as "aggression toward a lost love object," "retroflexed rage," "to kill the introjected object," and so on. Sometimes these themes are expressed almost literally in suicide notes. For example, a note left to his recently separated wife by a 31-year-old male stabbing suicide stated: "I'm trying to get you out of my blood."

Suicide notes often express feelings of great ambivalence about these relationships, where the sacrificial murder of the self appears to be the only way to express both how loved and hated the object was. To wit:

1. From a 31-year-old depressed female drug overdose suicide, recently separated from her husband: "Forgive me, I can't take it anymore. . . . Neither of us can take this anymore. I know you'll hate me for this. I think perhaps you'll never really understood what being inside you meant to me. . . . You tried harder with me than I

What lies behind us and in front of us
is nothing more than a grain of sand
in the ocean of eternity
when compared with what it is
that lies before us.

The luckiest of all are those for whom
that grain is beautiful,
and that ocean is boundless —
But even these people can never be happy
with their lives,
with what they have and have had,
If they are to always wonder about
what is still to come,
about what lies before them.

We must not be satisfied with our past,
accept our present, and
just curiously await our future . . .
For this curiosity about what is to come
prevents us from seeing the real value
in our past and our present.

Let us not just wish for the pot of gold
at the end of every rainbow,
but instead let us run to the end of each one
and look for that pot of gold.
Let us not just hope that the sun is shining
somewhere beyond the clouds,

but unstead let us push aside every one
so that the sun if it's shining
can come shining down on us.
And let us not just wander about what
does lie before us,
but instead let us go and find out.

And if the pot of gold is not there,
or we cannot find the sun, or
the future does not turn out to be
what it is we had hoped it to be . . .
We at least have the satisfaction of knowing
that we found out,
of knowing the truth for sure from that
moment on and never again
having to be curious,
and of knowing that what we do have
will never again have to be cheapened
by our wonder of what we could have.

Man cannot be happy if he waits in wonder
for his future to come to him . . .

Each of us must look for his future,
and go to it!

— CWH —

FIGURE 11.2. Excerpt from Craig Hunt's note to his parents.

ever had a right to expect. *So* [emphasis added] guilt is yours. I love you beyond words or comprehension. Don't hate me."

2. From a 46-year-old female who overdosed after an argument with her daughter about a traffic ticket:

I love you so much that I hate you.
I love you.

> Mom.
> You kill me.

3. From a 42-year-old divorced female with a diagnosed bipolar disorder who overdosed on Darvon: "No one killed me but Stanley [her ex-husband]."

Riddance Suicides

Often suicide notes blatantly paint the low self-esteem, worthlessness, hopelessness, and self-hate that drive the impulse to negate one's existence. Absolute cognitions tend to predominate in these notes, such as "My whole life has been a waste" and "I've been a fool all my life."

1. From a 44-year-old married male who suicided by propoxyphene overdose: "I don't want to burden you with a stupid funeral and putting plastic flowers on a hunk of dirt. Therefore my last wish is to donate my body to some medical research organization. I may at least do some good for somebody in death."
2. From a 30-year-old male gunshot wound suicide: "And now you don't have to worry about me. Just shove a ham bone up my ass and let the dogs run away with me."

Some of these notes reflect a Sisyphean struggle with life and the ultimate sense of exhaustion at never accomplishing one's objective:

3. From a 33-year-old, divorced male carbon monoxide suicide: "I'm just *too* tired. I have been fighting an uphill battle, alone, all my life. Every time I would get close to the top of the hill I would get kicked back down again."
4. From a 34-year-old married female with a history of depression and five prior non-fatal suicide attempts, who drowned herself while on a pass from her last hospitalization: "Even all small chores are a supreme effort . . . all my efforts have been hopeless . . . I feel utterly hopeless and unable to go on."

Respite Suicides

In the same vein, the pain of physical illness may be so extreme that in the absence of hope for change, death is seen as the great comforter. As noted previously, notes left by older suicides more often reflect these reasons for suicide:

1. From the note of a 67-year-old unmarried female written to her sister before she overdosed on sedatives: "Jane—Pain is so severe that I would rather be dead than live in misery."
2. From a 68-year-old female who overdosed on secobarbital: "For two days I have not been able to move my bowels. There's some obstruction. . . . The pain was terrible. I'm tired of all this pain and I know it will get worse—so I have to go. Took 30 seconals. Take trash out and garbage in refrigerator."

MULTIPLE AND ALTERNATIVE SUICIDE NOTES

A small proportion of note writers feel compelled to leave more than one note or, taking advantage of more modern technology, leave notes in the form of audiotapes and videotapes. In the only study to date comparing writers of multiple versus single notes, Tuckman and Ziegler (1968) found that those leaving multiple notes were more often divorced or separated persons whose notes were characterized by profound ambivalence (hostile and positive emotions). Their notes were used to explain to a parent or friend the reasons for the failure of their marriage, to rage at their spouse, and to express love and affection toward their children, while, concurrently admonishing them to obey their mother.

Some multiple note writers are more self-disclosing on their deathbed than at any point in their lives. Case 11.2 illustrates such a suicide note writer who apparently took advantage of his impending death to soliloquize about his intrapsychic pain.

Figure 11.3 displays the first and last notes (of five) written by a 54-year-old woman who died by a self-inflicted overdose of barbiturates and alcohol. The notes, leaving last-will-type instructions regarding the disposition of savings, dramatically illustrate the mental deterioration and loss of control as the effects of her ingestion become evident. (Note, in particular, the transposition of date and ZIP code, in addition to the handwriting on the second note.)

SUICIDE NOTES IN THE CONTEXT OF A LIFE

As mentioned previously, Shneidman's third turn of opinion about suicide notes (see Shneidman, 1993) viewed notes as invaluable within the context of a life history, wherein the note may illuminate important aspects of that life and, conversely, the life history can im-

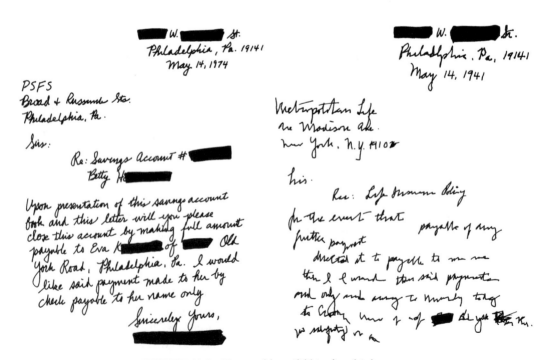

FIGURE 11.3. First and last (fifth) of multiple notes.

CASE 11.2. Multiple Note Writer

A 28-year-old single male was found in his bedroom, lying on his stomach, bed covers pulled over his head, with a washcloth in his mouth and a plastic bag tied about his head with a necktie. Known as a loner, sad, and quiet; he lived alone. His only brother had died 1 month earlier in a plane crash. As a child, he had polio; he still walked with a cane. Two weeks before his suicide, he fell and complained of head pains, necessitating treatment at a hospital.

His several notes, found next to his bed, are filled with symbolic images apparently activated by this experience. They suggest to the trained eye that he had or was developing a psychotic depression, as they are replete with statements of failure, worthlessness, delusional (and masturbatory) guilt, self-blame, and self-punishment.

Note A: "Dear Nana, This is goodbye. I climbed a mountain, but didn't know how to fly. I had a dream which turned into insanity; an empty negative insanity . . . Remember the few good things I have done during my abandoned life. I was like a wish that never came true . . . The sufferings of our family have largely been due to me. I can't assume that they will end because I have—They could have ended if I had come true."

Note B: (to a coworker) "I am leaving the world for it will be better off without me, considering what I have become—which is hardly even a shadow of humanity. He who climbs high risks a great fall. Well, I may not have climbed that high, but I certainly fell, again and again. . . .

As a child, I had recurrent thoughts of the perfect homicide. They had returned, to haunt me, to make me believe that I was evil. [A woman at work] said to me, 'You're eyes are really full of the devil.' This suprised me because I was trying to be so pure . . . to rid myself of evil, to shake free. The image of a crashing bird haunted me, flying higher and higher toward the sun, then falling to the ground."

Note C: (Unaddressed; after an acid trip) "That night was long. I believed I was Lucifer . . . I went home and indulged in an orgy of self-abuse. I now look at my hands and only see the damage they can do. For the last couple of years I have felt that I had a role in the Apocalypse. I had wanted to be one of the riders. Lately, I feel merely like the beast. I can only hope that in destroying myself, I will find peace—or, at least, an eternal sleep."

Source: Anonymous.

---

part special meaning to key words in the note. This reciprocal relationship between the suicide note and the life of the suicide places the note in its proper context as a signal of a suicidal life. It is unfortunate, then, that, most often, the discovery of a suicide note trails after the discovery of a suicide, rather than before the suicide occurs.

The important point here is that suicidal communications, be they threats, veiled messages, or suicide notes, all must be understood as idiographic messages; that is, they speak of the dynamics of the individual and may not share characteristics with others. These mes-

CASE 11.3. A Psychological Autopsy of Vincent Foster, Jr.

In the early evening of July 20, 1993, Vincent Foster, Jr.'s body was found next to a cannon in a park that once served as a Civil War battery on the Northern Virginia side of the Potomac River. His hand still gripped a 1913 Colt Army service revolver, an inheritance from his father. He was dead from a gunshot wound to the mouth. Foster, age 48, married and a father of three, was Deputy White House Counsel to and a childhood friend of President Bill Clinton, as well as law partner and friend of Hillary Clinton. He had been in the administration exactly 6 months from the day he arrived in Washington.

Foster's life was an autobiography of success and distinction: president of his high school class, first in his class in law school, top score on the Arkansas bar exam, partner and head of corporate litigation at a prestigious Little Rock law firm. He was listed as one of the "Best Lawyers in America" and earned over $300,000 a year. One of his partners in the law firm recalled that he "never saw [Foster suffer] a professional setback. . . . Never. Not even a tiny one."

Foster's commencement address to the University of Arkansas Law School in early May 1993 is a revealing record of what Vince Foster valued. Above all, he spoke of one's reputation (as having great integrity) and of the need to be in control of one's reputation. He viewed one's public image as a reflection of one's true self. And to this image he brought very high standards.

"The reputation you develop for intellectual and ethical integrity will be your greatest asset or your worst enemy. You will be judged by your judgment," he said. "Treat every pleading, every brief, every contract, every letter, every daily task as if your career will be judged on it."

Not content that his point was made, he went further:

"There is no victory, no advantage, no fee, no favor, which is worth even a blemish on your reputation for intellect and integrity. . . . Dents to [your] reputation are irreparable."

In this address Foster also focused on his family values, at once in apparent contradiction to his charge to be the complete lawyer: ". . . your children will grow up and be gone before you know it . . . God only allows us so many opportunities with our children. . . . Try not to miss one of them. The office can wait."

Foster's move to Washington had, indeed, caused just such a disruption in his life as his wife and youngest son had stayed in Little Rock so that his son could finish his senior year in high school and graduate with his classmates. In his address to the law school Foster now raised the question, "what motivates one with a comfortable practice in a prominent law firm to dislodge his family for a new job with longer hours, with half the pay, in a city that costs twice as much to live[?]" His answer spoke of duty, of responsibility to society, and of being an agent of change.

Four days after this speech, a chain of dents began. First, was what became known as "Travelgate." Suspecting financial mismanagement of the White House travel office, seven people were fired. Within the next few weeks, questions were raised about cronyism, about misusing the FBI, and so on, and outside investigations were being called for. Foster felt he had failed to contain the problem and that his reputation had been publicly blemished. He began looking for a lawyer.

That same week, President Clinton played golf at an all-white country club in Little Rock with his nominee for associate attorney general. Facing Senate confirmation, the nominee resigned from the club after a number of critical editorials in the *Wall Street Journal*. Foster, too, had to quit the club to avoid criticism.

On June 17, *The Wall Street Journal*'s lead editorial asked, "Who is Vincent Foster?" The editorial questioned his integrity and suggested that he might be being careless in the way he was handling a court order regarding a complaint against the health care reform task force holding closed meetings. Five more editorials followed over the ensuing weeks, the last appearing the day before Vince Foster's suicide and again questioning Foster's mores.

Friends recalled Foster as troubled. He commented that he had become a liability to the President. He looked "blue," "down," "frustrated," "out of sorts." He worried; he was introspective; he felt he was at the hub of things going wrong; he was wounded. When he had trouble sleeping one night, his wife counseled him to write out his complaints. This he did, perhaps about a week before his death. His list is that of a depressed, embattled person, replete with paranoid images of good (himself) versus evil (enemies), an obsessional denial of guilt, of no longer having control or power. Some time after writing this, he tore it into 27 pieces and put it in his briefcase.

> I made mistakes from ignorance, inexperience and overwork
> I did not knowingly violate any law or standard of conduct
> No one in the White House, to my knowledge, violated any law or standard of conduct, including any action in the travel office. There was no intent to benefit any individual or specific group
> The FBI lied in their report to the AG [Attorney General]
> The press is covering up the illegal benefits they received from the travel staff
> The GOP has lied and misrepresented its knowledge and role and covered up a prior investigation
> The Ushers Office plotted to have excessive costs incurred, taking advantage of Khaki [a White house staff member] and HRC [Ms. Clinton]
> The public will never believe the innocence of the Clintons and their loyal staff
> The WSJ [*The Wall Street Journal*] editors lie without consequence
> I was not meant for the job or the spotlight of public life in Washington. Here ruining people is considered sport.

Vince Foster had been described by others as a "pillar," as "The Rock of Gibralter," as "the spine." As he came to the end of his life, he was crumbling. He was in a much bigger pond with scavenger fish all around him and the rules of the game weren't those he had either known nor mastered. In the eyes of others, he believed he had failed. Perhaps he felt he could not return to Arkansas feeling disgraced and beaten. Perhaps he felt that leaving altogether was the only way to preserve a sense of himself.

On the day before his death he called his family physician in Little Rock and was prescribed by phone a prescription for trazodone (Desyrel), an antidepressant. He apparently took one 50 mg pill (only a third the recommended dosage) that night and went to bed. Names of two DC area psychiatrists were in his possession when he died, but they had never been called. At work the next day there were no signs of anything unusual. After eating lunch at his desk in the early afternoon, however, he left the office, never to return. His body was found around 6 P.M.; a bullet had passed through his mouth into his brainstem.

Note. Cf. Office of Independent Counsel (1997).

> *Ted, darling I loved you more than life itself. Forgive me I love you, I love you. You should have been better. I love you.*
>
> Nancy

FIGURE 11.4. A concluding suicide note.

sages and documented communications serve as the heartbeat of the psychological autopsy, giving life to the mirrored projections of others about the decedent.

As a final illustration (Case 11.3), we offer the case of Vincent Foster, Jr., White House Deputy Counsel and lifelong friend of President Bill Clinton. Foster's life was one of great success and stability, finally destroyed by his own unmeetable perfectionism. After a career of achievement and power in Little Rock, Arkansas, as a partner of Hillary Rodham Clinton in the Rose law firm, Foster came to Washington to serve in the White House. Six months to the day after arriving he was dead by his own hand. What the reader should pay particular attention to are the two documented communications near the end of his life: first, his commencement address to the University of Arkansas School of Law; and second, his handwritten note of lamentation, allegedly written at the request of his wife about a week before his death. Together, these statements dramatically provide first-person testimony to his tragic death.

SUMMARY AND CONCLUSIONS

As suicide notes reflect the writer's *last words*, it seems only appropriate to close with a note. Figure 11.4 shows the note of a 54-year-old married female who overdosed on her prescribed antidepressants. In a remarkable economy of words she writes to her husband expressing her love for him and her guilt over some unspecified wrong (her suicide?), closing with words designed to leave some guilt in his future. In this regard we perhaps need to remind ourselves of one final function of suicidal communications, that is, one of maintaining a connection to life and individuals through a memorial, a concrete lasting statement that outlives ourselves.

In Chapter 12, we move from ideation and communication to actual attempts at suicide and the various methods people use, as well as the meanings of these methods.

FURTHER READING

Gutheil, E. (1988). Dreams and suicide. *American Journal of Psychotherapy, 2*(2), 283–294. Reprinted in *American Journal of Psychotherapy*, 1999, 53(2), 246–257, with Commentary by T. Gutheil (pp. 258–259). This classic article presents seven cases in which suicidal communications are presented through dreams, indicating both "the patient's intentions, but also usually . . . hints as to the deeper mental mechanisms involved." Although dated in its reliance on the death instinct, this article captures the luxury of the era in its psychodynamic analysis of patient communications.

Leenaars, A. A. (1998). *Suicide notes: Predictive clues and patterns.* New York: Human

Sciences Press. Leenaars provides a theoretical and empirical review of suicide notes as personal documents of those who suicide. He, then, offers an analysis of a large sample of notes based on theoretical positions of 10 suicidologists and derives a unique system of categorizing themes commonly presented by those who leave notes. This work is more succinctly captured in Leenaars, A. A. (1992). Suicide notes, communication, and ideation. In R. W. Maris, A. L. Berman, J. T. Maltsberger, & R. I. Yufit (Eds.), *Assessment and prediction of suicide* (pp. 337–361). New York: Guilford Press.

Shneidman, E. S. (1993). *Suicide as psychache.* Northvale, NJ: Jason Aronson. In Chapter 6, Shneidman traces almost 50 years of interest in and conceptual formulations regarding suicide notes. In his career, the father of modern suicidology has had three distinct views of suicide notes, the latest of which embeds these last writings "in the context of a detailed case history of the individual.

Shneidman, E. S., & Farberow, N. L. (1957). The logic of suicide. In E. S. Shneidman & N.L. Farberow (Eds.), *Clues to suicide* (pp. 31–40). New York: McGraw-Hill. Based on a sample of over 700 notes, this study presents an analysis of the semantic confusion in the logic of the suicidal person and a sub-analysis of a comparison of genuine versus simulated notes to substantiate their findings.

12

Suicide Attempts and Methods

It is tempting to assume that the key to prediction and control of suicide is buried somewhere in the deceptively transparent observation that in order to kill yourself, you must first make an attempt.
—RONALD W. MARIS

On average, over their lifetimes about 10–15% of individuals making nonfatal suicide attempts eventually go on to kill themselves (see Chapter 1, Figure 1.1; Roy & Linnoila, 1990). Of course, it is also true that 85–90% of nonfatal suicide attempters never kill themselves. Depending on their age and sex, nonfatal suicide attempters outnumber suicide completers by at least 8 or 10 to 1. Although it is a little confusing, one could describe Figure 1.1 by saying *either* that "only" 10–15% of suicide attempters ever complete suicide *or* that "fully" 30–40% of suicide completers have made at least one prior nonfatal suicide attempt (depending on which set area A + B is taken as a proportion of). Prior suicide attempters are at a relatively high risk of completing suicide. The suicide rate in the United States is about 12 per 100,000 per year, but 15,000 per 100,000 (i.e., 15 per 100) for prior suicide attempters over their lifetime.

One commonly held belief about the psychosocial development of suicides is that some lifelong precursors (a family history of suicide; loss of a parent at an early age; isolation and/or inability to get along with other people; work, marital, or sexual problems; recurring episodes of depressive illness; alcohol and/or drug abuse; etc.) interact with acute stressors to "trigger" initial nonfatal suicide attempts (Clark, Gibbons, Fawcett, & Scheftner, 1989). The initial suicide attempt can be seen as having both benefits and costs to the attempter. On the positive side, nonfatal suicide attempts almost always get attention from family members, friends, and professionals. The attempter is usually allowed to assume a "sick role," and ordinary responsibilities are often temporarily suspended. Suicide attempts may even be cathartic or purging, with a short-term elevation of affect.

On the negative side, the attention resulting from a suicide attempt is sometimes stigmatizing and may make it more difficult for the individual to maintain a healthy identity. People may be sympathetic with suicide attempters, but they are also likely to be angry. Suicide attempts inconvenience and manipulate others. Many people believe that unlike physical illnesses, suicide attempts are intentional and to a degree unnecessary. After a period of recuperation, the attempter is expected to give up the "sick role" and to resume more normal, preattempt behavior and responsibilities. In short, suicide attempters incur costs. The

---

BOX 12.1. The Economic Burden of Suicide and Suicide Attempts

Suicidality costs society, and particularly the decedent's family, both directly and indirectly. Direct costs include both hospital and physician fees, costs for autopsies and criminal investigations, and so on. Indirect costs are estimated from years of productive life lost, assuming work until age 65, and the present value of lost earnings. Thus, indirect costs are age and gender specific. Palmer, Revicki, Halpern, and Hatziandreu (1995) using data from the United States estimated these costs as follows:

	Direct costs	Indirect costs	Total costs
Attempted suicide	$5,310	$ 27,979	$ 33,289
Completed suicide	$2,098	$394,968	$397,066

---

problems that were associated with the first suicide attempt tend to recur, in part because of the suicide attempt itself. As indicated in Box 12.1, moreover, suicidality has a real cost to society, as well.

Attempting suicide may become a conditioned reaction. The suicide attempter may learn to adapt to stress and life events by repeated self-destructive behaviors. However, subsequent suicide attempts may be made with more lethal methods (see "Suicide Methods," below). In part, this may be the case because the attempter is older and more hopeless. Furthermore, to get a positive response from significant others, the attempter may have to appear more dramatic and serious in his or her subsequent efforts. Of course, more lethal attempts may also provoke elevated anger and frustration from those individuals who are affected. Hospitalization may now be unavoidable. Community resources may begin to dry up, and supportive individuals may become increasingly impatient with the suicide attempter. Finally, perhaps after a few more nonfatal attempts, there may appear to be no way out of this progressively intolerable life situation except to complete suicide. The major problem with the stereotypical suicide career just outlined is that a large part of it is simply not true for the usual suicide completer (e.g., for older males).

NONFATAL ATTEMPTS VERSUS COMPLETIONS: COMPLEXITY OF THE RELATIONSHIP

The relationship between nonfatal suicide attempts and eventual suicide completion is complex. First, there is considerable comorbidity and interaction in the etiology of suicide. There are other major factors predicting completed suicide. In addition to prior nonfatal suicide attempts, they include the following (which are by now well-known): depressive illness; alcoholism and drug abuse; suicide ideation; use of lethal methods to attempt suicide; social isolation; hopelessness; being an older white male; a family history of suicide and/or mental disorder; work problems; marital and relational problems; stress, anger, and irritability; serotonergic disturbances; physical illness; and *repetition* and *interaction* of all these figures (usually over "suicidal careers" of 20–30 years).

A second problem is that most suicide completers make a relatively small number of attempts before completing suicide. Tables 12.1 and 12.2 reveal that in Maris's Chicago survey (Maris, 1981), 70–75% of all suicide completers made only one fatal attempt. If we fo-

TABLE 12.1. Number of Suicide Attempts Made by
Suicide Completers, Chicago

Number of attempts	%
1	70.0
2	13.8
3	4.8
4	3.9
5	3.5
6	0.0
7	1.1
8 or more	0.7
Don't know	2.2
Total	100.0

Note. N = 246.
Source: Adapted from Maris (1981). Copyright 1981 by Johns Hopkins University Press. Adapted by permission.

cus on older (over age 45) white males (who are "typical" suicides in many respects), then fully *88% made a single, fatal suicide attempt.* Thus, although nonfatal suicide attempts predict some suicides, they obviously do not predict about 85–90% of all completed suicides (depending on the age and sex of the attempters). Note in Table 12.2 that among suicide attempters in the Chicago sample, only females made a significant number of multiple suicide attempts before completing suicide. This is particularly true for younger females; 16% of completers in this group made five or more nonfatal suicide attempts before completing suicide.

Third, a clear reason why there are relatively few suicide attempts before completion (especially among men) is that lethal methods, particularly guns and hanging, tend to be used. Turning to contemporary (1996) data (National Center for Health Statistics, 1998) in Table 12.3, we see that firearms now constitute the method of first choice for *both* men and women (63.5% and 38.5%, respectively). Thus, in the United States suicide prevention is highly related to gun control. Hanging is the preferred second method for men, especially in jails, prisons, and hospitals. Women are still much more likely than men to overdose on drugs and medications (24% of all female suicides) and to use a broader panorama of methods.

Fourth, it is well-known that white males outnumber females in their suicide completion rates (4.4 to1 in 1996), females tend to exceed males in nonfatal suicide attempt rates and in rates of depressive illness (an important precursor of suicide). This suggests that the

TABLE 12.2. Number of Suicide Attempts Made by Suicide Completers by Sex and Age, Chicago

Number of attempts	Male (%)		Female (%)		Total (%)
	< 45 years	> 45 years	< 45 years	> 45 years	
1	79	88	50	71	75
2–4	19	10	34	26	20
5+	0	0	16	3	3
Don't know	2	2	—	—	2
Total	100	100	100	100	100
(*n*)	(55)	(90)	(44)	(77)	(266)

Note. N = 266.
Source: Adapted from Maris (1981). Copyright 1981 by Johns Hopkins University Press. Adapted by permission.

TABLE 12.3. Percentage of Completed Suicides by Method and Gender,
United States, 1996

Method	Male (%)	Female (%)
Firearms (E955.0–955.4)	63.5	38.5
Drugs/medications (E950.0–950.5)	5.5	24.0
Hanging (E953.0)	16.6	16.0
Carbon monoxide (E952.0–952.1)	6.0	6.7
Jumping from a high place (E957)	1.7	3.2
Drowning (E954)	0.9	2.0
Suffocation by plastic bag (E953.1)	0.7	3.1
Cutting/piercing instruments (E956)	1.4	1.3
Poisons (E950.6–950.9)	0.5	0.7
Other[a]	2.9	4.5
Total	99.7	100.0

Source: National Center for Health Statistics (1998).
[a]Includes gases in domestic use (E951); other specified and unspecified gases and vapors (E952.8–952.9); explosives (E955.5); unspecified firearms and explosives (E955.9); other specified or unspecified means of hanging, strangulation, or suffocation (E953.8–953.9); and other and unspecified means (fire, hypothermia, electrocution, aircraft crash, etc.) (E958).

social and psychiatric dynamics of at least some types of female suicides are different from those of male suicides. The suicide attempts of younger females more often involve changes in interpersonal relationships and family responsibilities, as well as motivations of revenge and perhaps of anger (see Chapter 6).

Fifth, in the Chicago survey, Maris (1981), inquired how long the time interval was between a suicide attempt and death, as well as who it was who discovered the suicide. Table 12.4 indicates, as expected, that 50–75% (depending on how the "don't know" responses would be distributed) of all suicide completers died within an hour after attempting suicide. The figures in Table 12.5 show that the persons responding to the attempts by suicide completers were more often police and firefighters (and by no one) and less often family members or friends than was true for nonfatal suicide attempters (the actual question was, "Who was primarily involved in trying to save the suicide attempter's life?"). These factors clearly contributed to their suicide attempts being fatal. One is reminded here of Weissman

TABLE 12.4. Time Interval between Suicide Attempt and
Completion, Chicago

Time interval between attempt and death	Completed suicides (%)
1 week or more	7
4–6 days	3
2–3 days	2
4–24 hours	3
2–3 hours	6
1 hour or less	15
Instantaneous death	34
Don't know	30
Total	100
(*n*)	(266)

Source: Adapted from Maris (1981: 284). Copyright 1981 by Johns Hopkins University Press. Adapted by permission.

TABLE 12.5. Types of Interveners in Suicide Attempts by Nonfatal Attempters and Completers, Chicago

Type of intervener	Suicide attempts by attempters (%)	Suicide attempts by completers (%)
Family member	48	26
Friends	19	6
Police officer/firefighter	5	21
Physician	6	6
Psychotherapist	0	0
Suicide prevention or crisis center worker	0	0
Other	3	2
None	11	33
Don't know	8	5
Total	100	100
(*n*)	(64)	(266)

Source: Adapted from Maris (1981: 283). Copyright 1981 by Johns Hopkins University Press. Adapted by permission.

and Worden's (1974) Risk–Rescue Scale, in which suicide outcome is conceived of as a joint product of the lethality of the attempt and the probability of effective intervention. It is interesting to note that virtually no interventions were reported by psychotherapists, crisis workers, or suicide prevention center workers for either attempters or completers.

SUICIDE METHODS

> Razors pain you;
> Rivers are damp;
> Acids stain you;
> And drugs cause cramp;
> Guns aren't lawful;
> Nooses give;
> Gas smells awful;
> You might as well live.
> —DOROTHY PARKER

The suicidal person has more to answer than the ultimate philosophical question, "To be or not to be?" Should the decision favor death over a continued painful existence, whether on impulse or carefully derived, the act of suicide requires some lethal method of self-destruction. Should some purpose other than extinction be sought, the act of self-harm still requires some means to effect that aim.

Richman (1991) has claimed that the suicide method can serve two functions. First, it most simply is a means to an end where it is the end that matters. From this perspective, the great variety of methods available within or near every household provides a treasure trove of self-destructive possibilities for the intended suicide. Second, Richman believes, the means may have a special meaning or symbolism (i.e., dynamic) of its own, as when an adolescent female ingests her mother's prescription medication at home after an argument with this parent.

From the early writings of Durkheim to the present, theorists have recognized that both psychological and cultural factors play a role in the "choice" of suicide method.

Whether viewed from a psychodynamic or social learning perspective, this choice is strongly influenced by a number of factors working both independently and in combination. They include the following:

- The accessibility and availability of the means.
- The user's knowledge, experience and familiarity with the means.
- The meaning, symbolism, and cultural significance of the means.
- Suggestion, contagion, or modeling factors.
- The potential suicide's state of mind.

Each of these is described in greater detail later on in this chapter.

In some respects these factors allow for a small measure of predictability with regard to the suicidal act. That is, knowing that one or more of the factors has importance or applicability to the potentially suicidal individual improves our guess as to what method might actually be used, if any. For example, knowing that a person at risk for suicide had a gun at home and was familiar and comfortable with its use might well concern us. Alternatively, hearing a threat to run in front of a moving car (a method of attempt most common to children and other impulsive individuals) from an obsessional adult giving no evidence of dyscontrol might lead to less concern for suicide risk.

Furthermore, it is with an understanding of these influences and that human behavior is characterized by learned habits that medical examiners and coroners often can make the distinctions necessary to differentiate and certify a suicidal from an accidental death. Where they lack this knowledge, behavioral scientists familiar with psychological autopsy procedures (see Chapters 3 and 21) can better make the discriminations necessary to decide the probable manner of death in otherwise equivocal cases. The distinguishing characteristics of the methods most commonly employed in suicides will now be described.

THE EPIDEMIOLOGY OF SUICIDE METHODS IN THE UNITED STATES

Annual compilations of mortality data in the United States, published by the National Center for Health Statistics, suggest a high degree of consistency in the methods used by Americans who suicide. However, over the last half century, a gradual shift has emerged toward the increasing use of firearms, which now accounts for three out of every five suicides and almost two-thirds (63%) of male suicides. In 1950, firearms were used by 43% of suicides in the United States; the 1996 proportion showed a 37% increase over the 1950 rate. Table 12.6 shows the percentage of suicidal deaths by method from 1960–1996.

TABLE 12.6. Percentage of Suicides by Method, United States, 1960–1996

Method	1960	1970	1980	1990	1996
Ingestion	12%	11%	10%	9%	10%
Gases and vapors	10%	9%	9%	7%	6.5%
Hanging	18%	14%	14%	14%	17%
Firearms and explosives	47%	57%	59%	61%	59%
Other	13%	9%	7%	8%	7.5%
Total	100%	99%	99%	99%	100.0%
(*n*)	(19,031)	(26,869)	(28,453)	(30,906)	(30,903)

Source: National Center for Health Statistics, annual mortality data, various years.

TABLE 12.7. Methods of Suicide by Race and Sex, United States, 1996

Method	M (%)	F (%)	W (%)	B (%)	WM (%)	WF (%)	BM (%)	BF (%)
Firearms	63.5	38.5	59	61	64	40	64	47
Hanging	16.6	16.0	15	18	15	12	19	12
Drugs	5.5	24.0	7	5	4	18	3	15
Gas	6.0	6.7	7	2	7	7	1	2
Other	8.4	14.8	12	14	10	22	13	24
Total	100.0	100.0	100	100	100	99	100	100

Note. M, male; F, female; W, white; B, black.
Source: National Center for Health Statistics (1998).

Suicide methods are usually grouped into eight major categories: drugs, [ingestion of] other solids or liquids, gases and vapors, hanging (strangulation and suffocation), firearms and explosives, submersion (drowning), jumping, and cutting (piercing and stabbing), and a residual ninth classification for all other types. However, as shown in Table 12.6, four methods—guns (firearms and explosives), hanging, drugs, and gases and vapors (particularly motor vehicle exhaust)—account for over 90% of all certified suicides in the United States.

Internationally, the leading method of suicide appears to be hanging (strangulation, suffocation). In an analysis of 1980 suicide rates by method in 30 countries, including the United States, the rate of hanging suicides was greatest in 21 of these countries, led by Hungary (24.53/100,000) (Lester, 1990). Outside the United States, the use of firearms and explosives was the leading method in only four countries (Australia, Canada, Israel, and Costa Rica); ingestion led in Denmark, England/Wales, and Scotland. Submersion (drowning) led all other methods in Iceland. We consider meanings of these various methods in the next section.

Table 12.7 presents methods of suicide data for the United States in 1996 by race and sex. These data affirm that firearms are used more frequently by males, although they are the most common method for female completers, also. Drugs are used more frequently by females and suicide by carbon monoxide is relatively uncommon among blacks compared to whites.

Table 12.8 gives a breakdown of the 1996 U.S. data for the four most commonly used methods by age groups. Some interesting patterns emerge in this analysis. In completed suicides firearms are most commonly employed by the elderly (elderly nonfatal suicide attempts are also more likely to be by firearms; see Frierson, 1991), hanging is more

TABLE 12.8. Methods of Suicide (Percentage) by Age, United States, 1996

Method	Age (years)							
	5–14	15–24	25–34	35–44	45–54	55–64	65–74	75+
Firearms	55.29	65.27	56.57	54.13	59.76	68.20	77.71	78.95
Hanging	40.61	22.74	23.04	18.52	12.52	11.48	8.21	7.86
Drugs	2.73	5.00	10.06	15.03	15.59	10.77	7.44	5.77
Gas	0.00	3.93	6.96	9.04	9.24	7.66	4.69	5.26
Other	1.37	3.06	3.47	3.28	2.89	1.89	1.95	2.16
Total	100.00	100.00	100.00	100.00	100.00	100.00	100.00	100.00

Source: National Center for Health Statistics (1998).

prevalent in younger than in older suicides, and the use of both drugs and gas peaks in middle age.

To interpret these trends we now return to the previous list of factors that influence choice of method and ask which of them, alone or in combination, best helps explain the demographic differences noted earlier.

FACTORS INFLUENCING CHOICE OF METHOD

Availability and Accessibility

For the most part, methods of self-destruction are readily available to all those intent on using them. Every home has knives and other instruments for cutting within easy reach; bodies of water and tall buildings are both available and accessible to practically anyone; speeding cars, which one may crash, fall out of, or jump in front of are ubiquitous in our society—and all methods can be lethal. Yet, as is apparent from the foregoing data, these methods are not equally used to bring about a suicidal death. Also, some of the most available methods are often among the more infrequently chosen.

When the range of alternatives is limited, the "ease of access" (attainability) and the "readiness for use" (availability) probably are most likely to define the choice of a particular method for suicide. Marzuk, Leon, Tardiff, and Morgan (1992) concluded from their study of suicides in the five counties of New York City that differences in suicide rates were due virtually entirely to differences in accessibility to lethal methods of injury. For example, Nowers (1997) reports that almost 40% of suicides in New York are ascribed to jumping from tall buildings. In a more specific context, suicidal death in a jail or prison setting is mainly predicted by the accessibility of method. These suicides are most likely to be by hanging (e.g., by torn clothing, bedsheet, shoelaces, tee shirts, or even the elastic waistband from underwear). In another study by Salive, Smith, and Brewer (1989), hanging accounted for 86% of all inmate suicides occurring over an 8-year period. The restricted circumstances of the jail or prison setting simply do not allow for significant use of alternative methods.

Varah (1981) has observed internationally that the method chosen is that which is most frequently available. For example, common agents of overdose ingestion in various countries are those found in almost every household: insecticide in Sri Lanka, acetic acid in Surinam, caustic soda in Peru, and paraquat in Trinidad and Tobago (cf. Hutchinson et al., 1999).

Thus, an actor's choice of suicide method must begin with it being either at hand or easily obtainable. But availability and accessibility are insufficient to define why an individual will use a particular method. Otherwise, we would expect that males and females, blacks and whites, those from the North and South, and so on, would be roughly equal in their use of available methods. Moreover, we would expect that the modal suicide methods chosen would be nearly universal (e.g., all police officer suicides would be by gunshot wound; all anesthesiologists would use lethal doses of drugs). That just does not happen.

Knowledge, Experience, and Familiarity

The range of possible alternative methods of suicide is also considerably narrowed by socialization (Marks & Abernathy, 1974). According to Marks and Abernathy, sociocultural norms help define acceptable and nonacceptable forms of behavior, including methods of suicide. If a method is available but not normatively appropriate, it will tend not be used. These norms of acceptability further define the likely prior experience a person will have had with particular methods. For example, individuals who dislike guns are far less likely to have a gun available, less likely to have had experience firing guns, and be more uncomfortable with the thought of using a gun. On the other hand, when there is a gun in the home, the risk of suicide in the home increases almost sixfold, ninefold if the gun is kept loaded (Kellerman, Rivara, Somes, & Reay, 1992).

Such suicide method socialization is accomplished through a variety of influences and has been documented in a number of studies that have examined variables such as occupation; geography, sex, race, and nationality.

Occupation

Occupation, familiarity, knowledge, and availability probably all combine to explain the more frequent use of revolvers by policemen (Friedman, 1967) and poisons by chemists (Li, 1971). In contrast, choice of method appears to be fairly equally distributed across social classes (Peck, 1986).

Geography, Race, Sex, and Nationality

Suicides by firearms are most frequently recorded in the southern United States. Marks and Abernathy (1974) demonstrated a statistically significant relationship between the degree of southern cultural influence in various regions of the United States and the use of firearms for suicide. However, race and sex may determine variations within regions with regard to preference for firearms (Taylor & Wicks, 1980).

Firearms, in general, are the preferred method of suicide among males, blacks, and Native Americans in the United States. Goss and Reed (1971) have demonstrated that among New York City males the choice of firearms varies according to age and religious affiliation. Blacks living in the tenement society of Harlem in New York City, where rooftop life is common, often jump from those rooftops when suiciding. Jumping is the modal method among blacks in New York City (Hendin, 1982). Varah (1981) has also noted the high frequency of jumping among suicides in Hong Kong, where the skyscrapers are available to people too poor to afford sleeping pills for overdosing. Farmer and Rohde (1980) have futher explored and explained differences observed internationally in the frequency with which various methods are used. Cultural differences have been noted as well in studies between immigrants and native-borns. For example, Asian Americans, perhaps maintaining the norms of their original cultures, more frequently use hanging as a suicide method; although with increasing acculturation and assimilation Asians are also increasing their use of firearms for suicide (McIntosh & Santos, 1982; Shiang, 1998).

Case 12.1 illustrates how factors of both accessibility and knowledge interact.

Meaning, Symbolism, and Cultural Significance

Hendin (1982) has noted that approximately 15% of suicides in Norway are by drowning, a prevalence seven times greater than that in the United States. According to Hendin (1982), "the sea is central to the conscious and unconscious life" (144) of Norwegians, a major theme and symbol in the art and culture of the country, and both personally and communally significant in terms of life, work and death styles. In contrast, the low rate of suicide by hanging in some countries is hypothesized by Farmer and Rohde (1980) to be due to its use in those countries as a form of capital punishment, "It is possible that this causes a death by hanging to be regarded with ignomy and loathing in those societies, and is not therefore adopted as the preferred way of suicide" (445)—unless suicide is also seen as a form of self-punishment. According to Clarke and Lester (1991), Durkheim similarly

---

CASE 12.1. The Arcane Case of Bob C.

Bob C., a 52-year-old married father of four grown children, had sold off several hundred head of dairy cattle during a government buyout program. After a few months of an unhappy retirement, he took a job as a regional salesman for the state agricultural college. His primary product was bull semen, which he marketed to area dairy farmers for artificial insemination of their herds. The bull semen was stored in 600 gallon containers and kept frozen by liquid nitrogen at temperatures of –320 degrees Celsius in the camper of his truck and could only be disseminated through a series of safety steps. Liquid nitrogen will flash-freeze anything with which it has contact in less than a second. As a farmer himself, Bob was well aware of the safe storage and handling of this product. In addition, he had completed a rigorous training program in safety procedures when he was oriented to this new job.

In the last several months of his life, Bob suffered several stressors. His wife was diagnosed as having and began chemotherapy for breast cancer, one of his sons announced his homosexuality, and several unpaid loans (from his farming days) were threatened with being called. Bob began to show signs of increasing strain and anxiety. His drinking increased markedly and he began having an affair with a woman he met during the several days per week he was on the road and away from home. He had recently told a friend that he was depressed, regretful of having sold his cattle, and scared his wife would learn of the affair. Normally a reserved and careful character, he began making mistakes in invoicing his customers.

On the day of his death Bob parked his camper to the side of a secluded country road and entered the rear of the truck. Positioning himself next to the container of liquid nitrogen, Bob placed the delivery hose to his mouth, turned three valves and flash-froze his larynx. When his body was found, it took 2 days to thaw sufficiently for an autopsy to be performed.

Source: Anonymous.

---

oberved that suicides by hanging were rare in England, because hanging was the traditional punishment for traitors and murderers.

Certain sites have become known as "suicide landmarks." For example, the Golden Gate Bridge, linking San Francisco with the cities of the East Bay area, is considered to be one of the world's leading active sites for suicides. The Golden Gate's cognitive association with images of grace and beauty, as well as its significance as a "gateway" to the Pacific, surely has an impact on the minds of intended suicides. So powerful is this association that between the years 1937 and 1979, 58 individuals traveled by automobile across the San Francisco–Oakland Bay Bridge (an equally high span from which to jump) in order to jump to their deaths from the more distant Golden Gate Bridge. About 58 people also suicided from the Bay Bridge during these same years (Seiden & Spence, 1982). Accessibility is also a key factor in the appeal of the Golden Gate Bridge as a favored site for jumping suicides (it has pedestrian walkways, whereas the Bay Bridge does not). Over 40% of the suicides from the Golden Gate Bridge had been on foot compared to less than 5% of those from the Bay Bridge.

Jukai, in Japan, provides a second suicide site example. Jukai is a dense forest which occupies the northern lava plateau around Mt. Fuji, the highest peak in Japan and the focus of much symbol and myth in Japanese culture. Jukai has recorded an average of 30 known suicides annually, considerably more than those observed from the Golden Gate Bridge. The number of annual suicides at Jukai apparently increased subsequent to its popularization in a mystery novel in the early 1960s, *Nami no Toh*, wherein the belief was stated that one cannot escape once having entered Jukai. Thus, its appeal was established by its symbolism (a wish to disappear), its location (a wish to belong to a larger group that shared the same site for their suicides), and imitation, among other factors specific to its history and mythology (Takahashi, 1988).

Meanings attached to particular methods may also be important as explanations for observed gender differences in the prevalence of these methods to complete suicide. Suicides by ingestion (of solids and liquids) have long been overrepresented in females (by approximately a 4:1 ratio; cf. McIntosh & Santos, 1982). Possible explanations for females' preference for ingestion as a method of suicide may include reference to a cultural concern for maintaining appearance and avoiding disfigurement, to the association between drugs and peaceful sleep or pain avoidance, and to an even more universal symbolic meaning—that is, the association between the wish to be pregnant and that of ingestion (Freud, as cited by Hendin, 1982).

Three studies, all with college students, have examined how different methods are perceived and their cognitive associations. Marks (1977) found that females associated painlessness and efficiency with drugs and poisons, whereas males associated masculinity and efficiency with firearms. Lester (1988a, 1988b) discovered that females were more concerned with issues of painlessness and less disfigurement in their hypothetical choice of a suicide method. Also, females more frequently than males endorsed the statement, "I am afraid of what might happen to my body after death." Irrespective of gender, suicide by gun was seen as "painful," "messy," and "masculine," whereas suicide by overdose was conceived of as "painless, "tidy," and "feminine."

Suggestion

Imitation and the influence of the media, ranging from newspaper and television news to the movies and publicized suicides of media stars, have increasingly been noted as part of the matrix of influences that suggest or model both suicide as a solution to life problems and specific methods to effect that solution (cf. Chapter 10). The literature on imitation effects (such as the "Werther effect") has been reviewed at length elsewhere (Berman, 1986b, 1988; Phillips, 1985). With particular concern for evidence of how specific methods may be modeled, Sonneck, Etzersdorfer, & Nagel-Kuess (1994) reported an abrupt decline in the incidence of subway suicides in Vienna immediately after the two largest-circulation newspapers curtailed drastically the publicity accorded these types of suicides. No similar decline was evident for any other type of suicide.

With regard to fictional presentations of suicide, Berman (1988) reported evidence of method imitation in an analysis of a large nationwide sample of suicides following broadcasts of three television movies about suicide. In the most elegant of these studies, Schmidtke and Hafner (1988) reported a significant increase in German railway suicides following broadcast of a six-episode television series about a 19-year-old male who suicides by jumping in front of a train.

Evidence for the effect of suggestion and imitation is illustrated by the case of the comedian Freddie Prinze. In the week subsequent to Prinze's 1977 gunshot wound suicide in Los Angeles County, there was a significant increase (from 6 to 13) in gunshot wound suicides in the county compared to the week preceding his death (Berman, 1987). The most plausible interpretation here is that of imitation of a particular method of suicide used by one (Prinze) whom others see as a model.

Suggestion may also occur in other, perhaps more subtle forms of interpersonal influence and transaction. For example, it is well known that the most lethal and frequently used suicide drugs (i.e., antidepressants) are those specifically prescribed to treat a predisposing psychopathology (e.g., depression). This iatrogenic effect may be due in part to the physician simply showing too little consideration for the possibility of suicide, either by providing a lethal quantity of pills to the patient or by not having awareness of the patient's possible hoarding behavior. This lack of consideration may reflect the professional equivalent of aiding and abetting a suicide. Richman (1991) gives a case example of an 80-year-old woman who consulted her physician because of insomnia. Behind this symptom was a series of traumatic life events which the woman would have confided to the physician had he just asked. But he did not. Instead, he simply supplied her with enough sleeping pills for her to kill herself on the next day. Similarly, there are a large number of clinical examples where a spouse (in a chronic, rageful, and conflictual relationship with his or her partner who is known to be suicidal) colludes by "carelessly" making a weapon available to be used in the spouse's suicide.

Family influences in suicide method determination may also be seen in suicides employing the same weapon that was kept at home subsequent to an earlier family suicide. In Case 12.2, this influence was presumed by the patient to be genetic.

State of Mind

Most of those who survive a suicide attempt do so because they use methods of low lethality, but why do they use such methods? It may be because their intent is not primarily to die but, rather, to manipulate others. The presumed lack of potential lethality of a particular suicide method may make it an attractive choice to those who do not really intend to die.

CASE 12.2. The Case of Bill F.

Bill F., a 31-year-old single male, sought psychotherapy to deal with his "suicide risk." Bill's presenting problem was stimulated by the recent suicide of his father, at the age of 51, by shotgun. Bill related that his paternal grandfather, as well, had shot himself to death, almost 20 years earlier, *using the same shotgun as Bill's father and at the same age of 51!* Bill's anxiety was bound by his obsession that 20 years hence, when he turned 51, he, too, would be compelled to take his life (as if there would be a "genetic unfolding or genetic determination" at this age) using the very same shotgun. The weapon, interestingly, had been presented to Bill by his mother after his father's funeral with the words, "I know your father would want you to have this" (cf. Chapter 1, Case 1.1, in which Hemingway's mother gave Ernest, as a Christmas present, the revolver with which his father had committed suicide).

As of our publication date, Bill F. is 46 years old and no longer in treatment.

Source: Anonymous.

For example, acetaminophen (Tylenol) is a commonly used drug in intentional overdose, accounting for more cases than either aspirin or ibuprofen in both children and adults (Veltri & Rollins, 1988). In a recent study (Myers, Otto, Harris, Diaco, & Moreno, 1992) 4 in 10 high school students misperceived the potential lethality of acetaminophen, instead perceiving little risk of medical danger.

Ingestion, the leading method of nonfatal suicide attempt, even when taken in lethal quantity, in general takes time to result in death. This allows for rescue or intervention (cf. Weisman & Worden's [1974] Risk–Rescue Scale). Methods that take time also allow for ambivalence to lead the potential decedent in a life-sustaining direction instead. Also, it may be that ambivalence is a significant factor leading to the choice of an overdose, because the individual realizes there will be time to reconsider. Berman, Leenaars, McIntosh, and Richman (1992) present the case of a 66-year-old highly ambivalent woman who attempted to slit her wrists (she "couldn't" follow through), then to turn the gas on in her apartment. Not being able to tolerate the wait, she tried to drown herself in her bathtub (but, again, "couldn't" do it). Next, she left her apartment to get her mail. In her mail she found a filled prescription of flurazepam (Dalmane, a sleep aid). She went to a neighborhood convenience store, bought a soft drink, then sat on a park bench and ingested some 50 pills. Expecting to die, she returned to her apartment to lie down on her bed. There she was met by the police, who had been called by a neighbor who had smelled escaping gas. She was taken to the hospital after she informed them of what she had done.

A further study assessing the state of mind of the suicide decedent is provided by Peck (1986). In his investigation of young, predominantly white midwestern suicides, Peck found that those who suicided by more passive and low-lethality means (e.g., alcohol and barbiturates [44%], carbon monoxide poisoning [37%]) were more likely to leave suicide notes than were those who chose more active and highly lethal means (firearms [26%], hanging [18%]). These differences were probably not merely a result of a differential need to communicate but were determined in part by the difference in time before unconsciousness. That is, lower-lethality methods give an opportunity to the suicide to share some last moments of thinking (or acting?).

Similarly, when the intent of a decedent is to conceal or disguise his or her suicide, methods difficult to certify as suicide may be viewed as advantageous. For example, unwitnessed drownings, some drug overdoses, and some single-driver, single-car crashes may be difficult to classify as suicides.

Perhaps the most significant illustration of how the decedent's state of mind may influence choice of suicide method is provided by examples of bizarre methods. It is reasonable that the more bizarre or unusual the suicide method was, the more likely that the decedent was seriously mentally disordered and even psychotic (e.g., schizophrenic suicides). When an individual's behavior conveys an absence of rationality concerning available choices of method, an absence of concern for pain, or a Herculean effort to inflict self-torture, the presence of a psychotic process should be suspected. However, the obverse does not hold. Psychotic individuals are well represented among those who suicide by more traditional suicide methods.

Psychopathology (particularly psychotic disorders) is perhaps inordinately represented among those who suicide by railroad train or subway train. Studies of individuals who have jumped into a subway pit ahead of a speeding train, placed their bodies across the tracks, or attempted to stop a moving engine with their outstretched arm have been found to have high rates of mental disorder (schizophrenia, bipolar, and other psychotic disorders) and histories of inpatient psychiatric hospitalization (Emerson & Cantor, 1993; Guggenheim & Weisman, 1972; Lindekilde & Wang, 1985).

Big-city newspapers are replete with case reports of unusual suicides and suicide attempts. Among those noted in the professional literature are cases of individuals who burrowed inside a mattress and asphyxiated (Nelson, McKinney, Ludwig, & Davis, 1983), injected poisonous snake venom (Yadlowsky, 1980), deactivated an hydraulic chassis supporting his car as he lay underneath, allowing his skull to be crushed (Boyer, 1975), and attempted to manually tear a permanent pacemaker from his chest (Rosenthal, Crisafi, & Coomaraswamy, 1980). Farberow's (1969) bibliography on suicide references a variety of reports of bizarre methods, including self-inflicted guillotining, self-crucifixion, igniting sticks of dynamite in one's mouth, swallowing Chinese firecrackers, and even "strangulation by tree root"! (see also Case 12.3).

A Final Statement on Factors That Influence Choice of Method

When an individual decides to end his or her own life, either by plan or on impulse, a wide variety of methods are available to accomplish suicide. However, it is also clear that a small number of determining parameters and motivational influences narrow the range of alternatives for methods of self-destruction. For example, Brent et al. (1988) have determined in their study of Pittsburgh suicides that the availability of a gun in the home and the potential decedent's familiarity with and knowledgablity of how to fire it are strongly related to the probable use of a gun for suicide. This is true even when other methods are equally available and accessible.

Card (1974) attempted to establish objective measures of the lethality of various methods of suicide based on their probability of ending in death (see Chapter 2). If human beings did not have specific cultural backgrounds, personality differences, ambivalence, subjectivi-

---

CASE 12.3. The Case of Joseph S.

Joseph S. was a 35-year-old divorced man living alone at the time of his death. He had a long history of psychosis and related psychiatric hospitalizations. For the past several years he had been maintained as an outpatient with injections of Prolixin. However, he would frequently discontinue his drug treatment and have to be rehospitalized. Joseph suffered from auditory hallucinations and religious fanaticism. He felt "one with God" and equally omnipotent. The voices commanded him to kill himself. In response to these voices he had already attempted suicide several times, by driving his car into a bridge abutment, cutting himself, and by setting himself on fire.

During one of his hospitalizations, Joseph boasted that he could communicate with and tame lions. For several days preceding his death, Joseph was observed to behave with greater agitation and argumentativeness, behaviors commonly noted when he went without medication. On the day of his death, he went to the county zoo, climbed over a 4-foot fence and through thick bushes in order to lower himself over a 30-foot wall into the lion compound. The local medical examiner ruled his death to be due to massive hemorrhaging from mutilation by one or more of the lions. At the scene near his body a crucifix was found. In his apartment police investigators found a bible opened to the Book of Daniel.

Source: Los Angeles Suicide Prevention Center.

ty and symbolic meanings, and psychopathology, choice of method would simply be determined by estimates of lethality. Because of the factors described in the preceding pages and the great individual differences in how these influences interact with one another, the term objective lethality has little relevance to the suicidal decision.

DISTINGUISHING CHARACTERISTICS OF SUICIDE METHODS

An unwitnessed death (cf. McDowell, Kothberg, & Kusbes, 1994) may still leave clues as to the manner in which the death occurred. For example, in trying to distinguish between a suicidal jump or an accidental fall from a tall building, one might be aided by evidence that the body landed feet first (Girard, Minaire, Castanier, Berard, & Perrincriche, 1980). In addition, autoerotic asphyxial deaths may be certified as accidents and not suicides by a number of site characteristics (see Chapter 6). Personality characteristics of individuals using certain methods of suicide also can help distinguish the manner of death. For example, Litman (1989), in reviewing 500 psychological autopsies, noted that individuals determined to have died by an accidental (vs. suicidal) gunshot wound were likely to have had a history of carelessness in handling guns.

Medical examiners and coroners tend to make assumptions or working hypotheses regarding methods. These assumptions may guide the type and amount of further investigation given a particular death. Some methods are assumed to be virtual "givens" as accidents, unless proven otherwise. Among these prototypical accidents are motor vehicle crashes and pedestrian–vehicular deaths. Suicide by automobile ("autocide") is a rare event. Running in front of a moving vehicle is most often a result of a tragic lack of caution or awareness. However, it also is a fairly common manner of attempted suicide by young children (Cohen-Sandler, Berman, & King, 1982b).

Other methods leading to death are initially presumed to be suicides, unless evidence exists to the contrary. Examples would include hanging (an exception would be autoerotic asphyxia; see Chapters 6 and 18) and carbon monoxide deaths. In contrast, cutting and stabbing fatalities are usually presumed to be homicides. Adelson (1974) studied 700 cutting and stabbing deaths and found 80% of them to be homicides and only 18% to be suicides. As noted in Chapter 18, most medical examiners assume Russian roulette deaths to be accidental deaths (Fishbain, Fletcher, Aldrich, & Davis, 1987). Some, however, argue that such deaths are suicides, given "the significant element of deliberate (e.g., 1 in 6 vs. 0 in 6) self-destruction involved" (Spitz & Fisher, 1980: 263).

Thus, data on suicide methods lead medical examiners typically to simply "bet the odds" (to interpret behaviors in light of their probabilities of being intended or unintended, etc.) in establishing initial working hypotheses. These bets are supported further by the specific characteristics attendant to each method of suicidal death.

Firearms

In the United States increasing rates of suicide have been linked to the increased availability of firearms (Centers for Disease Control and Prevention, 1996). Markush and Bartolucci (1984) demonstrated that total suicide rates showed significant statistical association to gun prevalence for all demographic groups except nonwhite females. Lester and Murrell (1980) also found a significant negative correlation between the strictness of state gun control laws and state suicide rates (the more strict the state law, the lower the state suicide rate). However, Rich, Young, Fowler, Wagner, and Black (1990) reported that any decrease in suicide by firearms may be offset by an increase in other methods. Interestingly, firearm suicide rates are highest in the Mountain region of the United States, but firearm prevalence is highest in the East South Central region (the Mountain region ranks second).

Guns are used in the majority of homicides and suicides. However, what is surprising is that the incidence of suicidal death by firearms is roughly 50% greater than that of homicidal death by firearms. In contrast to the high frequency with which guns are used in suicides and homicides, less than 2% of all accidental deaths in the United States are attributable to firearms. Thus, coroners and medical examiners tend to assume that a self-inflicted gunshot wound death was intentional. One exception to this rule, as noted previously, may be Russian roulette death, which commonly is "played" by a young male in front of others, while under the influence of alcohol or drugs (Fishbain et al., 1987). Several physical cues can give evidence of self-inflicted, intended death (i.e., suicide) by firearm. In Litman's (1989) review of 500 psychological autopsies, the type of wound and observations regarding the weapon were significant factors in 88% of those cases determined to be suicides, but none of the accidental firearm deaths. Among the factors considered were the following:

1. The location of the wound
2. The proximity of the weapon to the wound
3. The accessibility of the wound location
4. Ipsilaterality of the wound location to handedness
5. Trace metal residue on hand
6. Single wound
7. Removal of clothing

Wound Location

An individual intent on suicide by gunshot tends to aim the weapon at close range at a vital site, generally the head. Eisele, Reay, and Cook (1981), reporting on 223 firearm suicides, found that 75% of wound sites were in the head (see Figure 12.1), the majority of these (and 39% of the total) were to the right temporal region, consistent with most people being right-

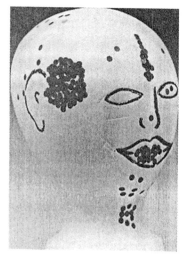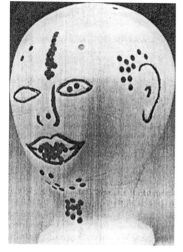

FIGURE 12.1. Approximate locations of 175 head and neck suicidal gunshot wounds. *Source:* Eisele, Reay, & Cook (1981: 48). Copyright 1981 by ASTM. Reprinted by permission.

handed. Nine percent of the total were to the chest-precordium area, 9% to the mouth, 5% to the left temporal area of the head, and 4% each to the neck and abdomen. Only 2 of 175 head and neck wounds were to the eyes. Males, who overwhelmingly comprise those who suicide by firearms, also are more likely than females to choose a more lethal wound site, such as the head. As noted earlier in this chapter, females' greater concern for possible disfigurement (although some may see this as a sexist comment) may account for their lowered lethality, even when using equally lethal means such as guns for suicide (Eisele et al., 1981); however, see Stone (1987: 714), who claims that both men and women prefer suicidal sites in the head, followed by the chest as the second most common site.

Proximity

Perhaps the "smoking gun" clue to a suicidal gunshot wound is evidence that the weapon was held proximate to or in contact with the wound site. Signs of contact would include residue (gunpowder stippling and/or soot, etc., at the wound entrance) singed hair, or the occasional impression of the outline of the gun barrel on the skin (DiMaio, 1999). The absence of residue "is a red light which warns of foul play" (Barnes & Helson, 1974).

Contact wounds are less likely in accidents or homicides, although some execution-style homicides involve contact or near contact wounds. Also, not all self-inflicted contact wounds are suicidal (cf. Adelson, 1974: 312). For example, Russian roulette deaths usually involve contact wounds.

Accessibility

An individual intent on suicide has little reason to be a contortionist. Suicidal wound sites are usually within easy reach. Few circumstances will allow a self-controlled range of more than 28 inches (or the length of the victim's arm) between muzzle and wound, unless some contraption specifically designed for such a purpose is used (Spitz & Fisher, 1980). One exception to this is the long-barrelled gunshot death accomplished by a toe-pulled trigger.

Ipsilaterality

The victim's right- or left-handedness is related to the possible range of fire. Suicide victims have a strong preference for ipsilateral wound sites (i.e., those located on or affecting the same side of the body as the dominant hand). In one study (Eisele et al., 1981) only 8% of right-handed suicides shot themselves on the contralateral side. All the left-handed victims' wounds were ipsilateral.

Residue

Firearm residue (e.g., primer trace amounts of antimony or barium) is often found deposited on the firing hand of the person who has discharged a gun (DiMaio, 1999, Ch. 12). However, not all weapons leave trace metals. In one study, positive residue tests for barium or antimony on the hand were found only 38% of the time, even when it was known by other evidence that the individual had in fact fired the gun (Reed, McGuire, & Boehm, 1990).

Single Wound

The overwhelming majority of suicidal gunshot wounds result from single shots. Multiple wounds have been found in roughly 1% of completed suicides, the majority of these involving .22 caliber handguns. These are low-energy weapons that may need a second shot to effect a mortal wound (Eisele et al., 1981). However, in our forensic cases it is not unheard of for a suicide to fire a gun once or twice into a nearby wall, ceiling, mattress, and so on, before firing a lethal head shot. This behavior may be related to getting one's courage up, hesitation, or "practice."

Removal of Clothing

Finally, on occasion suicide victims remove or reposition clothing away from the intended wound site.

Ingestion of Drugs

The drugs most often prescribed by psychiatrists to treat mental disorders (especially the tricyclic or tetracyclic antidepressants; the more recently developed selective serotonin reuptake inhibitors—such as Prozac, Paxil, and Zoloft—are much safer in overdose than the more sedating tricyclics) are those most used by our patients to attempt suicide. Among adolescents, drug overdoses may account for as much as 90% of parasuicidal behaviors treated in the hospital emergency room, with the great majority of these being of low lethality (cf, Garfinkel, Froese, & Hood, 1982).

Antidepressant overdoses are not all the same. Within the same class of drugs, symptom presentations may differ depending on the level of overdose. Tricyclic agents taken in doses greater than 1 gram, for example, will cause mild symptoms such as sinus tachycardia, increased tendon reflexes, extensor plantar responses, drowsiness, and delerium. Dosages over 2 grams, however, will produce severe consequences such as convulsion, coma, shock, respiratory depression, and abnormal electroencephalograms (EEGs) (Gallant, 1987). Signs of monoamine oxidase inhibitor overdose (anxiety, sweating, excitement, hyperventilation, and tachycardia) may not appear for 6 to 12 hours (Gallant, 1987).

It is common for overdose cases to present with symptoms of multiple drug overdose (including alcohol or drugs). In a study at the Massachusetts General Hospital (Wilens, Stern, & O'Gara, 1990), 75% of cases consecutively admitted to intensive care for tricyclic overdose had ingested other agents as well. Particularly when this combination included a neuroleptic, there was a markedly increased risk for conduction delays, ventricular arrhythmias, and cardiac-associated death. Similarly, trazadone (Desyrel), a relatively nonlethal tricyclic antidepressant even when taken in large doses, is potentially fatal when taken in combination with other drugs or alcohol (Gamble & Peterson, 1986). Racial differences have been noted in the use of analgesics, with whites being more likely to use prescribed propoxyphene (Darvon) and nonwhites, codeine obtained illicitly (Nelson, Litman, & Diller, 1983).

Illicit drug abusers have high rates of completed suicide (Grinspoon, 1986). Abusers who suicide are typically between 20 and 40 years old, male, multiple drug abusers (including concurrent alcohol abuse—Roy and Linnoila [1986] found that the typical alcoholic suicide had a mean age of 47 years and, on average, had been alcoholic for 25 years) and have comorbid diagnoses of depression, borderline personality disorder, or psychosis (Marzuk & Mann, 1988). When over-the-counter drugs are used, salicylates and acetaminophen are most commonly taken, the latter having the potential to have high lethality due to liver damage.

The great majority of nonfatal overdoses are with low suicide intent, low lethality, impulsive behaviors made by adolescent and young adult females, typically in response to conflict in their family or in an important relationship. Self-reported intent to die is generally much higher than that assessed by clinicians in these cases. Clinicians tend to believe the majority of these parasuicides are manipulative or punitive in intent (Hawton, Cole, O'-Grady, & Osborn, 1982). Similarly, significant others interpret the intent of the self-poisoner quite differently from what is reported as intended by the self-poisoner themself (James & Hawton, 1985) (see Box 12.2).

Hanging, Strangulation

Hanging is the second most frequent method of suicide in the United States, and, as noted earlier, is much more common worldwide. In the only known systematic review of deaths by hanging, Bowen (1982) noted that 155 of 201 cases (77%) occurring in North West London between 1956 and 1980 were suicides. Accidental hanging is rare, being comprised essentially of three types: children under the age of 2 who may strangle if caught in their own clothing or by attachments to their cribs, the experimenter (e.g., imitating others or recklessly using ropes), and the autoerotic (see Chapter 6).

Death by hanging generally is due to the compression or constriction of the neck which either obstructs the blood flow in the arteries of the neck, blocks the windpipe, or causes cardiac arrest. The resulting interference in the uptake or utilization of oxygen, together with the failure to eliminate carbon dioxide produces a subnormal level of oxygen in the blood supply. Loss of consciousness occurs virtually instantaneously. Complete arterial occlusion may occur even when the victim is sitting, kneeling, or in a lying position (Camps, 1976), as the tension on the rope needs only to be 7 to 8 pounds to block the carotid arteries (Picton, 1971). In 4 or 5 minutes, anoxic brain damage or death results (which makes hospital or jail 15-minute suicide watches not very effective). Prisoners in cells often tie or wear a piece of an undershirt (perhaps tearing off a tee shirt, pulling it over their head and affixing an arm hole to a door knob), a shoelace, a pants belt, a robe belt, a laundry bag string, and so on around a cell bar and their neck and then just lean forward while sitting or kneeling. Inpatient psychiatric patients may do much the same thing by using a door knob, a knot in a cloth from a door jamb, an overhead sprinkler pipe, and so forth. In one case a

---

BOX 12.2. Do People Who Take an Overdose Wish to Die?

Yes: Bancroft et al. (1979).

No: Bancroft et al. (1979).

Issue Summary:

The aim of this study was to clarify spontaneously offered reasons why parasuicides take overdoses and to compare these reasons with those ascribed by psychiatric judges. Forty-one patients who had been admitted to a hospital after a deliberate self-poisoning were interviewed and asked what their intent for death was. Psychiatrist judges were given both a transcript and recording of the interview and asked to make an assessment of suicide intent based on the Beck Suicide Intent Scale.

Almost all the patients spontaneously expressed that their overdose was motivated by a wish to die. In contrast, the psychiatrists judged only 12 patients (29%) to have suicide intent, more commonly ascribing reasons for overdose as "to frighten" or "to influence someone." *The patients never reported such reasons.* The researchers concluded that there was a tendency for self-poisoners to deny socially unacceptable reasons for overdose or that there was a tendency for others to mistakenly attribute them.

patient swallowed three cellophane-wrapped dinner rolls (which effectively countered CPR). In another case an electric bed was lowered onto the patient's neck, which was resting on the bed frame.

Jumping

Depending on the surface landed on, blunt-force trauma resulting from the impact of a fall or jump from heights greater than a few stories generally are lethal. In one series of cases reported by Lewis, Lee, and Grantham (1965), 4 of 11 people who jumped from four stories survived, but only 1 in 10 survived a jump from as high as six stories. Of course, should impact be blunted or cushioned in some way (e.g., by an awning), survival from even greater heights is possible. The survival rate for those who have jumped from the Golden Gate Bridge is 2%. The record height from which a jump from a bridge has been survived is 250 feet by a 24-year-old female in England (Lucas, Hutton, & Lim, 1981). Every city, state, and country has its "favorite" jump site: a bridge (e.g., the Golden Gate Bridge in San Francisco), a tower (e.g., the Eiffel Tower in Paris), or a building (e.g., the Empire State Building in New York; see Figure 12.2). Mount Mishara, in Japan, is reputed to be the most frequently chosen jump site in the world.

In the United States there are almost equal numbers of deaths by jumping from high places as there are falls. Thus, there is no a priori hypothesis regarding the manner of death in an unwitnessed fall or jump. The majority of jumpers are males (Prasad & Lloyd, 1983; Cantor, Hill, & McLachlan, 1989), who leaped from residential premises (e.g., apartment

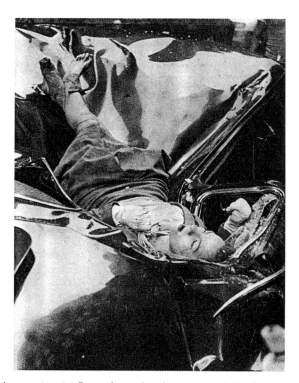

FIGURE 12.2. After plummeting 86 floors from the observation deck of the Empire State Building—visible in the metallic reflection at lower left—this young woman lies dead, the victim of suicide. *Source:* Despelder & Strickland (1996: 454). Photo © Robert C. Wiles.

buildings; apartment jumpers being disproportionately elderly males: Copeland, 1989) or other man-made structures (e.g., bridges), rather than natural sites. Younger jumpers often have psychiatric histories (Prasad & Lloyd, 1983) with reports of higher than expected rates of psychotic depression and/or schizophrenia (Cantor et al., 1989; Pounder, 1985; Salmons, 1984).

Kreuger and Hutcherson (1978) have provided evidence that some accidental falls are disguised suicides. Conducting interviews with survivors of rock-climbing falls, they reported that some decisions to suicide are impulsively made by climbers, who in addition to masking their intent thought they could achieve a heroic death in this manner (cf. Klausner, 1968).

Generally, jumpers leave evidence of their suicidal intent. For example, they may have no other reason to be at the site, have no history of reckless disregard for heights, or will leave valuables or folded clothing at the jump site. Also, there are typical distinguishing features of suicidal jumps (vs. accidental falls). For example, Girard et al. (1980) have noted that the typical suicide attempt involves a feet-first, vertical leap with relaxed muscles. Cooper (1973) has noted that jumpers can only jump as far out in the air as they could have jumped on the ground. Thus, a body found 30 feet from the base of a skyscraper would have had to be propelled by some external force. In spite of this, individuals high on PCP or LSD have been known to believe, and to attempt to prove, they could fly like Superman. When a jump occurs from a bridge into water and the force of impact is sufficient to render the individual unconscious or so restrain the individual's ability for self-rescue, the consequent death would be due to jumping (as opposed to drowning).

Gas and Vapors

Carbon monoxide has an affinity for hemoglobin in red blood cells. It binds with hemoglobin (producing carboxyhemoglobin), forcing out oxygen from these cells, producing a sort of internal asphyxia or tissue hypoxia (Picton, 1971). Carboxyhemoglobin causes the skin to turn a cherry red or bright pink. In Europe, carbon monoxide asphyxiation by home heating gas has been a common method of suicide. In the United States, the favored delivery system has been the automobile. In each, the environment must be sealed, keeping the gas within a closed space (e.g., a flat or a garage). Often, the decedent will have directed the fumes, for example, from an exhaust pipe directly into the interior of a car by a tube or vacuum cleaner hose attached to the muffler. As unconsciousness precedes death, carbon monoxide (CO) poisoning is presumed to be a painless method of suicide. This may be a significant factor in explaining the prevalence of this method in clusters of suicide among adolescents, as occurred in the 1980s in Plano, Texas (Coleman, 1987) and Bergenfield, New Jersey (Clarke & Lester, 1991). On inhalation of high concentrations of CO, saturation of the blood proceeds so rapidly that unconsciousness may occur suddenly and without warning.

Most of the literature on CO suicide has focused on this method from the perspective of prevention. In a series of studies Clarke, Lester, and their colleagues (Clarke & Mayhew, 1989; Clarke & Lester, 1987; Lester & Frank, 1989) have examined primarily the effect of detoxification of gas in homes (i.e., the conversion from domestic to natural gas) in England and Wales and changes in emission control laws for automobile exhaust in the United States. These changes have allowed for natural clinical trial experiments (pre- vs. posttoxicity) to examine consequent changes in the incidence of suicide using CO poisoning and in shifts to other alternative lethal methods.

Clarke and Mayhew (cited in Clarke & Lester, 1989) reported that as the level of CO was reduced to less than 1% in domestic gas in England and Wales between 1960 and 1976, suicides by gas decreased from 50% to 0.2% with no appreciable shift to other methods. However, in Scotland there was an increase in other methods during the years of detoxification.

After passage of emission-control standards for levels of CO in car exhaust in the United States, Lester and Frank (1989) found that rates of suicide by vehicular CO were lower in states in which car ownership and emissions toxicity were also lower. In addition, they reported that whites, females, white females, and the young were more at risk for CO suicides; which peaked in the winter months. In the United States, probably slightly under half of all CO deaths are intentional. In recent years there has been a decrease in unintentional CO deaths (Cobb & Etzel, 1991).

Cutting/Stabbing

As noted earlier, cutting and stabbing are uncommon methods for completed suicide but often are found in nonfatal attempts, in parasuicidal behaviors, and especially in self-mutilative acts (see Favazza, 1996). Suicidal deaths by cutting or stabbing have several descriptive characteristics. There are common wound sites (typically the neck, wrists, or chest), accessible to and consistent in the direction of penetration; the presence of multiple (repeated) penetrations; wounds made on bare skin rather than through clothing; the presence of hesitation marks; and the absence of other injuries and defense wounds (e.g., if one had been warding off an attacker, there typically would be cuts on the exterior surface of the forearm, hands, or fingers) (cf. Adelson, 1974; Camps, 1976; Spitz & Fisher, 1980). In addition, cutting is painful and does not lead to a quick demise. Thus, some suicides begin by cutting then switch to other methods, preferring not to wait to bleed to death. In contrast, many psychotic self-mutilators report feeling anesthetized (i.e., without pain) or even euphoric (Favazza, 1996).

Hesitation marks are trademarks of suicidal cutting. They are often found when death is due to some other method. These tentative "sawings" of the skin (multiple, superficial, parallel cuts of variable depth) may represent first tests of "courage" made by the suicidal individual. When found on the throat, they usually are on the side opposite that of the hand used to hold the incising instrument. Wrist cuts are usually found on the flexor surface of the wrist, opposite the dominant hand, and have systematic patterns. Horizontal cuts are typical; vertical cuts are rare (Adelson, 1974; Spitz & Fisher, 1980). One reason why wrist slashing is more common as a parasuicidal behavior (even when intent is high) is that wrist slashers have a tendency to turn their wrists outward, unknowingly protecting the very arteries they wished to cut (Cooper, 1973). Similarly, when the neck is cut, the victim has a tendency to throw his or her head back, causing the arteries and veins to be thrust back into the shelter of the windpipe. If death occurs, it is usually from slow bleeding of the tissues, complicated by asphyxia (Picton, 1971).

In Marks's (1977) study of sex differences in method preferences among college students, cutting was said to be the least acceptable method of suicide for men. Yet, in fact, among suicidal cutters (in contrast to the more impulse-driven, delicate wrist cutting by chronic nonfatal self-mutilaters), the prevalence rate of males approaches that of females.

Drowning

An unwitnessed drowning usually provides no clear evidence for determining how a body came to be in the water (Atkinson, 1978). After immersion, the recovered body will show few external signs of the manner of death. Internally, there will be evidence of anoxia, pulmonary congestion, and massive pulmonary edema which produces a white froth externally at the mouth and nose (Hendrix, 1972). Whereas drowning in fresh water occurs after approximately 4 minutes of immersion, in salt water drowning may take up to 8 minutes. This is due to differences between salt and fresh water in both osmotic pressure and the consequent fluid transfer in the blood plasma (Picton, 1971).

Overall, the great majority of deaths by drowning are accidents. The annual incidence of unintentional drownings in the United States averages about 10 times that of intentional drownings. In suicidal drownings, the medical examiner might look for signs of inappropriate dress, nonhazardous swimming conditions, or shallow water where self-rescue easily could have been accomplished. Thus, for example, adult drownings in bathtubs are usually first assumed to be suicidal *mutadis mutandis*.

Self-Immolation

Suicide by burning (self-immolation) is rare in the United States. But because it tends to be public behavior, it may receive undo media attention. This publicity may, in turn, lead to imitative behavior (see Zemishlany, 1987).

There appear to be three basic types of self-immolation suicides:

1. *Suttee (Sati)* is a Hindu custom of widow burning on the husband's funeral pyre. Historically, the needs of women in the patriarchy of the Hindu family were subordinated. Also, in British law, the wife was considered part of the husband's property. When widowed, remarriage was prohibited and celibacy was required. It was considered a courageous and noble act (an altruistic suicide) for the widow to escape this enforced life of misery by throwing herself on her husband's funeral pyre. Although declared illegal in India in 1829 (after as many as 2,300 Sati suicides in one year) isolated cases still occur (Inamdar, Oberfield, & Darrell, 1983). Indian women with insufficient dowries for marriage are sometimes mysteriously burned.

2. *Political protest* suicides by burning took place with some frequency in the United States during the 1960s in response to the war in Vietnam. In 1963 a Buddhist monk, Thich Quang Doc, publicly burned himself to death in Saigon. At least seven other monks followed this model that year in protest of the Diem regime. Reviewing cases publicized in the *New York Times* and the *London Times*, Crosby, Rhee, and Holland (1973) found almost 100 other cases of self-immolation reported between 1963 and 1971, almost all of which were meant as political protests. In an era of political volatility, these suicides were often by members of religious antiwar groups.

3. *Psychiatric* cases of self-immolation make up the bulk of the other burning suicides. The typical non-political protest burning appears to be by a mentally disordered, rigidly religious person who uses an easily available method (matches, lighters, and, perhaps, a flammable liquid) on impulse. Several case reports of suicide immolation in the literature (Andreasen & Noyes, 1975; Jacobson, Jackson, & Berkowitz, 1986; Scully & Hutcherson, 1983; Stoddard, Pahlavan, & Cahners, 1985) reflect individuals evidencing disturbed, often schizophrenic thought, impaired judgment, frequent histories of prior attempt, psychiatric treatment, and family psychopathology. One case reports a cluster of seven members of a religious cult who doused themselves with kerosene on a beach after the death of their leader (Takahashi, 1989).

Vehicular Suicide

Curren, McGarry, and Petty (1980) determined that over a 15-year period in the Miami area, 12 deaths of pedestrians run over by motor vehicles were in fact suicides (less than 0.5% of all suicides). However, the automobile, both ubiquitous and lethal in modern society, may be used for suicide in more cases than we can readily identify. The automobile, a symbol of power and speed, may hold special appeal to a depressed, helpless person. Some, especially those of a psychoanalytic persuasion, believe that some accident-certified vehicular fatalities in fact are suicides. For example, Litman and Tabachnick (1967) suggested that so-called vehicular accidents are often the result of immature management of hostile or angry feelings, poor stress tolerance, inner conflict, and interpersonal difficulties, and that accidents may be counterdepressive or counterphobic. However, empirical investigations of single-car, single-driver accidents have not been able to document that these factors lead to any significant use of the automobile as a method of suicide.

Schmidt, Shaffer, Zlotowitz, and Fisher (1977) investigated 182 single-car fatalities in Baltimore County over a 7-year period, finding only 3 to be possible suicides. In these three cases the drivers hit a fixed object, showed no evidence of having taken evasive action to prevent the accident, and drove cars with no mechanical defects. Murphy, Gatner, Wetzel, Katz, and Ernst (1974) could not document any of 24 single-vehicle deaths they studied to be suicides, nor could Tabachnick (1973), in a comparative study of 24 accident victims. In a more recent report, Connolly, Cullen, and McTigue (1995) "suspected" suicide in only 4.5% of 134 reexamined single road traffic deaths in County Mayo, Ireland.

Still, there is little question that vehicular suicides do occur and that personality factors can play a significant role in many accidents which occur under conditions of precipitant stress and excessive drinking. For example, individuals with personality disorders may be more likely than others to drive cars with mechanical defects (e.g., faulty brakes), which in turn causes their accidents. Huffine (1971) documented significant differences between single- and multivehicle accidents, which suggest that some of the former may have been suicides. In the former, drivers were more likely to have been males, white-collar workers, who had been drinking and driving at excessive speeds more often in good weather.

SUMMARY AND CONCLUSIONS

In this chapter we presented an overview and analysis of nonfatal suicide attempts and methods. The method chosen to carry out a suicidal behavior is, in part, determined by the individual's intent; that is, more lethal methods are chosen by those intent on dying. The method chosen also determines in part whether an individual will die as a consequence of its use; for example, adolescents intent on dying may not have sufficient knowledge or understanding of what amount of a particular drug will produce an overdose death. Thus, our understanding of suicide methods can teach us a great deal about suicidal individuals and the likely and intended consequences of their acts.

Most important, the more we can understand what determines the choice of suicide methods and the methods' relative lethality, the more we learn how to prevent suicide. A core concept in suicide prevention is that thwarting access to lethal methods, reducing lethality of methods, and so on (cf. Chapter 21), can be life saving.

The study of suicide methods, thus, is the study of a synergy between the means or mechanisms and the person who uses them. We now turn our attention to better understanding the suicidal person, specifically the relationship between suicide and mental disorders, which are so common to the suicidal condition.

FURTHER READING

Card, J. J. (1974). Lethality of suicide methods and suicide risk: Two distinct concepts. *Omega*, 5, 37–45. An older, but classic study, the first that attempted to establish the probability of death resulting from various methods of self-inflicted harm. Card also attempted in this study to follow up nonfatal attempters to determine the risk of completed suicide as a function of method used in the nonfatal attempt.

Maris, R. W. (1981). *Pathways to suicide: A survey of self-destructive behaviors*. Baltimore: Johns Hopkins University Press. Maris presents extensive interview data regarding a group of completed suicides in Cook County, Illinois, a group of nonfatal suicide attempters, and a group of natural deaths, both from Baltimore, Maryland. Multivariate analyses of hundreds of study variables produced an invaluable understanding of how these groups differ and led Maris to develop the concept that life histories are central to our understanding of completed suicide.

McIntosh, J. L. (1992). Methods of suicide. In R. W. Maris, A. L. Berman, J. T. Maltsberger, & R. I. Yufit (Eds.), *Assessment and prediction of suicide* (pp. 381–397). New York: Guilford Press. A nice summary of methods of suicide (lethality and factors affecting choice) and demographic characteristics (age, sex, and ethnicity) of those who select various methods for suicide.

National Center for Health Statistics (NCHS). (various years). *Vital statistics of the United States, mortality*. Washington, DC: U.S. Government Printing Office. The NCHS annually compiles and publishes mortality statistics for the United States. Included in these figures are data for suicide methods by age, sex, and race of suicide victim. These data are subject to a number of error factors but are considered the best available measures of completed suicide. Most important, temporal trends can be monitored with minimal concern that any sources of error will vary substantially from year to year.

Smith, K., Conroy, R. W., & Ehler, B. D. (1984). Lethality of suicide attempt rating scale. *Suicide and Life-Threatening Behavior, 14,* 215–242. Smith et al. developed an 11-point rating scale to assess the life threat posed by method used and circumstances of method usage (e.g., rescuability) in suicide attempts. This scale has value for clinicians to evaluate the lethality of both past attempts and current planned attempts among patients.

Weisman, A. & Worden, W. J. (1974). Risk–rescue rating in suicide assessment. In A. T. Beck, H. L. P. Resnik, & D. J. Lettieri (Eds.), *The prediction of suicide* (pp. 193–213). Bowie, MD: Charles Press. Weissman and Worden introduced the concept of rescuability into the literature of suicidology. Their effort established the importance of context in understanding suicide attempts and methods used.

PART III

MEDICAL AND PSYCHIATRIC ISSUES

13

Psychiatric Diagnoses and Suicidal Acts

Bryan L. Tanney

Extreme melancholia
Lunatic behavior
Depraved disposition
　　　—Premonitory and diagnostic signs of suicide, Sym (1637)

First, the diagnosis of mental illness is far from an exact science. . . . The requirement that mental illness not only be present but in addition be the cause of the dangerousness only compounds the difficulty, since the causal element may be difficult to establish even when it is possible to achieve consensus as to the presence of mental illness.
　　　—David F. Greenberg

The impact of mental ill health on the likelihood of suicidal behavior has long been a topic for reflection and discussion. Yet commentaries about etiology had little apparent impact as society's views of the act changed over the centuries through varying responses, from vilification, to acceptance, to even praise. By the late 1700s, there was a reemerging recognition that suicide might be a behavior of choice by an individual. In a renaissance of Greco-Roman beliefs, John Donne and others argued for the rationality of suicide (see Chapter 4). On the other side of this argument was a belief that the choice was misguided: either an irresponsible choice or one for which a person could not be made responsible. The latter view regarded the act as deviant and generated explanations such as "lunacy" or "madness." By the 19th century, for economic and political reasons, society had arrived at a belief in the value of each individual, though, curiously, without allowing free choice and autonomy. With this perspective, it became important to save individual lives and to make prevention of suicide an active focus for helpers of others. Persons at risk were offered places in "asylums" and, later, treatments were pressed on them. Their fellow inmates were not criminals or the poor and disadvantaged but mentally ill persons.

By the turn of the 20th century, those alienists who treated the aberrant, deviant, and ill had become psychiatrists and part of their domain was the treatment and prevention of mental illness, now including suicide. Beyond treatment, there were the beginnings of efforts to address prevention. These efforts focused on understanding the origins of psychopathology and then interrupting the causal pathways. Modern "scientific medicine" observed and classified, recognized the heterogeneity of mental disease, and began the search for specific and efficacious interventions. Suicide among asylum inmates became a focus for some of these investigations. It was only a short step for suicide (and suicidal behavior that was nonfatal) to be defined as a complication of mental disease. After all, everyone who was suicidal was in the asylum, the place where mentally ill persons resided. The study of suicide in some but not all mentally ill patients led to a half-century of brilliant, individual case studies in which the progress and process toward suicide was uncovered and analyzed. The driving theoretical model was Freudian psychoanalytic theory. Midway through the 20th century, virtually all our understanding of suicide and suicidal behaviors was based on the inner psychic mechanisms of persons who also had mental diseases. Today, we recognize this as a classic example of selection bias, shown by the tautology: Everyone who commits suicide must be mentally disordered because only suicidal people with mental disease had been the focus of examination and study.

Though we acknowledge problems inherent in that early selection bias, in this chapter we propose to examine and present evidence concerning the amount, type, and nature of the associations between suicide and mental diseases. Issues of the heterogeneity of suicidal acts and of the classification of both suicide and mental illnesses further complicate the subject matter to be examined. Individual case studies are now extremely rare, despite the considerable value of this ideographic approach. Knowledge is now derived from new methodologies. These new tools are given an overview and their results laid bare. Several mechanisms are proposed to explain these results, but our knowledge is incomplete and the proposed associations remain largely speculative. Three substantive reviews (Miles, 1977; Tanney, 1992; Harris & Barraclough, 1997) as well as summaries (Goldney, Positano, Spence, & Rosenman, 1985; Hirschfeld & Davidson, 1988) are recommended for those who wish to explore this evidence in fuller detail.

FRAMEWORKS FOR UNDERSTANDING

Mental Disease

There is no agreed-on definition of "Mental Infirmity" beyond a general statement that it reflects the absence of mental health. It is, however, significantly more than a "disorder of living." In all definitions, there must be a substantive impairment of one or several of the mental faculties of perception, thinking, feeling, behavior, or the physiological, neurological systems linked to these brain activities. Despite the fuzzy boundaries, there is substantial agreement that distinct and recognizable entities are present. Figure 13.1 illustrates the hierarchical structure of diagnosis, first identifying signs and symptoms, the syndromes, the disorders, and finally illnesses (diseases). The two most widely used systems for labeling and identifying mental difficulties have focused on different levels of organization (Table 13.1).

symptoms and/or signs
cluster into
clinically recognizable **syndromes**
that, when they impair normal functioning, are
disorders (dysfunctions)
and when causative mechanisms and natural history are known become
diseases/illnesses

FIGURE 13.1. Relationships of clinical observations in mental illness/disorder.

TABLE 13.1. Comparing Two Labeling Systems for Mental Illness/ Disorder

Item	International Classification of Diseases —Clinical Modification (CM)	Diagnostic and Statistical Manual of Mental Disorders
Current version	X (ten)	IV (four)
Sponsoring body	World Health Organization	American Psychiatric Association
Unit of study	Disorder–disease	Syndrome–disorder
Framework	Historical Pathophysiological	Multiaxial (five) Hierarchical
Suicidal acts	No entry	Not included *or* no entry
Mention of suicidal acts	Included in E codes ("due to . . .")	Symptom/sign in two disorders

The American Psychiatric Association system with its focus on disorders suggests the ongoing search by biomedicine for some structural abnormality as the organizing principle for mental problems (American Psychiatric Association, 1994). An alternative for this system might have considered the term "dysfunction" with its implication of disordered processes and not structures. The World Health Organization (WHO) system uses the term "disease" and considers mental difficulties in the same way as it does all illnesses in its body system or anatomy-based classification. With this clear biomedical approach, the International Classification of Diseases (ICD) expects that such parameters as etiology, pathology, course of illness, treatments, and complications can be specified for each disease (World Health Organization [WHO], 1992). Both systems have undergone numerous elaborations, and there are translations across the two systems in the form of the *Clinical Modification* of the *International Classification of Diseases* (Practice Management Information Corporation, 1992). It is important to recognize that most public health and epidemiology investigators use the WHO-sponsored system whereas most psychiatric and mental health clinicians employ the system based on the American Psychiatric Association's *Diagnostic and Statistical Manual of Mental Disorders,* or DSM. No useful or functional system based on pathology or on neurophysiological/neuropharamacological mechanisms has yet been proposed. Aware of the difficulties about naming, we use the term psychiatric diagnosis whenever possible to replace, or as a synonym for, either mental disorder or disease. This is done with the understanding that not all persons with such difficulties have had or will need the involvement of the specific professional discipline of psychiatry.

Reliability of diagnoses among trained clinicians is quite good, and is improved even further by the availability of structured interview schedules (e.g., Diagnostic Interview Schedule, Schedule for Affective Disorders and Schizophrenia, a simplified version of some DSM-IV diagnostic criteria called PRIME-MD, and the Present State Examination). In discussions of suicide, the DSM-III, DSM-III-R, and DSM-IV systems have an acknowledged problem. The diagnostic distinctions within the group of mood or affective disorders are still evolving in DSM because it is a cross-sectional diagnostic framework and many useful distinctions between mood disorders appear to be based on a longitudinal perspective involving order, recurrence, and timing of episodes. This unfinished business is important because mood disorders are believed to have a significant impact on persons at risk of self-harm. Later in this chapter, specific issues about the relationship between suicide and subtypes of mood disorders and between suicide and different features of these disorders such as severity, timing, and particular symptoms are presented. In its favor, the DSM system offers the possibility of making multiple diagnoses concurrently and historically along each of three independent axes. This allows for the possibility of coexisting or comorbid disorders, and we will see later that such occurrences are an important feature in the relationships between mental disorders and suicidal acts.

Suicidal Acts/Behaviors

The failure to establish a standard nomenclature for self-harming acts or behaviors remains a gigantic stumbling block to furthering our understanding. In this chapter, suicidal "acts" and "behaviors" are used interchangeably to include, at an operational level, both completed suicides and nonfatal suicidal behaviors, with the latter encompassing instrumental suicide-related behaviors, suicide attempts, and significant suicide ideation (O'Carroll et al., 1996). Although addressed elsewhere in this text, several issues of importance to our study of the linkages of mental disorders to these behaviors are reiterated here.

To some degree, completed suicides are underreported, and there are even significant doubts about the reliability of some of these adjudications. Specifying suicide as the mode of death rather than the other commonly used categories of natural, accidental, homicide, or undetermined, is a decision made by a medical examiner or coroner. In a large number of such determinations, wide variations in "diagnostic" criteria are recognized (Jobes, Casey, Berman, & Wright, 1991). Some authorities even insist on the presence of mental disorder before confirming suicide as a cause of death. Accurately identifying other acts of deliberate self-harm is even more difficult. The majority of persons who self-harm never reach medical care facilities, making it inappropriate to use hospital discharge data as a measure of the frequency of such behaviors in the general community. Various authors have suggested that more than three-quarters of actual acts of self-harm remain uncounted when we use medical care data bases (Meehan, Lamb, Saltzman, & O'Carroll, 1992). Community surveys have indicated that rates as high as 100 nonfatal suicidal behaviors for each completed suicide are feasible. In our efforts to establish associations to mental disorders, it is critical to realize that data about populations of persons who have performed suicidal acts are an incomplete sampling. (See also Box 13.1.)

A second major issue involves the relationship between different types of self-harm behaviors (Linehan, 1986). Beginning with David Rosen (1970), and most recently with Vietra (Vietra, Nieto, Gasto, & Cirera, 1992) and Beautrais et al. (1996), persons who have survived suicide attempts of high medical lethality have been used as close approximations of persons who complete suicide. Within these studies we find a clear assumption of a continuum or overlap between the two populations. Although there is agreement that overlap exists between the populations of completed and of all nonfatal suicidal acts, whatever their medical severity, the magnitude of this overlap remains controversial. It is usually estimated at 40 to 55% (i.e., about one-half of persons completing suicide will have a history of prior suicidal behavior; see Chapter 12). At present, it appears most prudent to separate the two

---

BOX 13.1. The Problem of Biased Sampling

Diagnosis is a clinical process requiring experienced mental health personnel, but many persons at risk of suicide never have such contact. As a result, much of the evidence for relationships between diagnoses and suicide are based on the limited subsample of those seeking or arriving for psychological/psychiatric assessment. Various estimates suggest that this subsample is less than one-third of the total group of persons with mental disorders.

populations and whenever possible to examine the associations of mental disorders to completed and to nonfatal suicidal acts separately. If there are congruencies in the associations, their number and strength may be a useful indication of the amount of overlap between the two populations of suicidal acts.

Finally, we come to the unresolved issue of whether suicide is to be understood from a categorical or a dimensional framework. Most of the literature reviewed in this chapter reflects the idea that suicide and its subsets are best regarded as unique entities that can be defined as present or absent through the use of specified criteria—a categorical approach. This may be only an artifact of measurement, as it was more convenient when examining associations between things if both were categorical for purposes of statistical analysis. Early in this century and partly reflected in Freud's elaboration of a "death instinct," there was a much stronger belief that suicidality might be an aspect of living present in everyone to some greater or lesser degree—a dimensional approach. This view of suicidality as a measurable trait has been reawakened by several important psychiatric groups since the 1980s (Black, Winokur, & Nasrallah, 1987; Mann, Waternaux, Haas, & Malone, 1999; Mehlum, Friis, Vaglum, & Karterud, 1994).

Interactions of the Frameworks for Understanding

The ICD classification does not specify diagnostic criteria for suicide, and suicidal acts and behaviors largely appear as disease modifiers or complications. Two of the DSM disorders (major depressive disorder, borderline personality disorder) include suicidal acts or behaviors and suicide ideation as part of the criteria used in specifying these diagnoses. Again, this illustrates the difficulty in studying the associations between mental disorders and suicidal acts. Friedman, Aronoff, Clarkin, Corn, and Hurt (1983) have demonstrated for borderline personality disorders that the diagnosis can still be made at an equivalent level of certainty even when the diagnostic criterion involving suicide is deleted. This certainly adds more confidence to studies examining this type of personality disorder and suicidal behaviors as independent entities. Several efforts have been proposed for making suicidal acts and behaviors a mental disorder to be included in future versions of DSM, under the category of "Criteria Sets and Axes Provided for Further Study." Table 13.2 suggests some underlying constructs of suicide which might contribute to the criteria used in defining such a disorder.

TABLE 13.2. Possible Defining Criteria: Signs and Symptoms of Suicidal Acts

Readiness
  Stressors (loss, disappointed, psychache)
  Arousal (perturbation, anxiety, anger)
  Lethality (planning and means)

Acceptability
  Hopelessness (constricted problem solving)
  Ambivalence

Supports
  Alone or lonely
  Worthless, guilty
  Invitations to help (help-seeking, help-inducing behaviors)

Failed protections
  Disinhibition (impulsivity, intoxication, aggression)
  Attachments

Such an opportunity would significantly advance our understanding of possible associations by allowing the examination of mental disorders and suicide as independent, although likely co-occurring, entities. At present, without defining criteria, taxonomy, or nomenclature for suicidal acts, the possibility of this occurring remains only faint speculation.

ESTABLISHING THE EXTENT OF THE ASSOCIATIONS BETWEEN MENTAL DISORDERS AND SUICIDAL ACTS

To demonstrate associations, beyond the ideographic studies of the first half of the 20th century, evokes the sciences of epidemiology and statistics and the study of groups of persons for the purpose of uncovering and understanding their commonalities. Specifically, the science of statistics is used to demonstrate that overlaps between populations are not random in origin. For our purposes here, large groups of persons with a specific defined problem (mental disorders or suicidal acts) are selected and then this group is investigated to see how many are also members in a group with the other specified defined problem (suicide attempts or mental disorders). It should be apparent that there will be problems in reliably making such comparisons because of the difficulty of constituting either of these population cohorts with any homogeneity. In fact, these problems of definition were a significant motivation for the development of the third and fourth revisions of the DSM classification of mental disorders.

Table 13.3 summarizes the available techniques for investigating such relationships. Prospective studies involve following persons in either group over time to ascertain if they

TABLE 13.3. Methods for Examining the Relationship between Suicidal Acts and Mental Disorders

Sample	Method	Outcome
I. Prospective studies		
A. General population	Suicide mortality	~1.5–2% annually
B. Clinical populations (28)/ specific disorders (30)	Record linkage to suicide mortality	~4.5% 4–20 × general population (rate = 37–673) (o/e = 9.8)
C. Suicidal acts (1)	Admission to psychiatric case register	—
II. Retrospective studies		
A. Completed suicides (19)	Linkage to psychiatric case register or known psychiatric contact/chart review	29%
B. Suicide attempters/parasuicides (2)	Chart review	70–90% psychiatric history
C. Completed suicides (16)	Follow-back/ "autopsy" study	79–100% mental disorders (median 93%)
III. Concurrent studies		
A. Medically serious acts (2)	Diagnostic interview	90.1% mental disorders (odds ratio = 17.4)
B. Suicide attempters/ parasuicides (9)	Diagnostic interview, questionnaires	91% mental disorders (DSM) 33% diagnoses (ICD)

Note. Numbers of studies in parentheses. Bibliography available from Tanney on request (e-mail: *tanney@calgary.ca*).

BOX 13.2. Temporal Linkages between Suicidal Acts and Psychiatric Diagnoses

There is an obvious, if not commonly invoked, caveat to studies that link suicidal acts and psychiatric diagnosis. In order to impute or assume any associations between the two populations, there must be a reasonable expectation that the event of membership in each group is somehow linked temporally, if not concurrent. It is certainly possible that events of psychiatric diagnosis, and episodes of suicidal acts could be independent occurrences over the lifetime of any person. To demonstrate that both events have occurred during a person's lifetime offers the weakest level of demonstration that there is any association of note between the disorders.

develop membership in the other group. Retrospective or follow-back studies specify a present group and examine their histories to determine whether there has been previous membership in the other group under investigation (Box 13.2).

Various measures from epidemiology and biostatistics are used to establish the degree of overlap between groups. These include, in ascending order of validity, percent of overlap, comparative rates, observed/expected (o/e) ratios (standardized mortality ratios), risk ratio (RR) and odds ratio (OR), and population attributable risk (PAR) calculations. Unfortunately, the fewest number of studies have been done with the most valid measures, with only one example of population attributable risk reported (Beautrais et al., 1996). In this chapter, efforts to utilize Venn diagrams to illustrate potential overlaps were abandoned because of the difference in order of magnitude of the various study populations. For example, completed suicides are as much as 100 times less common than nonfatal suicidal acts, and the yearly prevalence of mental disorders has been estimated at almost 150 times that of the number of nonfatal acts. Not wishing to distort the relative sizes of particular groups led to the decision not to use diagrammatic figures to illustrate such relationships. However, as discussed in the following sections, clear conclusions can be abstracted from the available data.

Prospective Studies

Figure 13.2 extrapolates from 16 studies of clinical psychiatric inpatients with mixed diagnoses to ascertain the proportional mortality by suicide when 100% of the study group have died from all causes. In the general population, suicide mortality is approximately 1.5 to 2% annually. In these clinical populations, 5.4% die by suicide. Measured by rates, ratios, or standardized mortality ratios, there is an excess mortality by suicide in persons with mental disorders variously estimated at 5 to 9.8 times the numbers expected in the general population. Table 13.4 summarizes these studies. It is useful to note that the actual excess of suicide in persons with mental disorders is even larger than indicated by these calculations. One must remember that the expected number of suicides in the general population, or the general population suicide rate, already includes all those persons dying by suicide who have been psychiatric patients. To illustrate, the extrapolated suicide mortality of mental disorder patients from Figure 13.2 is 5.4%. All these persons are also included in the general population mortality by suicide.

If it were possible to remove all those persons who die by suicide and who have had mental disorders from the general population rate, this latter number would be smaller and the ratio of mental disorder patients dying by suicide to general population persons (without mental disorders) dying by suicide would be even larger.

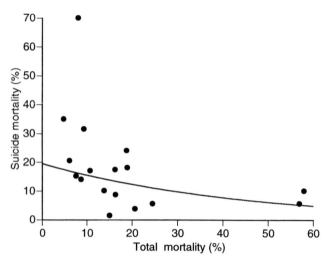

FIGURE 13.2. Proportional mortality by suicide in psychiatric patients. ($y = 3.7027 + 170.71/x$).
Source: Updated from Tanney (1992). Copyright 1992 by The Guilford Press. Adapted by permission.

TABLE 13.4. The Role of Mental Disorders in Suicide: Clinical Populations—Psychiatric Inpatients and Outpatients

Study	Number of suicides	Suicide rate[a]	Risk relative to that of general population
Inpatient only			
Copas & Robin (1982)	375	56 male, 33 female	4.6 times
Hesso (1977)	108	247	
Ritzel (cited in Hesso, 1977)	—	100	
Koester (cited in Hesso, 1977)	—	98	
Outpatient only			
Morrison (1982)	48	120	15 times
Hillard, Ramm, Zung, & Holland (1983)	22	111	
Mixed			
De Graaf (19823)	776	234	19.5 times
Farberow et al. (1971)	650	72	6 times
Evenson, Wood, Nuttall, & Cho (1982)	207	169[b]	5.7 times(males)
		99[b]	10–11 times (female)
Modestin & Hoffmann (1989)	72	209	20 times
	102	452	
Pokorney (1964)	117	165	4.5 times
Ciompi (1976)	107	—	4.7 times
Sletten, Brown, Evenson, & Altman (1972)	97	90	
James & Levin (1964)	75	119	5.3 times
Niskanen, Lönnqvist, & Rinta-Manty (1974)	71	140	
Pokorney (1983)	67 male	279	
Temoche et al. (1964)	66	37	3.9 times
Goldney, Positano, Spence, & Rosenman (1985)	46	222	
Borg & Stahl (1982)	34	—	4.5 times
Bolin, Wright, Wilkinson, & Lindner (1968)	27	177	
Fernando & Storm (1984)	22	333	
Haugland, Craig, Goodman, & Siegel (1983)	12[c]	—	> expected

Note. Bibliography available from Tanney on request (e-mail: *tanney@calgary.ca*).
Source: From Tanney (1992: 286). Copyright 1992 by The Guilford Press. Reprinted by permission.
[a]Per 100,000 patients admitted/treated at risk.
[b]Inpatient subsample only (*n* = 154).
[c]Accidents and suicides.

Retrospective Studies

Completed Suicides

It is feasible to examine the medical care history of persons who complete suicide. These data are much more accessible in countries, such as those in Scandinavia, that maintain a psychiatric case register. It is also possible to diligently search for any known psychiatric contact in local data bases. In 19 studies, some 29% of completed suicides were found to have a previous psychiatric/mental health contact and presumably a psychiatric diagnosis.

In one of the studies, which required being actively involved in mental health contact around the time of their death (past 6 months), only 12% of the community's suicides were connected (Spaulding, 1999). This information is exceedingly difficult to interpret with possibilities for overestimating and underestimating the extent of the relationship. Because we know that a significant number of mentally disordered persons do not seek or receive care from organized help-giving resources, or they receive it from informal or other professional support networks, the available information markedly understates the magnitude of the relationship in question. On the other hand, we do not know how many of those persons included in a psychiatric case register or with some contact had presented with a suicidal act and not necessarily a mental disorder.

It is essential to realize that a person presenting to a psychiatric resource with a suicidal act or behavior must receive a psychiatric diagnosis before discharge. This requirement of health records and demographic data base and financial utilization arbiters will lead to overestimates of the number of persons with psychiatric diagnoses who also have undertaken suicidal acts.

Suicide Attempters/Parasuicides

In general population surveys, persons with a suicide attempt in their lifetime were 2.6 (Canada) and 8.4 (United States) times more likely to also have had a psychiatric disorder at some point in their lives. In clinical studies, 70 to 90% of persons with nonfatal suicidal acts had a previous history of involvement with mental health resources. As discussed in Box 13.2, these lifetime data may inflate the amount of association. For example, an earlier suicidal behavior that resulted in the use of professional helping resources must generate a psychiatric record and diagnosis if mental health resources were accessed. In a retrospective study of the mental health of persons undertaking suicidal acts at some time in the future, this record of earlier involvement may artificially support the association. It has been suggested that data about other episodes of life distress are best used as evidence for the existence of suicidality as an enduring feature or trait in the lives of some individuals. In the U.S. study, it is noteworthy that 6.7% had a history of suicide attempt among all diagnoses and this is less than twice the figure of 2.9–4.3% in the general population.

Follow-Back (Previously Psychological Autopsy) Procedures

Follow-back procedures are interviews or extensive data collections about persons who complete suicide with the intent of establishing the presence and nature of any mental disorder immediately prior to death. Initially, the procedure was likened to an autopsy with its search for the pathology of mortality (Litman, Curphey, Shneidman, Farberow, & Tabachnick, 1963), but more recently an anthropological perspective has been introduced in an effort to acknowledge the multifactorial origins of suicide. These studies report from a diversity of international sites and span youthful, general, and elderly populations of completed suicides. The notable finding is the similarity of results across over four

TABLE 13.5. Frequency of Any Mental Disorder Diagnosis in
Completed Suicide: Data from Psychological Autopsy Studies

Diagnosis	% (median)	Range
Affective disorders	61	39–89
Substance abuse	41	19–63
Anxiety disorders	10	3–27
Schizophrenias	6	0–15.6
Axis II	42	29–57

Note. n = 16. Bibliography available from Tanney on request (e-mail: tanney@calgary.ca).

decades of investigation using this method. A mental disorder diagnosis could be established in almost 90% of the patients using this method (range 81–100). Using all mental disorder diagnoses whenever these have been reported, and not simply the principal diagnosis, Table 13.5 summarizes the different mental disorders reported by these studies. Of the more recent studies, a number have used case-control designs (Brent et al., 1993; Lesage et al., 1994; Shaffer et al., 1996; and Beautrais et al., 1996, whose study used a high lethality behavior population) with a similar conclusion that mental disorders are much more common in the persons who complete suicide than in appropriately selected controls. Lesage found that 37.3% of his early-adult, male case controls achieved a mental disorder diagnosis; Brent, 26.9%; Shaffer, 23%; and Beautrais, 20.4%. These frequencies for youthful populations are slightly or minimally above the usual childhood rates of mental disorder quoted at 17 to 23%. It does not appear that the follow-back method significantly overestimates the presence of disorder.

The methodology has also been challenged as a retrospective reconstruction with significant biases of recall and/or distortion of data. Beskow, Runeson, and Åsgard (1990) have well and capably answered many of these concerns. Shaffer et al. (1996) have allowed that best-estimate diagnoses (BEDs; Leckman, Sholonskas, Thompson, Belanger, & Weissman, 1982) from multiple informants using a nonblind conference realized a diagnosis rate of 91% whereas "parent-only informant" data identified only 59% of these young suicides as having mental disorders. The presence of Axis II diagnoses (personality disorders) in almost half of these suicides is an important finding and all the studies providing Axis II diagnoses acknowledge the extent and importance of Axis I/Axis II comorbidity.

Concurrent Studies: Medically Serious or Help-Seeking Acts

Vietra et al. (1992) and the Canterbury Suicide Project (Beautrais et al., 1996) both interviewed persons who had performed medically serious acts of self-harm, and they reported a high percentage, similar to the follow-back studies, with diagnosable mental disorders. Beautrais calculated an OR of 17.4 and also used a case-controlled comparison group in which only 20.4% achieved DSM-III-R criteria for at least one diagnosed mental disorder.

Concurrent diagnostic interviews of suicide attempters or parasuicides have been undertaken on several occasions. Subjects achieved scores on standardized measures of psychological distress comparable to those of mentally disordered, especially depressed, populations. They met criteria for mental illness based on signs and symptoms at levels well beyond chance expectations There is a major discrepancy in two recent reports that bears further investigation. Despite using the same definition of parasuicide to recruit the self-harming subjects, 91% of persons achieved a DSM mental disorder diagnosis in the Edmonton parasuicide study (Dyck, Bland, & Newman, 1999) whereas only 33% of the Euro-study parasuicides (Schmidtke et al., 1994) achieved an ICD diagnosis. Except for the European parasuicide study and another using the Present State Examination (also based on ICD criteria), the frequency of mental disorder diagnoses in those with nonfatal suicidal behaviors is not largely different from those with completed suicide.

Methodological Issues

Numerous methodological issues confound this search to understand the data relating suicidal acts and psychiatric diagnoses. Several are discussed here as examples of the difficulties in advancing science concerning the association relationship.

Recruitment/Selection of Psychiatric Study Populations

Harris and Barraclough (1998) quote an inpatient o/e ratio of suicides among mental disorder patients of 11 with an outpatient o/e ratio of 23. Morrison (1982) offers similar high suicide rate data for his extensive outpatient population. Blair-West, Mellsop, and Eyeson-Annan (1997) and Allgulander (1994) suggest that mood-disordered patients are often only admitted if they are severely ill, and especially if suicidal. If this were true, there should be more suicides in inpatient samples because more mood disorders are admitted. The data suggest both a beneficial effect of hospital treatment on suicide outcomes and a likelihood that inpatient samples of suicidal acts will be weighted toward a larger number of persons with mood disorders. In a further example of the impact of different populations being studied, Weissman's discovery of a significant association between panic disorder diagnoses and suicidal behavior in the general population Epidemiologic Catchment Area (ECA) study has not been widely replicated when treated samples of panic disorders are examined (see page 328 following).

For mentally disordered patients, we do not find the gender ratio—with a preponderance of male completed suicides—that is noted in the overall population. It is unclear whether females with mental disorders are at increased risk or whether males are at less risk. In the Finnish major depressive disorder, suicide follow-back study, Isometsa et al. (1994) remark that there are more males represented than expected if major depressive disorder is a female issue. Several authors investigating personality disorders found a relationship between mental disorder and suicidal behavior for females but not for males. There is now a widely held belief that gender data for suicidal acts should be reported and analyzed separately.

Temporal Linkages

Numerous studies (e.g., Isometsa et al., 1994; Goldacre, Seagroatt, & Hawton, 1993) demonstrate the increased risk of suicide soon after an inpatient stay (less than 1 month). This finding has generated long discussion about the effectiveness of hospitalization as a treatment modality, premature discharge, incomplete or inadequate linkage to follow-up, and even suggestions of lethal effects of hospitalization. Table 13.6 presents some evidence that suicide also occurs at different periods in the natural history of specific diseases. Deaths in persons dependent on alcohol occur later in their illness whereas deaths in those with affective disorders and schizophrenias occur early and evidence a steep decline with chronicity. In personality disorders, Sabo, Gunderson, Najavits, Chauncey, and Kisiel (1995) argue that suicidal behavior declines with time and is not linked to self-harm, whereas Mehlum et al. (1994) contend that suicidal acts are an enduring criterion for those with personality disorders.

TABLE 13.6. Suicide during the Course of Different Mental Disorders

Disorder	Number of studies with suicide occurring:		
	Early	Throughout	Late
Affective disorders	7	0	0
Schizophrenias	4	2	2
Anxiety disorders	1	5	1
Substance abuse/alcohol	0	0	4

Note. Bibliography available from Tanney on request (e-mail: *tanney@calgary.ca*).

Treatment Effects

Because there is no willingness to embark on placebo-controlled studies in the treatment of persons at risk and because effective treatments for mental disorders are available, the impact of treatment both for mental disorder and for suicidality must be considered in any discussion that follows the course of these populations. Worthy of note are the suggestions that Axis II comorbidity hinders the treatment of Axis I disorders (Pfohl, Stangl, & Zimmerman, 1984) and that many people with a history of suicidal acts are excluded from studies of treatment (Linehan, 1997), as well as discussion of the impact of treatment on hospital versus community samples. It is interesting that there is as much concern about the increased risk of suicide after hospital treatment as there are suggestions that hospitalization is the first and most important step in the treatment of a suicidal person with mental disorders.

Summary

It should not be surprising that the association between suicidal acts and mental disorders is validated in spite of all the aforementioned methodological and diagnostic difficulties. It makes inherent sense that most persons at risk for self-harm do not choose suicide actively but are instead under the influence of disturbances in thought, feeling, and behavior. Along with other consequences, these disturbances impair interpersonal and intrapersonal functioning, distort attitudes and values, and impair problem solving. Estimates are that a chosen death without any such disturbance—a "rational" suicide (see Chapter 19)—makes up no more than about 5% of all suicides. The critical issue for furthering our understanding of the suicidal act itself is the strength or weight of the mental disorder relationship, and this is a much more complex matter. Both quantitative and qualitative solutions can be argued. The first suggests that more mental disturbance will likely result in suicidal acts, whereas the latter holds that certain mental disorders are more important than others in furthering a self-harming outcome. We will examine the quantity contention through the study of comorbidity, but first we turn to the relationship of particular diagnoses to suicidal acts and to completed suicide.

SPECIFIC PSYCHIATRIC DIAGNOSES ASSOCIATED WITH SUICIDAL BEHAVIORS

Table 13.7 presents (1) the frequency of different diagnoses in psychiatric patients who die by suicide (prospective studies, B, in Table 13.3) and (2) the ranking of mental disorder diagnoses in populations of persons who die by suicide (retrospective studies, A, in Table

TABLE 13.7. Mental Disorder Diagnoses in Suicide: Frequency by Rank Score

Frequency (total rank score)[a]	Diagnostic classification used			
	ICD		DSM	
	General population (2 studies)	Clinical psychiatric patients (mixed) (19 studies)	Clinical psychiatric patients (mixed) (4 studies)	Clinical psychiatric patients (mixed) (3 studies)
1				
2				
3	AD			
4		AD	AD, Sc	AD, Sc
5				
6	SA			
7		Sc	SA, A	
	N	PD		PD
8	OP, SA, PD	SA, N		OP
9	Sc		OP, OM PD	A, OM
10		OB OP		
11				
12				
13	OB			
14				
15				

Note. AD, affective disorders; Sc, schizophrenias; OP, other psychoses; SA, substance abuse; N, neuroses; A, anxiety disorders; PD, personality disorders; O(B)M, organic (brain) mental disorders.
Source: From Tanney (1992: 290). Copyright 1992 by The Guilford Press. Reprinted by permission.
[a]Rank: 1, most frequent; 2, next most frequent; etc.

13.3). Harris and Barraclough (1998) have similarly generated o/e ratios for most mental disorders and Figure 13.3 illustrates them. Table 13.5 presented the follow-back studies (retrospective studies, C, in Table 13.3) in which the majority include data on *all* concurrent diagnoses. All these data sets indicate that affective or mood disorders followed by substance abuse are the most common disorders related to completed suicide. When psychiatric diagnoses are reviewed, similar findings are noted for persons undertaking nonfatal suicidal acts. Substance abuse and anxiety disorders are more common as presenting diagnoses with the mood disorders more common as a background, predisposing, or lifetime issues.

The core issue for any intervention that is prevention or treatment oriented is the identification of a specific at-risk diagnostic group (selected or indicated population). Before briefly discussing the particulars of risk status for individual disorders, this issue of relative risk across disorders demands further consideration. Until the decade of the 1990s, it was

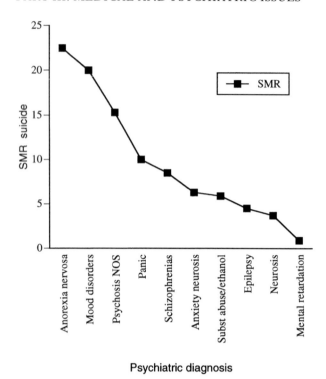

FIGURE 13.3. Psychiatric diagnoses and suicide. *Data source:* Harris & Barraclough (1998).

generally accepted and usually taught that the presence or history of affective/mood/depressive disorders was the most significant indicator among mental disorders that suicide risk would be increased (e.g., Goodwin & Jamison, 1990; Guze & Robins, 1970 [see Box 13.3]). This belief has now been strongly challenged without detracting from the absolute importance of depressive disorders. Inskip, Harris, and Barraclough (1998) calculated lifetime mortality risk for those with affective disorders, ethanol-dependent persons, and individuals with schizophrenia as 6, 7, and 4%, respectively. Blair-West argued that at most 2.5–3.5% of completed suicides could be associated with affective disorders. In a number of follow-up studies of psychiatric patients (Box 13.4) there is convergence toward a view that "risk did not vary very much with the type of diagnoses" (Allgulander, Allebeck, Przybeck,

---

**BOX 13.3. Various Labels Hinder Understanding
and Reflect Incomplete Knowledge**

Some of the confusion about the importance of mood/affective diagnoses may be an artifact generated by the competing diagnostic systems, the changes in nomenclature with the introduction of the DSM-III and finally the existence of subtypes of these disorders. The major subtypes, with approximate correspondences across classification systems (ICD and DSM), are as follows: manic–depressive disease = bipolar disorder (partial), primary depression = unipolar depression = major depressive disorder + (some) dysthymia, depressive neurosis = dysthymia, and reactive depression = adjustment disorder with depressed mood.

BOX 13.4. Impact of Specific Diagnoses on Suicidal Acts

P.I.-500 (United States):
[except for schizoaffectives] . . . suicide rates in the different diagnostic categories (schizophrenias and borderline personality disorder) varied little in either direction [from 9.6%].
—STONE (1987)

Psychiatric Case Register Diagnoses in Completed Suicides (Sweden):
Type of inpatient diagnosis has less to do with the magnitude of risk than generally believed.
—ALLGULANDER, ALLEBECK, PRZYBECK, AND RICE (1992)

Follow-Up of Psychiatric Inpatients Who Die by Suicide (England):
No significant variation among diagnoses for suicide smr's, though highest smr noted for Depression and affective psychoses among female patients from 29–365 days after discharge.
—GOLDACRE, SEAGROATT, AND HAWTON (1993)

& Rice, 1992: 323). Despite this apparent leveling of risk across diagnoses in epidemiological studies, it is still, however, critical to emphasize that affective disorders remain a preeminent clinical state associated with risk of a suicidal act. As discussed later in this chapter, the role of comorbidity seems a possible contender as an explanation for these disparate findings of clinical and epidemiological studies.

Mood/Affective Diagnoses

Numerous reports reaffirm and continue to support the importance of disturbances of mood in all suicidal acts, completed and nonfatal (Buchholtz-Hansen, Wang, & Danish University Antidepressant Group, 1993; Newman & Bland, 1991). In one of these reports (Beautrais et al., 1996), after accounting for intercorrelations, mood disorders were still by far the largest contributor to the likelihood of suicide behavior (OR = 33.4). Although four studies found no specific diagnostic subgroup associated to suicide, most of the investigations suggest a gradient of suicide lessening from secondary (comorbid) depression through primary unipolar depression, bipolar depressive disorder, and bipolar manic disorder. Table 13.8, comparing unipolar and bipolar disorders, clearly indicates that completed suicide is much more significantly linked to unipolar disorder. For suicidal acts that are nonfatal, persons with unipolar and bipolar depressions appears equally involved (Lester, 1993e). Asnis et al. (1993) commented that adjustment disorder is a highly unstable diagnosis characterized by high levels of suicide ideation, equivalent to that in major depressive disorder but with many fewer suicidal behaviors. In a further clarification of the influence of subtypes, the primary depressions linked to suicide are overwhelmingly unipolar–major depressive disorders and not dysthymia–adjustment disorder, with the exception that dysthymic persons with early onset appear to be at significant suicidal risk (Szadoczky & Fazekas, 1994). This last statement appropriately reflects the complexity and the numerous caveats in this evolving and critically important area.

Another important influence on the affective disorder and suicide linkage is the presence of specific components of the depressive disorders, particularly symptoms. As part of the outcomes of the NIMH Collaborative Depression study, three symptom clusters (anhedonia, hopelessness; anxiety, agitation, panic; aggression, impulsivity) have been put forward as more predictive of suicide than either diagnoses or syndromes (Fawcett, Busch,

TABLE 13.8. Suicide in Unipolar vs. Bipolar Depressions

Greater in unipolar	No difference	Greater in bipolar
Angst (1979)[a]	Tsuang (1978)[a]	Morrison (1982)
Berglund & Nilsson (1987)[a]		Buchholtz-Hansen et al. (1993)
Black et al. (1987)		
Dingman & McGlashan (1986)[a]		
Inskip et al. (1998)		
Lesage et al. (1994)		
Newman & Bland (1991)		
Perris & D'Elia (1966)[a]		
Roy-Byrne et al. (1988)[a]		

Source: Updated from Tanney (1992). Copyright 1992 by The Guilford Press. Adapted by permission.
[a]References available from Tanney on request (e-mail: *tanney@calgary.ca*).

Jacobs, Kravitz, & Fogg, 1997). Others have linked severity, agitation, insomnia, and self-neglect as well as hopelessness to an increased risk of suicide. Table 13.9 provides a clear indication that the severity of the disorder is associated with increasing likelihood of suicidal acts. The severity variable is usually understood as intensity, measured quantitatively as increasing numbers of diagnostic criteria fulfilled, but it may also be a reflection of duration of the illness. The combination of duration and intensity should probably be used to define a severity-of-illness variable for future studies. The symptoms of agitation, insomnia, and self-neglect are some of the outcomes of the biological aspects of depressive disorders. Related to hypothalamic hypofunction (see Chapter 16), they are part of a clinical syndrome that used to be called endogenous depression or melancholia. Three studies provide no clear data that this subset of symptoms is particularly linked to increased suicide risk. The contribution of cognitive dysfunctions, particularly hopelessness, has been convincingly argued as a strong predictor of a suicidal act in persons with affective disorders (Beck, 1986).

With respect to psychotic cognitions in depression—and this group of persons has sometimes been labeled "schizoaffectives"—three studies found no strong support for increased suicidality in persons with psychosis and affective disorder. Controversy surrounds the specific symptom of delusional thinking in unipolar depressions. At present, four studies support an association of suicide and delusional thinking in such depressions (Fawcett et al., 1987; Robinson & Spiker, 1985; Roose, Glassmann, Walsh, Woodring, & Vital-Herne, 1983; Wolfersdorf, Keller, Steiner, & Hole, 1987) with only one finding no relationship. Interestingly, that finding was in by far the largest study population followed for the longest amount of time (Coryell & Tsuang, 1982).

TABLE 13.9. More Severe Depression and the Likelihood of Suicidal Acts

Increased	Not increased
Bulik, Carpenter, Kupfer, & Frank (1990)	Corbitt, Malone, Haas, & Mann (1996)
Duggan, Sham, Lee, & Murray (1991)	Mann et al. (1999)
Fawcett et al. (1987)	van Praag & Plutchik (1984)[a]
Leon et al. (1999)	
Modestin & Kopp (1988)	
Patten & Carlson (1997)[a]	
Strakowski, McElroy, Keck, & West (1996)	
vanGastel, Schott, & Maes (1997)	
Vietra et al. (1992)	

[a]References available from Tanney on request (e-mail: *tanney@calgary.ca*).

It is also important to remember the impact of the age and gender structure of the population being studied. Conwell found that males with major affective illness were at special risk in his elderly psychological autopsy/follow-back study (Conwell et al., 1996). There is a striking leveling of the usual male–female (3–4:1) ratio of completed suicides in persons who have inpatient histories of mental disorder. It appears that this is largely due to the contribution of persons with affective disorders. We cannot at present discern whether this is an indication that females with affective diagnoses are at greater risk or that males are at significantly less risk than the general population.

Substance Abuse/Dependence

Toxicology data for completed suicides regularly indicate that between 40 and 60% are legally intoxicated at the time of death (Merrill, Milner, Owens, & Vale, 1992; cf. Chapter 15). Various speculations suggest that this abuse disinhibits rational protective systems against self-harm, or acts as a depressant which magnifies already disturbed emotional perspectives on a stressful situation. Clinical experience supports a profile of suicide among males characterized by an episode of interpersonal disruption and loss of support, alcohol abuse to significant levels, and a violent/highly lethal method of suicide.

Murphy and Wetzel (1990) have ably reviewed the issue of suicide in persons who are alcohol dependent. Risk ratios of 6 to 25 times compared to the general population or even psychiatric inpatient populations are reported for persons with alcohol dependency. Death by suicide in alcohol dependence commonly occurs later in the course of the disorder, and lifetime mortalities are variously reported at 1 to 6% (see Box 13.5). Persons with dual diagnoses (alcohol dependence plus another Axis I mental disorder) have much increased risks of suicide (see section "Comorbidity," following). There is controversy about the impact on suicide of other varieties of drug abuse. One review suggests an increased rate in other types of drug abuse (Harris & Barraclough, 1997). Dinwiddie (Dinwiddie, Reich, & Cloninger, 1992) suggests that persons using drugs of injection, cannabis, or solvents, while associated with an increased lifetime suicidal act incidence, do not experience significantly more risk than do persons with alcohol dependence. Others (Schuckit, 1985; Young, Fogg, Scheftner, & Fawcett, 1994) have suggested that there are subgroups of alcohol-dependent persons, based on characterological profiles, who are at increased risk of suicide.

Psychotic Illness

Schizophrenias and Paranoia

As discussed previously, there is no strong support for an increase in suicidal acts among persons with psychotic symptoms as part of a major mood disorder. For persons with se-

---

BOX 13.5. Substance Abuse/Dependence Impairs Appropriate Classification of Manner of Death

Diagnoses of alcoholism and drug addiction occur disproportionately often in undetermined deaths. It appears that these diagnoses may obscure a definite decision about the intent of a self-harming act for some authorities. The result is an underreporting of death by suicide in persons with such diagnoses.

vere mental illnesses primarily involving cognition, the relationships are much clearer. Of seven recent studies, six report that these psychotic illnesses, mostly schizophrenias, are associated with an increased risk of suicide (Addington & Addington, 1992; Fenton, McGlahan, Victor, & Blyler, 1997; Harrow, Westermeyer, Kaplan, & Butz, 1992; Heila et al., 1997; Nieto, Vietra, Gato, Vallejo, & Circha, 1992; Shuwall & Siris, 1994; but see Axelsson & Lagerkvist-Briggs, 1992). In particular, those with paranoid disorders and paranoid schizophrenia are highlighted as being at increased risk. These disorders are characterized by significant numbers of positive thought disorder symptoms, including delusions and hallucinations, thus confirming a similar finding of increased suicide risk in those persons with affective disorders who have delusional symptoms. Earlier studies of schizophrenia and suicide summarized in Table 13.10, did not indicate such a strong association. This may have been due to the study populations largely being drawn from long-term institutions with paranoid schizophrenia underrepresented. Fenton et al. reported that persons with a strong loading of negative symptoms of schizophrenia may in fact be relatively protected from suicide.

There is much discussion about the role of postpsychotic depression as an explanation for suicide in schizophrenia. Another explanation offered with significant support suggests that young schizophrenics may suicide soon after an episode of active illness as they confront the stigma and downward drift in their socioeconomic status associated with this chronic illness. This suggests in part that the suicide may have an illness (mal)adaptive component (Amador et al., 1996; Colton, Drake, & Gates, 1985). A third speculation suggests that some schizophrenics suicide during the active phase of their illness (Addington & Addington, 1992; Heila et al., 1997; Nieto et al., 1992). It is clear that there is much more to schizophrenia and suicide than a simple view that schizophrenics end their lives in response to command hallucinations urging or exhorting their death. A final speculation involves a potential suicidogenic effect of the early antipsychotic drugs. These reports were not confirmed and there are now several reports of a *protective* effect of the newer antipsychotics, such as clozapine, against suicide (Meltzer & Okayli, 1995; Reid, Mason, & Hogan, 1998).

Anxiety Disorders and Neurosis

Harris and Barraclough (1997) report o/e ratios for suicide in panic disorder and anxiety neurosis as 10 and 6.29, respectively. Beautrais and others partial out the intercorrelations with other disorders and usually suggest a much lower significance to the contribution of anxiety disorders in the matrix of suicide. This issue of mixing with other disorders and specifically identifying the impact of anxiety has been especially controversial in the study of panic disorders. After Weissman's report of an increased association of panic disorders with lifetime suicidal acts in the untreated, general-population sample of the ECA study, there was a marked flurry of activity to examine this finding (Weissman, Klerman, Markowitz, & Ouellette, 1989). At present, only three further studies support this finding

TABLE 13.10. Schizophrenias and the Frequency of Suicide: Controlled Studies

Greater in Schizophrenias	No difference	Greater in matched controls
Goldney et al. (1985)	Bolin et al. (1968)[a]	Fernando & Storm (1984)[a]
Roy (1986)[a]	Beisser & Blanchette (1961)[a]	
Wilson (1968)[a]		

Source: From Tanney (1992: 293). Copyright 1992 by The Guilford Press. Reprinted by permission.
[a]References available from Tanney (1992).

TABLE 13.11. Panic Disorders and the Likelihood of Suicidal Acts

Increased	No impact
If panic disorder only	
Coryell & Tsuang (1982)	Allgulander & Lavori (1991)
Harris & Barraclough (1997)	Andrews & Lewinsohn (1992)
Korn et al. (1992)	Beautrais et al. (1996)
Weissman et al. (1989)	Beck et al. (1991)
	Fava, Grandi, & Savron (1992)
If comorbidity was considered	
Johnson, Weissman, & Klerman (1990)	Anthony & Petronis (1991)
Lepine, Chignon, & Teherani (1993)	Cox, Direnfeld, Swinson, & Norton (1994)
Waern, Beskow, Allebeck, & Spak (1997)	Friedman, Jones, Chernen, & Barlow (1992)
	Henriksson et al. (1996)
	Hornig & McNally (1995)
	Korn, Plutchik, & van Praag (1997)
	Lecrubier (1998)
	Overbeek, Rikken, Schners, & Griez (1998)
	Rudd, Dahm, & Rajab (1993)
	Warshaw, Massion, Peterson, Pratt, & Keller (1995)

of a significant contribution. Four others do not, and there are now 12 reports that panic disorders are linked significantly to suicidal acts only in the added presence of mood disorders and/or substance abuse (Table 13.11). Of clinical note, Fawcett, Clarke, and Busch (1993) have reported anxiety and agitation as significant predictors of imminent suicide risk, in agreement with the characterization of the immediate presuicide state as a desperate one (e.g., Shneidman's "perturbation"). Anxiety symptoms related to posttraumatic stress disorder are also linked with increased suicide risk. It appears that the risk of increased completed suicide in persons with anxiety disorders and nondepressive neuroses is a lifetime issue, continuing even into old age (Allgulander, 1994).

Finally, it bears noting that obsessive–compulsive disorder may actually have little impact on suicidal acts and behaviors with some even hypothesizing a subtle protective effect.

Personality Disorders

The ECA study found that 5.9% of the population achieved a diagnosis of a personality disorder (Samuels, Nestandt, Romanoski, Folstein, & McHugh, 1994; see Table 13.12). This is quite a large number of persons in the general population and any associations to suicidal behavior among this group of diagnoses would certainly increase the overall visibility of suicide in the general community. Psychological autopsy/follow-back studies found that 31 to 57% of completed suicides qualified for an Axis II or personality disorder diagnosis. The

TABLE 13.12. DSM-IV Classification of Personality Disorders

Cluster A	Cluster B	Cluster C
Paranoid	Antisocial	Avoidant
Schizoid	Borderline	Dependent
Schizotypal	Histrionic	Obsessive–compulsive
	Narcissistic	

TABLE 13.13. Symptoms Associated with More Suicidal Acts in
Patients with Borderline Personality Disorder (BPD)

Symptom	No. of studies supporting effect
Severity of BPD	3/8
Self-mutilation	2/5
Dissociation	1/1
Impulsivity	1/1
Histrionic	1/2
Antisocial personality disorder	3/3

Note. Bibliography available from Tanney on request (e-mail: *tanney@calgary.ca*).

largest number of these were in Cluster B or Cluster C (11 to 41% for Cluster B and 10 to 28% for Cluster C). Brent reported an OR of 2.9 for any personality disorder and 8.5 for Cluster B traits, after controlling for Axis I disorders (Brent et al., 1993). The associations are similarly strong for non-fatal suicide acts. In the ECA study, 16.8% of personality-disordered persons reported suicidal behaviors or suicidal ideation versus 7.8% in the general population. In a study of adolescent inpatients, Brent et al. (1994a) reported that any personality disorder or trait had an OR of 2.1 for suicidal behavior. Modestin, Oberson, and Erni (1997) found that 71% of personality-disordered inpatients had histories of suicidal behavior versus 42% of those without personality disorder. Clusters B (especially) and C appear most important in establishing this relationship (Brent et al., 1994a; Mehlum et al., 1994; Modestin et al., 1997; Raczek, True, & Friend, 1989). Cluster B disorders, and especially borderline personality disorder (BPD), have been the subject of numerous further studies exploring their relationship to suicidal acts.

Nine studies report the outcome of completed suicide as 3 to 9% of patients with BPD (median, 6.5%). Table 13.13 elaborates the specific symptoms or associated features within the BPD diagnosis which contribute to the relationship between BPD and suicidal behaviors. Several individual features appear of value, but overall severity is not strongly supported as a feature predictive of suicidal behavior. In the DSM classification system, a person may have an Axis II diagnosis along with Axis I diagnoses, called comorbidity. Table 13.14 summarizes the effects of Axis II and Axis I comorbidity on the likelihood of suicidal acts in persons with personality disorders. There appears to be moderate support for the hypothesis (Blumenthal & Kupfer, 1986) that persons with BPD will only be suicidal in the presence of an Axis I diagnosis, usually major depressive disorder. In the Finnish nationwide follow-back study of completed suicides, 39% of deaths by suicide in personality-disordered persons, had co-occurring substance abuse and major depressive disorder (Isometsa et al., 1996). This study suggested substance abuse as a more important determinant than depres-

TABLE 13.14. Effect of Comorbidity on Increasing the Frequency of Suicidal Acts in
BPD/Axis II Patients

Study population	Comorbid diagnosis	Suicidal act	No. of studies supporting effect
Axis II	Axis I	Nonfatal SB	0/3
BPD	Major depression	Completed suicide	3/6
BPD	Major depression	Nonfatal SB	6/9
BPD	Substance abuse	All suicidal acts	5/8

Note. BPD, borderline personality disorder; SB, suicidal behaviors. Bibliography available from Tanney on request (e-mail: *tanney@calgary.ca*).

**BOX 13.6. The Structure of Our Classification
Systems Impacts Our Understanding**

In establishing personality disorder diagnoses, a categorical and not dimensional view of personality is used. Several authors (Brent, Malone, Holley, Razeck, Mehlum) suggest that a dimensional approach with a specific trait titled suicidality would be a valuable strategy to furthering our understanding of both personality disorders and suicide. The issue remains open.

---

sion in fashioning an outcome of completed suicide in patients with BPD. To further the complexity, they found depression more important than substance abuse when the outcome of other (nonfatal) suicidal acts was studied. Support for the hypothesized importance of an Axis I disorder in suicidal persons who have personality disorders is not unanimous. Four studies (Brent et al., 1994b; Malone, Haas, Sweeney, & Mann, 1995; Mehlum et al., 1994; Soloff, Lis, Kelly, Cornelius, & Ulrich, 1994) posit that suicidal behaviors in persons with BPD are independent and represent an enduring trait vulnerability (see Box 13.6). Several of these authors and others call for an increased weighting or importance of the suicide self-harm criterion in constructing the diagnosis of BPD. As illustrated by this group of mental disorders, the issue of comorbidity severely complicates our understanding of the associations between specific mental disorder diagnoses and various types of suicidal acts.

Other Psychiatric Diagnoses

Mental handicap and/or retardation have a particularly low rate of suicidal acts and completed suicide relative to other mental disorders.

Recent studies (Appleby, Mortensen, & Faragher, 1998; Hogberg & Innala, 1994) identify postpartum disorders as a particularly strong risk indicator for completed suicide. Persons with eating disorders are identified in 10 studies as at significant risk for completed suicide. Of interest, two recent reports (Coren & Hewitt, 1998; Korndorfer, 1999) do not find this increased suicide risk in studies using both record linkage and clinical follow-up methodologies.

Epilepsy is consistently reported as a neurological diagnosis linked to suicide (see Chapter 16). Rates of completed suicide in persons with seizures are estimated at 3–5%, with temporal lobe epilepsy being especially associated with elevated risk. Numerous explanations have been put forward including seizure-related behavior, psychotic phenomena, psycho/social stigmatization and postseizure depression. Our understanding is still largely incomplete.

COMORBIDITY

When DSM-III introduced diagnoses on three separate axes and allowed an opportunity to specify current and historical diagnoses, it quickly became apparent that different mental disorder diagnoses did occur together and even concurrently. This comorbidity is common with psychiatric diagnoses, one study finding that 95% of patients were affected by two or more disorders. Numerous technical issues are involved which together suggest that this is a complex and as yet incompletely understood area, but the size and impact of comorbidity as issues in our understanding of the mental disorder–suicidal act association should not be underestimated. In the early psychological autopsy studies, often only a single diagnosis was reported. In later studies using the DSM framework, the hierarchical organization of diagnosis and the opportunity to specify a principal or most responsible diagnosis encouraged a parsimony in reporting that diminished the recognition of some disorders in these studies of completed suicide. Our awareness of comorbidity has necessitated a reexamination or reconsideration of the impact of individual disorders and of their associations and linkages on the likelihood of suicidal acts. In the follow-back studies, an Axis I diagnosis found with another Axis I diagnosis occurred in 28, 42, 44, and 70% of studies that reported comorbid states. Cheng (1995) suggested that the OR for completed suicide if a person had two or more mental disorder diagnoses was 169.6; 56.6% of Beautrais et al.'s (1996) medically serious attempters had two or more disorders. For nonfatal suicidal acts, the Edmonton parasuicide study found 2.3 diagnoses per subject. Seventy-six percent of those with diagnoses had comorbid disorders (Dyck et al., 1999), similar to a Finnish study (Suominen & Henrikkson, 1996) in which 82% of those persons with nonfatal suicidal acts had comorbid mental disorders.

Table 13.14 summarizes comorbidity data for Axis I and Axis II diagnoses, with particular emphasis on Axis I disorders occurring in persons with BPD. The Finnish psychological autopsy study (Henriksson et al., 1993) found that 88% of those with mental disorders were comorbid for some combination of Axis I/Axis I or Axis I/Axis II diagnoses. It is notable that Axis II/Axis II comorbidity is uncommon but when it occurs as in the overlap of antisocial personality disorder and BPD, three studies found a significant association with suicidal behaviors.

There are two problems in assessing the impact of comorbidity on suicide risk: The first is establishing the independent contribution to risk by each individual disorder (A, B) and the other is estimating the actual amount of impact, whether cumulative in some way (A + B) or potentially interactive (A × B).

Important Diagnoses in Comorbid States

Several authors (Berglund & Nilsson, 1987; Black et al., 1987; Hagnell & Rorsman, 1979; Khuri & Akiskal, 1983; Martin, Cloninger, Guze, & Clayton, 1985) emphasized that secondary affective disorders (equivalent to comorbid) were more associated with completed suicide than were primary affective disorders. In the Finnish follow-back study (Isometsa et al., 1994), 85% of those with major depressive disorders evidenced comorbidity. In association with suicide, mood disorders are most commonly comorbid with substance abuse (Cornelius et al., 1995). Is it the depression or the comorbid disorder that contributes to suicide in those with mood disorders? Depression is regarded as the essential element in terms of contribution to comorbidity for substance abuse (Brent et al., 1993), panic disorders (Rudd et al., 1993), anxiety disorders (Bronisch & Wittchen, 1994), schizophrenia (Bartels, Drake, & McHugo, 1992), and bipolar disorder (Strakowski, 1996). Beautrais emphasizes this in her dissection using population attributable risk, finding that depression was overwhelmingly the most significant diagnostic entity. For personality disorders, there is disagreement whether substance abuse or depression is the more important single diagnosis, particularly as they occur together so often.

How Comorbidity Might Influence Suicide Risk

Comorbidity makes suicidal acts more likely. Although the quantitative impact is poorly examined, Lewinsohn found indications of a mathematical relationship where the likelihood of suicidal behaviors in his adolescent sample increased with the number of diagnoses

(Lewinsohn, Rohde, & Seeley, 1995). The Edmonton parasuicide study did not confirm this simple additive relationship, but Beautrais calculated that the OR for suicidal behaviors escalated from 17.4 for those with one disorder to 89.7 for those with two or more DSM-III-R mental disorder diagnoses. Cornelius et al. (1995) suggested a synergistic effect.

The mechanisms of comorbidity's cumulative impact on suicide may also involve patterns and temporal relationships between diagnoses. It has been proposed that Axis II disorders may impair adaptive capacities to master Axis I disorders and perhaps even increase vulnerability to them. The Edmonton parasuicide study described definite patterns of diagnoses associated with risk. Shaffer et al. (1996) has offered the idea of a developmental progression of mental disorder diagnoses likely to lead to suicide. Others have proposed specific sequences. Administering the K-SADS (Schedule of Affective Disorders and Schizophrenia for School-Age Children) diagnostic instrument to adolescents, Lewinsohn et al. (1995) made both current and lifetime diagnoses. They discovered that 60% of those with multiple diagnoses, were overlapping in time so that both concurrent, progressive, and sequential combinations are possible.

Examining the most frequent comorbid disorders linked to suicide, substance abuse and depression, offers some examples of these possible mechanisms. There is a moderately supported hypothesis that alcohol dependence might be part of the depressive spectrum of disorders. In this process, the comorbidity effect would simply be a severity factor. In the Edmonton parasuicide study, mood disorders were the lifelong substrate in these patients, even though anxiety disorders and substance abuse were more likely current diagnoses at the time of their self-harm behavior. This suggests a vulnerability or diathesis related to depression that is amplified by distress (anxiety) or by the disabling of mental resources (substance abuse intoxication). The entire range of possible association mechanisms is considered in the following section.

EXPLAINING THE RELATIONSHIP BETWEEN PSYCHIATRIC DIAGNOSES AND SUICIDAL ACTS

The evidence set forward in the earlier parts of this chapter supports the association or linkage of psychiatric diagnoses and suicidal acts (see Box 13.7). Table 13.15 summarizes spe-

---

BOX 13.7. Recognizing That Associations Cannot Direct Clinical Care

There is compelling information that persons with a variety of psychiatric diagnoses are more likely to engage in suicidal acts than are those without them. This knowledge should not be overgeneralized. It does *not* confirm or suggest that:

1. *All* suicidal persons are mentally ill (unless being actively at risk of suicide is defined as a mental illness). The multifactorial causation of suicidal acts is sufficient argument that mental disorder cannot be a "necessary" component for suicidal actions.
2. *All* mentally ill persons are actively at risk of suicide. A prudent clinician will estimate the risk of suicidal action in every new helping contact, but will also know that the largest majority of persons with psychiatric diagnoses, including depression, will not be suicidal in their lifetime. This flaw in overestimating the strength of statistical relationships is known as the "ecological fallacy."

TABLE 13.15. The Frequency of Suicidal Behaviors in Mental Disorders: A Summary

Mental disorder	Suicide	Nonfatal suicidal behaviors
Affective disorders	+++	+++
Bipolar depressed/mixed	++	
Major depression		
Unipolar	++++	
Psychotic/melancholic	++	
Dysthymia (neurotic)	++	
Adjustment disorder, depressed	+	++
Schizophrenias*	++	+
Paranoid	+++	
Other psychoses	+	
Substance abuse*	++	+++
Personality disorders*		
Antisocial	+	+++
Borderline	++	+++
Anxiety disorders		
Panic*	0	+
Obsessive–compulsive	–	–
Dissociative	0	+
Eating disorders	+	++
Developmental disorders	0	+
Organic mental disorders	–	0
Mental retardation	0	0
Affective disorders + substance abuse	+++++	+++++

Note. –, less than the general population; 0, equal to the general population; +, ++, +++, increasingly greater than the general population; no entry, no data; *, increase one "+" in presence of major depressive disorder.

cific relationships. Table 13.16 proposes seven possible configurations or explanations for the association and offers specific examples of each, several of which are discussed in the subsections below. It is assumed that any causative relation is unidirectional (i.e., that mental disorder may influence the development of suicidal acts) but not vice versa. In fact, speculation about the impact of suicidal thoughts and acts on mental functioning is warranted, but unexplored.

A. 1. Cause/Consequence: Direct

The simplest explanation of the association is a direct impact of mental disorder symptoms on the likelihood of suicide. Several examples are provided, the most challenging of which is the concept of time–event distortion. This intriguing hypothesis suggests that the biological origins of a specific vulnerability to suicide involve the temporal distortion of a person's experiencing of feedback in response to his or her actions. The defect involves a person's sense of the passage of time, known to be a (inferior) frontal cortex function. In particular, depressed and hopeless persons appear to experience a lengthening of objective time: their actions have an impact at a future time that appears more and more distant. On the opposite side of this disorder, persons with substance abuse and impulsivity, and perhaps BPD, experience a speeded sense of time in expecting that activity should be immediately followed by consequences. These persons cannot hold an adequate or realistic image of their own future.

TABLE 13.16. Explaining the Relationship between Psychiatric Diagnoses and Suicidal Acts

Mechanism	Examples
A. Cause/consequence	
1. Direct *Phenomenology sufficient to explain outcome*	• Depressive delusions, command hallucinations • Time–event distortion: elongated perception in helplessness, hopelessness; compression in impulsivity, BPD • Affect *and* aggression dysregulation in depression: decreased 5-HT functions in violent suicides
2. Indirect *Protective mechanisms impaired or vulnerabilities added*	Axis II disorder impairs resiliency / hardens treatment resistance → increases vulnerability to Axis I disorders
Threshold surpassed	• Mood disorders define baseline–threshold relationship (Vulnerability Index)
Baseline (trait suicidality)	• Dose-loaded for Cluster B disorders: more pathological personality traits, more suicidality
Trigger	• One phenotype of bipolar disorder activates a genetically based suicide factor • Major depressive, bipolar have suicidal acts early in episode

Release	• Anti-suicide protective systems masked by mental disorder:
	   Substance abuse disinhibits impulsivity
	   Depression dysregulates aggression threshold
	   More mental disorder immobilizes redundant systems

B. Complication	
1. Iatrogenic	• Mental health caregivers lacking intervention competency • Early discharge for community or 'managed' care • Stigma of mental disorder • *Not* behavioral toxicity of psychopharmacology (e.g., fluoxetine, phenobarbital, antipsychotics)
2. Illness adaptation	• Solution to chronic disorder (schizophrenias) • Rational suicide by mentally disordered ("slippery slope")
C. Co-occurrent/coexisting	
1. Equivalent	• Substance abuse as "indirect suicide" • Suicidal behavior/ideation as a defining criterion for major depression, borderline personality
2. Common origins	• Loneliness (Sainsbury) or isolation (Gove) → substance abuse and depression and suicide • Sexual abuse through posttraumatic stress disorder → suicidal acts and borderline personality • Problem-solving deficit (females) → substance abuse and depression and suicide
3. Independent	• *Unlikely* a chance occurrence

A. 2. Cause/Consequence: Indirect

Another straightforward explanation is a quantitative one that expands the comorbidity discussion. This hypothesis suggests that it is the intensity (severity plus duration of exposure) of disorder which either amplifies distress or renders efforts at coping impaired enough to be incompetent. In either scenario, protective factors or adaptive capacities inhibitory to suicide are eventually overwhelmed. A variety of potential mechanisms can be elaborated. The presence of mental disorders could elevate the baseline level of suicidality, add to its likelihood as a predisposing state or as a precipitating event when some threshold for action is approached, or alternatively lower the threshold for entry into the "suicide zone" (Maris, Berman, & Maltsberger, 1992) (Figure 13.4). The Vulnerability Index, defined as the quantity of risk that must be accumulated between baseline and threshold, is the critical measure. This quantitative hypothesis is supported or assumed by a significant body of research (Corbitt, Malone, Haas, & Mann, 1996; Lewinsohn et al., 1995; Vietra et al., 1992; Windle, 1994). Mann's suggestion (Mann et al., 1999) of a diathesis where mental disturbance, especially mood related, is necessary but not sufficient without the addition of some other factors of temperament is an example of the elevated baseline mechanism. His group suggests impulsivity–aggressivity as the additional temperamental variable, as have others (Nordstrom, Gustavsson, Edman, & Asberg, 1996).

Another baseline example is the dose-loading or intensity effect in Cluster B disorders where more pathological traits predispose to more suicidality. Other mechanisms may involve the creation of specific vulnerabilities or the impairment of protective mechanisms by trigger or release processes. The symptoms associated with particular mental disorders (specifically depression and substance abuse) may be themselves the specific vulnerabilities

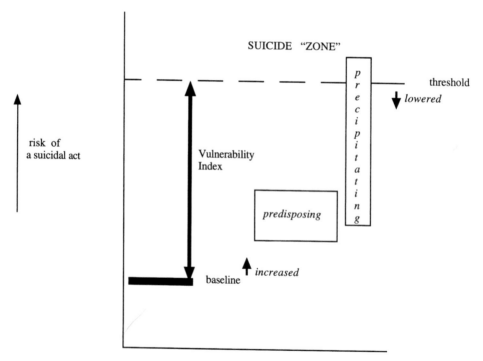

FIGURE 13.4. Sites of action (*italics*) for the contribution of mental disorders to the likelihood of a suicidal act.

which disturb the adaptive process or predispose a suicide solution. The release idea derives from a parallel to the suicide enzymes and the process of apoptosis found in molecular biology. It suggests that there are active suicide systems within each of us (trait suicidality) which are inhibited or checked by antisuicide systems. Mental disorders may mask these antisuicide systems or disable them in a number of ways such that the suicidality (read Freud's death instinct for those with a psychoanalytical passion) is released.

B. 1., B. 2. Complication: Iatrogenic, Illness Adaptation

Regarding suicidal acts as a complication of mental disorders offers two options. The first proposes that it is not the mental disorder but the social and treatment sequelae which lead a person to suicide. Suicide as a response to the unacceptable shame of stigma is one of the explanations for suicide in epilepsy. The other suggests that suicide is in fact an adaptive solution to illness experiences. The mental illness strains a given individual beyond his or her capacity to adapt and continue to function in a manner acceptable for that individual.

C. 2. Co-Occurrent/Coexisting: Common Origins

It is possible that mental disorders and suicidal acts are coincident occurrences neither directly nor indirectly related, but both deriving from a common precursor origin. In addition to the examples offered in Table 13.16, examination of a common paradigm for the evolution of suicidal behaviors in adolescents may be instructive. Depression, substance abuse, and conduct disorder presenting as academic difficulties, truancy, and other legal difficulties are all recognized as frequent accompaniments of suicidal behaviors in adolescents and youths (Jessor, 1991). In the most common linkage explanation, which follows the cause–consequence paradigm, suicidal acts and behaviors are seen to result or follow on from some matrixed interaction of these components (Figure 13.5B). One proposal has primary substance abuse behaviors leading to an inner experience of depression. When this affect further impairs the capacity to cope effectively, conduct and other behavioral disturbances are noted. Suicide represents either a maladaptive attempt at coping or a "giving up phenomenon" when internal resources are exhausted and external resources seem unavailable or unwilling to help. A number of similar hypotheses use different components in a variety of developmental progressions. Employing another linkage explanation, it is equally possible that suicide, whatever its outcome, is another direct component of coping. The spectral outcomes of conduct disorder, depression, substance abuse, and suicide would then interact dependent on their shared or independent origins (Figure 13.5A).

C. 3. Independent

Proponents of a suicidality trait, independent of mental disorders, include investigators of BPD and Mann et al. (1999), as well as Holley (1993). All acknowledge a relationship with mental disorder beyond chance occurrence, but not necessarily as some consequence or complication of mental disorder. Whether suicidality is viewed as a trait or as its own DSM disorder, this perspective is extremely worthy of further investigation.

Whatever the specific quantitative or qualitative contribution of mental disorders in a given individual, it can be indisputably concluded that the vast majority of suicidal acts occur as part of a disturbance within individuals and within their psychic/psychological/mind functions. In no way does this diminish the contribution of interpsychic and larger system

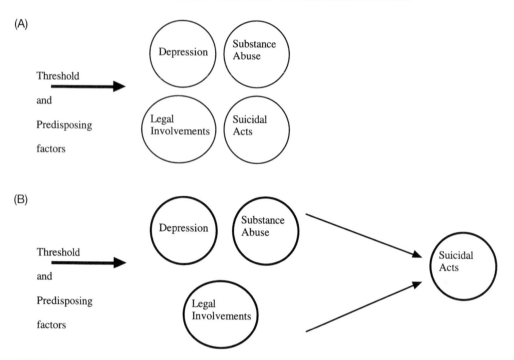

FIGURE 13.5. Suicidal acts in adolescence: Two models for development. (A) Concurrent/coexisting; (B) cause/consequence.

contributions to suicide, but it does affirm the work of a century of psychological and psychiatric investigations into the origins and meaning of suicidal acts and behaviors.

IMPLICATIONS FOR TREATMENT AND PREVENTION

Elaborating the psychiatric diagnosis–suicidal act associations is extremely important (see Chapter 21). Validation of mechanisms indicating a cause–consequence relationship either by direct or by indirect mechanisms (Table 13.16, A1 or A2) would strongly support both the prevention and treatment of psychiatric diagnoses as effective means of minimizing the morbidity and mortality of suicide. Treatment of mental disorders would be valid not only for the alleviation of distress and dysfunction but also as effective suicide prevention. It is important to realize that the exact mechanisms (risk processes) underlying the associations need not be specified for suicide to be reduced by the treatment and prevention of mental disorders. There are effective biological, psychological, and social treatments for the majority of the major and severe mental disorders. Unfortunately, there is substantial evidence that they are incompletely applied in the majority of communities. The issue becomes one of access or availability of mental health resources for those persons at risk in whom these associations are uncovered (Bland, Newman, & Orn, 1997; U.S. Public Health Service, 1999). Prophylactic or maintenance therapy for mental disorders is also validated because it will decrease the duration of exposure to the symptoms, substrate, or cofactor that generates suicidal acts. In the context of early treatment interventions, usually characterized as the task of recognizing that suicide ideation may be present, awareness of mental disorders current or historical becomes a mandatory item of inquiry in any suicide risk estimation. The

---

**BOX 13.8. Psychiatric Diagnoses Are Only One of
Several Important Factors in Suicide Prevention**

This chapter has highlighted abundant data and information affirming the contribution to be made by mental health clinicians in efforts to reduce the number of suicidal acts. The relative importance of psychiatric diagnoses/mental health issues in comparison to other strategies for prevention still needs to be addressed. There is real concern that societal stigma toward mental illness will compound with the taboo around suicide to minimize the use of this knowledge.

Rush Institute Group (Bush, Clark, Fawcett, & Kravitz, 1993; Clark & Fawcett, 1992) have championed this approach with their contention that all suicide helpers should have basic capacities to recognize severe mental illnesses, and further that specific risk estimation profiles may be uniquely constructed for different mental disorders.

A clear and rational explanation can now be offered for the need to develop effective and available mental health services as a cornerstone of any strategy a community adopts for the prevention of suicide. This has enormous implications for resources allocated to human services (see Box 13.8). The numbers of persons with mental disorders at any given time (6-month prevalence) were estimated in the ECA study as 17–23% of the general population (Myers et al., 1984). Estimates of the lifetime likelihood of experiencing a mental disorder would include almost one-half of the population. Using this criterion as a basis for planning the need for possible intervention, the sheer number of those who might be at risk would overwhelm any resource supply or delivery system. Tough decisions concerning the allocation of suicide intervention resources to specific disorders or whether those with psychiatric diagnoses should be a selected or an indicated target group for preventive interventions must be made.

SUMMARY AND CONCLUSIONS

1. There is an important and significant relationship between suicidal acts (completed and nonfatal) and mental disorders. Evidence from a variety of methods for population-based investigations has affirmed the findings of extensive, earlier literature based largely on clinical case study. The increased risk of suicide for persons with active mental disorders converges around 7 to 10 times that of the general population. The magnitude of this relationship is underestimated by a known undercounting of both suicidal acts and mental disorders, but also (to a lesser extent) overestimated by the selection of study populations in which the two entities are not independently defined. Other influences include gender, treatment exposures, cohort selection, and natural history of mortality in different disorders.

2. Different mental disorders have varying degrees of association to suicidal acts. Mood disorders, substance abuse/dependence, and the the forms of schizophrenia remain the most important Axis I diagnoses. Differences among these disorders in lifetime mortality due to suicide are now believed to be less marked than is widely believed. For Axis II diagnoses, Cluster B diagnoses and especially BPD are clearly associated with suicidal acts. Table 13.13 summarizes the relative frequency of suicide and of nonfatal suicidal acts in most psychiatric diagnoses.

3. The findings from comorbidity studies of a positive relationship between suicidal acts and the number of mental disorders (Axis I and Axis II) strongly suggests a role for

mental disorders in the causation of suicidal acts. Similar conclusions for the severity of specific disorders and likelihood of suicidal behaviors are equivocal. Major depression and substance abuse represent a lethal combination, although depression with almost any disorder significantly increases the likelihood of suicide. Depression appears to act as an underlying or distal risk factor while substance abuse and distress/anxiety are more proximal or immediate. Few available studies address the unique impact of a specific disorder by accounting for intercorrelations/ comorbidity. Some recent studies emphasize the importance of developmental progression or even sequencing of diagnoses in the trajectory of a suicidal act.

4. The nature of the linkages between mental disorders and suicidal acts is complex and remains largely speculative. A few are direct, where the mental disorder processes are sufficient to explain the outcome. A larger number are proposed as indirect mechanisms with both increasing vulnerability and/or diminished protection systems as possible pathways. Certain temperamental variables may be cofactors needing to be triggered or released by the mental disorders. Using these ideas as hypotheses, a variety of prevention and treatment interventions intended to minimize exposure to active mental disorders should be tested as suicide prevention strategies.

5. For the majority of suicidal acts, mental disorders may be a necessary but not sufficient element. The suicidal "process" (also called the trajectory of a suicidal act) is not, however, synonymous with mental disorder phenomenology. Establishing suicidal acts (or some agreed term) as a DSM-V diagnostic entity or exploring the utility of a trait suicidality construct would provide a strategy for further study of these linkages and relationships.

6. This chapter concludes with the assertion that suicidal acts are not only behaviors of individuals but also events that can be understood and explained within the infrasystems of that individual. Suicide is not only interpersonal and social but also intrapersonal. For those few individuals who decide for self-death as a rational, responsible choice, these acts are the price we sometimes pay as a society for protecting individual freedoms. To some, physician-assisted death is a modern paradigm for this point of view (see Chapter 19). Because we know that suicide is not a single beast, it is not appropriate to demand or expect such responsibility from all persons at risk. The evidence is coherent and convincing that mental disorders can have an impact on numerous faculties and competencies of "mind" to the extent that persons with such disorders are rendered not responsible for certain actions, even including their own self-termination.

FURTHER READING

Hagnell, O., Lanke, J., & Rorsman, B. (1981). Suicide rates in the Lundby study: Mental illness as a risk factor for suicide. *Neuropsychobiology, 7,* 248–253. This monumental work longitudinally interviewed 3,563 inhabitants of the Swedish community of Lundby. The team of psychiatrists has reported results in at least 30 publications. Fifty-seven percent of suicide completers had been in psychiatric care. Suicide among males with a psychiatric diagnosis was at least 2.5 times that of the general male population.

Tanney, B. L. (1992). Mental disorders, psychiatric patients, and suicide. In R. W. Maris, A. L. Berman, J. T. Maltsberger, & R. I. Yufit (Eds.), *Assessment and prediction of suicide*, New York: Guilford Press. An encyclopedic review of the links between individual psychiatric diagnoses and suicidal acts. It is written at a more introductory level and largely parallels the structure of this chapter.

Harris, E. C., & Barraclough, B. (1998). Excess mortality of mental disorder. *British Journal of Psychiatry, 173,* 11–53. A meta-analysis of 152 English-language reports on the mortality of mental disorder. Suicide is the most common cause of unnatural death, and extensive tables with SMR calculations are included. There is little commentary or interpretation offered, but the sheer volume of calculations is impressive.

Beautrais, A. L., Joyce, P. R., Mulder, R. T., Fergusson, D. M., Deavoll, B. J., & Nightingale, S. K. (1996). Prevalence and comorbidity of mental disorders in persons making serious suicide attempts: A case–control study. *American Journal of Psychiatry, 153,* 1009–1014. A sparkling example of good research methodology. A follow-back, case–control design is employed in which highly lethal suicide attempters serve as a proxy for suicide. The effort to define appropriate research questions leads to sophisticated analyses of the contribution of psychiatric diagnoses. This New Zealand work concludes that depression is the largest contributor (population attributable risk) after interrelationships are accounted for.

Mann, J. J., Waternaux, C., Haas, G. L., & Malone, K. M. (1999). Toward a clinical model of suicidal behavior in psychiatric patients. *American Journal of Psychiatry, 156,* 181–189. This meticulous work explores the association of mental disorders and suicide. It concludes that psychiatric diagnoses of depression and psychosis may act as stressors that overwhelm a vulnerability or diathesis to impulsive–aggressive behavior. The outcome is a suicidal act. Well referenced and broadly incorporating genetic and biological explanations, the argument is persuasive. One caution is that attempters are defined based on lifetime history.

14

Physical Illness and Suicide

with Mark J. Goldblatt

> It is a clinical maxim that medical illness is a risk factor for suicide . . . to the extent that suicide represents a confluence of factors that diminish a person's will to live, it seems indisputable that a medical illness with pain, disfigurement, restricted function, and/or fear of dependence would increase the risk of suicide."
> —THOMAS B. MACKENZIE AND MICHAEL K. POPKIN

Following the early research of Sainsbury (1955), physical illness has been identified as a risk factor for suicidal and for suicide behavior. Later studies have strengthened this finding (Robins, Murphy, Wilkinson, Gassner, & Kayes, 1959; Steward, 1960; Dorpat & Ripley, 1960; Dorpat, Anderson, & Ripley, 1968; Chynoweth, Tonge, & Armstrong, 1980). Diseases of the central nervous system (CNS) are most commonly implicated risk factors for suicide. Major depression is the psychiatric illness most commonly associated with suicide. The relationship between physical illness (in particular illness of the CNS), major depression, and suicide is complex. There appears to be some correlation between certain disease processes, with or without coincident major depression, and an increase in suicidality.

Every disease has unique features because of the anatomy, biochemistry, and physiology of the organ system involved and its interrelationship with other organ systems. Every individual who develops an illness has unique strengths and weaknesses that may contribute not only to the development of the illness but also to its maintenance and eventual resolution. An illness almost always results in a change in an individual's perception and relationship to self, family, friends, workplace, and society. Such changes in perception and relationships can contribute to suicidal behavior.

As illustrated in Table 14.1, there are a number of reactions to the development of a physical illness:

1. To what extent do these reactions relate to increased risk for suicidal behavior? What about increases in irritability, despondency, anger, frustration, hopelessness, helplessness, sense of withdrawal, sense of being separate and feeling out of place?
2. To what extent do these illnesses (and their treatment) cause changes in the biochemical and neurotransmitter milieu of the CNS? How do these illnesses affect

TABLE 14.1. **Reactions to Physical Illness**

1. Loss of sense of indestructibility (shattered omnipotence)
   - The world can suddenly be a dangerous and threatening place.
2. Loss of a feeling of connectedness to one's supportive interpersonal network and to one's body (a sense of disconnectedness).
   - Emotional, physical, social connections may be severed.
3. Failure of logic and reason when thinking about the disease which has taken over (illogicality)
   - Loss of competence and completeness of reasoning
   - Looking for a cause beyond "fate"
4. Loss of control over one's life and one's world
   - A feeling of helplessness leads to hopelessness, which can contribute to a depressive state

Data source: Cassell (1979).

oxygenation of the brain, sleep patterns, eating patterns, nutrient intake, and metabolism?

3. To what extent do these illnesses cause changes in real and perceived social networks and support systems? Are perceptions altered? Is cognitive processing of sensory input distorted? Is logic and rationality maintained when the individual cannot understand how or why he or she developed an illness? Has the patient constructed a separate world of the sick?

In this chapter, we review this association between physical illnesses and suicide, with particular attention to multiple sclerosis, epilepsy, cancer, spinal cord injury, HIV/AIDS, peptic ulcer disease, autoimmune disorders, diabetes mellitus, kidney disease, and terminal illness. Table 14.2 summarizes all the diseases, by organ system or disease process, that have been reported to be associated with an increased risk for suicide.

Albeit incomplete, Table 14.3 is an illustration of the factors that must be considered in characterizing an illness. Such a schema can help in understanding an illness's potential impact on an individual. One critical step is clarifying what is real from feared regarding these attributes of the disease process. Often patients fear the worst when informed of the development of a debilitating, chronic, painful, or socially unfashionable illness. How patients accept and understand their illness is absolutely critical regarding the extent to which they

TABLE 14.2. **Physical Illnesses Associated with Suicide**

Central nervous system	Gastrointesinal system
Multiple sclerosis	Peptic ulcer
Epilepsy	
Temporal lobe epilepsy	Genitourinary system
Spinal cord injury	Renal failure on dialysis
Delirium tremens	
Huntington's Disease	
	Cancer
Autoimmune disorders	Maxillofacial (head and neck)
Rheumatoid arthritis	Gastrointestinal
Systemic lupus erythematosus (SLE)	Pulmonary
Diabetes mellitus	
AIDS	
Cushing's disease	

TABLE 14.3. Characteristics of Physical Illnesses That May Predispose
One to Suicide

---

1. Chronic in nature—lasts over time
2. Debilitating—interferes with activities of daily life
   - Poor health
   - Disruptive to daily life
   - Limitation in range of motion or activity
3. Painful—unresponsive to conventional treatments
4. Deteriorating over time; downhill course
5. Embarrassing—socially isolating
6. Stigmatizing to society
7. Cognitively impairing—affects judgment, memory, insight, orientation, abstraction
8. Apathy and decreased motivation
9. Dependency—on others, medications, regimens
10. Irritability
11. Inabilitiy to adjust or cope to the illness
12. Life-threatening complications

A physically challenged individual may first display signs and symptoms of
depression or dysthymia before becoming suicidal, but not always.

---

will cooperate and invest energy in their own treatment, stabilization, or recovery. An important maneuver is to instill and nurture a sense of hope in the future. Without a sense of hope and a plan for the future, patients with life-threatening or chronic illnesses can enter into depressive states. As Beck, Steer, Kovacs, and Garrison (1985), and others have demonstrated, maintenance of hope and a sense of a future are essential psychological constructs for the prevention of suicide.

Nevertheless, a number of physical illnesses have been shown to be highly correlated with suicidal behaviors. It is instructive to review some of the research literature addressing this connection in the hopes of gleaning salient factors that might be helpful for the development of a preventive approach to these patients.

MULTIPLE SCLEROSIS

Multiple sclerosis (MS) is a neurological disorder in which the myelin sheaths of the nerve fibers are destroyed. MS can affect any part of the CNS; including the optic nerves, brainstem, cerebellum spinal cord, and subcortical white matter. The age of onset is typically between 20 and 40 years. It is more commonly found in females. Patients with MS often present with complicated neuropsychological and emotional problems, such as cognitive dysfunctions and affective disturbances (Schubert & Foliart, 1993). Depression is the most common psychiatric illness associated with MS, with some studies showing that 40–50% of patients with MS experience depression during the course of their illness (Stenager et al., 1990). Other studies (Jensen, Knudsen, Stenager, & Grant, 1989) have shown that in patients with MS, depression was significantly associated with exacerbation of the physical or cognitive symptoms of the disease.

A review of the literature on the relationship between MS and suicidality reveals mixed results. Most studies seem to suggest that there is an increase in suicidal behavior associated with MS. Beginning with the 1949 study by Muller, who founded death rate from suicide of 2.6% in a population of 810 patients diagnosed with MS, which is somewhat higher than the rest of a population. A later review by Miles (1977) of studies that evaluated MS and suicide seemed to confirm this finding. Another study by Kahana, Leibowitz, and Alter (1971) found that 17% of all deaths in patients with MS were the result of suicide. This was nearly three times higher than would be expected in a control population.

Other authors have found a statistically significant (although modest) increase in suicidality in patients with MS. Stensman and Sundqvist-Stensman (1988) concluded that "there seems to be an increased risk of suicide among multiple sclerosis patients and this might be the tip of the iceberg, indicating insufficient psychosocial adjustment among persons with this diagnosis" (151). However their data was limited by the small number of MS patients involved in the study and the fact that there were only a total of two suicide that were recorded.

In a report to the American Association of Suicidology, Berman and Samuel (1990) noted the problem of depression in patients with MS, and the difficulty determining how MS and major depression are related. "It has not been determined, however, whether depression precedes multiple sclerosis, is reactive to multiple sclerosis, or is an intrinsic part of the illness, i.e. a clinical manifestation of demyelination" (268). These authors emphasize the effect of comorbid depression and the chronic progression of the underlying illness as significant risk factors for suicide.

A number of other studies have also documented some increase in the suicide rate for patients with MS (Sadovnick, Eisen, Ebers, Wilson, & Platy, 1991; Stenager, et al., 1992; Long & Miller, 1991). Although these authors present a compelling argument about the association between MS and suicide, there are problems with the data. First, these studies are not comparable with each other because of the issue of possible "contamination" with the use of medications and because of the role of comorbid illnesses, such as major depression. Second, only Kahana's study used a matched control group. Third, none of these studies differentiates between male and female patients—a critical factor when looking at suicide rates. Finally, certain medical therapeutic agents such as antihypertensives, antiepileptics, and steroids may themselves be associated with psychiatric disturbances, because these agents themselves can be associated with behavioral and sleep disturbance, mood lability, and even psychosis.

Of note is that suicide is an option only for less disabled patients and thus usually those with a shorter disease duration (Sadovnick, Ebers, Wilson, & Paty, 1992). A Danish study found that the standard mortality ratio (SMR; which compares the ratio of observed suicides to the number expected based on sex- and age-adjusted national statistics) of suicide in patients with MS was 1.83. It was highest for males and for patients with onset of MS before age 30 years, and those diagnosed before the age of 40 years. The SMR was highest within the first 5 years after diagnosis (Stenager et al., 1992). An explanation for the increased suicide mortality among young male patients with MS who suicide within 5 years of diagnosis may be associated with a lack of social support, which is hypothesized to assist patients with the burden of not being able to fulfill ambitions and cope with the illness.

In contrast to the previous studies, Schwartz and Pierron (1972) reported on a review of 408 death certificates between 1955 and 1975 which listed MS as a cause of death. Four deaths were explicitly reported as suicide. The frequency of suicide obtained here was about the same as the percentage of deaths attributed to suicide as compared to deaths from all causes in the United States. Unfortunately, a major problem with relying solely on death certificates is that coroners often avoid listing suicide as a cause of death. The underreporting may be as high as 30–40% (Jobes, Berman, & Josselson, 1987).

The association between MS and suicide is complex. In addition, it is difficult to monitor suicide attempts in patients with physical illnesses. Whitlock (1986) highlighted the issues of comorbidity, medication complications, and the nonuniform manner of reporting suicide rates in the literature. "The existence of physical diseases cannot be taken on as incontravertible evidence that illness was the sole or even the most important factor leading to suicide" (151). In discussing a study of over 1,000 suicides in England from 1968 to 1972, Whitlock observed that there were only six suicides in patients with MS.

> Faced by the prospect of lifelong, progressive disability with ultimate confinement to a wheelchair, double incontinence and recurrent urinary tract infections, it is surprising that suicide among multiple sclerosis suffers is a relatively rare event—a further indication that what might be called rational grounds for taking one's life contribute only slightly to the frequency of suicide among patients with serious physical illnesses. (157)

In summary, we find the reported data to be equivocal. There is probably an increased risk for suicide among those diagnosed with MS, although the evidence is not consistently robust. The clinical picture is complicated by the increased incidence of affective illness in this population, which could adversely effect the risk of suicide. Coping with the ravages of this illness and accompanying loneliness are probably also significant contributors to suicidality in this population.

Closely related to the disabilities found in the late stages of MS are the cerebral palsies—neurological disorders which leave individuals unable to control their limbs or have control over muscle groups. The Elizabeth Bouvia controversy (Box 14.1) was one of the first instances in the United States in which an obviously severely physically impaired individual challenged her caregivers (and society, generally) to assist her with ending her own life, because "the struggle is not worth it." This sensational case raised ethical, moral, legal, religious, and medical questions about the right to die, and whether this can be seen as a suicide act. Is it a rational decision? What are the criteria to determine whether it is rational and therefore acceptable? Must the desire to remain alive be rational? Is it irrational to want to end one's pain and suffering?

BOX 14.1. Elizabeth Bouvia: "My Life Is Not Worth Living"

Background: Elizabeth Bouvia, born in May 1957, had been paralyzed since birth by cerebral palsy and was confined to a wheelchair because of a lack of control over her arms and legs (quadriplegia). Beginning at age 10, she spent the next 7 years in an orthopedic hospital. Despite these challenges, she grew up and attended college. She subsequently started graduate school but eventually dropped out because of difficulties with her physical limitations. After her husband left her in the fall of 1983, she signed herself into a psychiatric unit and decided that she wanted assistance to end her life.

The request: At the age of 26, she decided that "my life is not worth living." She informed her California physicians that "the struggle is not worth it," and asked them to assist her in dying. Because she was physically unable to kill herself, she asked her physicians to let her starve to death, administering only painkillers and hygienic care while under their hospital care.

The controversy: In 1984, this was one of the first cases of a request for a physician-assisted death. Does she have the right to die? Should physicians be involved in voluntarily ending her life? Does society have a responsibility for her life? To facilitate her death? Is this a suicide?

EPILEPSY

Epilepsy is the abnormal electrical discharge from neurons in the CNS leading to seizures or other abnormal cognitive states. The research into the relationship between patients diagnosed with epilepsy and suicide is quite limited. However, there appears to be an increased incidence of suicide in this population associated with factors relating to personality and psychological factors.

Mackay (1979) found an increase in self-poisoning among epileptics as compared to the nonepileptic population. The epileptic group showed an increased frequency of personality disorders, with a relative lack of alcohol excess when compared to the nonepileptic self-poisoning group.

In their review of the mortality literature for epileptics, Matthews and Barabas (1981) found that on average 5% of deaths in patients with epilepsy were due to suicide, compared to 1.4% in the general U.S. population. A later review by Mendez, Lanska, Manon-Espaillat, and Burnstine (1989) found that epileptics have a risk of completed suicide four to five times higher than that of nonepileptics. They found that those with complex partial seizures of temporal lobe origin have an especially high risk. When compared with the control group, patients with epilepsy showed more evidence of borderline personality disorder with multiple impulsive suicide attempts and more psychotic disturbances including command hallucinations. They showed a similar frequency of depression as the control group and a decreased frequency of adjustment disorders. These authors suggested that suicide attempts by patients with epilepsy appear to be associated primarily with interictal psychopathological factors, such as borderline personality disorder, and psychosis rather than with specific psychosocial stressors, seizure variables, or anticonvulsant medication.

In a large study of over 9,000 patients with epilepsy in Stockholm, Nilsson et al. (1997) found an SMR of 3.6, with an excess mortality rate for injuries and poisoning (SMR 5.6). Of note is that the SMR for suicide was 3.5.

The pharmacological management of epilepsy is less time intensive and often less difficult than managing the psychosocial aspects of the disorder. Issues related to self-esteem, disruptions of daily life, alcoholism and substance abuse, depression, and suicide are often the most challenging and important components of management. These limited studies suggest a slightly higher rate of suicide in patients diagnosed with epilepsy. Personality factors associated with psychological impairments seem to contribute significantly in this group.

CANCER

In an early study, Sainsbury (1955) estimated that malignant neoplasm was present 20 times more often in a sample of suicide victims than would be expected in the general population. In a study of suicide and accident victims over age 50, Whitlock (1978) found that cancer was significantly more common among those who took their own lives. Large-scale epidemiological studies have found patients with cancer to be at significantly higher risk for suicide than the general population (Louhivuori & Hakama, 1979; Marshall, Burnett, & Brasure, 1983; Fox, Stanek, Boyd, & Flannery, 1982).

In contrast, however, autopsy evidence of completed suicides shows that some individuals believed they had cancer when they actually didn't or that their cancer was worse than it actually was (Murphy, 1977). Overall, however, the literature is ambiguous. Some studies have found patients diagnosed with cancer appear to commit suicide most frequently in the advanced stages of the illness at a point at which the prognosis is poor (Farberow, Shneidman, & Leonard, 1963; Marzuk, 1994; Boland, 1985a, 1985b; Louhivuori & Hakama,

1979). Other investigators have found that the risk for suicide, especially in males, was greatest soon after diagnosis (Fox et al., 1982). This may reflect the fear that many people have of the disease and the pain or dependency it may bring. Suicide for this population may be an attempt to take control of their lives at a time at which they fear the loss of control and its consequences the most.

Farberow et al. (1963) related suicide in cancer patients to "the fundamental psychological organization of the patient." They also noted the importance of the sense of control for these patients as outlined in Table 14.3.

In an early study, Campbell (1966) showed that male patients with cancer of all ages had a greater risk of suicide than the general population. However, this increased risk was not found for female patients. Other authors found an increased risk of suicide in both men and women diagnosed with cancer (Louhivuori & Hakama, 1979). They found that the excessive risk was confined to the first 5 years of follow-up and was greater for those patients with nonlocalized disease. Others (e.g., Marshall et al., 1983) have confirmed this association between patients with cancer and risk of suicide. Allebeck, Bolund, and Ringback (1989) found that suicide rates were highest in the first year following diagnosis with cancer. Patients with cancer of the lungs and upper airways, as well as those with cancer of the gastrointestinal tract (GIT), had higher suicide rates than those patients with cancer at other sites. However, these differences in suicide rates were not statistically significant. In another study, Allebeck and Bolund (1991) found that the suicide risk for hospitalized cancer patients were highest during the first 2 years following the diagnosis of cancer and dropped off to approach normal population rates after a lapse of 5 years from diagnosis. They concluded that the increase in suicide risk attributable to cancer is real but small.

Fear of cancer plays an important role in the formulation of suicidal actions. Dorpat et al. (1968) noted the presence of a severe and morbid fear of cancer in the completed suicide they investigated. In their study, 65% of those who suicided in association with their severe fear of cancer showed no evidence of malignancy on autopsy. Brown and Pisetsky (1960) emphasize the effect of the patient's belief that he or she is a victim of cancer when the physical diagnosis has not been made. Conwell, Caine, and Olsen (1990) describe eight situations in which the victims' belief that they had cancer played a major role in the decision to end their lives. As an alternate explanation, Whitlock (1978) described the possible paraneoplastic effect that tumors may have on suicidality; that is, alteration in mental function (including cognitive impairment, mood alteration, or hopelessness) may arise from the effect of the tumor itself and effect suicidality.

In summary, literature on the subject seems to indicate that the incidence of suicide in males with cancer is increased in the immediate period following diagnosis, and extending perhaps for as long as 5 years. The data for women are suggestive in this direction, but not conclusive (Allebeck et al., 1989; Storm, Christiensen, & Jemsen, 1992). There is some evidence to suggest that the patients who underwent chemotherapy were at highest risk, implying either that chemotherapy induces an organic mental disorder (including organic mood disorders) conducive to suicide or that the use of chemotherapy is correlated with a poor prognosis and an attendant sense of hopelessness.

Data indicating that the risk of suicide is directly related to the severity of the disease favor the latter explanation. Risk of suicide appears to be higher among patients with disseminated as opposed to local cancers (Storm et al., 1992). GIT cancers confirm the greatest risk of suicide for men, whereas lung and upper airways cancers were associated with greater rates in both genders. Cancers of the head and neck have an 11-fold increase in suicide rates, as opposed to cancer generally which has a relatively modest twofold increase. The reason for the much higher rates among head and neck cancer patients is unclear but may relate to the association with alcohol and tobacco use, facial disfigurement following surgery, and a loss of voice.

SPINAL CORD INJURY

Assessing the risk of suicide associated with spinal cord injuries (SCI) is complicated because many of these injuries are a result of dangerous risk-taking behaviors or strenuous athletic activities. Persons who sustain such injuries may have a higher likelihood of engaging in impulsive, possibly self-destructive, behaviors than those in the general population. These individuals might be expected to have an increased risk for suicidal behaviors, independent of their SCI. The data indicate that once injured, the patient with SCI is at increased risk of suicide. Death from suicide occurs two to six times more often than in the general population (Frisbie & Kache, 1983; Geisler, Jousse, Wynne-Jones, & Breithaupt, 1983; Nyquist & Bors, 1967). Why do patients with SCI carry a higher risk of suicide? This relates to the impact of the sudden devastating injury on an individual's self-concept and self-esteem, as well as to the high incidence of major psychiatric disorders in the SCI population (including alcohol and drug abuse, psychosis, and depression). Each of these disorders can lead to suicide attempts, which in and of themselves can cause SCI. In addition, there are the acute and chronic effects of head injury in this group of patients, including postconcussive syndromes and posttraumatic brain injury.

Case 14.1 highlights the issues of multiple adjustment to a chronic, debilitating SCI, including a loss of mastery and control over one's immediate surroundings, adjustment of lifelong coping mechanisms and strategies, self-awareness and identity, and the need to balance new stresses and demands with a sense of hope.

Death from suicide occurred far more frequently during the first 3 years following injury (Wilcox & Stauffer, 1972). The rates of suicide appear to be related to the type of injury. Individuals with complete quadriplegia had a suicide rate four times greater than in the general population. Those with incomplete paraplegic had a rate three times greater; those with incomplete quadriplegia was more than twice the general population; and those with complete paraplegia was one and a half times the rate of the whole population (Geisler et al., 1983). Others have found that suicide in SCI appears related to age or severity of illness (Nyquist & Bors, 1967).

In a conflicting report, Hopkins (1971) found that suicide in patients with SCI tended to occur 5 or more years after the initial injury. This differs from the National Spinal Cord Injury Statistical Center (NSCISC), which reported that 80% of all suicides occurred within 3 years of the injury (Ducharme & Freed, 1980). One study that tried to identify factors that lead to increased risk of suicide in SCI found that the variables that strongly related to suicide or postinjury despondency were expressions of shame, apathy, helplessness, and a history of preinjury family fragmentation. Other factors that were more moderately related were injury not caused by a falling object; active involvement in the cause of the SCI; preinjury history of alcohol abuse, drug abuse, depression, or despondency; and a postinjury history of alcohol abuse, anger, destructive behavior, and other suicide attempts (Charlifue & Gerhart, 1991).

A number of movies have featured life dilemmas facing the chronically physically ill. One of the first was *Whose Life Is It, Anyway?*, a 1970s movie about a 30-year-old sculptor who, as a result of a car accident, suffers a severe SCI, leaving him a quadriplegic. The movie depicts the protagonist, Ken Harrison (played by Richard Dreyfuss), in the hospital and bed-ridden. He becomes depressed, despondent, and suicidal as he fully comprehends his limitations and what the future will be like for him. He decides to sue the hospital (a

CASE 14.1. Failing to Adapt to Adversity

A 24-year-old single white male was not wearing his protective helmet when his motorcycle spun out of control and he hit a patch of oil on a highway. He was flung from the motorcycle and sustained a spinal cord injury in the cervical spine area that severed his spinal cord. This left him with the loss of function in both legs and with only a small degree of function in one hand. Although he could lift his arms using his shoulder muscles, he was unable to grasp utensils or lift himself out of his wheelchair. Despite doing well with his rehabilitation and adjustment to being confined to a wheelchair, he was having great difficulty adapting to a new set of demands and expectations since he left the rehabilitation unit. Prior to his injury, he was not very psychologically minded and, in fact, had expressed disdain for those who were "weak-willed." He had been an athlete and a marathon runner. His prior employment was one in which he was highly rewarded and respected for being assertive, energetic, and organized. He now found himself spending a large part of his day trying to negotiate routine activities of daily life—eating, dressing, grooming, bathing, urination, and defecation.

At the point that signs and symptoms of depression were identified, he was referred to a psychiatrist and put on medications. Nevertheless, his physical condition continued to deteriorate and he lost interest in restructuring his life to respond to his new set of physical limitations. One day his wheelchair hit a crack in the sidewalk, and he was propelled forward from his wheelchair, sending him face down onto the sidewalk. He was unable to brace his fall and he sustained lacerations to his face and scalp. The next day, while no one knew of his whereabouts, he drove his wheelchair into a neighbor's backyard swimming pool and drowned.

writ of habeus corpus) to allow him to starve to death under their care. The movie depicts the intervention of his girlfriend, his physicians, psychiatrists (for the plaintiff and defense), and the legal profession. Although he wins his day in court (he has the right to starve himself to death), the movie ends without a clear resolution of his fate.

AIDS

Suicide following HIV or AIDS diagnoses may be better documented than for other illnesses because of the generally better statistics kept on these patients. AIDS-related suicides are likely to be attributed to the psychosocial turmoil attendant to learning that one has a highly lethal and communicable disease. In addition, recent evidence suggests that the HIV may affect CNS function early in the course of the illness and in so doing predispose seropositive individuals to catastrophic reactions by compromising memory, mood, or impulse control (Grant et al., 1987). As seropositive individuals develop AIDS, the associated stigma attached to this diagnosis may drive some to suicide. With disease progression, virtually 100% of patients will develop subacute encephalitis (Gabuzda & Hirsch, 1987). This may be marked by cognitive deficits, memory loss, depression, personality changes, or psychosis. Any of the symptoms might increase the risk of suicide.

BOX 14.2.   "Whose Life Is It, Anyway?"

1. **Partial character list:**
   - Ken Harrison (quadriplegic in car accident)
   - Pat (Ken's girlfriend)
   - Dr. Clare Scott (female internist who treated Ken)
   - Dr. Emerson (chief MD on Ken's treatment team)
   - John (orderly, in punk rock band)
   - Mrs. Boyle (social worker and occupational therapist)
   - Judge Wyler (judge who heard Ken's case for habeus corpus plea)
   - Carter Hall (Ken's lawyer)

2. **Key point:** Who decides life and death (not necessarily actually being dead or alive)? Power is a main issue here (who decides life and death).

3. Humor is a psychological defense against death, dying, and difficult life situations. Still, Ken's humor is childish and maddening at times; you almost want to shake him and say "grow up!"

4. Ken was rigid. He told Mrs. Boyle (SW) that he couldn't change. But his mind need not be his enemy (as he claims). Long life is a succession of compromises (although usually not as severe as Ken must make). Is Ken in denial?

5. The argument presented is that if one is depressed, then you cannot decide (rationally) to commit suicide or euthanasia. However, there are tests to measure clinical levels of depression (it need not only be the clinical judgment of psychiatrists).

6. Note the "Catch-22": if one wants to kill one's self, then he or she must be crazy, and if he or she is crazy, then this person cannot make rational choices.

7. The Valium injection (10 mg IV) by Dr. Emerson was both a bad thing (i.e., an abusive, coercive act) and a good thing (Ken decided afterwards that he should end his relationship with Pat). A dramatic (and symbolic) device was the breaking of the vase and then the orderly, John, picked up the broken pieces (also symbolic).

8. Death and sexual references. Why is Ken always making sexual jokes? Does sex equal life (Freud thought so). Is all energy sexual energy? If one is not sexually alive, is that person essentially dead?

9. Note that only Ken's brain is alive versus the more normal euthanasia situation in which the brain of the patient is dead (flat EEG) but the body is alive.

10. Contrast Ken's situation with that of the little girl who was also in kidney dialysis (she had a future).

11. Mercy killing of animals versus of human beings. What are the differences? Ken says "if I were a cat or a dog, you'd put me to sleep."

12. It is not clear what Ken decides to do at the end of the film (ambivalence). Although he wins the trial and the right to starve himself to death, will he actually follow through? The film closes with a shot of Michelangelo's hand (a sculpture). Ken tells Clare he is sure he wants to die, in fact that he is already dead in a sense. Dr. Emerson tells Ken after the trial that "we will not even feed you, if you want to stay at the hospital." But will he actually do it, now that he can control his life?

13. Law on assisting suicide: 1990, U.S. Supreme Court, *Missouri v. Parents of Nancy Curzon* (court decided hospital does not have to allow patients to starve themselves to death, even if they or their guardians want it).

In a study of New York City residents, Marzuk et al. (1988) determined that the relative risk of suicide in men ages 20 to 59 who were diagnosed with AIDS was 36 times that of comparable men without the diagnosis. This high rate of suicide most likely results from a complicated mix of stressors, including the direct effect of HIV on the brain, the increased likelihood of substance abuse as a comorbid problem, the perception of a grim prognosis (though this has changed dramatically with new treatments), and the stigma attached to the illness.

In addition to being a potential risk factor for suicide, contraction of AIDS may be a means of suicide. Four cases have been described wherein alcoholic homosexual males consciously sought infection with HIV as a means of suicide (Flavin, Franklin, & Frances, 1986; Frances, Wikstrom, & Alcena, 1985).

PEPTIC ULCER

Several studies have noted the increased risk of suicide associated with peptic ulcer disease (PUD). Early studies showed that men but not women with PUD had a greater number of deaths from suicide than the general population. Data from this study implicated mental illness among sufferers of PUD as a possible cause of the increased suicide rate. They show that the increase appeared to be unrelated to any surgical treatment for the illness, but the study population did show a greater number of nonpsychotic mental disorders. No data was presented on drug or alcohol abuse in this group (Viskum, 1975).

This finding was confirmed in a later study in which both male and female patients who had undergone surgical procedures for treatment of PUD showed almost a fourfold increase in suicide risk. Again, in this group, one-third had a diagnosis of alcoholism and a significant increase in psychiatric hospitalization compared with the survival group (Knop & Fischer, 1981). Others have found that the relative risk of suicide in male alcoholics in Sweden was 10 times that of the general population. However, the suicide rate among those with PUD with or without gastric surgery was 30 times that of the general population. In other words, PUD in men conferred a risk of suicide in this population beyond that associated with alcoholism alone (Berglund, 1986). It therefore appears that there is an increased risk of suicide in males conferred by PUD, and it is independent of the risk associated with alcoholism. The data for women with PUD are inconclusive.

AUTOIMMUNE DISORDERS

Rheumatoid Arthritis

The limited literature on rheumatoid arthritis and suicide seems to suggest that there may be a modest increase in the risk of suicide associated with this illness. In an early Veterans Administration hospital study, Pokorny (1960) found that 6 of 44 suicides among patients who had bone or joint disease, not otherwise specified, compared to 2 of 44 ex-patients who served as controls. Another study (Dorpat et al., 1968) found increased prevalence of rheumatoid arthritis in a series of consecutive suicides (15%), when contrasted with its prevalence in the study's nonmatched control population (2–3%). The authors felt that this increased suicide risk reflected years of pain and progressive disability as well as increasing isolation from other people. However, they did not specify whether any of these patients were taking steroids or other immunosuppressive agents, which could suggest another risk factor on the basis of cognitive impairment.

Systemic Lupus Erythematosus

There is an approximately fourfold increase in suicide risk among these patients. This increase probably results from the effects of the disease on the CNS. These effects can include acute psychosis, cognitive impairment, and depression. Additional complications such as organ failure (e.g., in chronic renal failure) and steroid-induced psychosis or mood disorder probably contribute to the higher than expected suicide rate.

DIABETES MELLITUS

The literature regarding diabetes mellitus and suicide is not very robust. Several studies show a modest increase in the suicide rate (Entmacher, Krall, & Krenczer, 1985; Teutsch et al., 1982; Turnbridge, 1981). This is somewhat surprising given the increased rates of cognitive dysfunction (Perlmuter et al., 1984; Ryan, Vega, & Drash, 1985) and mood disorders (Popkin, Callies, Lentz, Colon, & Sutherland, 1988) that are found in diabetics. Underreporting on death certificates may be one factor. Another factor may be the difficulty in recognizing suicidal behavior in this population. Self-directed discontinuation of insulin therapy is one of the two most common causes of diabetic ketoacidosis (DKA). Cohen et al. (1960) found that such omissions of insulin therapy accounted for 25% of all DKA episodes. Similarly, deaths from hypoglycemia may represent the consequence of intentional insulin overdose (Stearns, 1959). Findings of Turnbridge (1981) seem to support this explanation. This study showed that although no suicides were identified in the diabetic group, patient neglect was contributory in 27% of deaths, and personality factors and domestic difficulties which may have delayed medical attention were relevant in 25% of cases.

Diabetes probably does increase the risk for suicide. Treatment regimens should also address psychosocial issues. The goals of treatment for patients with insulin-dependent diabetes mellitus is to promote their well-being while preventing complications associated with their illness (Jacobson, 1996). These issues are not unique to diabetes mellitus and can be viewed as relevant to most chronic physical illnesses that have a potentially debilitating course over a patients' lifetime. Table 14.4 outlines many psychosocial issues relevant to the care of patients with diabetes. Failure to address these issues can predispose a patient toward suicidal behaviors.

TABLE 14.4. **Psychosocial Issues Relevant to Diabetes Care**

The patient's and family members' expectations, attitudes, and goals for treatment
Past experience with illness in general and diabetes in particular
Current affective state
Extent of grief or acceptance of the diagnosis
Readiness to learn and make behavioral changes
Extent and sources of current stress
Emotional reactions to key issues related to diabetes (e.g., ideals for weight, intolerance
    of regularity, fear of needles, fears about hypoglycemia, fear of complications)
Psychiatric illness, especially depression and eating disorders
Key people in the patient's life
Reactions to and relationships with members of the health care team
Cultural factors affecting the perception of the meaning of illness and its treatment.
Financial issues, especially insurance coverage

Source: Jacobson (1996). Copyright 1996 by Massachusetts Medical Society. All rights reserved. Reprinted by permission.

KIDNEY DISEASE

There is an increased rate of suicide for patients on renal dialysis (Abram, Moore, & Westervelt, 1971). This risk may be particularly high in young persons who suffer graft failure after renal transplantation and are forced to resume dialysis (Washer, Schröter, Starzl, & Weill, 1983). However, the magnitude of the relative risk, although undoubtedly significant, has been difficult to ascertain precisely (Levy, 1979). As Di Biance (1979) pointed out, this is at least partially because the definition of suicidal behavior is a point of disagreement among researchers in the field. For some clinicians, deaths related to nonadherence to a medical regime is considered suicide; for others, lethal noncompliance must be accompanied by symptoms of depression to be judged suicide.

Since hemodialysis and peritoneal dialysis became widely available for patients with chronic renal failure, there have been some reports of higher than expected suicide rates. Patients' requests for stopping therapy which, of course, results in death, have been referred to by some as veiled suicide and by others as rational suicide. Whether decisions to terminate treatment are recorded as suicide is unclear.

Chronic renal disease is complicated by uremic encephalopathy, hypertensive encephalopathy, hemodialysis disequilibrium syndrome, and dialysis dementia, all of which can present with confusional of states and contribute to increased suicide risk.

TERMINAL ILLNESS

It is incorrect to assume that terminal illness necessarily increases suicidality. Brown, Henteleff, Barakat, and Rowe (1986) found that 77% of the terminally ill who were questioned in a hospice setting had never wished for death to come early. All of those who had desired death were found to be suffering from severe clinical depression. Suicide in the terminally ill may have more to do with psychosocial factors than with the state of the illness per se. Marzuk (1994) identified three trends that inaugurated a renewed interest in suicide among terminally ill patients (vs. those with chronic debilitating disorders): (1) many terminally ill patients were becoming more chronic due to earlier diagnoses and improved palliative care; (2) the public's interest in voluntary euthanasia, rational suicide, and physician-assisted suicide had rapidly increased; and (3) the development of blood tests to diagnose terminal illness (e.g., Huntington's Disease and AIDS) at an early, asymptomatic phase had increased the concern about suicide potential in these populations.

Suicide in this population needs further study in consensus among investigators as to what exactly constitutes "terminally ill" (e.g., less than 1 year to live) and what is meant by suicide in his population group and active or willful use of lethal means to end one's life, as opposed to more passive actions such as refusal of treatment, withholding nutrition, or removal from life support.

SUMMARY AND CONCLUSIONS

Most patients with acute or chronic physical illnesses do not commit suicide. For those who do, certain risk factors play an important role. These factors include the presence of preexisting psychopathology, the ability to manage stress (physical and emotional), and the ability to seek and benefit from social support. Other contributing factors are those risk factors associated with the illness itself, which may precipitate suicide. These include altered mental states secondary to depression, anxiety, or psychosis; altered states of consciousness (delirium) secondary to medications or decreased physical functioning (e.g., oxygenation of blood and cardiac output); and physical and mental deterioration, pain management, social isolation, and external pressures such as financial worries (Derogatis et al., 1983; Perry, 1990; Conwell et al., 1990).

Although the data are far from complete, it does appear that physical illness increases the risk for suicide and suicidal behavior. Certain illnesses confer greater risk of suicide than others. Table 14.5 presents a comparison of physical illnesses with increased risks for suicide as summarized by Kelly, Mufson, and Rogers (1999). Multiple sclerosis is associated with increased risk of suicide especially in the first 5 years. Patients with epilepsy have shown a slight increase in suicide risk. This appears related to personality factors and not the seizures themselves. Cancer, and especially the fear of cancer, has led to an increase in suicide, particularly in males and those with aggressive tumors. Spinal cord injury increases the risk of suicide and seems to be related to the individual's sense of self and high incidence of psychiatric disorders in this population. AIDS, and the fear of AIDS, increases suicide risk due to a complicated combination of physiological, psychological, and environmental stressors. Peptic ulcer disease and autoimmune disorders increase suicide risk to a limited extent.

It is evident that health care providers and mental health care providers need to be more cognizant of their patients' perception of their chronic or debilitating physical illnesses, because of the likelihood of increased risk for suicide and other suicidal behaviors in these patients. A responsible clinician needs to carefully explore the presence of other risk factors as well as protective factors in each patient presenting with a physical illness. Once the assessment is completed, the clinician must rely on clinical judgment to assign relative risk for suicidal behaviors. Based on this clinical judgment, the clinician then establishes a treatment plan, including risk management protocols.

The treatment plan may include the need for psychotherapeutic interventions, psychosocial interventions, psychopharmacology, or environmental changes.

Unfortunately most clinicians, especially physicians working with the chronically physically ill, have not been sufficiently trained in suicide assessment, treatment, or prevention. One of the explicit goals of the U.S. *Surgeon General's Call to Action to Prevent Suicide 1999* (U.S. Public Health Service, 1999) is to educate primary care providers about how to effectively assess and intervene with their at-risk patients, as well to prevent the emergence

TABLE 14.5. Medical Conditions with Increased Suicidal Risk

Illness	Increased risk (×)
HIV or AIDS	6.6
Huntington's disease	2.9
Malignant neoplasms	
All sites	1.8
Head and neck	11.4
Multiple sclerosis	2.4
Peptic ulcer	2.1
Chronic renal failure	
Dialysis	14.5
Transplantation	3.8
Spinal cord injuries	3.8
Systemic lupus erythematosus	4.3

Source: Harris & Barraclough (1994). Copyright 1994 by Lippincott Williams & Wilkins. Reprinted by permission.

TABLE 14.6. Implications for Suicide Prevention

- Educate primary-care physicians about the association between some physical illnesses and suicidal tendencies. Increase awareness, recognition, referral, and consultation.
- Educate physicians regarding the role of medications in promoting conditions that facilitate suicidal behaviors. Increase judicious selection and use of nonpsychotropic medications.
- Educate physicians regarding the appropriate selection and use of psychotropic medications for the treatment and prevention of psychiatric symptoms associated with suicidal behaviors when they present in primary care settings.

of self-destructive behaviors. Table 14.6 outlines three sets of activities that begin to address the recognized need to increase suicide awareness and intervention among physicians caring for the chronically medically ill.

FURTHER READING

Goldman, L. S., Wise, T. N., & Brody, D. S. (Eds.). (1988). *Psychiatry for primary care physicians*. Washington, DC: American Psychiatric Press. This text, a joint effort of the American Medical Association and the American Psychiatric Association, strives to educate primary-care physicians about the presentation, diagnosis, and treatment of psychiatric disorders as they present in primary-care settings. Chapters cover topics including suicide and violence, elder abuse, depression, and commonly used psychiatric medications.

Murphy, G. E. (1992). *Suicide in alcoholism*. New York: Oxford University Press. This landmark book reviews the research on the association between alcohol abuse and suicidal behaviors across the lifespan. Fifty case histories are presented which highlight the range of alcoholic behavior across the lifespan as well as the tragic tale of self-destructive behavior associated with alcoholism.

Hobbs, N., & Perrin, J. M. (Eds.). (1985). *Issues in the care of children with chronic illness*. San Francisco: Jossey-Bass. This massive edited volume covers the entire range of issues related to the care of children with chronic illness. Chapters cover all the major chronic childhood illnesses, including juvenile onset diabetes, sickle cell anemia, chronic kidney diseases, leukemia, asthma, cystic fibrosis, and congenital heart disease. Chapters are devoted to the special training of physicians, nurses, and social workers to care for chronically ill children. Other topics cover the toll these conditions have on healthy family functioning, and the need for the provision of mental heath services to address these children and their families.

Committee on Handicaps of the Group for the Advancement of Psychiatry. (1993). *Caring for people with physical impairment: The journey back* (GAP Report No. 135). Washington, DC: American Psychiatric Press. This book brings together the expertise of caregivers from a variety of backgrounds to examine the special needs of patients with physical impairments. Topics include an exploration of the experience of physical impairment as well as developmental considerations. A separate section addresses clinical applications, including caregiver reactions, coping strategies, and therapeutic transactions.

15

Alcoholism, Substance Abuse, and Suicide

David Lester

Dear Mom,

    I am going to try to die but please don't blame [wife's name] for [what] I do for she can't help it if she doesn't love me and don't let anyone hurt her. I ask this of all of you, please. If anything try to help her in every way you can for I love that woman with all my heart. I don't care if she is the biggest pig in the world, she is a good mother to the kids

    Please forgive me if you can't read this for I am very sleepy. don't let them put me back ware [*sic*] I was, if God doesn't let me die I just can't live this type of life. "P.S. If God won't let me die please don't let them put me back in that ward. [nickname]

           —Suicide note written by a 41-year-old white male alcoholic
               dead from a barbiturate overdose; Murphy (1992)

The relationship between alcoholism/drug abuse and suicidal behavior can be studied at two levels: the societal and the individual. At the societal level, the per capita consumption of alcohol or incidence of alcoholism are measured for a society and compared with the rate of suicide. This comparison can be made over time (Are years with more per capita alcohol consumed those with higher suicide rates?) or over regions (Do regions of a country with more per capita alcohol consumed have higher suicide rates?). This type of research is important because it can lend support for strategies that may reduce the suicide rate of a society by suggesting changes in the social policies concerned with the sale of alcohol and treatment of alcoholism.

On the other hand, studies at the individual level are important because they generate research findings that may aid in the prediction of suicidal behavior and provide guidelines for the treatment of suicidal individuals. In this chapter, research from both strategies is reviewed, and we begin by looking at societal-level research.

SOCIETAL-LEVEL RESEARCH

Almost all the societal-level studies have focused on the use and abuse of alcohol rather than drugs, and all have looked at the impact of alcohol use and abuse on completed suicide

TABLE 15.1. Correlations between Suicide Rates and
Alcohol Consumption, 1950–1972

Belgium	0.76*
Canada	0.95*
Czechoslovakia	0.92*
Denmark	−0.11
Finland	0.56*
Luxembourg	0.37*
Netherlands	0.79*
New Zealand	−0.26
Norway	0.67*
Sweden	0.86*
Switzerland	−0.85*
United States	0.81*
West Germany	0.66*

Source: Lester & Yang (1998). Copyright 1998 by Nova Science Publishers. Reprinted by permission.
*Statistically significant.

(rather than on attempted suicide) because of the availability of good epidemiological data on completed suicide. Many of the studies of the association between alcohol use and suicide have looked at the variation in these variables over time. For example, Skog (1995) found a positive association over time in Portugal between alcohol consumption and suicide. An increase in per capita alcohol consumption of one liter was accompanied by a 1.9% increase in the male suicide rate. For the United States from 1936 to 1970, Lester (1993a) found that alcohol consumption, along with the size of the military (an indicator of wartime) and unemployment, were significantly associated with (and explained 91% of the variance of) the suicide rate.

This association is not always found for every group in a society. In Norway from 1911 to 1990, Rossow (1993) found a positive association between alcohol consumption and completed suicide for men but not for women. In Finland from 1950 to 1991, Makela (1996) found that alcohol consumption was associated only with the suicide rates of men ages 15–34 and 35–49.

The results also vary by country. Lester and Yang (1998) studied the association between alcohol consumption and suicide rates from 1950 to 1972 in 13 countries. The association was positive and statistically significant for 10 countries, negative and statistically significant for 1, and not significant for 2 (see Table 15.1).

Norstrom (1995a) predicted that the association between alcohol consumption and suicide will vary depending on the level of consumption. If the level of alcohol consumption is high (as in France, Denmark, and Portugal), fluctuations at this level may have less effect on the suicide rate than if the level of alcohol consumption is low (as in Sweden, Norway, and Hungary). In line with his prediction, he found that the association between alcohol consumption and suicide was weaker in France than in Sweden.[1]

Can social policies concerning alcohol affect the suicide rate? Wasserman, Varnik, and Eklund (1994) found that the restrictive alcohol policies in the early years of perestroika (1985–1988) in the Soviet Union were accompanied by a decline in the male suicide rate in the Soviet republics. Skog (1993) explored the results of a "natural" experiment in which the consumption of alcohol declined in Denmark in 1916 and 1917 as a result of price in-

---

[1]Supporting this hypothesis, Lester and Yang (1998; see Table 15.1) similarly found the association to be weaker in Denmark than in Sweden and Norway.

creases due to a shortage of the raw materials caused by a wartime blockade. The suicide rate decreased, especially among alcoholics.

Studies have also been conducted over regions. Lester (1993b) found that U.S. states in 1970 with more restrictive alcohol polices (e.g., more seizures of illegal grain mash, a higher price for alcohol, higher states taxes on alcohol, a greater proportion of the population living in "dry" areas, state monopolies on sales, and a lower minimum purchasing age and fewer retail outlets) had lower suicide rates. This positive association is not always found. For example, Skog (1995) found that the association between alcohol consumption and suicide over the regions of Portugal was negative. Although the association has not been studied in enough nations to enable the generality of the associations to be assessed, it seems likely that associations will be positive for the majority of nations.

Regional studies sometimes permit the investigation of the association of suicide rates with alcohol abuse and alcoholism treatment, because these measures can be obtained by region. For example, Lester (1998) found that the suicide rates of the U.S. states in 1974 were associated with the per capita consumption of alcohol but not with membership in Alcoholics Anonymous (AA) or mortality from cirrhosis of the liver. Changes in alcohol consumption from 1974 to 1983 (but not changes in AA membership or cirrhosis mortality) were positively associated with changes in the suicide rate. Thus, the average per capita alcohol consumption in the society rather than the prevalence of alcohol abusers appeared to be the important variable in the association with suicide rates. This finding lends support to a social policy of restricting alcohol sales as a way of reducing the suicide rate.

INDIVIDUAL-LEVEL RESEARCH

Measurement Issues

Research at the individual level faces several problems regarding focus. For suicidal behavior, investigators may study fatal suicidal behavior in which the individual dies (commonly called completed suicide) or nonfatal suicidal behavior in which the individual survives (commonly called suicidal ideation and attempted suicide).[2] Some investigators study the prior occurrence of nonfatal suicidal behavior in people, whereas others try to predict nonfatal suicidal behavior in the future. Those studying completed suicide may study predictors of the behavior retrospectively (after the people complete suicide) or prospectively (in follow-up studies of potential suicides). Regarding the measurement of substance abuse, some investigators study the "use" of alcohol and drugs, whereas others study their excessive and addictive use.

Combining these different operational definitions of suicidal behavior and substance use and abuse results in a variety of research designs, not all of which are of equal merit. It would seem that predictive studies of suicidal behavior are of more value than studies looking at prior suicidal behavior. Furthermore, although attempted suicide is a more common behavior than completed suicide (perhaps 8 to 10 times more frequent) and involves a large cost for medical treatment, it may be more important to predict completed suicide than nonfatal suicidal behavior.

Finally, it should be noted that far more research has been conducted on suicide and alcohol abuse than on suicide and drug abuse. To illustrate this, PsycLIT was searched for articles on suicide and drugs for 1991–1997 (see Table 15.2). It can be seen, for example,

---

[2]Some suicidologists prefer to call attempted suicide parasuicide or deliberate self-harm (O'Carroll et al., 1996).

TABLE 15.2. Research on Suicide and Drugs and
Alcohol, PsycLIT 1991–1997

Suicide and alcohol	352 entries
Suicide and cocaine	23 entries
Suicide and heroin	13 entries
Suicide and crack	7 entries
Suicide and inhalants	5 entries
Suicide and tranquilizers	5 entries
Suicide and PCP	3 entries
Suicide and lsd	2 entries
Suicide and hallucinogens	1 entry

that, whereas 352 citations were found for suicide and alcohol, only 13 were found for suicide and heroin. Thus, relatively little is known about suicide and drugs other than alcohol.

Alcohol and the Suicidal Act

Many suicidal individuals consume alcohol in the hours immediately before their suicidal act. For example, Suokas and Lönnqvist (1995) found that 62% of suicide attempters had drunk alcohol prior to or at the time of their attempt. Virkkunen and Alha (1971) found that 15% of Finnish completed suicides had consumed alcohol immediately prior to their deaths, and Welte, Abel, and Wieczorek (1988) found that 33% of completed suicides in Erie County (New York) had done so. Welte et al. (1988) found that the suicides with alcohol in their blood were more often male, ages 21–60, left no suicide note, had made no prior suicide attempts, had tranquilizers in their body, completed suicide in the evening or at night, used a firearm, and were found in their car. Welte thought that these results suggested greater impulsivity in the suicides with alcohol in their blood. Attempted suicides are also found frequently to have consumed alcohol (Hawton, Fagg, & McKeown, 1989).

Alcohol intoxication may also play many roles in suicidal behavior, from making it easier psychologically for the suicidal person to carry out his or her suicidal plan to increasing the lethality of ingested medication. Steele and Joseph (1990) have documented that alcohol ingestion has cognitive consequences, an "alcohol myopia" that includes a reduction in the range of perception and less ability to engage in inferential thought. Rogers (1992) noted that alcohol myopia is very similar to the cognitive state described by Shneidman (1987) as characterizing suicides involving constriction and dichotomous thinking. Rogers argued that alcohol intoxication increases the risk of suicide via the mediating effect of this alcohol myopia.

SUICIDAL BEHAVIOR IN SUBSTANCE ABUSERS

Substance abuse is itself sometimes viewed as a suicidal or self-destructive behavior. For example, Menninger (1938) included substance abuse in his category of "chronic suicide," because he felt that substance abuse may be motivated in part, consciously or unconsciously, by suicidal impulses. Alternatively, perhaps, suicide and substance abuse may be expressions of the same underlying variable, such as social disorganization or an oral personality.

Substance abusers appear to have a higher incidence of suicidal behavior than nonabusers. It may be that substance abuse disrupts the social relationships of people and impairs their work performance, leading to social isolation and social decline; that it increases their impulsivity and lowers their restraints; or that it increases their self-deprecation and depression, tendencies that may increase the probability of suicidal behavior (Kendall, 1983).

Alcoholism may also make the self-destructive medications (such as antidepressant drugs) often used for suicide more lethal to the body, and alcohol itself may be used in conjunction with medications to provide a more lethal concoction. Furthermore, the substances that can be abused are also those that can be used to commit suicide. Thus, people have committed suicide by overdosing on such drugs as heroin and cocaine (Sperry & Sweeney, 1989). It should also be noted that in the planning and the execution of a suicidal action, individuals often use alcohol and other drugs to achieve a state of mind in which it is easier to carry out their suicidal plan.

Roy and Linnoila (1986) have also explored the reasons that alcoholism and suicide may be associated. First, Roy and Linnoila noted that evidence from animal studies indicates that alcohol causes changes in the turnover of several neurotransmitters in the brain. A review of physiological research into suicide (Lester, 1988) concluded that serotonin is the neurotransmitter most likely to be involved in suicidal and depressive behavior, and alcoholism may have an impact on suicidal behavior by lowering serotonin levels in some regions of the central nervous system.

Second, Roy and Linnoila, like Kendall, noted that depression and depressive disorder are common in alcoholics as well as in their relatives. In addition, alcoholism itself also produces depressive symptoms. Thus, it may be that concomitant depression is the mediating factor in producing the higher suicide rate in alcoholics. Two other mediating variables may be the experience of a personality disorder (commonly noted in substance abusers who are suicidal) and the experiences of stressful life events.

The association between depression and alcoholism is especially important. Alcoholism is associated with depression, depression is common in the relatives of alcoholics, and alcoholism is common in the relatives of depressive patients (Goodwin, 1973). Depression is a powerful associate of (and predictor of) suicide, and if the association between alcoholism and suicide is simply a result of the mediation of depression, then alcoholism will never be as powerful a predictor of suicide as depression. In addition, alcoholism itself can produce depression. Thus, future research must compare and contrast the relative power of depression and alcoholism in predicting suicide.

The following sections address two issues:

1. Can substance abuse be a predictor of suicidal behavior?
2. Will the useful predictors of suicidal behavior differ in substance abusers and nonabusers?

First let us turn to the incidence of suicide in substance abusers.

Alcohol Abuse and Completed Suicide

Many studies have reported an excess of alcoholics among completed suicides. For example, Wihelmsen, Elmfeldt, and Wedel (1983) found an excess of alcoholics among Swedish completed suicides, and Boyer et al. (1992) found that suicides were more likely to have an Axis I diagnosis of alcohol/drug dependence than were people in the general population or those dying in motor vehicle accidents.

Many recent studies have also reported an excess of completed suicides among alcoholics (e.g., Klatsky & Armstrong, 1993). Indeed, Beck and Steer (1989) found that alcoholism was the strongest single predictor of subsequent completed suicide in a sample of attempted suicides.

TABLE 15.3. Lifetime Risk for Suicide in Alcoholics

Country	Annual rate	Lifetime risk
	Untreated	
Iceland	0.12%	2.25%
United States	0.05%	0.90%
	Former outpatients	
Canada	0.11%	1.99%
Netherlands	0.13%	2.37%
United States	0.28%	5.39%
	Former inpatients	
Austria	0.39%	7.34%
Canada	0.42%	7.97%
Denmark	1.05%	20.01%
Iceland	0.12%	2.30%
Norway	0.17%	6.79%
Sweden	0.36%	6.79%
Switzerland	0.24%	4.48%
United Kingdom	0.48%	9.23%
United States	0.13%	2.55%
West Germany	0.85%	16.14%

Source: Calculated by Lester from figures in Murphy & Wetzel (1990). Lifetime risk is annual risk × 19.

Murphy and Wetzel (1990) reviewed previous research and estimated the lifetime risk of suicide in U.S. alcoholics to be 2% to 3.4%. They noted that the annual and lifetime risk varies from nation to nation and may also depend on the level of treatment received by the alcoholics. Estimates of annual and lifetime risk of suicide for alcoholics in several nations are shown in Table 15.3. These estimates are not strictly comparable because (1) nations may differ in the treatment facilities available for alcoholics, and (2) alcoholics in inpatient versus outpatient treatment may differ in the severity of their alcohol abuse. However, these estimates do give some idea of the risk of suicide in alcoholics in the nations.

Roy and Linnoila (1986) provided estimates that are considerably higher than those provided by Murphy and Wetzel. Roy and Linnoila argued that, on average, about 18% of alcoholics subsequently complete suicide and that 21% of suicides are alcoholics.[3] Thus, not only is the suicide rate substantially elevated among alcoholics, but suicide is a cause of death for a substantial percentage of alcoholics. Roy (1993) described the typical alcoholic suicide as male, white, middle age, and unmarried, with a long history of drinking. Unemployment, living alone, and poor social support are common. Most important, comorbidity (a concomitant diagnosis of another psychiatric disorder, especially an affective disorder) increases the risk of suicide.

Alcohol Abuse and Attempted Suicide

A high rate of attempted suicide has been reported in alcoholics (e.g., Gomberg, 1989). In a community survey, Weissman, Myers, and Harding (1980) found that 24% of alcoholics had attempted suicide, as compared to 5% of those with other diagnoses. Cornelius, Sal-

---

[3]Roy and Linnoila (1986) found that studies with longer follow-up periods found a higher percentage of deaths in alcoholics to be from suicide.

loum, Day, Thase, and Mann (1996) found that 40% of a sample of alcoholics with major depression who were hospitalized had attempted suicide in the prior week and 70% had attempted suicide at some point in their lives.

In addition, attempted suicides also have a high incidence of alcohol abuse. For example, Petronis, Samuels, Moscicki, and Anthony (1990) found that those who had attempted suicide in a community sample more often abused alcohol (and incidentally cocaine) than did those who had not attempted suicide.

Thus, the research indicates that, in general, alcohol abusers are at increased risk for completing and attempting suicide and that attempted and completed suicides have a higher than average incidence of alcohol abuse.

Drug Abusers

Not only are studies of the association between suicidal behavior and drug abuse relatively rare, but also the study of suicidal behavior in drug abusers is complicated by the fact that many drug abusers abuse many drugs and also abuse alcohol (polydrug abuse). For example, Grella, Anglin, and Wugalter (1995) found that clients in treatment who abused both heroin and cocaine/crack were more likely to abuse alcohol than were simple heroin addicts. In a study of deceased persons in New York City with cocaine in their bodies, other opiates were found in 39% of the bodies and ethanol in 33% (Tardiff, Gross, Wu, Stajic, & Millman, 1989). Thus, it is important that researchers tease out the effects of the drug abuse and the alcohol abuse on suicidal behavior separately. Unfortunately, this is rarely accomplished.

An increased suicide rate has been reported in some studies of drug abusers. For example, O'Donnell (1969) found an increased suicide rate in narcotic addicts and Watterson, Simpson, and Sells (1975) found a similar association in opioid addicts.[4]

A high percentage of the deaths of addicts are from suicide: 7% of the deaths in a sample of cocaine abusers (Tardiff et al., 1989), 11% of deaths in persons taking methaqualone (Wetli, 1983), and 31% of the deaths in a group of young drug addicts (Tunving, 1988).

Paralleling this association, samples of completed suicides are found to have a higher proportion of drug abusers. For example, Marzuk et al. (1992b) found that 22% of suicides under the age of 60 in New York City in 1985 had cocaine in their systems, whereas 12% had both cocaine and alcohol. The presence of cocaine was associated with Hispanic ethnicity, the use of firearms for suicide, alcohol use, and an age in the range of 18–30.

Similar associations have been found in reports of nonfatal suicidal behavior. For example, drug abusers have also been found to have high rates of attempted suicide (e.g., Hatsukami, Mitchell, Eckert, & Pyle, 1986). Farberow, Litman, and Nelson (1988) found that suicidal ideation was associated with alcohol and drug abuse in adolescents in the community, and that substance abuse added significantly to the ability to predict suicidal ideation in a multiple-regression analysis.

Special Groups

There are several groups for whom the association of suicidal behavior and alcoholism has been especially noted. For example, both suicidal behavior and alcohol abuse have a high prevalence on some Native American reservations (Lester, 1997a).

---

[4]Not every substance is necessarily associated with increased risk of suicidality. For example, Vega, Gil, Warheit, Apospori, and Zimmerman (1993) found that, while use of tranquilizers in seventh- and eighth-grade male adolescents was associated with the greatest increased incidence of suicidal ideation, use of the PCP was associated with the greatest increased incidence of suicide attempts.

In studies of police officers who completed suicide, the presence of alcohol abuse is frequently observed. For example, Lester (1993c) studied 92 suicides among New York City police officers in 1934 to 1939 and found that alcohol abuse was common. The suicides who abused alcohol were younger, more often patrolmen, less often depressed prior to the suicide, more often had a history of problems at work, and more often had interpersonal conflicts precipitating their suicidal actions. Cantor, Tyman, and Slater (1995) found that alcohol abuse played a role in 35% of the suicides among Queensland (Australia) police officers from 1871 to 1992.

Conclusions

It is clear that substance abuse (both drug abuse and alcohol abuse) appears to be associated with suicidal behavior—with both completed suicides and nonfatal suicidal behavior. It should be remembered that this association is not found in every study, only the majority of studies, and that it is not always found in every subgroup of the sample (e.g., men and women or every ethnic group). Nevertheless, the association appears to be robust.

In many groups of individuals, suicidal behavior and substance abuse are found with a high incidence along with other symptoms. For example, Swift, Copeland, and Hall (1996) found that women who were substance abusers in Australia had a high incidence of eating disorders, suicidal behavior, self-mutilation, and experience of physical and sexual abuse. Similarly, Chandy, Blum, and Resnick (1996) found that female teenagers who had been sexually abused had a higher incidence of suicidal behavior, eating disorders, and drug use than those who had not been abused. Thus, the association between substance abuse and suicidal behavior may be part of a larger clustering of traumatic experiences, symptoms, and behaviors.

Several questions need to be addressed in future research. First, how does the increased risk of suicidal behavior in substance abusers compare with the increased risk when other psychiatric symptoms or syndromes are present? For example, is the risk of suicidal behavior in substance abusers greater if the individual has already attempted suicide or if the individual has a major affective disorder? How should these symptoms/syndromes be rated in relation to one another? In the classic suicide prediction scale devised by the Los Angeles Suicide Prevention Center (Whittemore, 1970), affective disorder is given a higher rating than alcoholism.

Other questions that must be addressed include the following: Are different abused substances associated with different risks for subsequent suicidal behavior and is the increased risk of suicide identified in the research to date found for all groups (by gender, race, psychiatric status, etc.) or only for some of these groups?

PREDICTING SUICIDE IN SUBSTANCE ABUSERS

In the previous sections, we have demonstrated the association between suicidal behavior and substance abuse. The next question to address is what variables predict suicidal behavior in substance abusers.

Many studies have compared substance abusers with a history of attempted suicide and those with no such history. Lester (1992a) reviewed the findings of these studies and Table 15.4 shows his summaries for alcohol abusers and Table 15.6 for drug abusers. It should be noted that all these studies have focused on previous attempts at suicide. Similarly, many studies have compared substance abusers who have completed suicide with those who have

TABLE 15.4. Predictors of Attempted Suicide in Alcohol Abusers

Alcohol abuse symptoms

Delirium tremens absent (1)
Delirium tremens present (1)
Began drinking earlier in life (4)
Severe alcoholism (5)
Type of alcoholic (using Jellinek classification (1)
More often members of Alcoholics Anonymous (1)
Less often on skid row (1)
At least one alcoholic parent (2)

Psychiatric symptoms

More psychiatrically disturbed (4)
Any psychiatric diagnosis (1)
More neurosis (2)
More anxiety/panic attacks or disorders (4)
More paranoia and aggression (1)
More socially withdrawn (1)
More antisocial behavior when young and adult (3)
Major depression/depressed (4)
Used psychotropic drugs in past (1)
Multiple diagnoses (1)
More psychiatrically disturbed relatives (1)
If antisocial personality disorder, more violence (1)

Demographic characteristics

Less often married (1)
More often separated/divorced (1)
More deteriorating social status (1)
Younger (2)

Note. Number of studies shown in parentheses.
Source: Lester (1992b). Copyright 1992 by The Guilford Press. Reprinted by permission.

not, and Tables 15.5 and 15.7 show Lester's (1992) summary of the results of these studies are for alcohol and drug abusers, respectively.

Several features of this information are noteworthy. First, many of the variables identified as predictive of suicide are similar to those identified for nonabusers. For example, psychiatric disturbance is predictive of subsequent suicide in all individuals, not simply substance abusers. Second, many of the variables that may differentiate suicidal abusers from nonsuicidal abusers have been identified by only one or two groups of investigators. The usefulness of these variables as predictors must therefore be considered suspect until this research can be replicated by others. Third, the major lacuna in the information is for variables that might predict completed suicide in drug abusers; only one study was located that addressed this question. Fourth, the most fruitful predictor variables may turn out to be those related specifically to the substance abuse, as these variables are unique to the substance abuser. Thus, they may add to the predictive power of variables common to all of those for whom we wish to predict subsequent suicidal behavior.

So far, no research has explored the usefulness of these variables in predicting subsequent suicidal behavior; perhaps this chapter may stimulate such a study. Motto (1980), however, has addressed the problem of predicting suicide in alcohol abusers. He inter-

TABLE 15.5. Predictors of Completed Suicide in Alcohol Abusers

---

Alcohol abuse symptoms

Late stages of alcoholism (1)

Psychiatric symptoms

More depressed/hopeless (1)
More prior suicidal behavior (2)
Higher neuroticism scores (1)
More affective disorder (1)
If prior suicide attempt, more precautions taken (1)

Demographic and social characteristics

Older (1)
Younger and active alcoholics (1)
Male (1)
Married (3)
White (1)
Employed (1)
Worse financial and marital situation (1)
Last-born (1)
More often from broken homes (1)
More self-critical (1)
More attached to mothers (1)
Better physical health (1)
More often raised by nonparent (1)

Note. Number of studies shown in parentheses.
Source: Lester (1992b). Copyright 1992 by The Guilford Press. Reprinted by permission.

viewed 3,006 depressed or suicidal individuals admitted to a hospital and coded the responses to 186 questions. Of this sample, 978 individuals met the criteria for alcohol abuse and could be followed up for 2 years. The alcohol abusers were divided into two groups: one for identifying the variables that predicted completed suicide, and another for cross-validating the variables. Motto identified 11 predictor variables (shown in Table 15.8). In the cross-validation study, this risk scale identified 60% of the suicides and 36% of the nonsuicides as being at high risk. Motto noted that the degree of differentiation was not as precise as he would wish. It is also noteworthy that none of the 11 variables identified by Motto included information about the alcohol abuse. Future investigators need to apply the methodology described by Motto to validate the usefulness of the variables identified in Tables 15.5 and 15.7 for predicting completed suicide in substance abusers.

More recent studies have not been as detailed as Motto's or prospective. However, occasionally findings do support the proposition that different scales are needed to predict suicide in alcoholics. For example, Heikkinen et al. (1994) found that the recent stressors differed for alcoholic and depressive suicides, with the alcoholic suicides experiencing separations and family discord, financial trouble, and unemployment whereas the depressed suicides had experienced more somatic illness, and the same difference has been reported for adolescent suicides (Marttunen, Aro, Henriksson, & Lönnqvist, 1994). Fawcett (1993) found that alcohol abuse predicted suicide in depressed patients in the first year of follow-up but not suicide after this 1-year period.

TABLE 15.6. Predictors of Attempted Suicide in Drug Abusers

Drug abuse symptoms

Oral abuse (rather than intravenous) (1)
If heroin addict, glue sniffer (1)
Used LSD and cocaine (1)
More blackouts from drug use (1)
Used alcohol (2)
Used hashish and heroin less (1)
Experienced withdrawal from barbiturates (1)
More often drug-dependent (1)
Polydrug users (2)
In opiate abusers, heavy use of amphetamines/barbiturates
    and sedatives/inhalants (1)
In opiate abusers, less use of marijuana (1)
In opiate abusers, more severely addicted (1)

Psychiatric symptoms

More psychiatrically disturbed (5)
Psychiatric disturbance in mother (1)
Sociopathy (1)
History of hyperactivity (1)
More learning disabilities/temper tantrums/accident
    proneness (1)
In opiate abusers, sibling alcoholic/depressed (1)
In opiate abusers, father psychiatrically disturbed (1)
More neuroticism and introversion (1)
Higher depression score (1)

Demographic and social characteristics

More often from broken homes (1)
More parental conflict (1)
More asthma and other illnesses (1)
White (2)
Female (2)
More often raised in foster homes/orphanages (1)
Parental physical abuse (1)

Note. Number of studies shown in parentheses.
Source: Lester (1992b). Copyright 1992 by The Guilford Press.
Reprinted by permission.

TABLE 15.7. Predictors of Completed Suicide in Drug Abusers

More psychiatric disturbance in relatives (1)
More alcohol abuse (1)
Less intravenous drug use (1)
More prison sentences (1)

Note. Number of studies shown in parentheses.
Source: Lester (1992b). Copyright 1992 by The Guilford Press. Reprinted by permission.

TABLE 15.8. Predictors of Completed Suicide in Motto's Study of Alcohol Abusers

1. Prior suicide attempt	More than two
2. Seriousness of present attempt—intent	Unequivocal/ambivalent weighted toward death
3. Attitude toward interviewer	Negative/mixed
4. Financial resources	Over $1,000
5. Type of residence	Small or medium hotel/large apartment house/no stable residence
6. Intelligence	High intelligence
7. Emotional disorder in family	Opposite-sex parent
8. Present state of health (subject's view)	Other than good
9. Physical health past year	Minor impairment/getting worse
10. Number of moves past year	None
11. Job stability past 2 years	Any change

Source: After Motto (1980, p. 233). Copyright 1980 by The Guilford Press. Adapted by permission.

Differential Prediction

Many years ago, in discussing the problem of predicting suicide in general, Lettieri (1974) suggested that it would be useful to devise scales specifically tailored for different sociodemographic groups. He presented separate scales for young and old men and for young and old women. Lettieri's work suggests that in the present endeavor, for example, a scale could be developed to predict suicide in male alcoholics that would differ from a scale designed to predict suicide in female alcoholics. Different scales might be designed for substance abusers of different ages, for individuals with different psychiatric diagnoses, and for individuals abusing different drugs.

Data supporting these possibilities exist. For example, male alcoholics appear to have much higher suicide rates than female alcoholics. It has been argued that alcoholism in women is less disturbing to their lives, because they are less likely to hold jobs and because their alcoholism is probably less disruptive of their families' lives than is the alcoholism of men (Rushing, 1969). Thus, perhaps female alcoholics experience less stress than do male alcoholics, and thus are less likely to commit suicide. Male and female alcoholics also differ quite considerably in social–psychological characteristics, such as family history of psychiatric disorder, developmental experiences, and drinking behavior (Linnoila, Erwin, Ramm, Cleveland, & Brendle, 1980). Overholser, Freiheit, and DiFilippo (1997) found that suicidal intent in a sample of adolescent psychiatric inpatients who had attempted suicide was predicted for the girls by depression and hopelessness scores but by alcohol abuse and depression scores for the boys.

Male alcoholics are frequently diagnosed with sociopathy whereas female alcoholics are frequently diagnosed with affective disorder. Persons of these psychiatric subtypes have different reasons for suicide. For example, the sociopathic individual who commits suicide is more likely to have experienced a disruptive childhood and recent social disruptions than is the individual with an affective disorder who commits suicide (Robins & O'Neal, 1958), and these differences may account for the differences in the backgrounds of male and female alcoholic suicides. Therefore, it may prove quite useful to have separate predictive scales for suicide for male and female alcoholics.

Murphy (1992), in his detailed examination of alcoholic suicides, classified the sample by sex and by age of onset of the alcoholism. The male suicides with onset of alcoholism before age 25 survived an average of 25 years before killing themselves (on the average at age 46). These men tended to come from families in which the parents also abused alcohol. Only 60% had serious medical problems as a result of the alcoholism, although 95% had serious symptoms of addiction (such as a history of benders). Forty percent were single, divorced, or separated at the time of their suicide, and 72% of those who were or had been married were physically abusive to their wives.

The men whose onset of alcoholism was between 25 to 44 years of age were almost all married, with most of them still being married. This group expressed more guilt about their addiction than did those with earlier onset. Two-thirds were diagnosed as having an affective disorder, and the same proportion had serious medical problems as did those with earlier onset.

A small group of the men had late-onset alcoholism, and they completed suicide soon after the onset, after an average of only 4 years. None of these men were abusive to their wives, and none had experienced problems with the police. Nearly all had comorbid depression.

The women in the sample had been alcoholics for a shorter period than were the men (only 14 years on the average), had fewer medical problems, and showed less abusive behavior. All had attempted suicide in the past. What struck Murphy most about the women in the group who were married was the lack of support and interest on the part of their husbands. These women lacked careers and seemed to live in social isolation, to some extent self-imposed. Murphy's study suggests that groups distinguished by sex, age, and the age of onset of the alcohol abuse differ considerably and confirms Lettieri's suggestion that different predictive scales may be necessary for the different groups and that the etiology of suicidal behavior may differ in the groups.

Murphy compared the alcoholics who completed suicide with both alcoholics in the community and alcoholics in treatment. The suicides had heavier levels of recent drinking, more often had a major depressive disorder, and were more often unemployed and living alone.

It has also been noted that alcoholic suicides tend to be older. Barraclough, Bunch, Nelson, and Sainsbury (1974) found that their alcoholic suicides had been abusing alcohol for about 25 years and had an average age of 51. Suicide may be more common in these middle-age alcoholics because of the higher incidence of physical disease resulting from their alcoholism (Goodwin, 1973). It may be also that middle age is the period of most stress for alcoholics. This may be the time that their marriages break up and during which they experience severe job difficulties. It is found, for example, that alcoholics who complete suicide are less likely to be married than are both other suicides and nonsuicidal alcoholics. Again, then, different predictive scales may be in order for young, middle-age, and elderly alcoholics.

BIOCHEMICAL INDICATORS OF SUICIDE IN ALCOHOLICS

There has been a tremendous growth in studies of the biochemistry of suicide in recent years, and there have been many claims that biochemical predictors of suicide will soon be discovered. Because there is also much research into the biochemistry of alcoholism, the possibility exists of identifying biochemical predictors of suicide in alcoholics. It must be borne in mind that biochemical research on suicides is primarily carried out because many suicides are depressed, and thus study of the suicidal person promises to further knowledge about the biochemistry of *depression* (cf. Maris, 1986). Such knowledge is welcome because there is no sound biochemical theory of depression at the present time.

Lester (1988d, 1992b) reviewed the biochemical research on suicides and identified several replicable results: Suicide was associated with abnormal responding on the dexamethasone suppression test, lower levels of 5-HIAA in the cerebrospinal fluid, lower levels of serotonin in the central nervous system, and a lower epinephrine–norepinephrine ratio in the urine. The first two findings have been confirmed by meta-analyses of the data (Lester, 1992c, 1995) and implicate the serotonergic system in suicide. Serotonin has also been implicated in assaultive aggression (van Praag, 1986; see Chapter 17) and aggressive/impulsive behavior (Brown & Goodwin, 1986).

Roy and Linnoila (1986) have recently reviewed some of the biochemical research on alcoholism. They concluded that the serotonergic system may be involved in Type II alcohol abuse (alcoholism associated with an early onset, a genetic predisposition, antisocial personality traits, and the seeking of alcohol for its euphoric effects). Thus, Roy and Linnoila infer an association between the serotonergic system and impulsive behavior (see also Weiss & Coccaro, 1997).

The conclusions to be drawn from this research would seem to be that we are a long way from having a clear idea of the biochemical causes of depression, suicide, impulsive behavior, or assaultive behavior. It is unlikely that a specific biochemical predictor of suicide will soon be discovered because the potential predictors appear to be associated with a wide variety of other pathological behaviors.

IMPLICATIONS FOR PREVENTING SUICIDE

It is obvious that substance abuse increases the risk of suicidal behavior, and, therefore, treatment of substance abuse should reduce the incidence of suicidal behavior. For example, Caplehorn, Dalton, Haldar, Petrenas, and Nisbet (1996) found that heroin addicts in a methadone maintenance treatment program were less likely to die from suicide (or from a heroin overdose) than were addicts no longer in the program.

Murphy (1992) identified seven risk factors for suicide in alcoholics from his study:

1. Current heavy drinking
2. Major depressive disorder
3. Little or no social support
4. Unemployment
5. Living alone
6. Suicidal thoughts or communication
7. Serious medical illness

In one study of the first six of these risk factors, using a score of four or more risk factors as the criterion, Murphy identified 69% of white male alcoholic suicides correctly and had only 1% false positives in alcoholics currently living. In a replication sample, replacing little or no social support with age and using three or more risk factors as the criterion, Murphy identified 76% of the alcoholic suicides currently and 19% of the living alcoholics were false positives.

Murphy (1992), in his discussion of suicide in alcoholics, notes that treatment of the underlying psychiatric disorder is critical in preventing suicide in alcoholics, and the same would be true for substance abusers. Murphy also reviewed the treatment options available; options presented in Chapter 21. The evidence suggests that a good proportion of substance abusers are depressed, and thus treatment of the depression would seem to be imperative, especially as the depressive lifestyle may itself have contributed to the development of the alcohol and drug abuse.

However, as in the case of John Berryman (see Case 15.1), treatment failures are

CASE 15.1. An Alcoholic Who Completed Suicide

John Berryman was a poet who committed suicide at the age of 57. Famous suicides have the advantage for study in that they are often the subject of biographies that describe their lives in much greater detail than the life of an ordinary person who completes suicide.

The role of alcohol in the production of creative works has often been discussed (Goodwin, 1988). Among noted U.S. authors who abused alcohol and who killed themselves are Hart Crane, Ernest Hemingway, and John Berryman. Here we look briefly at the life and death of John Berryman, a U.S. poet and winner of the Pulitzer Prize and other literary awards, who jumped to his death in 1972 (Haffenden, 1982).

Berryman's early life was marked by the death by suicide of his father when Berryman was 14. Lester (1989) has found that loss was common in the early years of suicides, particularly in the age range of 6–16, and such a loss seems to sensitize the individual to later loss in life (Lester & Beck, 1976). That Berryman's father completed suicide assumes even greater importance because Berryman himself completed suicide when he was also middle age and under stress. Berryman seems to have identified with or modeled himself on his father, at least in this respect.

Berryman fits Murphy's (1992) group of alcoholic suicides with onset 25 to 44 years of age. Like the men in Murphy's sample, he married several times and was married at the time of his suicide. He was not violent toward his wives (unlike those with early onset of alcoholism). Affective disorder was common in Murphy's group of alcoholic suicides, but Berryman was never diagnosed as having an affective disorder, although the periods when he worked to exhaustion may have been manic-like episodes. Unfortunately, in the 1960s, those in charge of Berryman's treatment may not have considered this possibility.

Interestingly, Berryman had received treatment for his alcoholism, but he relapsed. It is obvious that treatment of alcohol and drug abusers could prove useful in preventing their suicidal behavior, but it is easy to find examples of those for whom treatment did not lead to improvement in their mental health.

John's Life

John Berryman was born on October 25, 1914, in McAlester, Oklahoma, and a younger brother followed in 1919. John's childhood began uneventfully except for a little sibling rivalry. John was raised as a Catholic, and the family was devout.

In 1924, John's father had trouble at his bank job moved the family to Florida where he failed as a restauranteur. John's mother fell in love with their landlord, and John's father shot himself. Later John called his father's suicide the turning point in his life, a turning point toward psychological instability.

Within a few months of the suicide, John's mother married the landlord, and her sons took his name. The family moved to New York City. John was an outstanding student, and he went to Columbia University where, despite a patchy performance (he flunked a course and had to drop out for a semester) he began to draft poems which were published in *Columbia Review*.

(cont.)

CASE 15.1. (*cont.*)

Two themes became apparent in his college years. First was John's need for women in his life and his distress when the relationships failed. Second, once John decided to apply himself to his studies, he overdid it. Working throughout the night to the point of exhaustion became a general pattern in his life. Women, work and breakdown characterize most of John's later life.

John's career involved many moves and he was often unemployed or appointed only for temporary positions (weeks or months at a time). Thus, he faced job insecurity for much of his life. He studied for two years in England and returned to the USA in 1938 where he remained unemployed for a year. He spent one year as an instructor at Wayne State University, three years at Harvard University, and eight years in various capacities at Princeton University where he taught occasionally and was supported by fellowships. In 1954, John was appointed to teach at the University of Iowa, but he was dismissed after a drunken altercation. In 1955, he began teaching at the University of Minnesota, and he remained there for the rest of his life, eventually becoming a Regent's Professor of Humanities in 1969.

Though John was awarded many prizes and fellowships which helped support him and his family, he was turned down for others and faced the uncertainty each time he applied for a fellowship as to whether it would be awarded him. He was in financial straits for much of his life, except toward the end, and never owned a house until after his third marriage.

John's work never was easy. For example, at Wayne State University, he sank into a cycle of alienation, bouts of work, followed by starvation and social withdrawal. Throughout his life, John was productive, getting his poems and critical essays published quite successfully. However, writing inevitably involves many rejections too. The rejections upset John terribly, probably because of his doubts about his own merits as a writer. As his career progressed, the honors came faster: Rockefeller Fellowships, Guggenheim Fellowships, a Pulitzer Prize, and so on. However, as his career progressed, his aspirations increased. Once it was enough to have his poems accepted for publication. Then the books of poems had to be praised, and finally he needed to be the greatest living American poet. What would have once thrilled him soon ranked as a bitter disappointment because of what he did not achieve. Toward the end of his life, John doubted more and more the quality of his work, and he sought the praise of his friends for his latest poems.

John married three times, but there were numerous other loves and sexual conquests. As his life progressed, John threw himself into alcohol. By 1949, his day was filled with drug use including vitamins, an anti-spasmodic, dexedrine, martinis, nembutal and sherry—all this while smoking heavily!

After his first two wives left him, he met and married Kate Donahue in 1961, in her early twenties, whose father had been an alcoholic, the ideal wife for an aging alcoholic. They remained married until John's suicide.

John arrived in Minnesota in 1954. There his health deteriorated and his drinking increased steadily. After his second divorce, he was frequently hospitalized for brief periods. Eventually he was diagnosed as an alcoholic and during his third marriage was treated on several occasions for alcoholism.

CASE 15.1. (*cont.*)

He entered treatment for alcoholism in 1966 and 1967, but not seriously until late 1969. He was diagnosed as an alcohol and drug abuser. A list of drugs used revealed: sleeping pills since 1949, nerve pills since 1955, phenobarbital since 1959, Haldol, Vivactic and Tuinol since May 1969, Serax since November 1969, Thorazine since May 1969, Nembutal in 1961, and Librium occasionally. He also smoked five packs of cigarettes a day.

He had great trouble staying off alcohol and had to be readmitted several times. He joined Alcoholics Anonymous and worked hard at fighting the craving. In 1970, one doctor diagnosed him as having a cyclothymic personality (with swings from depression to elation). Another felt that John was not psychotic when sober, but that he had a fear of insanity and of committing suicide.

John's Suicide

In 1971, John was still married to Kate, but Kate was now a school teacher. Their marriage had severe problems, and it was likely that Kate might leave him. John's confidence in his ability to write well had gone. He was beginning to recognize that he no longer had the perseverance to finish any major work. He also began to lose confidence in his teaching ability.

On Wednesday January 5th, 1972, he left the house intending to kill himself. His note read "I am a nuisance." However, he returned home. On Friday January 7th he left again, telling Kate "You won't have to worry about me any more." He took the bus to the University and walked to the Washington Avenue Bridge. At about nine in the morning, he climbed over the railings and jumped without looking back. He fell one hundred feet, landing near the pier of the municipal coal docks, rolling fifteen feet or so down the embankment.

Discussion

John suffered from tremendous insecurity about his self-worth. The weak and sickly kid at school had developed into an abrasive and self-absorbed adult. Was he any good as a teacher, as a poet, as a son, husband or father, or as a lover? Despite the successes of his life (teaching jobs at good universities, acclaim for his poems, and three marriages), he continued to be plagued by doubts, and to alienate those who wanted to be close to him. At the age of 57, rather than reaping the rewards from his earlier successes, he seemed to be facing failure. His poetry was perhaps no longer good. His craving for alcohol was as hard to fight as ever, and his marriage was disintegrating. Sexual liaisons would probably become rare.

He could have continued the struggle and sought to improve himself. But his past attempts had not proved successful. Perhaps he had lost hope that future efforts would succeed? Rather than face a continuing decline, John chose the solution that his father had chosen 45 years earlier.

frequent. Often clients do not respond to the treatment; nor do they always continue the treatment regime (e.g., taking the appropriate medications) once released from inpatient care. It has been much easier to document the impact on lowering suicide rates of social policy changes, in the present case from lowered per capita consumption of alcohol, than of improvements in individual treatment techniques.

SUMMARY AND CONCLUSIONS

This chapter has indicated clearly that substance abuse is associated with an increased likelihood of suicide, a conclusion that makes sense if we agree with Menninger's (1938) view that substance abuse itself is a self-destructive (and, in some sense, suicidal) behavior. Thus, substance abuse may be considered a predictor for suicide. Despite this, many previously devised scales for predicting suicide do not include substance abuse. For example, Lettieri (1974) included alcoholism only on his scale for predicting suicide in older females. Thus, much research needs to be done to pinpoint the groups for which substance abuse is a useful predictor and its interaction effects with other predictors.

This chapter has also indicated a large number of possible variables that might predict completed suicide in alcoholics and in drug abusers. Far more research has been conducted on alcoholics than on drug abusers. For alcoholics, 1 alcohol abuse symptom, 6 psychiatric symptoms, and 13 demographic and social variables were identified as potential predictors of completed suicide in at least one study (see Table 15.5). In contrast, only four variables were identified as predictors of completed suicide in drug abusers, but these were derived from only one study (see Table 15.7). Thus, much more research is needed to identify potential predictive signs of completed suicide in drug abusers. In addition, these potential predictive signs for completed suicide need to be validated (and cross-validated) in future research. Despite the enthusiastic reports in the biochemical literature about the potential of biochemical variables to predict suicide, this chapter has found little evidence for any reliable and useful predictors at the present time. If useful biochemical predictors of suicide are ever identified, it will not be for many years.

It appears that the more effective predictors of suicide in alcohol and drug abusers are similar to those in those who do not abuse alcohol or drugs. For example, in Table 15.5, the predictors of completed suicide in alcohol abusers included depression, hopelessness, and the presence of an affective disorder—all variables that predict suicide in general. Indeed, it has been difficult to identify unique predictors of suicide in alcoholics. The suicide note reproduced at the beginning of this chapter is one from a sample from Murphy (1992), and a recent research study by Leenaars, Wenckstern, and Lester (1999) found no differences between the content of the notes from alcoholics who committed suicide and the notes of non-alcoholic suicides. As a result, Leenaars et al. (1999) could draw no conclusions about the suicides of alcoholics in particular as opposed to suicides in general.

Although it is obvious that adequate detection and treatment of substance abuse in individuals might prevent suicide, the best evidence for the prevention of suicide by tackling the problem of substance abuse comes from the study of social policies. For example, Norstrom (1995b) estimated that a 25% decrease in the overall per capita consumption of alcohol in Sweden would halve the mortality from liver cirrhosis, accidents, and suicide. The same decrease in mortality from these three causes could be achieved by a 36% reduction in the consumption of alcohol by the heaviest drinkers (i.e., the top 5%).

In conclusion, this chapter has established a program for future research rather than revealing already validated knowledge about suicide in substance abusers. It is hoped that it will stimulate scholars to pursue this interesting and important topic for the understanding and prediction of suicide.

We have noted previously that alcohol may play a role in the etiology of suicide through its effects on neurotransmitter levels in the central nervous system, particularly the serotonergic system. In Chapter 16, the role of neurotransmitters in the etiology of suicide is explored in detail. In addition, the medications (developed, in part, as a result of this expanding field of investigation) that have been found to be helpful for suicidal individuals are reviewed.

FURTHER READING

Motto, J. A. (1980). Suicide risk factors in alcohol abuse. *Suicide and Life-Threatening Behavior, 10,* 230–238. This is the best study done to date on trying to predict suicidal behavior in alcoholics, with a large sample and cross-validation. It should serve as a model for future research on this issue.

Murphy, G. E. (1992). *Suicide in alcoholism.* New York: Oxford University Press. This, the only book on suicide and substance abuse, presents an excellent review of the literature and details on 50 alcoholics who completed suicide. Murphy also provides suggestions for treatment.

Ojehagen, A., Berglund, M., & Apel, C. P. (1993). Long-term outpatient treatment in alcoholics with previous suicidal behavior. *Suicide and Life-Threatening Behavior, 23,* 320–328. This report analyzes the importance of prior suicidal behavior for the treatment of alcoholics in long-term treatment.

Petronis, K. R., Samuels, J. F., Moscicki, E. K., & Anthony, J. A. (1990). An epidemiological investigation of potential risk factors for suicide attempts. *Social Psychiatry and Psychiatric Epidemiology, 25,* 193–199. A follow-up study of over 13,000 community residents examined the predictors of suicidal behavior over the next 2 years. Both alcohol and cocaine use contributed to the prediction of subsequent suicidal behavior, whereas marijuana and sedative use did not.

Rogers, J. R. (1992). Suicide and alcohol. *Journal of Counseling and Development, 70,* 540–543. This article examines the role of alcohol in facilitating the suicidal action, whether or not the suicidal individual is a substance abuser. It discusses implications for practitioners and ethical considerations.

Wasserman, D. (1993). Alcohol and suicidal behavior. *Nordic Journal of Psychiatry, 47,* 265–271. This article discusses the role of alcohol in suicidal behavior and suggests techniques for assessment and treatment for alcoholics at risk for suicide.

16

The Biology of Suicide

> Most of the available biological evidence in the study of suicide comes from examining the serotonergic system in both completed and attempted suicide, but additional evidence exists that indicates the involvement of other neurotransmitter systems. Indeed, the neurobiology of suicide, just as suicide itself, has become multidetermined. . . . Taking all evidence together, it is likely that suicide is not the result of a single factor but, rather, the outcome of several factors operating simultaneously at a given moment in life.
> —VICTORIA ARANGO AND MARK D. UNDERWOOD

The biology of suicide is a rapidly expanding field of great interest and activity (Stoff & Mann, 1997). There has been a veritable explosion of research and findings in the scientific fields of human genetics, molecular genetics, neurochemistry, neurophysiology, neuroendocrinology, and neuroanatomy in the last 20 years. Ground-breaking techniques and new technologies are being discovered and applied to the biology of suicidal behaviors at an unprecedented pace. Our understanding of the brain, its integration, organization, structure, composition, and function is taking flight. The 1990s have been referred to as the "decade of the brain," in part because of the important recognition that this second most important organ in our bodies has attained regarding its role and function in regulating behavior, mood, affect, and perception.

The neuroscience of suicidal behaviors has only recently been recognized as a distinct specialty, in part due to its dependence on the earlier foundations set by the related areas of epidemiology, neuroanatomy, neurophysiology, neurochemistry, molecular biology, and neuroendocrinology. These related fields have become established as we have developed more sophisticated techniques for statistical analysis of data, better surveillance mechanisms, more advanced laboratory techniques to analyze biological material (cerebrospinal fluid, brain and spinal tissue, blood products), and more powerful radiological and investigative tools, such as magnetic resonance imaging (MRI) and positron emission tomography (PET). We can now visualize the process of thinking as well as the effect of medications and other psychoactive substances on specific regions of the brain.

There has been a remarkable confluence of epidemiological, clinical, and laboratory findings with sophisticated biological and radiological imaging findings. Clinical lore and axioms about at-risk populations are now being confirmed by exact measurements of cerebrospinal fluid (CSF) metabolites and blood products, and through radiological imaging techniques, to name but a few.

TABLE 16.1. Types of Neurobiological Studies
Related to Suicide

Genetics

Twin studies—monozygotic versus dizygotic
Family studies
Adoption studies

Populations at risk

Suicide ideators
Suicide attempters
Suicide completers
Depressed patients
Criminals (aggressive/impulsive)

Biochemical/anatomical studies

Postmortem brains—receptor site and quantification
    of chemicals
CSF studies of neurotransmitter metabolites
Platelet receptor binding studies
Animal models—anatomical lesions; chemical
    interruption of neurotransmitter production

Radiological studies

SPECT (functional)
PET (using ligands)
MRI (structural)

It is beyond the scope of this chapter to review exactly how the currently available psychotropic medications work (Nemeroff, 1994). It is also beyond the scope of this chapter to review issues such as genetic predisposition to response to certain classes of drugs (DeVane, 1994) or gender differences in absorption, metabolism, and excretion of psychotropic medications (Yonkers, Kando, Cole, & Blumenthal, 1992).

The purpose of this chapter is to highlight some of the more promising areas of investigation identified at this time. Table 16.1 lists some of the more common types of neurobiological studies related to suicide that will be discussed. The neurosciences, and specifically the neurobiology of suicide, are rapidly evolving areas of intense scientific activity. Our level of understanding of the mechanisms of central nervous system (CNS) action are becoming more sophisticated with every new finding and with the development of new investigative techniques in the fields in neurochemistry, molecular genetics, radiology, and human genetics. Hence, the findings presented here may well be challenged and refined over time.

THE GENETICS OF SUICIDAL BEHAVIOR

There has been a great deal of progress in the scientific investigation of human and molecular genetics as it relates to the transmission and expression of disease. The goal of understanding diseases and behaviors from a molecular or human genetics perspective is multifold: (1) to develop better screening approaches; (2) to develop better prevention techniques; (3) to investigate the possibility of definitive preventive interventions at the molecular, cellular, or pharmacological level; and (4) to better understand the interrelationship

between biology and environment (nature vs. nurture) as they affect the expression of behavioral disorders.

Evidence that an illness or behavioral disorder may have a genetic component comes
from many different types of studies, including surveillance studies of populations at risk,
clinical studies of families, twin and adoption studies, and molecular genetic studies.

As noted in Chapter 2, suicide is a multidimensional, multidetermined, and multifactorial behavior. Risk factors that are statistically associated with suicidal behaviors include biological, psychological, and social factors. Biological factors include physical illness and al-
terations in neurotransmitter function in the CNS (especially of serotonin). Psychological
factors include the presence of a major psychiatric disorder (including alcoholism and other
drug abuse) and personality traits (i.e., impulsivity). Social factors include unemployment,
stressful life events, and certain family environmental exposures (childrearing; psychological, emotional, physical, or sexual abuse).

Risk factors such as a family history of psychiatric illness and/or suicidal behaviors cut
across the three domains of the biopsychosocial model (cf. Figure 2.6). To what extent are
any, some, or all of these risk factors influenced by genetic predisposition? Is impulsivity a
learned trait or an inherited biological tendency which gets expressed under certain environmental conditions? Which biological risk factors place an individual at increased risk for
suicide? We review some of the most influential studies that attempt to answer these questions by studying families, twins, and adoptees.

Family History of Suicide

The first question often asked is whether suicidal behaviors are "inherited." There is some
confusion about the many ways of "inheriting" a behavior—by learning, by genetic transmission, by environmental influences, and so on. The first attempts to answer this question
raised as many questions as they answered.

Pitts and Winokur (1964) found that among 748 consecutively admitted psychiatric inpatients, 37 (4.9%) reported a possible or definite suicide in a first-degree relative (i.e.,
sons, daughters, siblings, or parents). In 25 of these 37 cases (68%), the diagnosis was an
affective disorder. The statistical probability of this distribution's occurring by chance was
less than .02. Pitts and Winokur estimated that 79% of the suicides of the first-degree relatives were associated with probable affective disorder.

Murphy and Wetzel (1982) reviewed the literature and found that 6–8% of those who
attempted suicide have a family history of suicide. They studied 127 patients hospitalized
after attempting suicide and found that when they examined them by psychiatric diagnosis,
the personality disorder group had as high a family history of suicide as the affective disorder group. Seventeen percent of those with a primary diagnosis of primary affective disorder had a family history of suicide, and 17% had a family history of suicide attempts.

Roy (1983), in his review of the existing literature, noted that a family history of suicide had been found in a small but meaningful number of studies. Roy examined the medical charts of 243 psychiatric inpatients who reported 274 suicides among their first- and
second-degree relatives.

Almost half (118, 48.6%) of these patients had attempted suicide, more than half (137,
56.4%) had a depressive disorder, and more than a third (84, 34.6%) had recurrent affective disorder. Regardless of the primary diagnosis, the great majority (84.4%) of all the patients with a family history of suicide had had a depressive episode at some time in their
lives. During the 7½-year study, 7 (2.8%) of the 243 patients committed suicide.

Tsuang (1983) found that the first-degree relatives of the 500 psychiatric inpatients in
his study had a risk of suicide almost eight times greater than the risk in the relatives of nor-

mal controls. The risk of suicide was significantly greater among the first-degree relatives of depressed patients than it was among the relatives of either patients with schizophrenia or those classified as manic. Among the first-degree relatives of the 29 psychiatric patients who had committed suicide, the suicide risk was four times greater than the risk in the relatives of patients who did not commit suicide. Here the suicide risk was equally high among the relatives of both patients classified as depressed and as manic.

In an often quoted study, Egeland and Sussex (1985) reported on the suicide data obtained from the study of affective disorders among the Older Order Amish community of Lancaster County in southeast Pennsylvania. Of the 26 suicide victims among these Amish over the 100 years from 1880 to 1980, 24 were diagnosed with a major affective disorder. Twelve of the suicide victims had a diagnosis of a bipolar disorder, and 12 had unipolar affective disorder. A further case met diagnostic criteria for a minor depression.

Almost three-quarters of the 26 suicide victims were found to cluster in four family pedigrees, each of which contained a heavy loading for affective disorders and suicide. Interestingly, the converse was not true, as there were other family pedigrees with heavy loadings for affective disorder but without suicides; a family loading for affective disorder was not in itself a predictor for suicide. Egeland and Sussex (1985) concluded: "Our study replicates findings that indicate an increased suicidal risk for patients with a diagnosis of major affective disorder and a strong family history of suicide. . . . The clustering of suicide in Amish pedigrees follows the distribution of affective illness in the kinship and suggests the role of inheritance" (918).

Shaffer, Gould, and Trautman (1985) reported psychological autopsies on 20 adolescent suicide victims in Louisville, Kentucky. They found that significantly more of the suicide victims, as compared to the controls, had a family history of suicide. Shaffer et al. subsequently performed psychological autopsies on a consecutive series of suicides under 19 years of age occurring in the New York City area. In a preliminary report of the first 52 suicide victims, they noted that 20 (38%) had a relative who had either committed or attempted suicide.

In summary, these and other studies suggest that individuals at risk for suicidal behaviors have a higher than statistically expected family history of an affective disorder (depression or bipolar illness) and/or a suicide (Shaffer, 1974; Mitterauer, 1990; Malone, Haas, Sweeney, & Mann, 1995; Linkowski, deMaertelaer, & Mendlewicz, 1985). Whether these observations confirm a genetic inheritance is not proven, because of the possible role that a positive identification with parents and siblings and subsequent mimicking behavior might play in later expression of an affective disorder or suicidal behavior.

Twin Studies

The twin study method may help to address the question of whether a predisposition for suicidal behavior may be genetically transmitted independent of a psychiatric disorder. Identical twins come from one egg (monozygotic, MZ) and share the same genes, whereas fraternal twins come from two eggs (dizygotic, DZ) and share only 50% of their genes. If suicide is a genetically transmitted behavior, then concordance for suicide should be found more often among identical twins (MZ) than fraternal (DZ) twins.

Haberlandt (1967) pooled the data from twin studies from different countries and found that among 149 pairs of twins in which one twin had killed him- or herself, there were nine sets of twins in which the other twin had also killed him- or herself; all these twins were found among the 51 MZ pairs (18%). In an additional five pairs of the 51 MZ twin pairs (10%), the other twin had attempted suicide. No DZ twin pairs were found in which both twins had committed suicide.

Four of the nine MZ twins concordant for suicide revealed an affective disorder in the twins or their relatives (Juel-Nielsen & Videbech, 1970). Zair (1981) reported suicide in identical male twins widely separated in time, but in both twins the suicide occurred during a depressive episode. Also, both parents of the twins had been treated by psychiatrists for depression with electroconvulsive therapy (ECT) and antidepressants.

Roy, Segal, Centerwall, and Robinette (1991) studied 176 twin pairs (62 MZ and 114 DZ) in which one or both twins had committed suicide. They found that 7 of the 62 MZ twin pairs were concordant for suicide compared with 2 of the 114 DZ twin pairs (11.3% vs. 1.8%); thus, the MZ twin pairs showed a significantly greater concordance for suicide relative to the DZ twin pairs. The presence of psychiatric disorder in the twins and their families was examined in a subsample of 11 twin pairs (9 MZ and 2 DZ). Two of these 11 twin pairs were concordant for suicide, and both were MZ twin pairs: "Nine of the 13 suicide victims had a history of a diagnosed depressive disorder that had been treated with antidepressant medication; three had bipolar disorder. Two others had experienced a schizophrenic illness and had received neuroleptic medication. Nine of the 11 co-twins (eight surviving co-twins and one suicide victim) had received psychiatric treatment from a psychiatrist" (31–32).

Roy (1992) subsequently combined his 176 twin pairs with the 149 twin pairs reviewed by Haberlandt (1967), the 73 twin pairs (none of which were concordant for suicide) reported by Juel-Nielsen and Videbech (1970), and the 1 concordant MZ twin pair reported by Zair (1981), yielding a total of 399 twin pairs: 129 MZ twin pairs (17 of 129, or 13.2%, concordant for suicide) and 270 DZ twin pairs (2 of 270, or 0.7%, concordant for suicide). He concluded that "these combined data further demonstrate that MZ twin pairs show significantly greater concordance for suicide than do DZ twin pairs (Fisher's exact test, $p = .001$)" (576).

In a second study, Roy, Segal, and Sarchiapone (1995) examined suicide attempts among living co-twins whose twin had committed suicide. They hypothesized that if genetic factors play a part in suicidal behavior, then significantly more living MZ than DZ co-twins would themselves have attempted suicide. They then collected a group of 35 twins in which one twin had committed suicide and interviewed the living co-twin about whether he or she had ever attempted suicide. "We found that 10 of the 26 living MZ cotwins had themselves attempted suicide compared with 0 of the 9 living DZ cotwins ($p < 0.04$). We concluded that, although MZ and DZ twins may have some differing developmental experiences, studies show that MZ twin pairs have significantly greater concordance for both suicide and attempted suicide" (1076).

In summary, the twin data presented here suggests that genetic factors related to suicide may largely represent a genetic predisposition for the psychiatric disorders associated with suicide. However, these studies leave open the question of whether there may be an independent genetic component for suicide, perhaps related to impulsivity. Future studies of the surviving co-twins of twin suicide victims and their family members are needed to investigate possible genetic and biologic markers for impulsivity.

Adoption Studies

The strongest evidence for the presence of genetic factors in suicide comes from the adoption studies carried out in Denmark by Schulsinger, Kety, Wender, and Rosenthal (1979; Kety, 1986). The strength of the adoption strategy is that it is the best way to tease apart "nature" from "nurture" issues. This is because individuals separated at birth, or shortly afterward, share their genes—but not subsequent environmental experiences—with their biological relatives. In contrast, adoptees share their environmental experiences through childhood and adolescence with their adopting relatives but share no genes.

The Psykologisk Institut has a register of the 5,483 adoptions that occurred in greater Copenhagen between 1924 and 1947. A screening of the registers for causes of death revealed that 57 of these adoptees eventually committed suicide. They were matched with 57 adopted controls for age, sex, social class of the adopting parents, and time spent both with their biological relatives and in institutions before being adopted. Twelve of the 269 biological relatives (4.5%) of these 57 adopted suicides had themselves committed suicide, compared with only 2 of the 269 biological relatives (0.7%) of the 57 adopted controls ($p <$ .01). None of the adopting relatives of either the suicide group or the control group had committed suicide.

These results are important because the suicides were largely independent of the presence of psychiatric disorder. Schulsinger et al. (1979) found that 6 of the 12 (50%) biological suicide relatives had had no contact with psychiatric services and thus presumably did not suffer from one of the major psychiatric disorders commonly found among suicide victims. They proposed that there may be a genetic predisposition for suicide independent of, or additive to, the major psychiatric disorders associated with suicide.

Wender, Kety, Rosenthal, and Schulsinger (1986) went on to study the 71 adoptees identified by the Psykologisk Institut's psychiatric case register as having suffered from an affective disorder. They were matched with 71 control adoptees without affective disorder. Significantly more of the biological relatives of the adoptees with affective disorder had committed suicide than had those of the controls. In particular, adoptee suicide victims with the diagnosis of "affect reaction" had significantly more biological relatives who had committed suicide than did controls. This diagnosis is used in Denmark to describe an individual who has affective symptoms accompanying a situational crisis (often an impulsive suicide attempt). These findings led Kety (1986) to suggest that a genetic factor in suicide may be an inability to control impulsive behavior, which has its effect independent of (or additive to) that of psychiatric disorder. Affective disorder and/or environmental stress may serve "as potentiating mechanisms which foster or trigger the impulsive behavior, directing it toward a suicidal outcome" (Kety, 1990: 132).

The existing family, twin, and adoption studies suggest that there may be genetic factors in suicide. In many suicide victims, these will be the genetic factors involved in the genetic transmission of bipolar disorder, schizophrenia, and alcoholism. However, the Copenhagen adoption studies strongly suggest that there may be a genetic factor for suicide that is independent of, or additive to, the genetic transmission of affective disorder. Kety's (1986) suggestion that this may be an inability to control impulsive behavior is compatible with the data that diminished central serotonin turnover may be associated with poor impulse control.

BIOCHEMICAL INVESTIGATIONS

In recent years, increasing attention has been paid to the biology of suicide (cf. Maris, 1986), with particular emphasis on the examination of two neurotransmitters (serotonin and dopamine) and of the hypothalamic–pituitary–adrenal (HPA) axis. This research has pointed to a number of biochemical features that may be common to the seemingly disparate group of psychiatric disorders with which higher incidences of suicide are associated; it may also provide the basis for developing specific treatment approaches for some suicidal patients.

Table 16.2 lists the currently known neurotransmitters that have been found to be associated with psychiatric disorders. The three neurotransmitters associated with affective disorders and suicidal behaviors are dopamine, norepinephrine, and serotonin.

TABLE 16.2. Neurotransmitter Classes Associated with
Psychiatric Illnesses

Acetylcholine (Ach)

Dopamine (DA)

Excitatory amino acids (EAA) (e.g., glutamate)

Gamma–aminobutyric acid (GABA)

Lithium/mood stabilizers (PI; phosphoinositol cyclic AMP)

Norepinephrine (NE; noradrenaline)

Serotonin (5-HT; 5-HIAA as the metabolite)

Serotonin

Evidence has been accumulating of decreased serotonin levels in three groups of patients: depressed patients, suicide attempters, and suicide victims. The role of serotonin as a unifying factor in suicidal behavior was originally proposed by Äsberg and colleagues, who reported an association between suicidal behavior and low levels of CSF 5-hydroxyindoleacetic acid (5-HIAA), the principal metabolite of serotonin in depressed patients (Äsberg, Träskman, & Thorén, 1976).

They reported a bimodal distribution of levels of 5-HIAA in the lumbar CSF of 68 depressed patients. Äsberg et al. (1976) noted that significantly more of the depressed patients in the "low" CSF 5-HIAA group had attempted suicide in comparison with those in the "high" CSF 5-HIAA group. Subsequently, a number of other studies have reported that low CSF levels of 5-HIAA are significantly associated with suicidal behavior in depressed, personality-disordered, and schizophrenic patients, although there have been some negative reports as well (for a review, see Äsberg, Nordstrom, & Träskman-Bendz, 1986b). Although CSF levels of 5-HIAA are an imprecise indicator of serotonin levels in the brain, these data have led to the suggestion that reduced central serotonin metabolism may be associated with suicidal behavior (Roy & Linnoila, 1988, 1990; Roy, Nutt, Virrkunen, & Linnoila, 1987).

Äsberg (1980) has reported that only 15% of those with high CSF 5-HIAA attempted suicide in contrast to 40% of patients with low levels. Decrease in CSF 5-HIAA is more correlated with suicide attempts and most specifically to violent ones than to reported depression (Äsberg, Bertilsson, & Martensson, 1984; DeLeo & Marazziti, 1988; Träskman, Äsberg, Bertilsson, & Sjostrand, 1981). In studies of a schizophrenic population, lower serotonin levels are found more frequently in those with previous suicide attempts (Braunig, Rao, & Fimmers, 1989). Individuals with low CSF 5-HIAA who have attempted suicide are reported to be 10 times more likely to die by suicide than those not found to have the decreased levels of 5-HIAA (Äsberg, 1986). Those found to have low CSF 5-HIAA are not only prone to more violent suicide attempts but also to more frequent (Äsberg, Nordstrom, & Träskman-Bendz, 1986; Cohen, Winchel, & Stanley, 1988) and less premeditated ones (Äsberg, 1986).

Träskman et al. (1981) carried out the first follow-up study of patients who had attempted suicide and who had had a lumbar puncture for determination of CSF levels of 5-HIAA. They found that within a year of leaving the hospital, 21% of the patients who had both a suicide attempt and a CSF level of 5-HIAA below 90 nmol/liter had committed suicide. Hence, among patients who had made a suicide attempt, those with low CSF levels of 5-HIAA were 10 times more likely to die of suicide than the others.

Roy et al. carried out a 5-year follow-up study of suicidal behavior among depressed patients who had earlier determinations of CSF levels of monoamine metabolites (Roy et al., 1986; Roy, DeJong, & Linnoila, 1989). Patients who reattempted suicide during the follow-up period had significantly lower CSF levels of both the serotonin metabolite 5-HIAA and the dopamine metabolite HVA. The findings were most striking among depressed patients with melancholia. Over 50 percent of those melancholic patients who had attempted suicide and had a CSF level of 5-HIAA below 80 pmol/ml reattempted suicide during the follow-up period. Two-thirds of those melancholic patients who had attempted suicide and had a CSF level of homovanillic acid (HVA) below 100 pmol/ml reattempted suicide during follow-up.

Three (25%) of the 12 depressed patients who had made a past suicide attempt and who had a CSF level of 5-HIAA below 80 pmol/ml committed suicide during the first year of follow-up. This 25% is similar to the 21% rate of suicide reported by Träskman et al. (1981) as occurring within a year of leaving the hospital among their previous attempters with a CSF level of 5-HIAA below 90 nmol/liter. These follow-up results suggest that among depressed patients who have previously attempted suicide, these measures may be predictive markers of an increased risk of further suicidal behavior.

Exactly what role serotonin (as measured by its metabolite 5-HIAA) plays in the initiation, modulation, maintenance, or regulation of aggression, impulsivity, affect, self-destructive behaviors, addictions, thought processing, and assessment of sensory input remains under study. It is most likely that serotonin is involved along the pathway from genetic predisposition and environmental stimulus to expression of psychiatric disorders and suicidal behaviors.

Dopamine

A number of studies have pointed to the coupling of serotonin and dopamine systems in various regions of the brain. High-order correlations between CSF HVA, the principal metabolite or breakdown product of dopamine, and 5-HIAA in depressed patients have been reported in several studies (Aber-Wistedt, Wistedt, & Bertilsson, 1985; Äsberg, 1986). The role of dopamine in suicidal patients with personality disorders has been inferred from studies on the use of dopamine receptor blockers to decrease suicidal behavior in such patients. Montgomery and Montgomery (1982) reported on the use of flupenthixol, a dopamine receptor blocker, in patients with personality disorders (mainly borderline or histrionic) who had a history of multiple suicide attempts. They raised the possibility that the effect of reducing suicidal behavior in personality disorders is mediated via the dopamine system. They also noted lower levels of CSF HVA in depressed patients with a history of suicidal acts. More recently, Soloff et al. (1986) reported that haloperidol, an antipsychotic medication, decreased suicidality in borderline patients. Thus, blocking postsynaptic dopamine receptors appears helpful in decreasing suicidality in personality-disordered patients.

Neuroendocrine Measures

The HPA axis has been a major focus of research in depressive disorders. We monitor the activity of this endocrine axis by measuring a number of hormones and steroids in blood and urine. Elevated 24-hour urinary free cortisol and dexamethasone nonsuppression are common features of depressed patients. Suicidal behavior has been reported to be associated with elevated 24-hour urinary 17-ketosteroids (Bunney & Fawcett, 1965; Fawcett, Scheftner, Fogg, et al., 1987). Nemeroff, Owens, Bissette, Andorn, and Stanley (1988) have reported decreased corticotropin-releasing factor (CRF) receptor activity in the brains of suicide victims, suggesting that elevated CRF may also play a role in suicidality in depression. Cortisol and dexamethasone have been reported to decrease serotonin or 5-HIAA levels in the frontal cortex of rats, perhaps by stimulating alternate synthetic pathways (Green & Curzon, 1968). Conversely, enhanced postsynaptic serotonin activity or sensitivity has been implicated in increased cortisol levels in depressed patients. Hence, cortisol and serotonin activity in the brain may be linked particularly in depressed patients with suicidal tendencies.

In depressed subjects, cortisol levels are highest in those with psychotic features—a subgroup that has been reported to be at increased risk for completing suicide (Schatzberg, Rothschild, & Stahl, 1983). Several groups have reported that psychotic patients with depressive symptoms demonstrate not only extremely elevated plasma cortisol levels but also high plasma dopamine levels (Rothschild et al., 1987). Others have reported generally higher CSF HVA and 5-HIAA in psychotic depressives (Ägren & Terenins, 1985; Äsberg, 1980, 1986; Äsberg et al., 1984; Äsberg, Eriksson, Martensson, et al., 1986a; Äsberg, Nordstrom, & Träskman-Bendz, 1986b), although low HVA and 5-HIAA levels have been reported in a subgroup of older psychotic depressives with suicidal ideation (Brown, Linnoila, & Goodwin, 1992).

In summary, the role of elevated CSF HVA or 5-HIAA in suicidal behavior in psychotic depressives has not been well studied, but findings to date suggest that low or high extremes in serotonin or dopamine (i.e., low 5-HIAA/HVA or high 5-HIAA) may each play a role in different suicidal psychiatric patients.

Studies of Monoamine Oxidase Activity

Some studies indicate a lower level of monoamine oxidase, one of the brain enzymes that break down neurotransmitters into their metabolites, in individuals who have been suicidal or suffered psychiatric disorder (such as depression), but these studies fail to control for severity of depression and other psychiatric disturbance. Lester (1992d) reviewed these studies of monoamine oxidase and concluded that on the whole there is no evidence to support a lower level of monoamine oxidase in those individuals who are suicidal.

Studies of Norepinephrine and MHPG

The brain amine norepinephrine breaks down into 3-methoxy-4-hydroxyphenylglycol (MHPG), which can be measured in both the CSF and in the urine. Although CSF levels of MHPG do not appear associated with suicidal behaviors, studies lack comparison of controls matched for level of depression, anxiety, and other indicators of psychiatric disturbance (Lester, 1992d). Ägren (1983) reported a negative relation of urinary MHPG levels to severity and lethality of previous suicide attempts and current or recent suicidal ideation.

CSF Studies in Violent Suicide Attempters

Low CSF 5-HIAA levels have been found to be particularly associated with violent suicide attempts. In fact, Träskman et al. (1981) reported that CSF 5-HIAA levels were significantly lower only among those patients who had made a violent suicide attempt (hanging, drowning, shooting, gasing, several deep cuts), and that levels were not reduced among those who had made a nonviolent suicide attempt (overdose). Banki and Arato (1983), studying 141 psychiatric patients suffering from depression, schizophrenia, alcoholism, or adjustment disorder, found that levels of CSF 5-HIAA were significantly lower among the violent suicide attempters in all four diagnostic categories.

Brown et al. (1992) have reviewed the research on impulsivity, aggression, and affect as it relates to self-destructive behaviors and suicide. Violent attempters (e.g., jumping, neck slashing, hanging, and shooting) are found more frequently in those with lower CSF 5-HIAA levels who also have alcoholism, adjustment disorders, major depression, personality disorders (Brown et al., 1982), and schizophrenia (van Praag, 1983). The same low levels of 5-HIAA are reported in the CSF of violent criminal offenders (Linnoila et al., 1983).

Patients with low 5-HIAA levels seem prone not only to more violent suicide attempts but also to attempts that are less premeditated (Äsberg et al., 1976b) and more frequent (Äsberg, Thorén, & Träskman, 1976a; Cohen et al., 1988). In addition to increased suicidal behavior, there is a significant inverse correlation between CSF 5-HIAA and overt aggression (Äsberg, Nordstrom, & Träskman-Bendz, 1990; Brown et al., 1982; Cohen et al., 1988; Lidberg, Tuck, Äsberg, Scalia-Tomba, & Bertilsson, 1985; Lidberg, Äsberg, & Sundquist-Stenmann, 1984; Linnoila et al., 1983; Träskman-Bendz, Äsberg, & Schalling, 1990) including murder (particularly impulsive homicide) and to increased anxiety (Äsberg et al., 1984). The relation appears to relate to overt behaviors (e.g., hostile acts and suicide attempts) and not to self-reported affective states (e.g., thoughts of suicide or hostile feelings) (Äsberg et al., 1984). The relation of low serotonin to both depression and expressed anger, social dominance, and fearlessness (Äsberg, 1986) supports the literature from Freud to the present (Äsberg et al., 1984), associating anger with depression.

The incidence of suicide among murderers in some European countries is higher than in any other risk group, exceeding in some instances 30% (Äsberg et al., 1984). In Äsberg et al.'s (1984) study of murderers, low 5-HIAA levels, comparable to those of suicide attempters, were found in those who killed someone with whom they had an intense relationship, such as a paramour or spouse. It is this group that also is most likely to commit suicide after the homicide. Parents who attempt suicide after killing their own children have also been found to have lower CSF 5-HIAA levels (Lidberg, Äsberg, Sundquist-Stenmann, 1984).

Postmortem Anatomical and Neurochemical Studies

CSF 5-HIAA determinations are an imprecise way to measure serotonin levels and activity in the living brain. A much better approximation of actual activity level of neurotransmitters at the time of suicidal behavior is to conduct careful neurochemical studies on the brains of suicide victims soon after they have died.

A large number of studies in postmortem brain tissue from suicide victims have been carried out (see Table 16.3) examining the serotonergic, noradrenergic, and dopaminergic

---

TABLE 16.3. Brain Areas Involved in Suicidal Behavior

Brainstem

Dorsal raphe nucleus (DRN)

Prefrontal cortex (PFC): dorsolateral and ventral

Frontal cortex (FC)

Temporal lobe (TL)

Locus coeruleus (LC)

Hypothalamus

Hippocampus

neurotransmitter systems. The few studies that have examined norepinephrine, dopamine, or the dopamine metabolite (HVA) have tended to be negative (Stanley, Mann, & Cohen, 1986). Studies of the serotonergic system have generally found decreases in presynaptic serotonin nerve terminal binding sites, of which we currently know six. More recent studies of postmortem brain tissue have suggested that these abnormalities are more pronounced in the ventral prefrontal cortex than in the dorsolateral prefrontal cortex.

Similarly, postsynaptic serotonin receptors, such as the 5-HT1A receptor and the 5-HT2A receptor, appear to be increased in number in the prefrontal cortex of suicide victims. The explanation for the increases in these subtypes of postsynaptic serotonin receptors is uncertain, but one possibility is compensatory upregulation (i.e., increased proliferation) in response to reduced serotonin neuron activity overall (Mann, 1998). These receptor changes appear to be more pronounced in the ventral prefrontal cortex. A preponderance of altered serotonin receptor binding measures in the ventral prefrontal cortex would suggest that this brain region is of particular importance in relation to the risk for suicide. Mann (1998) postulates the following:

> The ventral prefrontal cortex is involved in the executive function of inhibition and injuries to that area of the brain may result in disinhibition. Reduced serotonergic input into this part of the brain may result in impaired inhibition and a greater propensity to act on powerful feelings such as suicidal or aggressive feelings. Lifetime externally directed aggression is more frequent in suicide attempters and vice versa. Both behaviors are associated with reduced serotonergic function. Aggression is also associated with ventral prefrontal lesions; this area of the brain may mediate a more universal restraint mechanism that is suboptimal in some suicidal patients, as well as in association with aggression. (26)

Mann, Stanley, McBride, and McEwen (1986) reported that norepinephrine levels in the prefrontal cortex are increased and that beta-adrenergic binding is decreased. They conclude that such noradrenergic overactivity may have resulted in the depletion of norepinephrine from the smaller population of nonadrenergic neurons found in suicide victims. Studies of chronic stress in rodents report depletion of norepinephrine. There is evidence of hyperactive stress response systems reported in depression. Thus, these biochemical findings could potentially be a result of the stress preceding a suicidal event in a serious psychiatric illness.

Taken together, these postmortem neurochemical and receptor studies tend to support the hypothesis that diminished central serotonin metabolism (as evidenced by reduced levels of serotonin and 5-HIAA, and upregulation of the postsynaptic serotonin-2 receptor) is associated with suicide. (Åsberg, 1986; Braunig et al., 1989; DeLeo & Marazitti, 1988; Mann et al., 1986; Stanley & Mann, 1983; Stanley & Stanley, 1990; Stanley, Virgilio, & Gershon, 1982; Träskman-Bendz et al., 1990). The development of a noninvasive biological test to measure CNS neurotransmitter functioning seems like a logical, yet challenging, next step. However, there may well be clinical, ethical, legal, and moral reasons not to use such screening measures. See Box 16.1 for a look at the pros and cons of the controversy.

PSYCHOPHARMACOLOGY OF SUICIDAL BEHAVIOR

The psychopharmacology of suicidal behavior is based on the premise that the majority of individuals who are at highest risk for suicide are those who have one or more of the following underlying psychiatric or behavioral disorders: depression, anxiety, panic, impulsivity, aggression dyscontrol, alcohol or other drug (e.g., cocaine) abuse or dependency, bipo-

---

BOX 16.1. Controversy: Developing a Biological Test to Predict Risk for Suicide

Argument: The development of a simple blood test, saliva assay, or urine analysis as a screening measure for CNS neurotransmitter functioning would identify individuals at risk for the development of suicidal behaviors.

Pros:
1. Blood tests are simpler, faster, and cheaper than psychiatric interviews.
2. Problems can be identified before they occur.
3. Biological tests will pinpoint which neurotransmitter system is malfunctioning.
4. Such tests could be used to monitor response to drug treatment, and assess degree of recovery.
5. It is a more efficient and effective approach to preventing suicidal behaviors than waiting for a problem to occur and then treating the individual.

Cons:
1. Screening the entire population becomes expensive, because of the low base rate of suicidal behaviors in the general population.
2. It is stigmatizing to label someone, based on a single biological test, as being at-risk for suicide, especially in advance of any symptoms.
3. Many factors contribute to the development of suicidal behaviors, not just a change in neurotransmitter levels.
4. We lack specific medications, interventions, or therapies to prevent the development or expression of suicidal behaviors in all individuals at risk, so why label people with a problem we can't fix.
5. The number of false-positive individuals who are screened and referred for further evaluation or treatment might overload the available resources for those truly in need of such services.

---

lar illness, or schizophrenia. A second premise is that these disorders and dysfunctions involve a biochemical alteration in the brain that is amenable to the introduction of a psychotropic medication which is designed to correct the resulting imbalance of neurotransmitters.

The most frequent psychiatric disorders associated with suicide attempts and suicide are major depression, schizophrenia, bipolar affective disorder, and alcohol abuse. The most common complaints heard in a primary-care setting that are associated with subsequent suicidal behaviors include insomnia (sleep disturbance), irritability, anhedonia (apathy), emotional lability, anxiety, restlessness, depression, fatigue, and general decreased energy (Goldman, Silverman, & Alpert, 1998).

Large-scale empirical studies of consecutive suicides emphasize the correlation between mental illness and suicide (Robins & Murphy, 1959; Dorpat & Ripley, 1960; Barraclough, Bunch, Nelson, & Sainsbury, 1974). Robins and Murphy (1959) reported that 94% of 134 cases of completed suicide were found to have psychiatric diagnoses at the time of death. Just over 50% of these were due to primary depression, and almost 33% were associated with chronic alcoholism.

The underlying approach to medicating individuals at increased risk for suicidal behaviors is to ameliorate, alleviate, or reduce those symptoms that "facilitate," or "contribute" to the expression of suicidal behaviors. However, much controversy remains about the possibility that certain "therapeutic" medications may, in fact, increase the propensity toward the expression of suicidal behaviors (Mann & Kapur, 1991). Another recent suggestion is that certain medications may, in fact, prevent the onset of suicidal behaviors in at-risk individuals (Baldessarini & Jamison, 1999).

Not everyone can or will benefit from the administration of pharmaceuticals to alleviate target psychiatric symptoms or suicidal behaviors. What follows is a review of the evolving state of the art regarding the more common medications in current usage, as well as the related clinical issues associated with the prescribing, administration, and monitoring of psychopharmacological agents.

The Art and Science of Prescribing Medication

Goldblatt and Schatzberg (1990) outline general management approaches for patients undergoing psychiatric treatment, especially those with suicidal ideation and/or plan. The following factors in the patient's history and presentation are particularly important to note from a clinical, research, theoretical, and forensic (liability) perspective:

> (1) extent of a current plan or thoughts about hurting oneself; (2) overall psychopathology—psychotic depression, unipolar and bipolar depression with hopelessness, schizophrenia with command hallucinations, and substance abusers while intoxicated; (3) strength of social supports; (4) history of past suicide attempts and their outcomes; (5) current stressors, including degree of losses; (6) availability of means to follow through with suicidal plans; (7) quality of the therapeutic alliance between the patient and clinician; (8) strength of alliance between the patient's family and the treating clinician; and (9) degree of patient's communication about his or her depression, dysphoria, and suicidality. (429)

Concerns about the inappropriate use of prescribed medications by the patient take on profound importance when medicating potentially suicidal patients, because many of the psychopharmacological medications available today are potentially lethal when taken in overdose, in inappropriate dosages, or in combination with other drugs (especially benzodiazepines and alcohol). The physician must avoid the oversupplying of potentially lethal medications while conveying a clear message to the patient about trust, mutuality of effort and activity, and goals of treatment with the use of medication (Goldblatt, Silverman, & Schatzberg, 1998). Goldblatt and Schatzberg (1990) suggest the following:

> This begins with a careful review of the adequacy of previous medication trials vis-à-vis dosage, duration, clinical response, and the patient's history of compliance. The physician should attempt to follow a plan of prescribing relatively small total amounts, while ensuring adequate daily doses and allowing for periodic increases. . . . The patient should receive a 1-week supply at their initial appointment, to cover the amount of medication needed, including dosage increase. In the face of no side effects, dosage should be increased weekly until the patient demonstrates a persistent clinical response, or until maximum levels are obtained. (p. 430)

They highlight the importance of regular assessments of clinical signs and symptoms in order to evaluate responsiveness to the medication. They acknowledge that for some patients, hospitalization may be required to achieve the goals of safety and security while undergoing an adequate trial of medications. They recommend frequent contact to ensure compliance and adherence to a drug regimen.

The use of psychopharmacological agents should never be seen as monotherapy. In fact, the largest study ever completed on therapeutic interventions for depression found that psychopharmacology in combination with psychotherapy yielded the highest percentage of

TABLE 16.4. **Commonly Used Classes
of Psychotropic Medications with Implications
for the Treatment of Suicidal Behaviors**

Antianxiety agents (anxiolytics)

Benzodiazepines
Beta-blockers

Antidepressants

Monoamine oxidase inhibitors (MAOIs)
Tricyclic/tetracyclic antidepressants (TCAs)
Selective serotonin reuptake inhibitors (SSRIs)
Atypical/novel agents

Antimanic agents (mood stabilizers)

Anti-epileptics
Lithium

Antipsychotic medications (neuroleptics)

Major tranquilizers

Sedatives/hypnotics

Barbiturates
Nonbarbiturates
Atypical/novel agents

successful outcome (National Institute of Mental Health Extramural Collaborative Study of Depression). Table 16.4 lists the currently available classes of psychotropic medications most often used in treating patients expressing suicidal ideation or behavior.

Psychiatric Illness

Many psychiatric diagnoses are associated with self-destructive behaviors (cf. Chapter 13). Although subject to reanalysis, a number of studies have indicated that affective illness (major depression, bipolar illness, and schizoaffective disorder) is the most common diagnosis among suicide completers, accounting for up to 60–70% of suicidal deaths (Bulik et al., 1990). According to Slaby and Dumont (1992):

> If other illnesses with a strong depressive component are included, such as depressions associated with dysthymic disorder, cyclothymic disorder, narcissistic personality, and borderline personality disorder, the number may be as great as 80%. Many of those affectively ill are dually diagnosed. They self-medicate the mania or depression with drugs or alcohol, thereby decreasing judgment, increasing hopelessness, decreasing self-esteem, and enhancing the risk of impulsive self-inflicted death, particularly if the means to do so are available (189).

Slaby, Lieb, and Tancredi (1985) have identified the most common psychiatric diagnoses associated with self-destructive behaviors (see Table 16.5).

Risk of suicide for individuals with affective illness is estimated to be 30 times that of those not suffering from the disorder (Bulik et al., 1990). Approximately 15% of individuals with major depression take their own life (Guze & Robins, 1970; Bulik et al., 1990). Ten to 15% of schizophrenics are estimated to die by suicide during the first 10 years of the illness (Cohen, Test, & Brown, 1990), or, put another way, suicide of schizophrenics occurs at a rate 20 times that of the normal population (Breier & Astrachan, 1984). Lifetime

TABLE 16.5. Differential Diagnosis of Self-Destructive Behavior

Adjustment disorders

Anxiety disorders

Bipolar disorder

Brief reactive psychosis

Delusional (paranoid disorder)

Depressive disorder

Impulse control disorder

Organic mental disorders associated with physical disorders or conditions

Personality disorders

Posttraumatic stress disorder

Psychoactive substance-induced organic mental disorders

Schizoaffective disorder

Schizophrenia

Source: Slaby, Lieb, & Tancredi (1985).

prevalence of suicide of those with schizophrenia is 15% (Cohen et al., 1990; Haas, 1997) and the incidence of suicide is increasing among young schizophrenics.

Panic disorder, which occurs in about 1.5% of the population at some time during their life, carries a high risk of morbidity and mortality if not identified early and treated aggressively. Panic attacks that do not meet the diagnostic criteria for panic disorder are even two to three times more prevalent (Weissman, Klerman, Markowitz, & Ouellette, 1989). Of those with panic disorder approximately 20% make a suicide attempt, and of those with panic attacks about 12% (Weissman et al., 1989).

Patients with major depression alone have at least a 15% lifetime risk of suicide (Guze & Robins, 1970). The presence of severe hopelessness, suicidal ideation, history of previous suicide attempts (Fawcett, Scheftner, Fogg, & Clark, 1990; Fawcett, Clark, & Busch, 1993), and severe anxiety (Fawcett, 1992) are strong correlates of potential suicide, both early and late, in a depressed patient. The link between depression and suicidal thoughts or behaviors is well established.

Suicide risk is five times higher in delusional than in nondelusional depressions. Robins (1986) reported that 19% of 134 subjects who committed suicide had also been psychotic—a finding that has been confirmed by others. Roose, Glassman, Walsh, Woodring, and Vital-Herne (1983) found that delusionally depressed patients were five times more likely than nondelusionally depressed patients to commit suicide. These patients are among the most difficult to treat because they hide the degree of their cognitive disturbance, become distant, and are difficult to assess for true suicidal risk.

Antidepressants

Although a number of antidepressants have been found to be effective in the treatment of obsessive–compulsive disorder, panic disorder, nicotine addiction, and eating disorders (especially bulimia), we focus mainly on their role in the treatment of depression and particularly suicidal ideation and intent.

Since the 1950s, tricyclic antidepressants (TCAs) and monoamine oxidase inhibitors (MAOIs) have been the pharmacological mainstay of the treatment for major depressive disorders. Most of the known antidepressants are mediated by both the norepinephrine and serotonin receptor systems (Stahl, 1996). These drugs can effect different parts of the cycle of neurotransmitter production, release, receptor binding, reuptake, and resynthesis.

The National Institute of Mental Health (NIMH) Extramural Collaborative Study of Depression revealed that substantial undertreatment of depressed patients was common, even in academic medical settings (Isaccson & Rich, 1997). The generally low dosages of medications prescribed and the variability of treatment regimens were attributable to individual medical practitioners' decision making and prior training (Keller, Lavori, Klerman, 1986). Fewer than half of the medication trials that "refractory" depressed patients received were reported to be adequate in dosage or duration (Schatzberg et al., 1983).

Although most of the currently available antidepressants have been developed to target specific neurotransmitter receptor systems, none are without side effects attributed to their blockade or enhancement of other receptor systems in the CNS or peripherally. For example, although the TCAs nonselectively enhance both noradrenergic and serotonergic activity, they also significantly antagonize (or block) histaminic, cholinergic, and alpha-adrenergic receptors. Hence, one class of antidepressants affects at least five different neurotransmitter systems—all to varying degrees as evidenced by clinical response. It is the side-effect profile of some of these antidepressants that have linked them with controversies concerning enhancement of suicidal behavior secondary to antidepressant use.

Of note is that the "gold standard" by which all newer antidepressants are measured in terms of clinical efficacy and adverse effects remains the compound imipramine, one of the first TCAs used. Table 16.6 lists the currently available classes of antidepressants organized by their primary mode of action or chemical structure.

TCAs

If patients are not responding to a course of antidepressant medication, the clinician must assess whether an adequate trial has been achieved. The response to TCAs is often slower than one might wish—up to 6 weeks even when therapeutic levels are prescribed initially. Quitkin, et al. (1984) concluded in their review of a series of studies on TCAs in depressed patients that relatively few patients demonstrate significant improvement after only 2 weeks of therapy, and many require as long as 6 weeks to respond. The necessary time course for treatment response remains in considerable debate. Waiting 6 weeks for a response is often not tolerated or tolerable for patient and physician alike.

If only a limited clinical response is noted with a TCA after 6 weeks, the physician should consider increasing the dosage, because some patients metabolize medication rapidly and may require higher doses to respond. Obtaining plasma levels may be helpful for adjusting the dosage of TCAs or for determining the adequacy of a full trial. For nortriptyline, a curvilinear relationship has been described, with a critical peripheral blood level range of 50 to 150 ng/ml. representing a "therapeutic window"; blood levels above and below this range are frequently associated with poorer responses (Äsberg et al., 1971).

For some patients, adding lithium carbonate or liothyronine (a thyroid hormone) to a TCA can bring about a clinical response. If these additions do not result in a response within a few weeks, the physician is faced with the option of either changing the medication within the same class of drug, moving onto another class of antidepressant, or considering ECT.

TABLE 16.6. Classes of Antidepressants and
Representative Examples

Atypical/combination Antagonists

Mirtazapine
Nefazodone
Trazodone
Mianserin

Dopamine and norepinephrine reuptake inhibitors

Buproprion

Monoamine oxidase inhibitors (MAOIs)

Phenelzine
Tranylcypromine
Isocarboxacid

Selective norepinephrine reuptake inhibitors

Desipramine
Nortriptyline
Maprotiline

Selective serotonin reuptake inhibitors (SSRIs)

Citalopram
Fluoxetine
Fluvoxamine
Paroxetine
Sertraline

Serotonin and norepinephrine reuptake inhibitors

Venlafaxine

Tertiary amine tricyclics

Amitriptyline
Doxepin
Imipramine
Clomipramine
Amoxapine

MAOIs

MAOIs block the intraneuronal action of monoamine oxidase, the enzyme that degrades various neurotransmitters, including norepinephrine, dopamine, and serotonin. MAOIs have been reported to be particularly effective in refractory depressed patients and atypical depressives. Clinicians frequently worry that suicidal patients on MAOIs may kill themselves by ignoring their special tyramine-restricted diets or by taking unprescribed additional medications. Among other food items, this diet restricts the ingestion of figs, red wine, blue cheese, and preserved meat. Although case studies of adverse reactions after ingesting these foods have been reported in the literature, they are relatively uncommon. Generally, the potential headaches, pain, and other symptoms associated with the subsequent hypertensive reactions frighten even suicidal patients, so that this becomes an unattractive method of self-harm. Rather, MAOIs are often effective for some suicidal depressives and should be strongly considered.

Three MAOIs are currently available in the United States. Phenelzine and isocarboxacid are more calming and anxiolytic; tranylcypromine is more stimulating. Distressing side effects of dizziness and orthostasis can be effectively treated by maintaining adequate hydration (especially in the summer months), by the use of elastic stockings, or by increasing salt intake.

It appears that this is an effective class of antidepressant in patients with whom the physician has enough of an alliance and who are able both to cooperate and to comprehend the physiologic consequences of monoamine oxidase inhibition and potential hypertensive crises. A 10- to 14-day drug-free period is recommended when changing between an MAOI and a TCA. Although a briefer drug-free period may be sufficient going from a TCA to an MAOI, a 10- to 14-day drug-free period is probably safer.

Selective Serotonin Reuptake Inhibitors

A major advance in the pharmacotherapy of depression arrived with the development of fluoxetine, the first of many selective serotonin reuptake inhibitors (SSRIs) released in the late 1980s and 1990s. The advantages were the relatively low adverse-effect profile, ease of administration (once daily dosing), single-dosage dosing, and virtually no risk of mortality due to overdose. Here was a drug which purportedly was an "activator" and even an "enhancer" of potential and creativity (Kramer, 1993). As time went on, the pharmacologists learned more about the multiple clinical actions of SSRIs on the serotonin receptor systems, and clinicians documented its clinical effectiveness in various populations across a wide range of related disorders (e.g., panic disorder, obsessive–compulsive disorder, and bulimia).

It is the possible adverse effects of agitation, insomnia, anxiety, panic, and akathisia that have been implicated in cases of violent behavior erupting in patients being treated with SSRIs, particularly fluoxetine (Teicher, Glod, & Cole, 1990). A literature exists suggesting that it is the chemically induced akathisia that may enhance the subjective report of irritability and agitation associated with some forms of acting-out behaviors, possibly including homicide, suicide, and domestic violence (Healy, 1998). Yet there exists another literature which seriously questions the possibility that the SSRIs enhance, promote, or facilitate violence behaviors (Mann & Kapur, 1991).

Shortly after fluoxetine was introduced to the market, a small number of case reports (e.g., Teicher et al., 1990) noted the emergence of suicidal ideation in patients taking fluoxetine. A great deal of publicity in the mass media surrounded such reports, and some observers hypothesized that fluoxetine may trigger emergent suicidal and homicidal ideation in a small proportion of patients taking this medication. Further study has suggested that there is no "increased risk of suicidal acts or emergence of substantial suicidal thoughts among depressed patients" associated with the treatment of fluoxetine (Beasley et al., 1991: 685).

The American College of Neuropsychopharmacology Task Force's review of suicidal behavior and psychotropic medication concluded:

> New generation low-toxicity antidepressants, including SSRIs, may carry a lower risk for suicide than older TCAs. There is no evidence that antidepressants such as the SSRIs, for example fluoxetine, trigger emergent suicidal ideation over and above rates that may be associated with depression and other antidepressants. What is clear is that most patients receive substantial benefit from treatment with this drug and related antidepressants. (Mann, Goodwin, O'Brien, & Robinson, 1993: 182)

Nevertheless, controversy remains regarding whether the use of SSRIs, and particularly fluoxetine, results in no increased risk for suicidal behaviors (Isacsson & Rich, 1997). In fact, a number of treatises and malpractice lawsuits have emerged that challenge whether these antidepressants are as safe as initially reported (Healy, 1998; *Forsyth v. Lilly*, 1999).

SSRIs have well-established efficacy for major depression, obsessive–compulsive disorder, panic disorder, and bulimia. These indications relate directly to the fact that SSRIs cause desensitization of 5-HT$_{1A}$ receptors, leading to more serotonergic neurotransmission in the prefrontal cortex, basal ganglia, limbic cortex/hippocampus, and hypothalamus. The stimulation of 5-HT$_2$ receptors by the SSRIs leads to possible adverse effects of agitation, akathisia (restlessness, pacing, fidgetiness), anxiety, panic attacks, insomnia/myoclonic jerks, and sexual dysfunction. SSRIs' stimulation of 5-HT$_3$ receptors leads to possible adverse effects of nausea, gastrointestinal (GI) distress, and diarrhea. Thus, the least preferred uses for SSRIs could include patients with major relationship problems in which the development of sexual dysfunction could be problematic, patients in whom nocturnal muscular contractions (myoclonus) are present, patients with persistent insomnia and agitation, patients with preexisting GI problems, and those with secondary refractoriness or loss of efficacy with long-term treatment.

Atypical/Combination Medications

This group of medications consists of drugs that do not fit easily within the previously discussed classes of medications, because of their unique chemical structures, modes of action, or target neurotransmitter effects.

Because of its ability to boost levels of norepinephrine and dopamine, bupropion may be preferred in patients with retarded depression, patients with hypersomnia, nonresponders to serotonergic antidepressants, nontolerators of serotonergic drugs, patients with cognitive slowing/pseudodementia, and those preferring to avoid sexual dysfunction. Bupropion's least preferred uses could include those patients with seizure disorders or those who are seizure prone.

At low doses, venlafaxine may function more as an SSRI than as a dual serotonin and norepinephrine reuptake inhibitor, because its serotonin reuptake properties are more potent than its norepinephrine reuptake properties. Venlafaxine has generally fewer drug interactions than the SSRIs. Rather than switch to another agent or augment with a second agent when a patient has an inadequate response to venlafaxine, one can simply increase the dose and turn it into a dual-action antidepressant, almost like adding bupropion to an SSRI. The preferred profile for medium to high doses of venlafaxine may be patients who fail to respond to SSRIs, to low doses of venlafaxine, or to various other antidepressants and melancholic, severely depressed, and hospitalized patients.

Nefazodone, with its 5-HT$_2$ blocking effects and serotonin reuptake inhibition, offers possible benefits for depression with anxiety, agitation, and sleep disturbance, for prior SSRI-induced sexual dysfunction, for inability to tolerate SSRIs, and for SSRI responders who lose their response.

Mirtazapine has dual actions on both norepinephrine and serotonin via its 1-adrenergic blockade, coupled with postsynaptic blockade of both 5-HT$_2$ and 5-HT$_3$ receptors. Thus, the possible preferred uses would be depression associated with anxiety, agitation, insomnia, panic, weight loss, and severe depression. It can also be a useful alternative for patients intolerant of SSRI-induced sexual dysfunction, agitation, nausea, and GI disturbance.

Case 16.1 illustrates some of the difficulties that are associated with the treatment of a behavior that results from a biopsychosocial etiology. Each factor, biological, social, genetic, environmental, and psychological, may have initially effected his baseline serotonergic activity as he grew up, and contributed to fluctuations throughout his life. These factors surely influence how we might view his current situation and how to resolve his symptoms.

CASE 16.1. Suicidal Behavior: A Biopsychosocial Disorder

John is a 32-year-old white male who apparently was born with a bio-chemical predisposition to low levels of serotonin. In his mid-20s, he de-veloped a major depressive disorder that was successfully treated over a 9-month period with a selective serotonin reuptake inhibitor (SSRI) and individual psychotherapy. John had some side effects of sexual dysfunc-tion and akathisia, which persisted throughout the course of treatment. He recovered and went on to get married and start a new job. Recently, he has again become irritable, pessimistic, restless, and short-tempered. As a result, his job status is being threatened because of decreased produc-tivity and increased absenteeism. He has returned to a former preoccupa-tion with episodic heavy alcohol drinking, and his 6-year marriage is fail-ing (due to his social withdrawal, displays of anger, and lack of interest). When his wife threatens a separation unless he reenters psychiatric treat-ment, he becomes more isolated, hopeless, and angry. He begins to con-template suicide as a real alternative to feeling hopeless and helpless. He now believes that suicide would put an end to his psychological pain and overall feelings of despair. He is reluctant to go back on medications and thereby admit that he is vulnerable to recurrent depressions. He feels that he has no one to turn to because no one can understand his pain or feel his dysphoria.

Many patients with depressive symptoms will first attempt to treat themselves through the use of alcohol or other drugs (legal or illegal). Such exposure to mood-altering drugs can fa-cilitate a worsening of the depressive symptoms or lower one's inhibitions, resulting in an impulsive self-destructive act.

For many individuals with a depression complicated by suicidal ideations or intent, the treatment of choice often is to adapt a biopsychosocial approach—in direct response to the biopsychosocial etiology of the disorder. Specifically, John would most likely benefit from a combination of an antidepressant medication (and even an initial trial using the SSRI which was successful previously), individual therapy (possibly utilizing a cognitive-behavioral ap-proach), interventions for those environmental factors that may be causing unusual stress in his life (job, career decisions, marital relations), and an appraisal of his social skills (ability to make and keep friends, problem-solving abilities).

Mood Stabilizers

Closely related conceptually to the antidepressants are that class of pharmaceuticals known as mood stabilizers or antimanic drugs (e.g., lithium carbonate, valproic acid, and carba-mazine). These drugs have entered the psychiatrist's pharmacopoeia serendipitously. For example, the fascinating history of the discovery and first use of lithium by Cade in the 1950s deserves a careful reading (Goodwin & Jamison, 1990). Lithium is a naturally occur-ring salt that was found to have calming effects and mood-stabilizing functions in agitated patients, many of whom were initially believed to be suffering from schizophrenia and oth-er psychotic disorders of unknown origin.

Today lithium remains the drug of choice in the initial stabilization and treatment of manic disorders. It also has been found to have a mild to moderate antidepressive effect. As compared to the SSRIs, lithium has not incurred the same notoriety (e.g., possibly being in-volved in the facilitation of violent behaviors in prone individuals). In fact, it has been hailed as not only a major discovery for the treatment of manic–depressive illness but also as a preventive measure for suicidal behaviors. A number of studies have shown that the continuous use of lithium in at-risk individuals lowers their frequency of suicidal actions.

Antianxiety Medications/Anxiolytics

Symptoms of anxiety, agitation, irritability, sleep disturbances, and panic are often reported or observed in patients with a primary diagnosis of depression, bipolar affective disorder, and substance abuse disorders, not to mention in the primary anxiety and panic disorders. All of the previously discussed diagnoses are associated with increased risk for suicide. Thus, it is not surprising that anxiolytics and sedative/hypnotics have been used in the treat-ment of patients with these disorders and especially those acknowledging the intense onset of suicidal ideations, intent, or plans.

Follow-up studies of patients with panic disorder, dating back to 1982, have reported significantly increased rates of premature deaths, most resulting from suicide (Coryell, Noyes, & Clancy, 1982; Coryell, 1988; Allgulander & Lavori, 1991). Weissman et al. (1989) reported that 20% of community members surveyed who met criteria for a diagno-sis of panic disorder reported a history of suicide attempts (odds ratio for suicide attempts compared to other disorders was 2.62). In addition, 12% of those who experienced panic attacks but who failed to meet full criteria for a diagnosis of panic disorder were reported to have a history of suicide attempts. A reanalysis of the data found that 7% of respondents with uncomplicated panic disorder reported a history of suicide attempts (odds ratio = 5.4) (Johnson, Weissman, & Klerman, 1990).

These findings have been criticized from a methodological perspective (Appleby, 1994; Clark & Kerkhof, 1993), as well as from a clinical perspective, because of the presence of comorbidity (particularly depression); this may have accounted for the high prevalence of suicidal ideation and attempts in the cohort reporting panic attacks and panic disorder (Fawcett, Scheftner, Fogg, & Clark, 1990; Beck, Steer, Sanderson, & Skeic, 1991). Never-theless, other studies have also found an increased rate of suicide attempts in patients with panic disorder (Lepine, Chignon, & Teherani, 1993; Korn et al., 1992).

Hence, many clinicians now see panic attacks as one of several contributing clinical states associated with an increased risk of suicidal behaviors when they present in conjunc-tion with other psychiatric disturbances, particularly major affective disorder (Appleby, 1994; Clark & Fawcett, 1992). This underscores the importance of rapid, appropriate treatment for patients with panic attacks and panic disorder, especially when they occur in association with other psychiatric disorders. The initial treatment of panic disorder and panic attacks is either with alprazolam or with low doses of antidepressants such as imipramine, desipramine, phenelzine, or fluoxetine.

The use of anxiolytics and sedative/hypnotics are not without their own history of con-troversy. These drugs have been implicated in suicide attempts and lethal overdoses. In combination with other drugs, especially alcohol, they can be lethal. They also have abuse potential and can foster dependency through increasing tolerance with chronic use. This is especially true of the benzodiazepine class of drugs. In addition, in high doses, they have been shown to impair eye–hand coordination, alter consciousness, impair judgment, and af-fect short-term memory.

So, why use them? First, they are specifically found to be helpful to relieve those symp-toms often associated with the escalation or expression of suicidal states—agitation, irri-tability, sleep deprivation, and aggressive/impulsive tendencies. Second, they are used often to alleviate the adverse effects of the antidepressants—side effects such as uncomfortable levels of activation, anxiety, akathisia, and sleep disturbances. This class of drugs has been implicated in inaugurating violent outbursts in at-risk individuals. Medications such as alprazolam and triazolam have been prescribed to patients in close proximity of episodes of unpredictable violence.

On the other hand, Fawcett, Clark, and Busch (1993) believe that it is the agitation/aggression/impulsivity component of the depression and/or of the suicidally prone individual that predisposes an individual to act in a self-destructive manner. For Fawcett and others (Busch, Clark, Fawcett, & Kravitz, 1993), the use of adequate doses of anxiolytics is the treatment of choice to assist the patients through a suicidal crisis. By chemically sedating patients through the lowering of their subjective level of anxiety and by ensuring regular sleep patterns, one may well eliminate risk conditions that predispose to imminent self-destructive behaviors.

Successful treatment presumably decreases suicidal risk. However, it has also been suggested that benzodiazepines induce behavioral disinhibition that results in suicide attempts. One study of a small number of patients noted an increased suicidality with alprazolam in patients with a personality disorder (Gardner & Cowdry, 1985a). Other studies, however, concluded that there is no evidence to suggest that therapeutic benzodiazepine treatment of anxiety or panic disorder is associated with an increased risk of suicidality (Jonas & Hearron, 1996; Smith & Salzman, 1991). Overall, the successful treatment of panic, anxiety, and other anxiety-related syndromes appears to be associated with a decreased risk of suicidal behavior.

Antipsychotics/Neuroleptics

The spectrum of schizophrenic disorders predispose individuals to increased risk for suicide (Haas, 1997). Depressions with psychotic features (delusional depressions) and the acute manic phase of bipolar affective disorder also carry increased risk for suicide. These disorders and psychological states of disordered thinking (hallucinations, delusions, poor reality testing, disorientation, poor judgment) are amenable to the use of antipsychotics (neuroleptics).

Although schizophrenic disorders are primarily considered to involve difficulties with cognition and thinking rather than with mood, suicide is a serious and unfortunately common complication of this disorder. More than 20% of patients who have been hospitalized for schizophrenia will attempt suicide at some time. The majority of schizophrenic suicides occur among outpatients, usually soon after discharge from the hospital (Caldwell & Gottesman, 1992).

The illness is debilitating, and a patient may be easily demoralized by the cycles of decompensation and recompensation. However, interventions aimed at reducing psychosis and at alleviating distress and depressive/negative symptoms should help to decrease the likelihood of untoward outcomes.

Some schizophrenic patients who commit suicide demonstrate increased agitation or psychosis at the time of their suicidal action. In this subgroup, adequate treatment with antipsychotic medication is essential. Depression in the schizophrenic population is particularly difficult to define or study. The consensus in the literature is that suicidal schizophrenic patients are more likely than nonsuicidal schizophrenic patients to be depressed. However, it is often difficult to distinguish depression from the chronic and debilitating "negative symptoms" of schizophrenia. Initially, it was believed that antidepressant treatment of the symptoms resulted in an exacerbation of the schizophrenic condition. However, more recent studies have argued that some of these symptoms respond to treatment with TCAs or alprazolam. In severe cases, ECT and lithium carbonate can also be considered.

For patients who do not begin to improve on an adequate dose of an antipsychotic medication, a different antipsychotic drug can be tried, or a switch can be made to one of the newer antipsychotics: clozapine, risperidone, or olanzepine. Pragmatically, more than 2 weeks without response in a markedly psychotic patient and 5–6 weeks in a patient with milder symptoms generally indicate a consideration of a change in medication regimen. Shifting the chemical class of antipsychotic would be a reasonable strategy, but this has not been well studied.

Clozapine, risperidone, and olanzepine are new additions to the treatment armamentarium for schizophrenia. They are structurally different from the more common antipsychotics. In early studies, clozapine has been shown to decrease suicidality in neuroleptic-resistant schizophrenic patients and has been associated with improvement in depression and hopelessness (Meltzer & Okayli, 1995). Although more studies are needed to assess the role of the "atypical antipsychotic medications" in suicidal patients, these new drugs have already proven to be highly valued for their improved response in treatment-refractory psychosis. Sometimes the addition of a different class of drug, such as lithium or a TCA, may be effective. Depot preparations (long-acting injectable medications) ensure compliance in patients who are not responding, especially those who do not seem to be responding to adequate doses.

The risk of developing a permanent and disfiguring movement disorder (tardive dyskinesia) as a result of conventional neuroleptic medication makes the long-term use of these drugs worrisome. It is currently not possible to predict which patients will develop tardive dyskinesia. However, the best available data suggest a rate of development of dyskinesia of about 3% to 4% over the first 4 or 5 years of exposure. Elderly women and patients with affective disorders appear at greater risk than do schizophrenic patients (Gardos & Casey, 1984).

Special Cases

For some suicidal patients, combining the therapeutic effect of different drug classes may help prevent suicide. For example, there is a clear need for neuroleptic augmentation of antidepressant medication for treatment of the delusionally depressed patient (Roose et al., 1983; Spiker et al., 1981). Recent evidence also suggests that rapid reduction of anxiety in a hospitalized depressed patient may prevent suicide (Fawcett et al., 1993; Busch et al., 1993). Bipolar depressed patients often receive mood-stabilizing medication in conjunction with antidepressant treatment to prevent the development of mania.

Borderline personality disorder (BPD) is associated with suicidal ideation and self-destructive (sometimes suicidal) behavior. BPD is characterized by impulsivity; unstable and intense interpersonal relationships; inappropriate, intense anger; identity disturbance; affective instability; self-destructive acts; and a chronic sense of emptiness. Suicide may be a higher risk for the patient who is suffering from major depression and also has this form of personality disorder (Corbitt, Malone, Haas, & Mann, 1996). Patients with BPD may actually experience an increase in suicidal behavior during treatment with antidepressants (Gardner & Cowdry, 1985b; Soloff et al., 1986, 1987). In the famous case study report linking fluoxetine with increased suicidality, two of the six hospitalized patients who experienced increased suicidality during fluoxetine treatment carried a diagnosis of major depression and BPD, and two others may also have had characteristics of BPD (dissociation, multiple personality) in conjunction with major depression (Teicher, Glod, & Cole, 1990). In contrast, mildly symptomatic research volunteer subjects with BPD without comorbid major depression did not report an increase in suicidal ideation or behavior during treatment with fluoxetine (Salzman, Wolfson, & Schatzberg, 1995). Regardless of whether antidepressant treatment actually increases the risk of suicidality in a patient with BPD, the role for antidepressant treatment needs to be clarified with further studies.

Soloff et al. (1986) reported that haloperidol, a neuroleptic, produced significant improvement on a broad spectrum of symptom patterns, including depression, anxiety, hostility, paranoid ideation, and psychoticism, in borderline patients. On a composite measure of overall symptom severity, haloperidol was found to be superior to both amitriptyline and placebo, with no difference noted between amitriptyline and placebo. Goldberg et al. (1986) also reported a therapeutic benefit of thiothixene over placebo in treating some selected symptoms of BPD. The mean daily dosage was lower than that used in outpatient schizophrenics.

Although there are at least two studies that have indicated that phenothiazines are helpful in reducing suicidal and other symptoms in borderline patients, there is still much debate about how and whether to use them (Gunderson, 1986). This area requires further study.

Two other treatment strategies that may be helpful in BPD patients are MAOIs and anticonvulsants. The MAOIs may be most useful in treating anxiety with related depression in patients with personality disorders. Cowdry and Gardner (1988) noted that carbamazepine was effective in decreasing the self-destructive behavior of borderline patients, compared to other drug regimens; however, self-destructive behaviors in this group were by no means eliminated. Still, further studies on this approach appear warranted. Recent studies on the effects of SSRIs on BPD patients are encouraging, but more work needs to be done to clarify their potential role for these patients.

Alcohol and drug abuse/dependence and affective disorders are commonly associated with suicide. The lifetime risk for suicide is approximately 15% for patients with alcoholism as compared to 1% in the general population. Alcohol misuse increases the risk for suicidal behavior for both alcoholic and nonalcoholic populations, being associated with 50% of all suicides, and 5–27% of suicides in alcoholics (Murphy, 1992).

Alcoholics who attempt suicide have a greater incidence of preexisting lifelong psychiatric diagnoses of major depression, panic disorder, phobic disorder, and generalized anxiety disorder (Roy et al., 1990). In some instances, posttraumatic stress disorder or an anxiety disorder is present and the individual is self-medicating that psychiatric disorder.

Serotonin represents a possible link between alcoholism and depression. Sellers, Naranjo, and Peachey (1981) have reported that serotonin reuptake blockers reduce alcohol consumption in heavy drinkers. Serotonin activity may provide a link between suicidality in alcoholic and depressed patients. Eventually, SSRIs may be included in an overall approach to the treatment of alcohol-related disorders. However, at this point there is no substitute for treatment programs aimed at abstinence, vocational rehabilitation, and psychoeducation.

Use of Medications and the Prevention of Suicide

As we learn more about the role of medications in the treatment of major depression, mania, and schizophrenia, new observations suggest that certain medications, such as lithium, clozapine, and the SSRIs, may in fact be preventive for suicide as well as therapeutic for the underlying symptoms associated with these psychiatric disorders. An argument has arisen that suggests that the use of these pharmaceuticals may be indicated in all individuals expressing suicidal ideation and intent, regardless of any specific psychiatric symptoms they may report or exhibit. The converse is that all patients with diagnosable major depressive disorder, bipolar affective disorder, or schizophrenia should be medicated not only to treat their primary symptoms but to prevent the expression of suicidal behaviors. However, not all suicidal behaviors are known to be linked to a psychiatric disorder or biochemical abnormality, for which medication may well serve as a first-line treatment of choice. Box 16.2 presents some of the pros and cons for prescribing medications to prevent suicide.

Carl Salzman (1999: 373) has cogently reviewed the existing literature regarding the question of whether the use of antidepressant medications can prevent suicide. His analysis follows:

> Although it is plausible to assume that reduction of depressive symptoms will secondarily prevent suicide, there are relatively few controlled studies regarding the efficacy of antidepressant treatments in preventing suicide. There is controversy regarding the available evidence for antidepressant efficacy. One interpretation of the data strongly indicates that antidepressant medication is more effective than placebo in reducing suicidal ideation, although it is not as clear that medication reduces suicide attempts (Malone, 1997). Another opinion holds that the value of antidepressants in preventing suicide has not yet been established (Montgomery et al., 1992).
>
> No trials of tricyclic antidepressants have been undertaken that specifically demonstrate their ability to prevent suicide. For example, Avery and Winokur (1978) found no significant difference in suicide attempts between those who received antidepressant medication and those who did not receive treatment. Black, Winokur, Mohandoss, Woolson, and Nasrallah (1989) also reported no significant difference in the risk of suicide between patients who were acutely treated with adequate antidepressants and those who did not receive antidepressant treatment, but these studies may not be representative of clinical patients, since suicidal patients are usually excluded from clinical trials (Malone, 1997).

BOX 16.2. Controversy: Are Medications Necessary to Prevent Suicide?

Argument: *If* suicide is (1) a self-inflicted violent act, (2) impulsive by nature, (3) highly associated with mood disorders, *then* all suicidal individuals should be placed on the newer medications that are believed to be effective for aggression, violence, and impulsivity.

Pros:
1. Medications are easy to administer and monitor.
2. Medication dosages can be easily adjusted and tailored to address certain symptoms.
3. Medications are relatively safe.
4. Medications are cheaper than psychotherapy.
5. Medications are becoming more selective for neurotransmitter systems and specific behaviors.

Cons:
1. Taking medications can be stigmatizing for some patients.
2. Medications can be expensive, especially if used over long time periods.
3. Medications may lose their efficacy over time, resulting in increasing dosages to achieve the same effects. There are no accepted criteria for knowing when to safely stop medications for suicidal behaviors.
4. Some medications can cause longterm neuromuscular disorders (tardive dyskinesias) or potentiate agitation and restlessness (akathisias).
5. Most studies suggest that it is a combination of medications plus psychotherapy that works best to reduce symptoms, at least for depression. Medications alone do not address an individual's social and psychological contributions to their illness.
6. No medication as yet seems to be sufficiently "clean" or specific in its selectivity for specific symptoms or target behaviors.

Data regarding the effect of SSRI antidepressants in preventing suicide are slightly more positive but still equivocal. These studies (for review, see Malone, 1997) suggest that there may be a more rapid reduction in suicidal ideation with SSRI antidepressants as compared with nonserotonergic antidepressants, which is apparent at about 2 weeks. By 4 to 6 weeks of treatment, however, there are no longer any differences between SSRIs and other classes of antidepressants, thus suggesting that the serotonergic antidepressants may be more useful in reducing suicidal behavior only during the early phases of treatment. Other studies, however, concluded that the SSRI antidepressants were "equivocal" in preventing suicide (Montgomery & Montgomery, 1982, 1984; Schifano & De Leo, 1991; Freemantle, House, & Song, 1994).

Because placebo-controlled trials of antidepressant treatment in the suicidal depressed patient are unethical, only retrospective reviews of treated versus untreated (or inadequately treated) patients can be used to assess the overall efficacy of treatment in preventing suicide. Three studies clearly indicate that the incidence of suicide in depressed patients is greater in those who are not taking antidepressants than in those who are adequately medicated. Isacsson, Bergman, and Rich (1994; Isacsson & Rich, 1997) found that less than half of the patients who committed suicide in a San Diego study were prescribed antidepressants and commented that "more suicides might be averted by decisively treating depressed patients with antidepressants than by not treating them to avoid antidepressant overdoses." (Isacsson, Bergman, & Rich, 1994: 6) They found that 8% of 283 suicide victims and only 12% of those with a diagnosis of major depression were on antidepressants at the time of death. Of these, only 4% showed lethal levels of antidepressants, usually combined with toxic levels of other drugs. These studies suggest that more aggressive treatment with antidepressants will be effective in preventing suicide.

Isacsson, Boethius, and Bergman (1992; Isacsson, Holmgren, Wasserman, & Bergman, 1994) also published similar data from a population of people committing suicide, in Sweden, finding that of patients who committed suicide only 15% had received antidepressant treatment during the previous 3 months. Marzuk et al. (1995) reported virtually identical data from a population of suicide patients in New York City. Eighty-four percent of these patients were not taking an antidepressant (or neuroleptic) medication. These authors agree that "the potential of these drugs [antidepressants] to prevent suicide has not yet been realized" (Isacsson, Rich, & Bergman, 1996: 1659; Marzuk et al., 1996).

There are related and intertwined corollary issues regarding antidepressants and the emergence of suicidal behaviors. If it remains unproven that the use of antidepressants actually prevents the expression of suicidal tendencies, then is it possible that they might facilitate the expression of suicidal behaviors under certain conditions? The two conditions most often discussed are the increased risk of suicidal behavior during the early recovery phase from a major depressive episode and whether certain classes of antidepressants (i.e., SSRIs) cause agitation, activation, and unwarranted irritability and restlessness in individuals sufficient to promote the onset of suicidal tendencies. Some clinicians hold that for certain patients, suicide risk increases as patients start to recover from their depressive symptoms (Clark & Fawcett, 1992; Himmelhoch, 1987). However, there are few data to support this belief (Goldney et al., 1997).

A storm of controversy began in 1990 with the publication of a scientific case report suggesting that fluoxetine, an SSRI, might increase or even cause suicidal behavior in treated patients (Teicher et al., 1990). Mann and Kapur's review (1991) concluded that this class of antidepressants was not associated with an increase in suicidal ideation or behavior, except in a small number of patients with dual diagnoses or with idiosyncratic responses. Subsequent reviews mainly failed to confirm this initial case report observation (Tollefson et al., 1994; Beasley et al., 1992; Fava & Rosenbaum 1992; Wirshing et al., 1992). Nevertheless, such publicity has left an indelible mark on the public's perception of the safety of these drugs, and especially on depressed patients who otherwise might well benefit from treatment with fluoxetine or another SSRI.

Of note is that the newer classes of antidepressants seem to carry a lower risk of fatality from overdose than the older TCAs (Kapur, Mieczkowski, & Mann, 1992; Molcho & Stanley, 1992). In summary, factors of patient education, compliance, adherence to drug regimens, adequate and consistent dosing over time, and therapeutic response seem to be the critical factors in lowering the emergence of suicidal behaviors in depressed patients being treated with antidepressant regimens.

Similar arguments and investigations have been put forward for the role of lithium (a mood stabilizer) (Goodwin & Jamison, 1990; Barraclough, 1972) and certain "novel" antipsychotic medications (Meltzer & Okayli, 1995) in the prevention of suicide. The argument is that when adequately medicated, the symptoms most associated with the onset of suicidal behaviors (i.e., delusions, agitation, akathisia, restlessness, and hallucinations) are sufficiently reduced to lower the potential for suicidal action.

Electroconvulsive Therapy

Clinical wisdom and experience suggest that ECT is an established and effective treatment for conditions in which suicidal ideation or intent are associated with an underlying psychiatric disorder, especially with affective disorders. ECT has been found to be more efficacious, efficient, and effective when compared to the more standardized treatment modalities using antidepressant medications (Tanney, 1986, 1992).

Even though no specific biological mechanism has been demonstrated to explain the effectiveness of ECT, there are documented changes in brain biology following ECT (New York Academy of Sciences, 1985). These changes in biological parameters seem mostly to effect 5-HT$_2$ receptor density and neurotransmitter activity at the synapse.

Nevertheless, there has been virtually no systematic study of the direct effect of ECT on suicidal ideation, intent, or plan. Rather, most reports in the literature discuss ECT's benefit in the relief of morbid depressive symptoms, which, in turn, lessen or eliminate the presence of suicidal ideation or intent.

Tanney (1986) summarizes the existing literature at the time which identified the major indications for the use of ECT: (1) major affective disorder; (2) depressive psychoses; (3) depressive disorders—psychotic, involutional, postpartum, manic–depressive, depressed; (4) depressive psychosis, depressive mood states, and depressive delusions; and (5) manic–depressive/depressed. Other endorsements for its efficacious use included manic excitement, catatonia, and some types of schizoaffective disorders.

Of note is the remarkable agreement that ECT is "the treatment of choice" for affective disorder. But what of its effectiveness in reducing suicidality? Tanney reports that five of six controlled studies provide support for ECT in reducing suicidal behaviors in a range of depressed patients. This may be attributed to the rapid response of depressive disorders to ECT, hence decreasing the period of risk for suicidal preoccupations and subsequent behaviors. If one entertains the possibility that a certain amount of suicidal behavior may be spontaneous, impulsive, or situationally reactive, then any intervention that quickly lowers this behavioral predisposition toward self-destruction is destined to be seen as efficacious and preventive.

Avery and Winokur (1977) found that those with a history of suicide attempts or suicide thoughts are markedly improved at discharge when treated with ECT (56% for those with attempts; 54% for those with thoughts) compared to no treatment (26% and 29%, respectively), or to adequate antidepressant drug therapy (23% and 14%). Six months after treatment (Avery & Winokur 1978), there were no suicides in the ECT group compared to 10% for those patients who had received antidepressants. As noted earlier, the literature remains unclear regarding whether antidepressant medications are efficacious in reducing suicidal ideation, intent, or attempts (Paykel, 1972; Robin & Langley, 1964). As already discussed, determining efficacy is confounded by problems with ascertaining and ensuring patient compliance to following treatment recommendations, adequate dosing, and the measurement of treatment responsiveness in the study populations.

SUMMARY AND CONCLUSIONS

The State versus Trait Debate

Slaby (1994a: 144), while acknowledging the role of psychological and social factors in the etiology and maintenance of suicidal behaviors, has summarized the biological research to date as follows:

> Åsberg (1986) and others have specifically demonstrated that, regardless of diagnosis, violent suicides and suicide attempts are often associated with changes in the metabolism of the indoleamine serotonin. Indoleamines and catecholamines and their metabolites in the cerebrospinal fluid of suicide attempters and the brains of completers, and receptor binding, and measures of cortical and thyroid-releasing hormone in attempters have been studied to support this hypothesis (Slaby, 1993).
>
> The results of these investigations indicate that impulsive violent behavior, be it self or other directed, is associated more with disturbances of serotonin (5-hydroxytryptamine) metabolism in the brain than with mood disorders. Serotonergic mechanisms are involved with fight-or-flight behavior, sexual drive, and affect (Linnoila et al., 1983; Träskman-Bendz, Åsberg, & Schalling, 1990), which at times may be manifested as impulsive and self-destructive behavior. Serotonergic aberrations have been reported with suicide, homicide, assaults, rape, and eating disorders (Cohen, Wichel, & Stanley, 1988). Serotonergic dysfunction has also been found in obsessive-compulsive disorder, schizophrenia, and panic disorder (Van de Kar, 1990). Many healthy people also show a decrease in cerebrospinal fluid levels of 5-hydroxyindoleacetic acid (Åsberg, Nordstrom & Träskman-Bendz, 1990), supporting the multifactorial theory of suicide.

The most compelling data thus far indicate a relative deficiency of serotonin (5-hydroxytyramine [5-HT]), or its metabolite (5-HIAA) in the CNS of suicide victims. Postmortem studies reveal decreased presynaptic inhibitory 5-HT receptors and increased postsynaptic 5-HT receptors in the prefrontal cortex. 5-HIAA, the major metabolite of serotonin, is reduced in the CSF of depressed patients and is even further reduced in depressed patients who are suicidal or have attempted suicide. This finding is particularly robust in patients who have attempted suicide by violent means (e.g., with firearms).

Compared with those who have died by other causes, suicide victims have (1) increased beta and decreased alpha-1 adrenoreceptors and (2) reduced numbers of corticotropin releasing-factor receptors in the frontal cortex. These findings suggest dysregulation of CNS adrenergic function and the HPA axis, respectively, but they may represent the neurophysiology of depression rather than being specific to suicidal behavior (Åsberg et al., 1990).

The serotonergic correlations with suicide appear to be equally strong regardless of the associated psychiatric disorder. Therefore, the serotonergic abnormality in the brain of suicide victims may be related to the predisposition to suicidal behavior rather than to the psychiatric illness that may have triggered it (Nordstrom et al., 1994). Twin studies show a roughly sixfold greater concordance for suicide in MZ than in DZ twins. However, such findings may represent inheritance of predisposing psychiatric illnesses rather than a specific genetic susceptibility for suicide, although heritability of suicide per se cannot be ruled out. Mann (1998: 27) summarizes the research as follows:

> The serotonergic changes are more likely to be related to the vulnerability of suicidal behavior based on the observations that the level of serotonergic system activity shows considerable stability over time, and is under substantial genetic control.
>
> Therefore, the serotonergic system fulfills the criteria for a biochemical trait. In contrast, the noradrenergic system is more state dependent, under less genetic control and, perhaps, reflects responses due to the acute stress of the psychiatric illness or in relation to the suicidal act. The stress of feeling desperate and suicidal may result in excessive noradrenergic activity and consequent depletion in that stress-response neurotransmitter system. With regard to that possibility, studies of the stress systems, including the hypothalamic pituitary adrenal axis (HPA), are of great interest because corticotrophin releasing hormone and corticosteroids can modulate both noradrenergic and serotonergic activity. Major depression is often associated with hyperactivity of the HPA axis, and suicidal patients may exhibit even greater hyperactivity. Thus, there is evidence from studies of both the HPA axis and brain noradrenergic indices consistent with the presence of chronic stress responses that may contribute to the risk for suicide. If this hypothesis can be confirmed, relief of stress effects may help to enhance therapeutic interventions. . . .
>
> These findings suggest that decreased serotonergic functioning is associated with suicidal behavior independent of the psychiatric diagnosis. This is consistent with the concept that predisposition to suicide includes a biological vulnerability, which is in part genetically determined. Moreover, decreased brain serotonergic function may be related to a tendency toward physical aggression or violence, of which suicide is one manifestation (Brown et al., 1982; Coccaro et al., 1989; Mann, 1995; Virkkunen, De Jong, Bartko & Linnoila, 1989). Whatever determines aggression to be outwardly or inwardly expressed is not known at this time. However, both types of violence often coexist in the same individual, such as cases of multiple homicides followed by suicide.

Approximately one-third of violent individuals have a history of suicidal behavior, whereas 10–20% of suicidal individuals have a history of violent behavior toward others (Mann, 1995). Individuals with major depression and personality disorders who have a history of suicidal behavior also have a greater lifetime history of aggression and impulsivity. Criminals who have a history of suicidal behavior also have a history of more severe aggression than do criminals who do not have a history of suicidal behavior. Thus, there may be a fundamental predisposition to more impulsive behavior, whether it is self-directed, in the form of suicidal behavior, or externally directed, in the form of aggression against property or other persons.

Reduced serotonergic function appears to be associated with impulsive aggression and has also been reported to predict recidivism in murderers. This relationship is analogous to that between serotonergic function and suicidal behavior and leads to the more general hypothesis that serotonergic function supports a restraint mechanism and a deficiency of serotonergic function results in greater impulsivity and aggression that also includes self-directed aggression in the form of suicidal behavior.

To the extent that suicidal behaviors are associated with affective disorders (major depression, dysthymia, bipolar affective disorder, depression with psychotic features) and to the extent that antidepressants have been shown to be effective in alleviating these symptoms and disorders, one can conclude that antidepressants are, by and large, therapeutic and even preventive for suicidal ideation, intent, plans, and attempts. Nevertheless, until we better understand the basic biochemistry and genetics of suicidal behaviors, we can only

TABLE 16.7. Implications for Suicide Prevention

Understanding of the role of neurotransmitters will result in the development of
- Better diagnostic tests to diagnose presence of disorder
- Better screening tools and techniques
- Better medications(sensitivity and specificity)

Understanding of the human genome and the role of nature and nurture (biology and environment) on the development, expression and maintenance of suicidal behaviors and predispositions will result in
- Better diagnostic tests
- Better screening tools and techniques
- Development of interventions (biopsychosocial) for individuals at risk
- Better understanding of pathogenesis of suicidal behaviors
- Clarification of trajectories for suicidal behaviors
- Better understanding of the anatomy, physiology, and neurochemistry of suicidal behavior

conclude that antidepressants are but one component in an overall treatment strategy that addresses the entire biopsychosocial paradigm that we currently understand to contribute to suicidal behaviors.

Implications for Prevention

Advances in human and molecular genetics will result in the accurate identification of those individuals with familial loading for psychiatric illness and/or predilection for suicidal behaviors. Neurobiological measures or testing may ultimately improve the clinician's ability to detect high-risk patients. These measures currently involve measurement of CSF 5-HIAA, but, in the future, newer techniques involving functional brain imaging of serotonergic activity and candidate gene markers hold promise. Given the rapid advance in PET and SPECT imaging of serotonergic function *in vivo*, and the identification of genes associated with serotonin production, we now have the tools for developing neurobiological tests to detect patients at high risk for suicide. Such tests may facilitate the testing of treatment interventions that may ultimately reduce the rate of suicide through the judicious use of medications or the early identification and intervention with individuals found to be at high risk. These future screening mechanisms are not without their own set of potential problems, as suggested in Box 16.1.

From a neurobiological perspective, the best hope we currently have to prevent suicide is to accurately identify those at risk (by better understanding human genetics, biology, and environmental interactions), and to offer them the opportunity to benefit from the expanding armamentarium of psychotherapeutic medications that have been found to be efficacious in the treatment of those psychiatric disorders and impulsive behaviors most often associated with suicidal behaviors. Through scientific advances we hope to understand better the role that neurotransmitters play in the development, onset, and perpetuation of suicidal behaviors. Table 16.7 suggests some benefits that might derive from research advances in the neurobiology of suicide and suicidal behaviors that may well lead to more effective approaches to suicide prevention.

In Chapter 17, the concluding chapter in Part III, we turn specifically to the topics of violence and aggression.

FURTHER READING

Effects of Medical Interventions on Suicidal Behavior. (1999). *Journal of Clinical Psychiatry* [Special issue] 60(Suppl. 2). This 122-page special issue contains 16 articles as well as an "Introduction" and "Conclusion" by the leading researchers in the field. This is a state-of-the-art review of the neurobiology of suicide risk, including articles on genetics, screening instruments, role of medications in the treatment and prevention of suicidal behaviors (lithium, antidepressants, anticonvulsants, antipsychotics), ECT, and suicide risk in different patient populations. Recommendations are made about next steps for research, clinical interventions, and best-practice options for medicating individuals at increased risk for suicide.

Faraone, S. V., Tsuang, M. T., & Tsuang, D. W. (1999). *Genetics of mental disorders: A guide for students, clinicians, and researchers*. New York: Guilford Press. This highly readable volume offers clinicians, students, and researchers a comprehensive introduction to the basic knowledge they need to evaluate reports of genetic research, understand implications for treatment, and communicate genetic information to clients and families. The book illuminates the complex interplay of genes and environmental factors involved in the causation and expression of frequently encountered disorders including schizophrenia, bipolar disorder, depression, and Alzheimer's disease. A wealth of charts, definitions, and clinically relevant examples aid in rendering technical concepts accessible to readers without extensive training in genetics.

Schatzberg, A. F., & Nemeroff, C. B. (Eds.). (1998). *Textbook of psychopharmacology* (2nd ed.). Washington, DC: American Psychiatric Press. Covering both basic science and clinical practice, this new edition of the definitive psychopharmacology text has been thoroughly updated and expanded to keep up-to-date with the explosive growth in the field. Four major sections include such topics as the principles of psychopharmacology with the necessary background in neurobiology and pharmacology. A section on clinical psychobiology and psychiatric syndromes reviews the data on the biological underpinnings of specific disorders. An entire section on psychopharmacological treatments provides specific information about drug selection and their prescription.

Stoff, D. M., & Mann, J. J. (Eds.). (1997). *The neurobiology of suicide: From the bench to the clinic, Annals of the New York Academy of Sciences, 836.* This edited volume is the result of a conference titled, "Suicide Research Workshop: From the Bench to the Clinic," held in Washington, DC, in November 1996, and sponsored by the National Institute of Mental Health and the American Suicide Foundation. The workshop presented the most current research in suicide from preclinical, clinical, neuroscience, and treatment perspectives.

Yudofsky, S., & Hales, R. E. (Eds.). (1997). *Textbook of neuropsychiatry* (3rd ed.). Washington, DC: American Psychiatric Press. Written and edited by an internationally renowned group of experts including 39 new authors, the third edition has been extensively revised to provide psychiatrists, neurologists, neuropsychologists, internists, and residents with the latest developments in research, clinical practice, and diagnostic technology. With the addition of new chapters, increased emphasis has been placed on molecular and intracellular aspects of neuropsychiatry and the role of functional imaging in neuropsychiatric disorders. In addition, this text is lavishly illustrated with tables and figures, including many full-color images.

17

Aggression, Violence, and Suicide

Robert Plutchik

Good creatures, do you love your lives
And have you ears for sense?
Here is a knife like other knives,
That cost me eighteeen pence.

I need but stick it in my heart
And down will come the sky,
And earth's foundations will depart
And all you folks will die.
—A. E. HOUSMAN

Considerable clinical experience suggests a relation between suicide, or self-directed violent behavior, and violence directed toward other people. Early psychoanalytic theory considered suicide to be violence turned toward oneself. Later psychoanalysts have seen the relationship as more complex. For example, Menninger (1938) has said that suicide involves both the wish to die and a wish to kill. Gutheil (1996) suggests that suicide expresses identification of the individual's ego with someone else, a giving up on oneself because of repudiation by this important figure, and consequent turning of the aggression toward the self. Consistent with these ideas, he believes, are the common suicidal wish fantasies: to be reborn into a happier life, to punish others, to escape, or to rejoin. Samy (1995) suggests that suicidal impulses tend to develop around developmental crises: the appearance of genital sexuality, problems of separation and individualization, and inadequate coping with parental aggression. Chessick (1992) interprets Freud's concept of a death instinct as the basis of war, homicide, and suicide.

Possibly consistent with the psychoanalytic view is the claim that aggressive moods in populations during wartime are associated with a reduction in suicide, and that in small religious communities where aggression is severely condemned, depressions are relatively frequent (Jakubascik & Hubschmid, 1995). All these psychoanalytically derived views based largely on clinical evidence imply a complex relation between suicidal impulses and violent impulses directed at others and, most important, that they should not be considered in isolation from one another.

Another framework also contributes to the recognition of an intimate relation between suicide and violence toward others. Shneidman (1985) has pointed out that among the many factors associated with suicides are frustrations and anger, both of which can lead to

407

aggression. Some of the elements he lists are (1) unendurable psychological pain, (2) frustrated psychological needs, (3) feelings of helplessness–hopelessness, (4) ambivalence, and (5) anger.

Despite these ideas, most theories of suicide have nothing explicit to say about aggression in general (Lester, 1992a). Conversely, most theories of violence or antisocial behavior have little to say about suicide (Stoff, Breiling, & Maser, 1997).

TERMINOLOGY

It is of some interest that despite the ever-increasing number of diagnostic categories found in the *Diagnostic and Statistical Manuals* (DSMs) issued by the American Psychiatric Association there is no explicit diagnosis for either suicide or aggression. Neither term is found in the index for DSM-IV. The closest DSM-IV comes is the category of impulse-control disorders, which include intermittent explosive disorder (defined by two symptoms), kleptomania, pyromania, pathological gambling, and trichotillomania. Suicidal thoughts are mentioned only as a possible symptom of depression, dysthymia, or borderline personality disorder. Because of these omissions, several authors have suggested the need for a diagnostic nomenclature for the various forms of violence and suicide (Eichelman & Hartwig, 1993; Lopez-Ibor & Carrasco, 1993; O'Carroll, 1993).

Even a casual examination of the relevant literature reveals a certain amount of confusion and inconsistency in the use of terms. For example, even though Moyer (1986) and others have identified a variety of types of aggressive behavior (e.g., predatory, intermale, fear-induced, territorial, maternal, irritable, and instrumental), these distinctions are seldom made when discussing aggression. It is not always clear whether aggression refers to an impulse, a feeling, an emotion (e.g., anger), or a violent act directed against a person or object. Sometimes aggression refers to antisocial behavior and sometimes to criminal behavior, which are not necessarily the same. Suicide has been described as being on a continuum from thoughts to mild self-harming behavior to serious attempts to kill oneself to death (see Chapter 2; Pfeffer, 1986). And the term "parasuicide" has been defined as any acute, intentional, self-injurious behavior that creates the risk of death (Kreitman & Foster, 1991). This definition includes the range of behavior from superficial cuts or swallowing a few aspirins to shooting oneself. Sometimes the word "aggression" is used to refer to suicidal behavior and sometimes to violence toward others. One conclusion with which most writers agree is that both suicide (Lester, 1992a) and violence (Ferris & deVries,1997) are multidetermined. Aggression, in whatever form it is expressed, is determined by the interaction of many variables, environmental, situational, and hereditary. In an effort to be consistent I distinguish between suicidal impulses and suicidal behavior directed toward oneself. A similar distinction is made between aggressive impulses and violent behavior directed toward other people.

EMPIRICAL DATA ON THE RELATIONS BETWEEN SUICIDE AND VIOLENCE

A number of studies have examined the statistical relation between violence directed toward oneself and violence directed toward others. Using homicide rates in the United States as a measure of violence, Holinger, Offer, Barter, and Bell (1994) reported that homicide and suicide rates in adolescents and young adults have tended to rise and fall in parallel ways from 1930 to the present. Using data from the National Center for Health Statistics for the period 1900–1979, Holinger (1987) reported a correlation of .33 between homicide and suicide rates. These findings are inconsistent with the earlier report by Henry and Short (1954), using less reliable data, of a generally inverse relation between homicide and suicide.

Clinical studies with psychiatric populations have generally confirmed the positive correlation between suicide or suicidal behavior and violence toward others. Plutchik and colleagues have published a number of studies that revealed a moderate positive correlation (of the order of magnitude of .5 ± .1) between self-report measures of suicide risk and violence (Apter, Plutchik, Sevy, Korn, & van Praag, 1989; Apter, van Praag, Plutchik, Sevy, Korn, & Brown, 1990; Apter et al., 1991; Botsis, Plutchik, Kotler, & van Praag, 1995; Greenwald, Reznikoff, & Plutchik, 1994; Plutchik, van Praag, & Conte, 1989). Garrison, McKeown, Valois, and Vincent (1993) report similar findings in 3,764 South Carolina high school students; those who reported severe suicidal behaviors also had the highest levels of aggressive behavior toward others.

This has also been reported for psychiatric inpatients as well (Convit, Jaeger, Lin, Meisner, & Volavka, 1988). Cairns, Patterson, and Neckerman (1988) evaluated 1,120 assaultive and violent juveniles and found that suicidal adolescents were most likely to be diagnosed as having a conduct disorder. Inamdar, Lewis, Siomopoulos, Shanok, and Lamela (1982) found that among 51 hospitalized adolescent psychotic patients, 67% had been violent, 43% suicidal, and 27% both violent and suicidal. Similarly, Pfeffer, Newcorn, Kaplan, Mizruchi, and Plutchik (1989) found four subgroups among 129 adolescent psychiatric inpatients: suicidal-only patients, assaultive-only patients, both suicidal and assaultive patients, and neither suicidal nor assaultive patients. Hillbrand (1992) found that of 50 habitually aggressive men in a psychiatric forensic facility (see also Box 17.1), 15 men (30%) made suicide attempts.

In a study of more than 4,156 patients in Missouri mental hospitals, Altman, Sletten, Eaton, and Ulett (1971) found that suicidal thoughts were the highest single predictor of homicidal ideas and vice versa. It is interesting that depression was a significant predictor of suicidal thoughts but not of homicidal ideas. This observation suggests the possibility that certain variables correlate with violence directed toward oneself but not with violence directed toward others. Other variables may correlate with other-directed violence but not with suicidal acts. This idea, of differential actions of variables on suicide and aggression, provides the basis for a model of their interrelations to be described later in this chapter. Finally, based on a study of 5,128 incident reports in a mental hospital, it was found that for all diagnostic groups, a positive correlation existed between assaultive and suicidal behavior (Evenson, Sletten, Altman, & Brown, 1974).

BOX 17.1. Crowding and Violence in Prisons

Other evidence of a connection between violence and suicide comes from the literature on the effects of crowding in prisons (Cox, Paulus, & McCain, 1984). A major review indicates that population increases in prisons are associated with increased rates of suicide, disciplinary infractions (violence), psychiatric commitment, and death. Decreases in prison populations are associated with decreases in assaults, suicide attempts, and death rates. The authors of this review suggest that the underlying reasons for these effects of crowding are the increases in uncertainty, goal interference, and cognitive load.

Studies with Adolescents

Many other studies have confirmed the positive correlation between suicide attempts or completions and measures of violence directed toward other people. For example, in 51 adolescents hospitalized for one or more suicide attempts, the multiple attempters had higher levels of aggression than did the single attempters on the Multidimensional Anger Inventory (Stein, Apter, Ratzoni, Har-Even, & Avidan, 1998). In another study, a group of 136 adolescent inpatients were assessed using the Schedule for Affective Disorders and Schizophrenia (SADS). It was found that conduct-disordered patients had the highest suicidal behavior scores and that a measure of violent behavior correlated positively with suicidal symptoms (Apter, Gothelf, Orbach, & Weizman, 1995). A similar investigation evaluated 60 adolescents diagnosed with conduct disorder, most of whom had high aggression ratings. Conduct-disordered symptom counts correlated with suicide attempts and self-injury (Young, Mikulich, Goodwin, & Hardy, 1995). When 43 adolescent suicide victims were compared with 43 community controls, it was found that the suicide victims had greater scores on a measure of lifetime aggression. The authors of this study conclude that impulsive violence is a risk factor for completed suicides (Brent, Johnson, Perper, & Connolly, 1994).

A group of 219 homeless adolescents were evaluated using the Diagnostic Interview Schedule for Children and other measures. Severe aggression was found in 62% of the adolescents and conduct disorder in 55%. Severe aggression toward others was found to be correlated with attempted suicide (Booth & Zhang, 1996). In another study of 93 homeless adolescents in Los Angeles, California, it was found that the individuals had a high prevalence of conduct disorder with violence, and that almost half the group had attempted suicide (Greenblatt & Robertson, 1993).

It is evident that many of the studies cited deal with adolescent patients. In contrast is an investigation that surveyed 2,062 female and 1,702 male high school students. Eleven percent of the students reported serious suicidal plans, 5.9% reported making a mild attempt, and 1.6% reported serious attempts that required medical care. It was found that as the severity of the suicidal behavior increased, violent behaviors and cigarette use also increased (Garrison et al., 1993).

In a 25-year prospective study of 456 male and 496 female African Americans, it was found that violence and drug use were risk factors for suicidal behaviors. Females who reported highest assault behavior in adolescence were more likely to report suicide attempts (Juon & Ensminger, 1997).

One final study of the relation between violence and suicide is cited (Feinstein & Plutchik, 1990). Structured clinical rating scales covering 10 areas related to suicide and violence were constructed for use in a psychiatric emergency room (ER). Ninety-five ER patients were evaluated with the scales, 50 of whom were discharged after the visit and 45 of whom were admitted to the inpatient psychiatric wards of the hospital. The admitted patients were found to differ significantly from the discharged patients on every one of the 10 scales. The scales are shown in Figure 17.1. Scores on the scales were also found to predict suicide precautions on the wards, harassment of other patients as assessed from nursing notes, and indicators of violence on the wards. The scales were also found to have high internal reliability and high sensitivity and specificity. They appear to be helpful to clinicians in identifying patients in need of hospitalization and may also serve as limited predictors of hospital functioning.

These studies that have been cited are quite consistent in revealing a positive correlation between various measures of suicidal behavior or suicide itself and measures or diagnoses of violent behavior. From a theoretical point of view the following conclusions about violence are suggested:

Current Violent Thoughts (during interview)
4   Expresses intense wish to kill someone specific.
3   Reveals command hallucinations to injure someone.
2   Expresses ambivalent wish to kill someone specific.
1   Expresses nonspecific feelings of rage and belligerence.
0   Reveals no homicidal ideas.

Recent Violent Behaviors (during the past several weeks)
4   Showed serious assaultive behavior (e.g., tried to strangle, stab, or shoot someone).
3   Beat up someone badly (e.g., broke bones or required hospitalization).
2   Slapped or pushed or punched someone (no serious outcomes).
1   Broke things in house or elsewhere.
0   Showed good control of his (her) behavior.

Past History of Violent/Antisocial/Disruptive Behaviors (lifetime history)
4   Has committed violent acts in the past (e.g., beaten up people).
4   Has been arrested for assaultive behavior.
3   Carries weapons (e.g., knife, gun, chain, razor, etc.).
3   Has access to weapons.
2   Has been arrested for automobile infractions.
2   Has a criminal record.
2   Chronic problems with authority (e.g., truancy, running away from home, family fights).
2   Has a history of impulsive or unpredictable behavior. (e.g., loses temper easily, overeats, sexual promiscuity, etc.).
2   Frequent changes of living situation as a child.
0   Has no past history of violence.

Current Suicidal Thoughts (during interview)
4   Expresses intense wish to kill self and has made a plan
4   Reveals psychotic or delusional ideation or hallucinations to kill or injure self
3   Expresses intense wish to kill self and has made no plan
2   Expresses ambivalent wish to kill self
0   Reveals no suicidal ideas

Recent Suicidal Behaviors (during the past several weeks)
4   Made a serious suicidal attempt (e.g., tried to kill self by gunshot, ingestion, hanging or jumping).
3   Made a suicidal gesture (e.g., superficially cut wrist or ingested two pills).
3   Made a specific suicide plan.
3   Attempt made with little chance of discovery by others.
2   Had no interest or hope for the future.
0   Has no suicidal plans or attempts.

Past History of Suicide (lifetime history)
4   Mother, father or sibling has committed suicide or made a suicide attempt.
3   Has (or had) a diagnosis of major affective disorder or psychosis.
3   Has made one or more previous suicide attempts.
2   Current attempt is an "anniversary" reaction.
2   Has a serious medical illness or disability.
0   Has no past history of suicidal ideas or attempts.

Support Systems/Stresses
3   No family, friends, social agency, or psychiatrist available.
2   Has tenuous connection with family, friends, social agency, or psychiatrist.
2   Has had many recent life stresses (e.g., job, family, children, health, etc.)
1   Has a family which is marginally willing or able to help.
0   Has a family strongly committed and able to help.

Ability to Cooperate
3   Refuses to cooperate with interview and treatment plan.
2   Unable to cooperate with interview and treatment plan.
1   Wants help but motivation is weak.
0   Actively seeks treatment; willing and able to cooperate.

Substance Abuse
3   Is intoxicated.
3   Is in withdrawal.
3   Is a compulsive long-term drug abuser (includes alcohol or other drugs).
2   Is an occasional drug abuser (alcohol or other drugs).
1   Recreational use of drugs.
0   No abuse of any drugs.

Reactions During Interview
4   Assaultive behavior against a person (or object) in the environment.
3   Challenges authority (e.g., curses, yells, screams).
2   Shows approach–avoidance behavior toward interviewer.
1   Shows motoric activity (e.g., pacing, smoking, fidgeting, etc.).
1   Seems very impatient.
0   Calm, seated, responsive to questions.

FIGURE 17.1. Violence and suicide assessment scale. Copyright 1986 by Robert Feinstein and Robert Plutchik.

1. The presence of violence as well as its degree is always an inference from various kinds of evidence. The law distinguishes between accidents that result in assaults and assaults that are premeditated.

2. On a comparative scale, violent acts are relatively rare events and are therefore difficult to predict. Any given act of violence requires the simultaneous occurrence of a large variety of background variables plus a triggering stimulus in the environment.

3. By their very nature, violent acts are the vectorial result of a variety of forces that are acting simultaneously. The emotion of anger and the impulse to destroy conflict with the various control and inhibitory mechanisms that each human being possesses. The violent outcome occurs when the control mechanisms are inadequate to the task.

4. There are at least six classes of variables that interact to influence the occurrence of a given act of violence. These are (a) past history variables, (b) family variables, (c) constitutional and medical variables, (d) personality variables, (e) environmental variables, and (f) chance events.

5. Of considerable importance is the fact that there are a number of variables that have been found to be negatively correlated with the occurrence of violence (Plutchik, van Praag & Conte, 1989). These are (a) a high number of symptoms of depression, (b) a high number of symptoms of anxiety, (c) previous outpatient psychiatric care, (d) a history of drug addiction (in contrast to alcohol addiction), and (e) the personality traits of timidity and trust.

The implication of these ideas is that there are certain factors that increase the likelihood of violence and others that decrease it. The exact values of these variables at any given moment determines the probability of an act of violence.

NEUROPHYSIOLOGICAL EVIDENCE OF A POSITIVE RELATION BETWEEN SUICIDE AND VIOLENCE

Over the past two decades a number of studies have indicated that levels of serotonin in the brain or serotonin metabolites in the cerebrospinal fluid correlate with aggressive behavior (Chapter 16). The most consistent finding (with occasional exceptions) is that low levels of serotonin or its metabolites tend to be associated with violent behavior directed at oneself (suicide) or others (Roy, 1994). Recent studies dealing with these and other neurophysiological measures tend to support a connection between aggressive impulses and neurochemistry. For example, certain plasma neuropeptide levels were measured in 38 suicide attempters. (Neuropeptides are substances produced by nerve cells which have a variety of functions, one of which is neurotransmission. More than 50 kinds have been identified.) Personality and temperament scales were also administered. The plasma neuropeptide levels correlated positively and significantly with irritability in the patients (Westin, Engstroem, Ekman, & Traeskmna-Bendz, 1998). In a related study, 97 patients diagnosed as having a personality disorder underwent a biochemical challenge test to assess level of serotonergic activity. It was found that patients with a history of suicide or self-mutilation attempts had the largest deficits in serotonergic functioning (New, Trestman, Mitropoulou, & Benishay, 1997).

Another attempt to study this problem compared patients with compulsive personality disorder with patients diagnosed as having other types of personality disorders. A standard challenge test was used (prolactin response to fenfluramine) to indirectly measure serotonin function. The authors reported that the patients with the highest aggression scores had the lowest prolactin responses, thus supporting the idea of an inverse relation between aggression and serotonin levels (Stein, Trestman, Mitropoulou, & Coccaro, 1996).

Several similar studies may be cited. Virkkunen and his collaborators describe a series of studies that indicate that criminal offenders who tend to show violent behavior while intoxicated have a low brain serotonin turnover rate. (Turnover rate is a measure of how long it takes before a substance is rendered inactive.) For alcoholic fathers who have committed violent crimes, it was found that their sons have very low concentrations of serotonin metabolites in their spinal fluid. Offenders who have a tendency toward hypoglycemia also have low levels of serotonin metabolites in their spinal fluid and were more likely to commit violent crimes under the influence of alcohol (Virkkunen, Goldman, Nielsen, & Linnoila, 1995). A comparison of platelet and whole blood serotonin of 29 depressed patients and 27 controls showed no differences between the groups. However, current hostility and lifetime history of aggression were positively correlated with platelet serotonin content (Mann, McBride, Anderson, & Mieczkowski, 1992). The problem posed by this apparent inconsistency with the previously cited literature concerns the relation between whole blood serotonin levels and brain levels of serotonin, a point that has not been fully elaborated. Mann and Kapur (1991) also point out that cases have been reported in the clinical literature of paradoxical suicidality during antidepressant treatment. Laboratory studies have shown that the use of serotonin uptake blockers (e.g., fluoxetine [Prozac]) causes an initial decrease in serotonergic function followed, after continued administration, by a normal level of activity. These investigators conclude that the initial changes in serotonin function are a result of a change in threshold for activation of the neurobiological regulators of suicide or violence. This raises the possibility that Prozac and similar substances may produce temporary increases in aggressive impulses.

It is important to recognize that serotonin levels are not the only physiological influences on the threshold for aggression. A number of medical reports have suggested that the lowering of cholesterol levels by medications has been related to an increased risk of suicide or accidental death in such patients. How this may be related to serotonin levels, diet modifications, or brain neurochemistry is unknown (Conroy, 1993; Wardle, 1995).

The fact that serotonin or cholesterol levels may have some limited or partial relation to the expression of suicidal or violent behavior suggests that they represent risk factors for aggression. But psychologists, sociologists, and psychiatrists have been identifying risk factors for aggression for a long time. To the extent that multiple risk factors exist, it implies that some kind of interactions must take place between them in order to influence the threshold level required for overt aggression to appear. In view of this likely conclusion, the next section reviews some of the recent literature on risk factors for suicidal behaviors, followed by a section on risk factors for violent behavior directed toward other people.

RISK FACTORS FOR SUICIDAL BEHAVIOR

Since the last century, investigators have focused on a risk-factor approach toward the goal of predicting suicide (see Maris, Berman, Maltsberger, & Yufit, 1992). Over the years a number of demographic variables, such as age, sex, race, and nationality, and medical variable, such as illness and psychosis, have been found to be related differentially to suicide rates. This approach, though useful, has some problems connected with it. For one thing, broad sociological variables have little value for prediction of individual behavior. Second, it tends to assume that some variables such as psychosis, because they are found relatively frequently in a suicidal population, are somehow more important than others for predicting suicide outcome. Third, it ignores the fact that large numbers of people have many suicide risk factors and show no signs of suicidal thinking or behavior.

In a recent review of the literature, Plutchik (1995) listed 41 factors that were found to be correlated with the risk of suicide attempts in his own research and that of his colleagues. Table 17.1 presents these factors.

A review of the recent published literature adds some additional variables to the list. These include EEG alpha asymmetry (Grace, Tenke, Bruder, & Rotheran, 1996); low self-esteem (Milling, Campbell, Bush, & Laughlin, 1996); low family support (Yuen, Androde, Nahulu, & Makine, 1996); cynicism (Nierenberg, Ghaemi, Clancy-Colecchi, & Rosenbaum, 1996); family conflicts (Arieli, Gilat, & Aychek, 1996); neuroticism, psychoticism, interpersonal aversiveness, anhedonia, hostility, and antisocial traits (Nordstroem, Schalling, & Asberg, 1995); low cholesterol levels in the blood (Wardle, 1995); stressfulness of life (Linsky, Bachman, & Straus, 1995); low blood glucose (Linnoila & Virkkunen, 1992); and frequent mobility and high assault behavior in adolescence (Juon & Ensminger, 1997).

In addition, several papers have added the following risk factors: exposure to family violence (Botsis et al., 1995), poor reality testing and sexual conflicts (Box 17.2) (Plutchik, Botsis, & van Praag, 1995), and dysthymia and self-debasement (Greenwald et al., 1994).

This list of 62 risk factors that has been compiled is itself surely incomplete. As new personality, situational, family, and historical variables are used in research, additional risk factors are likely to be found. One may ask, however, what practical or preventive implications stem from these findings?

TABLE 17.1. Risk Factors for Suicide Attempts or Suicides

1. Schizophrenia	32. Alcohol abuse
2. Depression	33. Drug abuse
3. Other mental illnesses	34. Family history of alcoholism
4. Personality disorders	35. Severe impairment in physical health
5. Hopelessness	36. Paranoid thinking (ideas of reference)
6. Number of life problems	37. Homosexual life style
7. Recent psychiatric symptoms	38. History of previous suicide attempts
8. History of violent behavior	39. Recent loss of a close attachment
9. Accepting attitudes toward suicide	40. Job problems
10. Impulsivity	41. Low CSF 5-HIAA (low dietary intake of tryptophan)
11. Number of family problems	
12. Number of physical symptoms	42. EEG alpha asymmetry
13. History of family violence	43. Low self-esteem
14. Coping style of avoidance	44. Low family support
15. Coping style of help seeking	45. Cynicism
16. Persistent feelings of anger	46. Family conflicts
17. Persistent feelings of resentment	47. Neuroticism
18. Trait anxiety	48. Psychoticism
19. Defense mechanism of regression	49. Interpersonal aversiveness
20. Defense mechanism of displacement	50. Anhedonia
21. Suspiciousness	51. Hostility
22. Rebelliousness	52. Antisocial traits
23. Aggressive behavior in one's mother	53. Low cholesterol blood levels
24. Rejection by one's father	54. Stressfulness of life
25. Feelings of isolation and loneliness	55. Low blood glucose
26. Suicidal threats or attempts in close friends or relatives	56. Frequent mobility
	57. High assault behavior in adolescence
27. Strong sex drive	58. Exposure to family violence
28. A large number of medical and neurological disorders in members of one's family	59. Poor reality testing
	60. Sexual conflicts
29. Early loss of mother or father	61. Dysthymia
30. Easy access to weapons	62. Self-debasement
31. Previous psychiatric treatment	

**BOX 17.2. An Example of How to Identify Risk and
Protective Factors for Suicide and Violence**

The Botsis et al. study (1995) was concerned with the relations between suicide and violence
risk and a number of clinically important variables. The clinical variables were self-esteem, ego
strength, reality testing, depression, sexual drive, sexual inhibition, and impulsivity. Data were
obtained from 45 male and 34 female psychiatric inpatients. Results showed that depression,
impulsivity, and poor reality testing correlated significantly with both the suicide risk and violence risk measures. The strength of the sexual drive correlated with violence risk but not with
suicide risk, while sexual inhibition correlated with suicide risk but not violence risk. Ego
strength and self-esteem correlated negatively with suicide risk but not at all with violence risk.

These results suggest that both risk factors and protective factors in relation to aggression
exist in all individuals. Whether or not an aggressive impulse will be expressed in some form of
overt behavior depends on the interaction of the risk and protective variables. Small variations
in any one of a large number of variables may have a major effect in determining whether the
aggressive impulse will be expressed in overt behavior. Another way to say this is that the subjective weight of a particular factor for a given individual may be more important than the objective weight for that factor obtained as an average from a group of individuals. This idea is
consistent with the concepts of chaos theory in mathematics where it can be demonstrated that
small changes in a variable can have major and often unpredictable effects.

First, as has often been pointed out, risk factors are not necessarily causes of an event
but may simply be associated in some way. For example, truancy or drug use or even low
serotonin levels in the brain do not cause suicide because large numbers of people have
these conditions who never contemplate or act suicidally. Second, the fact that a variable
(e.g., depression) correlates highly with suicidal behavior in a group of patients does not
mean that depression necessarily has anything to do with the suicidal behavior of a particular individual (O'Carroll, 1993). Third, it is evident that large numbers of risk factors interact or perhaps summate to contribute to a suicidal act. Because it is impossible for clinicians
to have information available about all these variables, it is not surprising that the possibilities of prediction are limited. The most reasonable conclusion is that the more risk factors
that apply to an individual, the greater the probability of a suicidal act. Prediction is limited
because, as has often been noted, the low base rate of suicide in the general population
makes accurate prediction impossible (Plutchik & van Praag, 1990; Pokorny, 1992).

RISK FACTORS FOR VIOLENCE DIRECTED TOWARD OTHER PEOPLE

There has been a parallel attempt to identify risk factors for violent behavior (up to and including homicide) directed toward other people. Interestingly, overall homicide rates in
United States have been quite comparable to suicide rates. For example, in 1980, the suicide
rate for the total U.S. population was 11.4 per 100,000 people while the homicide rate was
10.8 per 100,000 people. In 1995, the suicide rate was 11.0 while the homicide rate was 8.8
(*Statistical Abstract of the United States*, 1997). Much variation, however, exists as a function of age, sex, race, and geographic area. Both homicide and suicide rates are much higher in males than in females, and great variation exists in such rates both between and within states. These observations suggest that different factors influence suicide and homicide in
the United States.

In a review of the research literature carried out by my colleagues (Plutchik, 1995), we identified 37 variables that are risk factors for violent behavior directed at other people. Table 17.2 shows these variables.

A review of the recent published literature adds a number of variables to the list. These include suicide attempts in close family members (Brent, Bridge, Johnson, & Connolly, 1998), multiple suicide attempts (Stein et al., 1998), panic plus comorbid depression (Korn, Plutchik, & van Praag, 1997), family discord (Rutter, 1994), toxic social context and school failure (Dishion & Patterson, 1997), association with deviant peers (Thornberry & Krohn, 1997), attention-deficit/hyperactivity disorder and genetics (Carey & Goldman, 1997), younger age and maleness (Peterson, Zhang, Santa Lucia, & King, 1996), sexual abuse (Garnefski & Diekstra, 1997; Booth & Zhang, 1996), compulsive personality disorder (Stein et al., 1996), conduct disorder (Apter et al., 1995), societal stress (Linsky et al., 1995), elevated levels of serum testosterone and low levels of cortisol (Bergman & Brismar, 1994), use of amphetamines and cocaine (Moss, Salloum, & Fisher, 1994), low cholesterol produced by drugs (Conroy, 1993), hypoglycemia (Linnoila & Virkkunen, 1992), platelet serotonin content (Mann et al., 1992), coming from a divorced family (Workman & Beer,

TABLE 17.2. Risk Factors for Violent Behaviors Directed toward Other People

1. Schizophrenia	35. Recent stresses
2. Alcohol abuse	36. Low CSF 5-HIAA
3. Drug abuse	37. Social conflicts over resources
4. Borderline personality disorder	38. Suicide attempts in close family
5. Antisocial personality disorder	39. Multiple suicide attempts
6. Troubled early school experiences	40. Panic plus comorbid depression
7. Violence in one's own family	41. Family discord
8. Previous trouble with the law	42. Toxic social context
9. Poor impulse control	43. School failure
10. Strong sex drive	44. Association with deviant peers
11. Previous suicidal behavior	45. Attention-deficit/hyperactivity disorder
12. Many soft neurological signs	46. Genetics
13. Fire setting	47. Younger age and maleness
14. Sadistic behavior toward animals or people	48. Sexual abuse
15. History of previous psychiatric hospitalization	49. Compulsive personality disorder
16. Episodic dyscontrol	50. Conduct disorder
17. Total number of life problems	51. Societal stress
18. Loss of mother at an early age	52. Elevated levels of serum testosterone
19. Loss of father at an early age	53. Low levels of corticol
20. Medical and neurological problems in one's immediate family	54. Use of amphetamines
21. Easy access to weapons	55. Use of cocaine
22. History of menstrual problems	56. Low cholesterol blood levels
23. Homosexuality	57. Hypoglycemia
24. High testosterone levels	58. Platelet serotonin content
25. Previous arrests and convictions for violent crimes	59. Coming from a divorced family
26. Neurological abnormalities	60. Presence of seizure disorders
27. Deviant family environment	61. Frequent menstrual problems
28. Impulsivity	62. Number of behavioral problems in oneself
29. Instability	63. Number of behavioral problems in first-degree relatives
30. Suspiciousness	64. Depression
31. Rebelliousness	65. Disturbed reality testing
32. Resentfulness	66. Strength of one's sexual drive
33. Defense mechanism of regression	67. A history of previous suicide attempts
34. Defense mechanism of displacement	68. A history of suicide attempts in one's family

1992), and the presence of seizure disorders (Tardiff, 1981). Estimates of the percentage of psychiatric patients of varying diagnoses who show violent behavior range from 3% to 20% (Troisi & Marchetti, 1994). From a purely clinical standpoint, violent behavior has been reported to be associated to varying degrees with dementias (such as Alzheimer's), chromosomal/genetic disorders (such as Klinefelter's syndrome), neurological disorders such as epilepsy, and metabolic disorders such as Cushing's disease (Stowe, 1994).

Some research done at the Albert Einstein College of Medicine, also adds the following variables as risk factors for violence: presence of frequent menstrual problems (Plutchik et al.,1989); number of behavioral problems in oneself or in first-degree relatives (Botsis et al., 1995); depression, disturbed reality testing, and strength of one's sexual drive (Plutchik et al., 1995); and history of suicide attempts and history of suicide attempts in one's family (Grosz et al., 1994).

It thus appears that the research and clinical literature has identified more than 60 variables as having some relation to violence or antisocial behavior. Here, too, as is the case with regard to suicide, it is not possible to make causal statements about any of the variables. Some appear to be of very low effect, some seem to function only in the presence of other variables, and some would seem to be part of the definition of violence (e.g. conduct disorder). The studies vary greatly in terms of sample size, populations evaluated, control groups used, age of sample, length of follow-up, and statistical methods, yet despite these differences, certain variables have been replicated in different studies (alcohol abuse, violence in one's family, etc.). Here, too, as is the case with suicide, it is not possible to say that one variable is a more important risk factor than another for the individual because violence is often triggered by apparently minor events superimposed on a predisposing background. However, for a large sample it is possible to say that, on average, some variables correlate with the possibility of suicide or violence more than do others. Perhaps surprisingly, research has shown that some little studied variables correlate with suicide or violence risk as much as or more than do well-known variables. Thus, it has been reported that "disturbed reality testing" correlates as highly with suicide risk as does depression, and that "sexual drive" correlates as highly with violence risk as does impulsivity (Plutchik, Botsis, & van Praag, 1995). Only by expanding the range of variables studied will such interesting possibilities be discovered.

Also of interest is the observation that has been often made that stressors seem to have a cumulative effect. Many studies have shown that as the number of stressors experienced by an individual increases, rates of assault and violence increase (see, e.g., Linsky et al., 1995). This general concept is well-known in medical epidemiology where, for example, the risk of cardiovascular disease is a function of the total number of risk factors an individual possesses.

Examination of Tables 17.1 and 17.2 reveals that there are many overlapping variables listed; at the same time, some variables appear to be risk factors for suicide and not for violence toward others, whereas other variables appear to be risk factors for violence toward others but not toward oneself. This raises the question of how to account for such observations. Before considering that question, we examine a phenomenon that has been discussed in recent years: the issue of *protective* factors.

It has often been noted that individuals may have many risk factors for suicide and may not make any attempts, and that many individuals grow up in communities that exhibit all the predisposing factors for antisocial behavior and yet never act violently toward others. To account for such observations it has been suggested that certain variables exist in a particular person's life that protect him or her from expressing aggression either toward the self or others.

In 1983, Garmezy described protective factors that are associated with "stress resis-

TABLE 17.3. Protective Factors That Decrease the Risk
of Suicide or Violence

---

 1. Large social network
 2. Marriage
 3. Calm mood state
 4. Happy mood state
 5. Trait anxiety (for violence risk only)
 6. Social supports
 7. Replacement' as a coping style
 8. Overcoming shortcomings as a coping style
 9. Denial as a defense mechanism (for suicide risk only)
10. Repression as a defense mechanism (for violence risk only)
11. Father's sociability
12. Mother's sociability
13. Father's acceptance
14. Mother's acceptance
15. High ego strength
16. High self-esteem (for suicide risk only)
17. Religiosity

---

tant" children. These included (1) high self-esteem, (2) a confident sense of one's ability to handle problems, (3) a belief in the predictability of one's environment, (4) a warm and cohesive family, and (5) a satisfying school environment. Other examples of possible protective factors are attitudes of pacifism and impulse control in the family and expectations of obedience to parental authority (Hill, Soriano, Chen, & La Fromboise, 1994), parental monitoring of activities (Smith & Krohn, 1995), and positive parent–child attachments (Catalano et al., 1993).

In a series of studies, Plutchik and his associates have identified at least 17 protective factors (Plutchik & van Praag, 1994). These are (1) presence of a large social network, (2) presence of social supports, (3) willingness to seek help from others, (4) tendency to cope with problems by overcoming shortcomings, (5) use of denial as a defense mechanism, (6) use of repression as a defense mechanism, (7) ego strength, (8) assertiveness as a trait, (9) sociability in father and mother, (10) acceptance in father and mother, and (11) timid personality trait. It is of some theoretical and practical interest that research has revealed at least 68 risk factors for the expression of aggression but only about a dozen or so protective factors. I hope that future research will change this imbalance. Some details of the method for identifying risk and protective factors will be presented in the next section (see Table 17.3)

A THEORETICAL MODEL OF THE RELATIONS BETWEEN SUICIDE AND VIOLENCE TOWARD OTHERS

During the past decade, my colleagues and I at the Albert Einstein College of Medicine developed a theoretical model of the relations between suicide and violence that has guided our research (Plutchik & van Praag, 1990). The assumptions of the model are presented here along with an illustration of a study that was based on the model.

1. Aggressive impulses are defined as impulses (inner states, tendencies, dispositions, or motivations) to injure or destroy an object or person. An individual may have aggressive

impulses without showing violent behavior. In our terminology, aggression refers to a theoretical inner state and violence refers to an overt act.

2. There are various kinds of life events that tend to increase aggressive impulses. These include threats, challenges, changes in hierarchical status, and loss of social attachments (Blanchard & Blanchard, 1984). It also includes physical pain, loss of power or respect, insults, and things not working out as expected (Shaver, Schwartz, Kirson, & O'Connor, 1987).

3. Whether or not the aggressive impulse is expressed in overt behavior depends on the presence of a large number of variables, some of which act as amplifiers of the aggressive impulse and some as attenuators of the aggressive impulse. The balance and vectorial interaction of these factors or forces at any given moment determines whether the aggressive impulse exceeds a threshold and is then expressed in overt behavior. We refer to these amplifiers and attenuators as Stage I countervailing forces. The term "vector" refers to a directional force. For example, if one variable impels an individual toward a violent act and another to a compassionate act, the vectorial summation of these two variables might be no action at all.

4. Overt action, however, requires a goal object toward which it is directed. The model assumes that some variables determine whether the violent behavior will be directed at oneself in a suicidal act, and that different variables determine whether the violent behavior will be directed toward other people.

5. An important idea that is part of the model is that the overt behavior at the end of the chain of events has a negative feedback function. It interacts with the initial triggers and tries to reestablish the kind of situation that existed before the provoking event occurred. For example, if someone insults you and you verbally or physically attack that person, causing him or her to withdraw, you reestablish the prior condition. We call this process a behavioral homeostatic feedback system, because it functions like an internal homeostatic mechanism, to keep social interactions within certain limits (Plutchik, 1980).

The general strategy of the research we carried out involved the identification of variables that could be related to measures of suicide risk or violence risk. We chose self-report instruments, because they are easy to administer and to score, and because there is now considerable evidence to show that patients often provide more valid information to a test or a computer than to an interviewer (see Plutchik & Karasu, 1991, for a review of this literature). We then administered these scales to various groups of psychiatric inpatients and determined the correlations between each scale and suicide risk. and also violence risk.

Initially, we did not attempt to select any particular diagnostic subgroup of patients. We believed, as has been shown by us and by others, that all psychiatric patients are at relatively high risk for suicide or violence and that a history of suicidality is frequently found in patients admitted for other reasons. Our experience has indicated that in different samples, anywhere from 20 to 50% more or less randomly selected patients have a history of one more suicide attempts, about the same number have a history of violent acts toward others, and about 25% have a history of both suicidal and violent acts (Plutchik et al., 1989).

Some of the scales we used were taken from the existing literature, and some were constructed by us. Reliability and validity measures were obtained, and a battery of scales was completed by each patient and each member of any control group used. Figures 17.2 and 17.3 show the suicide risk and violence risk measures that were used.

The following study illustrates the procedure (Plutchik et al., 1989). One hundred psychiatric patients were studied. They provided self-report data on 30 variables for each pa-

Name_____Date_____Age_____ Sex_____

Instructions: The following questions are about things that you have felt or done. Please answer each question with a simple YES or NO.

	YES	NO
1. Do you take drugs such as aspirin or sleeping pills regularly?		
2. Do you have trouble falling asleep?		
3. Do you sometimes feel that you will lose control of yourself?		
4. Do you have little interest in being with people?		
5. Do you feel that your future will be more unpleasant that pleasant?		
6. Do you ever feel that you are worthless?		
7. Do you feel hopeless about your future?		
8. Do you often feel so frustrated that you just want to lie down and quit struggling altogether?		
9. Do you feel depressed now?		
10. Are you separated, divorced, or widowed?		
11. Has anyone in your family ever tried to commit suicide?		
12. Have you ever been so angry that you felt you might kill someone?		
13. Have you ever thought about committing suicide?		
14. Have you ever told anyone you would commit suicide?		
15. Have you ever tried to kill yourself?		

FIGURE 17.2. The SR (Suicide Risk) Scale. Copyright 1988 by Robert Plutchik and Hope R. Conte.

tient. A correlation was obtained between each variable and the two measures of suicide risk and violence risk. Table 17.4 provides an illustration of some correlations that were obtained.

Because it was found that the suicide risk and violence risk measures correlated about .5, partial correlations were obtained. The results revealed certain variables that correlated significantly with suicide risk but not significantly with violence risk. Similarly, some variables were found that correlated significantly with violence risk but not significantly with suicide risk. Tables 17.4 and 17.5 illustrate these differential correlations.

Some measures have similar relations to the two outcome variables (suicide risk and violence risk), whereas others have differential relations to the two outcome variables. In the terminology of the model, Stage I aggression "amplifiers" are those variables that correlate significantly (although to different degrees) with either the suicide risk or violence risk measures. These variables increase the chances that the aggressive impulse will exceed a threshold level and become expressed in overt behavior. These variables summate in an algebraic sense to increase covert or overt levels of aggressive impulse. It is important to note that some variables correlate negatively with either suicide or violence. These "attenuators" variables also influence the outcome by summating with the amplifier variables in a vectorial sense. To varying degrees, attenuator variables cancel out amplifier variables. It is evi-

Name_____Date_____Age_____ Sex_____

Instructions: Please read each statement and indicate how often you do or feel each of the things described by placing a check (✓) in the appropriate space

	Never	Sometimes	Often	Very often
1. Do you find that you get angry very easily?				
2. How often do you feel very angry at people?				
3. Do you find that you get angry for no reason at all?				
4. When angry, do you get a weapon?				
5. Have you ever caused injury in a fight (for example, bruises, bleeding or broken bones)?				
6. Have you ever hit or attacked a member of your family?				
7. Have you ever hit or attacked someone who is not a member of your family?				
8. Have you ever used a weapon to try to harm someone?				
9. Are weapons easily accessible to you?				
	Never	Once	Twice	More than twice
10. How often have you been arrested for a nonviolent crime such as shoplifting or forgery?				
11. Have you ever been arrested for a violent crime such as armed robbery or assault?				
12. Do you keep weapons in your home that you know how to use?	NO_____		YES____	

FIGURE 17.3. The PFAV (Plutchik Feelings and Acts of Violence) Scale. Copyright 1985 by Robert Plutchik.

TABLE 17.4. Variables That Predict Suicide Risk but Not Risk of Violence

	Partial correlations	
Variables	Suicide risk	Violence risk
AECOM depression scale	.61	.11
PCL intrapersonal problems	.58	.18
PCL total number of problems	.51	.22
Hopelessness scale	.49	.08
Recent psychiatric symptoms	.50	−.14
Attitudes toward suicide scale	.39	.03
PCL health problems	.35	.09
PCL religious problems	.34	.07
Family violence	.25	.04
Coping style of help seeking	-.24	.02

Note. $r = .20$, $p < .05$; $r = .25$, $p < .01$; $r = .32$, $p < .001$. PCL stands for Problem Check List.

TABLE 17.5. Variables That Predict Risk of Violence but Not
Suicide Risk

Variables	Partial correlations	
	Suicide risk	Violence risk
Impulsivity	.22	.53
Trouble with the law	.17	.34
Menstrual problems	.08	.32
Recent stresses	.08	.25

Note. r = .20, p = .05.

dent that the amplifier variables are the theoretical equivalent of risk factors, whereas the attenuator variables are the theoretical equivalent of protective factors. The distinction is worth making in the sense that risk and protective factors refer to empirical observations, whereas amplifiers and attenuators are based on observations but have a more complex meaning within the theoretical model. Many studies have been carried out using this model, leading to the identification of many of the risk and protective factors cited in Tables 17.1 and 17.2.

SUMMARY AND CONCLUSIONS

This chapter has attempted to document the intimate but complex set of relations between aggression expressed toward oneself and aggression expressed toward other people. It has identified dozens of variables that are risk factors for suicidal behaviors and dozens more that are risk factors for violent behavior toward other people. It appears that there is considerable overlap between these sets of variables. Protective factors have also been described that reduce the likelihood of violent behavior to self or others. Finally, a theoretical model has been presented that attempts to understand why some people high on risk factors do not show aggressive behavior in any form, and why those who may have few risk factors become violent. The model assumes that risk and protective factors (or more generally, amplifiers and attenuators of the aggressive impulse) interact vectorially to determine a violent act. A separate set of variables differentially determines whether the violent act will be directed to oneself as a suicide attempt or toward others as violence or antisocial behavior.

Examination of the different amplifier and attenuator variables shows that although many factors are long-term situational or dispositional factors, there are others, such as feelings of anger, rejection by a parent, or presence of social supports, that may change transiently in unpredictable ways. Such changes make the vectorial sum representing the aggression level at a given point in time, relatively unstable and capable of fluctuating from day to day, or even moment to moment. This is why an apparently trivial event to an outside observer may sometimes appear to trigger a suicide attempt or a violent outburst. This is also why it is impossible to describe the relative importance of each variable as if its effects are forever fixed and why precise prediction will always be impossible. However, to the extent that an individual has a large number of amplifiers of aggression and a small number of attenuators, the probability of suicide or violence will be high. The aims of research should include the identification of both risk and protective factors, as well as the special (Stage II) variables that determine the direction of aggressive behavior. Such information should increase our ability to make reasonable judgments about the likelihood of aggressive behavior in individuals.

Another implication concerns the use of psychopharmacological agents in the treatment of suicidal patients. At present it is believed that antidepressant medication reduces an individual's depression, and in turn his or her risk of suicide. From the point of view of the model presented here, the new class of drugs—serenics—designed to reduce aggressive behavior, should have as large an influence on suicide as do antidepressant drugs. In fact, any intervention that changes the balance of forces may influence the risk of suicide or violence to others.

Another implication of the model is that it suggests a relation between the study of suicide and the study of emotions in general. For example, both suicidal behavior and emotional behavior function for the individual as a way of regulating interpersonal relations. Both represent transient efforts at adaptation to difficult emergency situations (Plutchik, 1980, 1994, 1997). For all the reasons given previously, it is important to see suicidal behavior and violent behavior as aspects of the same basic domains of life. Future research on either aspect of aggression should include measures of the other. Only then may we begin to truly see the whole picture.

In Part IV, Chapter 18 examines another set of variables (i.e., those related to indrect self-destructive behaviors).

FURTHER READING

Colt, G. H. (1991). *The enigma of suicide.* New York: Touchstone. A beautifully written review of the history of our ideas about suicide with many interesting cases. Ethical issues concerning suicide are also discussed.

Hollander, E., & Stein, D. (Eds.). (1995). *Impulsivity and aggression.* New York: Wiley. A major contribution to the literature on the relations between impulsivity, aggression, and suicide. Individual articles deal with the phenomenology, the neurobiology, the diagnosis, and the treatment of such disorders.

Maes, M., & Coccaro, E. F. (Eds.). (1998). *Neurobiology and clinical views on aggression and impulsivity.* New York: Wiley. Researchers contribute to our knowledge of the relations among aggression, suicidality, and other clinical conditions. Studies of animals, children, and genetics are included.

Mann, J. J., & Stanley, M. (Eds.). (1986). *Psychobiology of suicidal behavior* [Annals of the New York Academy of Sciences, Vol. 487]. New York: New York Academy of Sciences. An early and important book as key issues involved in the study of suicide and aggression. Methodological issues are discussed along with neurochemical studies, psychiatric syndromes, and treatment.

PART IV

INDIRECT SELF-DESTRUCTION, ETHICS, PHILOSOPHY, AND THE LAW

18

Indirect Self-Destructive Behavior

with Norman L. Farberow

I've always taken great pride in being one of the few people to face death and beat it.
—Evel Knievel

. . . when I put the gun to my head and was about to pull the trigger I was terrified. When I pulled it and heard the click, it was like an adrenaline high . . . it felt great!
—A Survivor of Russian Roulette

Both Evel Knievel and the young Russian roulette survivor appear to be gamblers. But, rather than placing their money at stake in a game of chance, their bet is on their continuation, on life versus death or severe injury. Each risks their very existence for the sake of an adrenaline rush, the counterphobic mastery of death, and/or status among those they wish to impress.

In this chapter we explore dangerous *risk-taking behavior* and *indirect self-destructive behavior* (ISDB). These may be defined as volitional acts that pose significant risk to life or limb. They span a continuum from high-risk sports to unprotected sex, drunk driving, and Russian roulette. While consciously accepting the odds of death and injury, the actors who gamble in these ways operate with defenses that defy describing these acts as suicidal in intent. They are either unaware of or in denial of any suicidal wish or goal; outcomes are either left in "God's hands" or often believed controllable by preparation, training, and a personal sense of mastery. Sometimes these beliefs appear to border on delusional. Concurrently, there is a recklessness or a reckless disregard of potential consequences, in spite of precautionary warnings.

Some of these behaviors are *chronic* and repetitive, with the risk for premature death increasing over the term of the behavior, for example, as in drug abuse or noncompliance with a prescribed medical regimen (such as diabetes treatment). At the same time, each has a certain degree of *acute* risk, with an increased risk of immediate death or injury attending each and every act (e.g., autoerotic asphyxia or Russian roulette).

As a starting point, we must distinguish ISDBs from behaviors more directly suicidal. Self-destructive behavior takes many forms. We are most familiar with and can most easily identify those behavioral manifestations that result in death, injury, or pain intentionally inflicted upon the self or that are voiced verbally in the form of threats that death is intended

427

or planned. For the most part such behaviors are overt and visible and frequently have as an important element in their manifestation a forceful communication of an unhappy, distressed state—so distressing that the person voluntarily intends to leave it.

In marked contrast, there are, however, a vast number of behaviors that are self-harmful, frequently injurious, self-negating, and self-defeating in which the individual engages but in which there may be no intention to die; in which there is often what seems like complete disregard of the painful and harmful effects of their behavior and in which the individual does not consider himself suicidal. These behaviors are called ISDBs to distinguish them from the direct forms of self-destruction.

Classification of suicidal behaviors assumes that direct and indirect forms lie on a somewhat linear continuum with one end occupied by completed suicide; that is, death by one's own hand, unequivocal and clearly intended, and often substantiated by a written note or by verbal declarations that death was the purpose of the individual's actions. Less direct or less lethal suicidal behaviors would include suicide attempts, parasuicides, threats to kill oneself, attractions to death, and continuous rumination about death.

At the other end of the continuum is a vast array of ISDBs that includes harmless errors, bungled actions, minor accidents, substance abuse and addictions, gambling, noncompliance with prescribed medical regimen, borderline or excessive risk taking, self-punishment, and self-mutilation.

ISDBs lie along the continuum between the two opposites poles. A convenient axis is the presence or absence of a physical condition that the person can use against himself. Such conditions are most often long-term or chronic illnesses which impair life functioning but do not prohibit it (e.g., diabetes, hypertension, asthma, ulcer, allergies, kidney disease, and others). Such illnesses can ordinarily be controlled with the patient exercising some measure of care in terms of medication, diet, and observation of a well-defined medical regimen. Accidents, congenital defects, with loss of limb or mobility, or sensory function would also belong in this group. In this group the individual engages in behaviors that are noncompliant and recognizably harmful (e.g., a diabetic bingeing on sweets, a dialysis patient disregarding his diet, and a Raynaud's patient continuing to smoke).

ISDBs have been considered for a long time. Durkheim (1897/1951) described them as a sort of embryonic form of suicide, which though "not methodologically sound to confuse them with complete and full suicide," must be recognized for their close relation to it. Freud (1920/1955) included ordinary mistakes, errors, minor accidents, bungled actions, slips of speech, and forgetting. Menninger (1938) developed the concept most fully, calling it focal suicide and including such behaviors as malingering, polysurgery, neurotic invalidism, impotence and frigidity, and psychosis. Meerloo (1968) called the behavior hidden suicide, and Shneidman (1968) coined the term "subintentioned" death for self-destructive behaviors that he felt the person did not consciously intend.

Farberow (1980) has presented us with a good working template for this discrimination, adapted for this discussion in Table 18.1. Based on his study of medically ill patients who behave in a manner to worsen their preexisting conditions (diabetics, Buerger's and Reynaud's diseases, hemodialysis, and elderly chronically ill), he compared the characteristics of direct and indirect self-destructive behaviors, noting similarities and differences.

The distinguishing characteristics of ISDBs lie in their dynamics, intentions, defenses, and social responses. In suicidal behavior, the motive force is either interpersonal (i.e., to change or influence others' behaviors) or intrapsychic (i.e., to escape a painful state). The underlying dynamics are defined by a negative sense of self and/or of one's existence, and these feelings are typically described by one or more mental disorders (e.g., depression). In ISDBs, psychopathology is less in evidence—in fact, the actor may often be described as overtly asymptomatic and the aim of the behavior is to seek pleasure, increase arousal, and

TABLE 18.1. Comparative Analysis of Suicide (Direct Self-Destruction) and Excessive Risk Taking (Indirect Self-Destruction)

	Direct self-destruction	Indirect self-destruction
Dynamics:		
Feelings	Inadequacy, low self-esteem, worthlessness, helplessness, hopelessness, "exhaustion," "psychache"	Boredom, nihilism, well-being, problem-free
Motives	Interpersonal: to effect change in others	Power and control (denial of inadequacy)
	Intrapsychic: surcease, escape, to end pain	Pleasure
Futurity	Low: future expectations blocked, tunnel vision	Low: immediate here and now gratification; intolerance of delay or postponement
Risk taking	Goal oriented: death or changed life or unknown	Process oriented: present excitement and/or pleasure
Coping mechanisms	Regressive: immature and passive–aggressive Constrictive: focus = loss	Denial Suppression of discomfort
Society's attitudes	Condemnatory: self-murder Countertransferential hate, anger, guilt, anxiety (in helper) Possible acceptance/glorification: terminally ill, to avoid torture, altruistic self-sacrifice	Condemnatory: Russian roulette, autoerotic asphyxia Countertransferential anger, frustration, resentment Possible glorification: death-defying dare-devils
Intervention	Society's right to intervene and prevent; assumption of impaired capacity to make rational judgment; social good outweighs individual right	No right to intervene

Source: Adapted from Farberow (1980). Copyright 1980 by The McGraw-Hill Companies. Reprinted by permission.

feel in power or in control. The suicidal person seeks death or is willing to harm the body to change his or her human condition. The person who engages in ISDB is willing to face the risk of death or bodily harm in order to overcome his or her anxiety about death, to experience heightened pleasure, and so on. In a sense, the suicidal person is attempting to escape dysphoria, whereas the indirectly self-destructive person is attempting to seek euphoria.

Both groups appear to have little investment in the future but for different reasons. The directly suicidal person feels a sense of loss, either anticipated or real, through rejection or abandonment. As a result, suicidal persons question their worth, feel helpless and hopeless, and try, as a goal of their suicidal behavior, to change their painful condition. People who engage in ISDB have little long-term focus because their investment is in the here-and-now, on arousal and pleasure.

Directly suicidal persons do not have mature coping skills. Rather, they operate with cognitive constriction and solve their problems by regressively acting out (against self and/or others). Often, the message to others is undeniable—I hurt and, either by your action or inaction, you will feel responsible. Those who engage in ISDB more clearly use denial as a defense and are narcissistically invested in pleasure with little apparent concern for affecting others negatively.

A major area of difference is in social attitudes and behaviors. With suicide, society has long had a stigmatizing attitude. Suicides have been and are condemned, seen as acts of disturbed, narcissistic individuals and to be prevented whenever possible. The only exceptions are under conditions of altruistic self-sacrifice and terminal illness with intractable pain. With ISDB, society respects the rights of the individual to make choices, may or may not intervene, and, with respect to adventure taking, may even glorify those who fail to survive.

The origin of self-destructive behaviors, both direct and indirect, was sought in an extensive historical and proactive study by van der Kolk, Perry, and Lewis-Herman (1991) by following 74 subjects with personality disorders or bipolar II disorders for an average of 14 years and monitoring them for self-destructive behavior. The behaviors were then correlated with independently obtained self-reports of childhood trauma, disruptions of parental care, and dissociative phenomena. The sample consisted of young adult patients from a university hospital, a probation department, and newspaper advertisements. Information was gathered by interview, self-report questionnaires, the Traumatic Antecedents Questionnaire, and the Dissociative Experiences Scale at both intake and in subsequent years. The investigators found that childhood sexual and physical abuse were significant predictors of self-cutting and suicide attempts. The nature of the trauma and the subject's age affected the character and the severity of the self-destructive behavior. In the follow-up, the subjects with the most severe histories of separation and neglect and those with past sexual abuse continued to be self-destructive. Cutting was specifically related to dissociation. It was concluded that childhood trauma contributed to the initiation of self-destructive behavior, but it was the lack of secure attachments that helped to maintain it. Experiences related to interpersonal safety, anger, and emotional needs may precipitate dissociative episodes and self-destructive behavior.

The psychodynamics of the two groups are markedly different. Litman (1980) states the fundamental difference succinctly by focusing on their intention. He says, "In contrast with [directly self-destructive] persons, who consciously seek to injure or kill themselves, victims of ISDB would probably admit responsibility without admitting intention" (28).

Litman argues that much of ISDB is *masochistic*. Describing the case of a patient who would drive his car recklessly for several hours after having a fight with his wife, he interpreted the patient's lack of caring as to whether he lived or died and the concurrent feelings of triumph and mastery that came with surviving each dangerous ordeal as "one of the essential psychodynamic features of masochism" (p. 30). Litman believes that many forms of ISDB are initiated as coping mechanisms to overcome depression through temporary pleasure (see Box 18.1). They, then, with repetition become habituated, some even addictive, for the sake of their immediate rewards. Similarly, thrill-seeking activities produce stress and the relief from stress, both of which are pleasurable, thus reinforcing and more likely to be repeated.

This dynamic may be most clearly seen in the abuse of alcohol or drugs (see "Alcohol and Substance Abuse," below), behaviors described by Menninger (1938) as forms of *chronic suicide*. Although a person may initially drink, for example, to reduce tension and/or increase a sense of well-being, long-term and increased reliance on alcohol for these short-term gains begins to affect performance, increases deleterious after-effects, negatively affects relationships, has detrimental effects on internal organs, reduces controls, exacerbates depression, and shortens life through premature natural death (cirrhosis of the liver), accidental death (drunk driving), or suicide.

THEORETICAL EXPLANATIONS OF RISK-TAKING BEHAVIOR

What motivates someone to consciously and volitionally behave in a way in which the outcome may be uncertain *and* may include the possibility of identifiable health problems (e.g., a sexually transmitted disease, disability, or even death)?

BOX 18.1. Are Indirect Self-destructive Behaviors Antidepressants?

Yes: Litman (1980).

Litman argues that ISDB has the psychodynamic function of denying or coping with mental pain which might otherwise lead to states of helpless depression; that is, ISDB is a defense against feelings of depression. All individuals have personal histories which are replete with events that made us feel weak, helpless, insecure, and unsafe. When, later in life, our sense of well-being and safety is threatened, these early experiences are reactivated and signal anxiety that becomes depression when the threat is overwhelming. Through ISDB "there is an experience of mastery and victory. . . . Essentially . . . the function of ISDB is to deny helplessness and replace it with coping mechanisms that enhance self-esteem."

No: Apter (1992).

Apter argues that it is human nature to need some level of excitement or arousal. The level of arousal we seek varies for each of us and determines the margin of safety we seek and the danger we are willing to confront. To be excited, Apter argues, is to expose oneself to enough danger (risk of trauma) to experience high arousal, while feeling protected (safe) through our level of skill, therefore confidence, appropriate training, trust in our equipment, the support of others, etc. Excitement, he illustrates, results from seeing a tiger in a cage. Without the protection of the cage, the tiger poses real danger; without the tiger, the cage would be boring.

Some have argued that risk taking is a part of normal adolescence (Baumrind, 1987). These theorists distinguish developmentally constructive risk taking (i.e., adaptive experimentation to build confidence, enhance competence, and develop initiatives, behaviors that play a role in developing autonomy and mastery, and skills essential for the transition to adulthood) from pathogenic, deviant, life-threatening risk taking that potentially jeopardizes health and life.

Positive risk-taking is constructive and essential for personal growth. Jessor (1992), for example, views behaviors such as smoking, drinking, illicit substance use, and risky driving as instrumental in gaining acceptance and respect among peers, establishing independence from parental authority, in coping with the anticipation of failure, and so on.

Biological theories attribute risk-taking tendencies to the influence of hormones and to genetic predispositions. Risk-taking behaviors have been observed to cluster within families, producing a higher than expected rate of physical injury among family members. This has led to speculation that genetics may play a role. Alcoholism, for example, has a strong familial loading. Children of alcoholic parents are more likely than children of nonalcoholic parents to have alcohol abuse problems in adulthood.

The rise in testosterone in males during adolescence has also been postulated to explain the initiation of increased risk taking. This is confounded by observations that asynchronous maturation in adolescence (i.e., physically maturing earlier than one's peers) promotes engaging in more "adult" behaviors sooner, partly because one tends to be more accepted by an older peer group. However, when cognitive development lags behind early physical development, judgment and inexperience make adolescents more vulnerable to untoward effects from increased risk-taking behaviors.

Psychological theories emphasize cognitive ability and personality characteristics. As noted previously, the perception of risk may be influenced by optimistic expectations and feelings of invulnerability. Risk takers may not appreciate potential long-term consequences relative to expectations of short-term gain. Condom use, for example, has been found to be highly related to peer pressure and ease of use to facilitate sexual intercourse, more so than its intended preventive function regarding the risk of pregnancy and/or sexually transmitted diseases.

One personality theory that has been widely studied is *sensation seeking* (Zuckerman, 1979). Zuckerman (1979) defines sensation seeking as a trait described by a "need for varied, novel, and complex sensations and experiences and willingness to take physical and social risks for the sake of such experiences" (10). People high in sensation seeking tend to perceive less risk (than those low in this trait) and anticipate more positive outcomes. High sensation seeking is correlated with risk-taking behaviors such as reckless driving, substance abuse, and delinquency. High sensation seekers are more likely to engage behaviors appraised by most persons to be moderately risky. They volunteer for experiments that offer new and unusual experiences (e.g., hypnosis or sensory deprivation) and are more likely to engage in activities and sports that have some degree of risk, such as parachuting, scuba diving, and bungee jumping, or vocations such as firefighting or emergency services. High sensation seekers have been shown to process novel or intense stimulation differently and have higher thresholds for pain.

Zuckerman has developed a personality test, the Sensation-Seeking Scale, to measure this trait. The scale has been factor-analyzed and is described by four subscales: Thrill and Adventure Seeking (TAS; the desire to engage in risky physical activities), Experience Seeking (ES; the desire to seek new experience through the mind and senses and through unconventional lifestyle and travel), Disinhibition (DID; the seeking of sensation through other people or partying, or social drinking, and sex), and Boredom Susceptibility (BS; an aversion for unchanging or unstimulating environments or persons). Table 18.2 illustrates some sample items from each subscale. Each is presented in a forced-choice, paired format.

A corollary to sensation seeking as a personality construct is thrill seeking. Farley (1986) has proposed that a cluster of characteristics make up a "Type T" personality style, one that describes people more likely to seek out and take risks. For some seekers of adventure and excitement, the outcome is creativity (T+), for others the outcome is destructive (T–).

Building on the work of Zuckerman and others, Farley believes that Type T personalities are primarily established by genetics. Some people are simply born with an unusually low level of arousability; they need higher levels of external stimulation to "turn them on." On the positive side, Type T personalities tend to be more creative and extroverted, prefer

TABLE 18.2. Illustrative Items from Zuckerman's Sensation-Seeking Scale

Subscale	Sample items (from Form V of the SSS)
TAS	"I sometimes like to do things that are a little frightening;" "I would like to learn to fly an airplane;" "I would like to try parachute jumping."
ES	"I like to explore a strange city or section of town by myself, even if it means getting lost;" "I have tried marijuana or would like to;" "People should dress in individual ways even if the effects are somewhat strange."
DIS	"I like 'wild' uninhibited parties;" "A person should have considerable sexual experience before marriage;" "I feel best after taking a couple of drinks."
BS	"I have no patience with dull or boring persons;" "I get very restless if I have to stay around home for any length of time;" "I usually don't enjoy a movie or play where I can predict what will happen in advance."

Source: Adapted from Zuckerman (1979). Copyright 1979 by Lawrence Erlbaum Associates. Adapted by permission.

variety in their sex lives, and have more experimental artistic preferences. They also think differently, moving with great ease from the abstract to the concrete and back. They can approach problems from different angles, think "outside the box," thus increase the likelihood of novel solutions and insights.

Destructive Type T personalities seek stimulation and thrills on the "dark side of the street." Unrestrained drug experimentation, drinking and driving, unsafe sex, and juvenile delinquency are all examples of negative outcomes for Type T personalities. Even among delinquents, those highest in Type T characteristics have been found to attempt to escape institutional detention four times (for females) to seven times (for males) more often.

As noted in Box 18.1, Apter (1992) similarly argues that there is a genetic predisposition to seek arousal. Barnard (see Klausner, 1968) termed this "eustress seeking," defining the motivating forces to be to escape the routine, the stable, the fixed, to obliterate boredom and ennui.

Normal avenues for such arousal seeking might be found in high-risk sports (mountaineering, sky diving), interests (bungee jumping, the running of the bulls at Pamplona), and occupations (firefighting, race car driving, stunting). Although death and injury do attend these behaviors, training, safety mechanisms, collaborative supports, and so on establish the protective frame.

HIGH-RISK SPORTS AND RECREATIONAL ACTIVITIES

A growing number of people are engaging, and seemingly deriving pleasure from, challenging thrill-seeking activities. These range from bungee jumping and skydiving to the media-sponsored X Games. It has been estimated that approximately 150,000 people skydive each year and more than 7 million bungee jumps occurred worldwide between the late 1980s and 1997 (Heath, 1997).

These activities are clearly sensation laden, and participants have been found to score high on sensation seeking. Malkin and Rabinowitz (1998) have summarized 13 studies using Zuckerman's Sensation-Seeking Scale, comparing enthusiasts of such activities (skydiving, mountain sports/rock climbing, hang gliding, skiing, canoeing/kayaking, and rodeo riding) with matched control groups. The results confirm typically higher scores on all scales except for Disinhibition. It should be noted, however, that these scales may be culturally biased in that they tap activities and behaviors engaged in by those who can afford them and have easy access to them via financial resources and geographic proximity. Thrill and experience seeking, therefore, may be derived in culturally biased forms.

Klausner (1968) relates some of the background of the concept of this type of stress seeking. Originally the idea of stress referred to pressure, and its image was that of coping with an evil arising from somewhere in the physical, interpersonal, or institutional environment. First conceptualized as a societal problem, it became predominantly individually centered when Selye's *Stress of Life* (1976) proposed the "adaptation syndrome" in the 1950s. The art of living was seen from the perspective of medical and psychological coping against stress with homeostasis as the sought after goal. The concept of stress seeking, introduced into this social and intellectual climate, challenged the image of coping and its underlying model of tension reduction with the recognition of tension seeking as a basic aspect of normal functioning. Stress seeking was introduced as a personality attribute, stimulated by social conditions, not intrinsically good or bad for the individual or for society but, like a drive, as something that met basic needs in the individual. Its definition was "behavior designed to increase the intensity of emotion or level of activation of the organism" (Klausner, 1968, p. 139).

Stress seeking in the individual was described as striving and effort, as pushing against the odds, as an excitation that was experienced as fearful or pleasant depending on the situation and its meaning for the individual. In this respect it differed from the risk taker who failed to plan or control for a situation, who left loose ends in his preparation, or who disregarded the threshold of danger. Societies generally encourage both individualistic and social stress seekers, indicating that stress seeking and its reduction have a social as well as a personality function. They may contribute to the constructive development of a society, often by participating in the high-risk aspects of exploration and development (e.g., outer space) as they test previously established limits. Society's problem is to encourage enough stress seeking to get the work of society done, while reining in the drive so that it does not become destructive. Society tries to control its stress seekers through its rules, regulations, and values but apparently gives wide latitude to the individual's attempts to conquer danger (e.g., Evel Knievel). Society applauds, supports, and often pays large sums of money to watch daredevils "entertain," but the admiration is often tinged with ambivalent feelings about the potentials for injury or death versus success.

Audiences also exercise some measure of control over the extent of stress seeking in terms of establishing norms of acceptable and nonacceptable violence (as in contact sports). For example, the state regulates who will and who will not hunt and when by dispensing licenses and determining acceptable periods of time. Peer judgment serves the same purpose as in parachute clubs and scuba clubs by granting memberships only to those whom the club judges to be stable enough and then to provide training in the rules, the required procedures, and the efficacy of the equipment used.

Why does man jump out of an airplane at several thousand feet depending on the correctly folded and processed layers of nylon and cloth to prevent inescapable death, or dive beneath the surface of the ocean with only the contrivance of compressed air fed by a mechanical valve between him and almost certain drowning, or subject himself to tremendous physical risk from cold, thin air and almost unimaginable physical rigors in mountain climbing? Blau argues that "the lure of the deep is compelling. Water covers five-sevenths of the earth's surface and can be considered 'the last frontier.' Exploration and adventure are a part of even the most elementary kind of diving. It is exciting and fulfilling" (Blau, 1980: 413).

It is impossible to obtain reliable statistics on the number of participants in high-risk sports or the frequency of fatalities and injuries that result from those activities (Delk, 1980). Some statistics are available, although rates are impossible to ascertain given a lack of accurate population estimates. For example, the North American Bungee Association estimated that between 1 and 2 million commercial jumps took place in North America between 1987 and 1993. Of these, there were 11 known significant injuries and 3 fatalities. In 1996 the U.S. Parachute Association reported 39 fatalities, whereas the U.S. Hang Gliding Association reported 7 fatalities. In contrast, there were five fatalities directly related to football during 1996 (National Safety Council, *Accident Facts* [various years]).

The little existing research on risky sports has tended to concentrate on the demographic aspects of individuals who participate in such high-risk sports as scuba diving (self-contained underwater breathing apparatus), parachuting, spelunking (cave exploration), auto racing, mountain climbing, and others. The available figures are mostly estimates and are difficult to verify because no official records are kept, particularly of nonfatal injuries Skydiving and scuba diving may be seen as prototypic high-risk sports. Blau (1980) reports that scuba diving has the highest fatality rate of any sport practiced in the world today but does not report a mortality rate. The Divers Alert Network reported 104 underwater diving fatalities in 1995 (National Safety Council, 1996), but insists that the figures must be viewed in respect to the estimated 9 to 11 million dives made each year.

Delk's (1980) study of 41 male skydivers indicated that a mean age of 28 years with occupations involving mostly mental activity had a mean number of 546 parachute jumps, of which the average number involving freefall was 531. Asked if and when they thought of death, 73% admitted that they did and that those thoughts took place mostly before a jump rather than during or after. Anxiety was moderately high during takeoff and climb, increased to the highest peak immediately before the jump, fell with the jump, then increased to a secondary peak at the point of the chute opening, and fell steadily thereafter. Pleasure, on the other hand, was low at the outset, rose to a sharp, high peak during freefall, declined below anxiety during the time of the chute opening, and then rose again to stay above anxiety. There is an inverse relationship between anxiety and pleasure, especially pronounced from the point of immediately before the jump to the point of the chute opening, all of which, including the freefall and hookup of chutists, takes less than 30 seconds. This means the fall of anxiety with the jump occurs rapidly and is accompanied by a rather intense state of pleasure. The experience has been likened to the sexual act, which involves a build up of neurovascular tension and is suddenly and explosively reduced with orgasm. The only part of the activity in which the anxiety rises above the level of the pleasure is at the point of the chute's opening. This signals the end of the skydive and freefall (Delk, 1980) It is as this point, when the skydiver delays in pulling the cord to extend as long as possible the pleasure of the fall, that deaths occur because the chute opens too late.

Parachuting is one sport in which there is a rapid reduction of self-induced heightened stress accompanied by intense pleasure. Selye (1976) says it is possible to become addicted to one's own stress hormones. This may be what happens with skydivers who become addicted and need a fix (a skydive) every few days. Although each high-risk sport has its own characteristic anxiety and pleasure curves, the stress-production–stress-reduction cycle appears to operate in all such sports. Other motivations that have been considered include reaction formation and counterphobic defiance in which danger is sought in order to overcome a fear of death and to gain a sense of mastery, power, and achievement. An important element is peer recognition and acceptance. The motivations for risk-taking behavior in scuba diving are similar to those listed for skydiving. Reaction formation and counterphobic defiance are reflected in the behaviors of divers who report that they are continually "testing" their own strength, their own worth, and their own bravery. Similar motivations might be found in certain high-risk occupations (see Box 18.2).

The protective frame is important in differentiating adolescent risk taking from that of

---

BOX 18.2. A Risk-Taking Vocation: Stunting

What motivates someone to risk life and limb at the office—even if the office is a movie set, a 70-foot waterfall, or the outside of a 500-foot skyscraper? Stuntmen (and women), no doubt, appreciate the monetary rewards (yes, they are paid well) and the acclaim and esteem of others and self. They are considered professional athletes by the insurance industry. Indeed, agility, speed, strength, the ability to play through pain, etc. are job requirements. They also appear to be sensation-seeking personalities; they must also be eager for varied experiences, relatively unconcerned about the negative consequences of their actions, and able to concentrate under conditions of risk to be disciplined and vigilant enough to maximize the odds of survival. ("Surviving is the one thing, above all others, that a stuntman is supposed to do. . . . Anybody can be a daredevil if he's crazy enough.")

Sources: Newman (1992); Piet (1987).

adults. Adolescents do not necessarily take more risks than do adults, but they do experience more negative consequences because they are less skillful or knowledgeable in perceiving risks and preventing these negative consequences.

This existence and quality of this protective frame also describe the differentiating threshold between what we might view as risk-taking behaviors and indirect life-threatening behaviors. In the latter, people are unrealistic in their perceptions and assessments of their ability to control danger. Their foolhardiness or abject recklessness is based in denial, psychopathology, ignorance, or an unconscious suicidal drive.

Related to this protective frame is an intriguing psychological construct commonly applied to explain adolescent risk taking (i.e., that of *invulnerability*). Adolescents ignore or underestimate the likelihood of negative outcomes because they view themselves as invulnerable to these threats. As a result, they focus primarily on the benefits of risky behaviors. Research evidence for this perceived invulnerability, however, is scant, inconclusive, and open to considerable interpretation. For example, is an adolescent's rationalization for unprotected sex, "I thought I couldn't get pregnant," a perception of invulnerability or naivete or a misunderstanding. Moreover, there is considerable evidence of perceived invulnerability among adults; that is, the risk of negative events faced by "me" is generally evaluated as significantly below that faced by "others."

As noted in Box 18.1, low self-esteem and depression are additional psychological variables often cited as associated with risk taking, although the research evidence for these has inconsistent. One area of risk-taking behavior which has been linked to underlying depression is pathological gambling.

PATHOLOGICAL GAMBLING

Pathological gambling is defined by the fourth edition of the *Diagnostic and Statistical Manual of Mental Disorders* (DSM-IV; American Psychiatric Association, 1994) as an impulse-control disorder in which the essential feature is persistent and recurrent maladaptive gambling that disrupts personal, family or vocational pursuits. Five of the following 10 criteria must be present to merit the diagnosis:

- The individual is preoccupied with reliving past gambling experiences, planning the next venture, or thinking of ways to get money with which to gamble.
- He or she must play with increasingly larger bets to achieve the desired excitement.
- He or she continues to gamble despite repeated efforts to control, cut back, or stop the behavior.
- He or she becomes restless or irritable when attempting to stop or cut down the behavior.
- Gambling relieves a dysphoric mood or is a way of escaping from problems.
- He or she chases his or her losses with increasingly larger bets in the attempt to recoup his or her losses.
- He or she lies to the family, therapist, and others to conceal the extent of involvement with gambling.
- He or she has resorted to antisocial behavior, such as forgery, theft, fraud, or embezzlement, to obtain money to gamble.
- He or she has jeopardized or lost a significant relationship, job, or educational or career opportunity because of gambling.
- He or she relies on others to provide money to relieve a desperate financial situation caused by gambling.

Pathological gambling has been estimated to be present in 1–3% of the general adult population. Typically the gambling begins in early adolescence in males and later in life in females. The course of development is generally slow, starting with social gambling and then followed by an abrupt onset that may be precipitated by a personal or social stressor. The gambling pattern may be regular or episodic, but the course of the disorder typically becomes chronic. It is marked by a progression in the frequency of gambling, the amount wagered, and a preoccupation with gambling and obtaining money with which to gamble. Gambling activity generally increases during periods of stress or depression. Custer's (1984) pioneer work in the study of the pathological gambler led him to posit three definable phases in the development and progression of the disorder. First, there is the winning phase, in which the gambler's initial luck may produce winning experiences, which lead to more and more excitement. Bets get higher and more frequent, eventually climaxing in a win of a large amount that nearly equals or exceeds the individual's annual salary. The losing phase that follows is difficult for the gambler to tolerate. The gambler begins to "chase" bets, that is, to bet more in order to recoup losses, a cardinal sin in gambling. Borrowing money becomes common, family and work problems multiply, the gambler loses time from work, the family is deprived of basic needs, and there is a growing alienation from spouse, parents, and children. Eventually there is a financial crisis in which a large sum of money must be raised or imprisonment becomes a threat. There is a bailout and the gambling stops for a while, but, typically, only for a while.

The desperation phase follows from the time of the first bailout. Frequently there are several bailouts and the rescuers drop away. Increased time and money spent on gambling produce alienation, panic follows, and the pace of gambling increases to a frenzy as the individual attempts to recoup his or her losses. This phase is characterized by an all-consuming intensity and "stupid gambling" and there is an apparent disregard for all other attachments—family, friends, and employment. Illegal activity begins, such as writing bad checks and even of committing nonviolent crime to obtain money.

The gambler's behavior becomes restless, irritable, and hypersensitive. Sleep is often disturbed, eating is erratic, physical and psychological exhaustion appears, feelings of hopelessness and helplessness may be expressed about debts, feelings of alienation, threats of divorce, and pariah status. At this point, depression, suicidal thoughts, suicide attempts, and/or criminal behavior may appear.

Bland, Newman, Orn, and Stebelsky (1993) conducted a survey of household residents in Edmonton, Canada, using the Diagnostic Interview Schedule and found among gamblers high rates of comorbidity with a high frequency of suicide attempts, youthful episodes of drunkenness, convictions for drunk driving, spouse abuse, child abuse, and long periods of unemployment. In particular, these researchers noted a high prevalence in gamblers of substance use disorders, affective disorders, anxiety, agoraphobia, and obsessive–compulsive disorders. All the social problems and every psychiatric disorder listed had a higher prevalence in the gamblers than in the nongamblers.

Depressive disorders were found in high incidence in pathological gamblers. A study by McCormick, Russo, Ramirez, and Tabor (1984) of 50 patients admitted successively to a gambling treatment program in a Veterans Administration hospital, using the Schedule for Affective Disorders and Schizophrenia (SADS), found that 76% of the patients were diagnosed as having major depressive disorder and 38% as having hypomanic disorder. A moderate to lethal potential for suicide was found in 48%, of which 12% had made a potentially lethal attempt. Three-fourths had missed more than 1 month of work due to gambling in the past 5 years compared to only 27% in a comparison group. It was hard to tell which came first, the gambling or the depression.

Gambling seemed to act as an antidepressant for many. The hypomanic symptoms included restlessness, racing thoughts, extreme distractibility, reduced need for sleep, and pressured speech. To many the gambling meant an almost total disruption of their lives. The casino offers opportunity for a 24-hour escape from real life, even an artificial alternative existence. Depression, loss of work, financial loss, and decreasing options led to a situation in which the gambler came to believe that the only chance for recovery lay in continued gambling. For the gambler, the behavior that caused the problem became the only solution (McCormick et al., 1984).

Gambling and suicide are often associated. Lester and Jason (1989) found that in seven suicides that occurred in the casinos in Atlantic City from 1982 to 1987, information indicated that six were clearly psychiatrically disturbed, with three of the seven suicides apparently gambling-related. Phillips, Welty, and Pearson (1997) recently reported findings of elevated numbers of suicides among both residents of and visitors to major gaming comunities; however, no direct data were presented linking gambling behavior to these observed deaths.

Social or environmental models of risk-taking behavior examine how interpersonal, group, and institutional contexts provide models, opportunity, and/or reinforcers for risk-taking. For example, parental modeling, permissive attitudes, familial conflict and a lack of cohesion and support have all been related to risk-taking behaviors. As peer influences increase through adolescence, so does peer influence increase as a factor in substance use, delinquency, and sexual behavior. These influences clearly interact with personality variables, such as locus of control; as those more dependent on external approval may be more moved toward risky behaviors by peer pressure.

In the yet larger social context, risky behaviors may be modeled from the media and influenced by cultural attitudes (e.g., ethnicity and religious affiliation). Consider, for example, the practice of religious snake handling. In a few fundamentalist churches in West Virginia—the last state in the Union where this practice is still legal—parishioners gather on weekends to show their faith in the Scriptures by singing hymns, dancing to rockabilly gospel, and passing hand to hand *poisonous* snakes. Devotees claim this practice is literally dictated by the Bible, in the Book of Mark, 16:18: "They shall take up serpents; and if they drink any deadly thing, it shall not hurt them."

Figure 18.1 presents a summary by Irwin and colleagues (Irwin & Millstein, 1986; Irwin & Ryan, 1989) of these biological, psychological, and sociocultural factors as a system of interacting, predisposing, protective, and precipitating factors that contribute to the onset of risk-taking behaviors.

Our discussion of Russian roulette toward the end of this chapter serves as an apt metaphor for other forms of ISDB. Each ISDB poses decidedly increased chances of disease or death; however, with a lower and unknown probability of negative outcome. For example, among the sexual risk-taking behaviors, each time someone decides to forego condom use when engaging in a sexual encounter with a partner of unknown HIV-seropositivity status, and each time a devotee of autoerotic asphyxia ties ligatures around his neck in the pursuit of heightened pleasure, figuratively, a gun with some loaded chambers has been aimed at his head. Similarly, when someone free-bases heroin or drinks excessively and gets behind the wheel of a car, the probability of finding the "fatal bullet" increases immeasurably.

SELF-MUTILATION

Probably the best known, the most widely investigated, and the most representative ISDB is self-mutilation—defined as deliberate alteration of body tissue without conscious suicidal content or intent (Favazza, 1996; Favazza & Rosenthal, 1993). It is known by many other

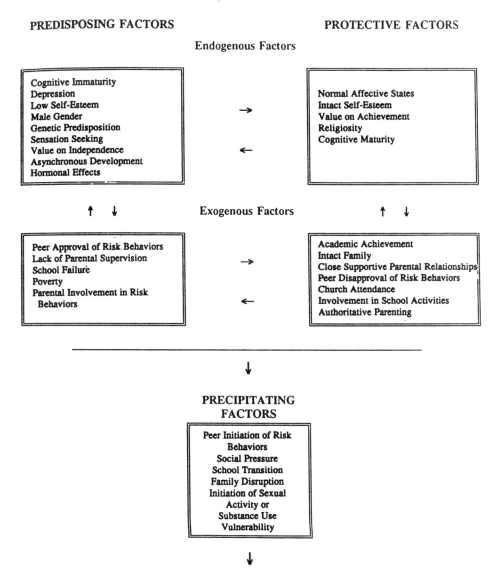

FIGURE 18.1. Factors contributing to the onset of risk-taking behaviors. *Source:* Igra & Irwin (1996: 47). Copyright 1996 by Kluwer Academic/Plenum Publishers. Reprinted by permission.

names, such as autoaggression, malingering, deliberate self-harm, symbolic wounding, intentional injury, self-injurious behavior, parasuicide, attempted suicide, and focal suicide. It has been considered both a symptom of mental disorders and a distinct syndrome.

The typical self-mutilator is female, adolescent or young adult, single, usually from a middle- to upper-class background, and intelligent (Suyemoto & Macdonald, 1995) The incidence of self-mutilation in adolescents and young adults has been estimated at around 1,800 per 100,000 (Favazza & Conterio, 1989) compared to estimates of 14 to 750 per 100,000 in the general population. Wrist cutting is the most common type, frequently by thoses with a history of sexual or physical abuse as children in families in which there was divorce, neglect, and/or parental deprivation. "It appears to be related to adolescent developmental issues such as separation and individuation. . ." (Suyemoto & Macdonald, 1995: 163).

From a review of over 250 books and articles and their own clinical experience, Favazza and Rosenthal (1993) concluded that a phenomenological classification was most suitable, and they proposed that the wide variety of behaviors could be categorized into three basic types: major, infrequent act resulting in significant tissue damage that usually occurred in psychoses or acute intoxications (examples are castration, eye enucleation, and limb amputation); stereotypical, fixed, rhythmic behavior that occurred without associated symbolism, found most frequently in mental retardation (about 14% prevalence in state schools for the mentally retarded in Texas) (examples are head banging, eyeball pressing, and finger biting); and superficial or moderate, with a prevalence ranging from 40 to 1,400 per 100,000—and as an associated feature of many disorders, these low-lethality behaviors result in relatively little tissue damage and occur repetitively (such as skin cutting, skin carving, skin burning, needle sticking, excoriation [skin picking], and scratching).

The most common diagnosis associated with self-mutilation is borderline personality disorder. Others are antisocial personality disorder, multiple personality disorder, posttraumatic stress disorder, anorexia nervosa, bulimia nervosa, episodic alcohol abuse, and kleptomania. The disorder has also been described as an addiction, with the act and the subsequent scar providing a special meaning and a sense of security When it appears in institutional inmates it is frequently purposive to gain a transfer to a more desirable location or to gain acceptance with the group. Significant predisposing factors have been found to be physical and/or sexual abuse in childhood, an early history of surgery, medical illness requiring hospitalization, parental alcoholism or depression, and residence in a total-care institution. The most common precipitants are real or perceived rejection and situations that produce feelings of helplessness, anger or guilt.

As with all ISDB, we must raise and answer the question, "Why does someone self-mutilate?" A number of explanations have been offered. Favazza and Rosenthal (1993) found that in the major self-mutilations, the acts seemed to occur most often in psychotic patients preoccupied with religious and/or sexual concerns. Occasionally, the actions are the result of hallucinatory commands. Among the stereotypical mutilations, with such disorders as Lesch–Nyhan, Tourette, and autism, the behaviors have been seen as an attempt to reexperience the comfort of hearing a mother's heartbeat when held in her arms, as an autoerotic response to understimulation, and as expressions of frustration, anger, and aggression.

The superficial or moderate self-mutilative behaviors have been regarded as a type of self-help behavior that provides a form of temporary release from psychological distress along with a sense of self-control. People who engage in this behavior have described relief from feelings of tension and depression, alleviation of feelings of loneliness and alienation, escape from feelings of depersonalization, enhanced sexual feelings, and euphoria. Psychological and sociological explanations include a projective identification process that provides a feeling of belonging to the major group in repressive total-care institutions, or a method of dealing with sexual conflicts, or a way of gaining revenge against significant others, a means of punishing oneself to relieve dysphoria, or a method for establishing a social identity of a "cutter" that is highly valued in some social subgroups.

The act of cutting seems to have special meaning for many self-mutilators. As the person experiences anger, depression, frustration, rejection, abandonment, and tension, the idea of cutting may occur and with it a sense of comfort. The experience of pain varies, with some persons describing absolute or relative analgesia for the event. For some the experience is accompanied by relief, as if they are reassured by the capacity to feel physical sensation, which assures them they are still alive. Others describe a feeling of empowerment when overwhelmed by feelings of helplessness. As the rage or tension becomes overwhelming, there is a transition into a state of depersonalization, described as "numb" and "unreal." The person becomes totally self-engrossed and withdrawn until the cutting ends the depersonalized state. The individual feels in control despite the withdrawal, for the extent and depth of the wounds are usually limited and the person stops when he or she has bled enough.

Suyemoto and Macdonald (1995) found eight models of explanation in the literature of self-cutting in females: behavioral (pain and caring are linked through early family experiences), systemic (cutting deflects attention from familial dysfucntion and maintains familial homeostasis), suicidal (self-mutilation is an active way to avoid suicide with mastery over death), sexual (cutting controls sexuality, avoids sexual feelings or actions, or may be a masturbation equivalent), expression (cutting stems from a need to externalize overwhelming anger, anxiety, or pain for more direct expression), control (makes the affect concrete, or provides punishment for affect perceived as out of control), boundaries (creates identity, differentiating the self from other), and depersonalization (a way to cope with the effects of dissociation and maintain a sense of self in the face of overwhelming internal emotion). Simpson (1980) feels that in many ways the act is antisuicidal, with the cutting used to end depersonalization or come back from an unreal preceding state. Grunebaum and Klerman (1967) have called wrist slashing a self-prescribed therapy.

Blood also seems to play a special role, especially in the self-mutilative practices that are not impulsive, such as flagellation, insertions of rings in nipples and genitalia, and tattooing. A journal, *Piercing Fans International Quarterly*, has been published to represent the "modern primitive" movement involving various constriction with corsets, piercing of various body parts, and skin branding. The actions assert control over the body and may lead to transcendent states of consciousness and enhanced sense of well-being. A professional body piercer claims that the

> act of being cut and surviving is a very strengthening and powerful experience for people. "To ask to be cut (not in a violent situation, but in a loving, supportive, trusting situation, and then bleed, and then end up with something beautiful . . . and then it heals and you have it and you're proud of it, that can be very empowering." (Ehrlich, 1991: 237)

Favazza and Rosenthal (1993) have proposed that a diagnostic category be considered for the next revision of the DSM entitled "repetitive self-mutilation," whose essential feature would be recurrent failure to resist impulses to harm oneself physically without conscious suicidal intent. The diagnostic criteria proposed are as follows:

- Preoccupation with harming oneself physically.
- Recurrent failure to resist impulses to harm oneself physically, resulting in the destruction or alteration of bodily tissue.
- Increasing sense of tension immediately before the act of self-harm.
- Gratification or a sense of relief when committing the act of self-harm.
- The act is not associated with conscious suicidal intent and is not a response to a delusion, hallucination, transsexual fixed idea, or serious mental retardation.

The diagnosis has to be differentiated from self-mutilative acts that occur in mental disorders, obsessive disorders, factitious disorders with physical symptoms, and stereotypical and habit disorders. When repetitive self-harm behaviors occur as responses to disturbing psychological symptoms or environmental events, they meet the criteria for an Axis I diagnosis. When they are found to coexist with Axis II disorders they are best regarded as an impulse disorder.

ALCOHOL AND SUBSTANCE ABUSE

As noted earlier alcohol and drug abuse typically begin in adolescence as alcohol and drug experimentation, to experience "kicks," to prove oneself in front of or gain acceptance from peers, to reduce discomfort, to get a "buzz" on, and so on. These behaviors must be considered normative and adaptive for the development of identity and social competence. Adolescents who never try cigarettes or take a drink are more socially isolated and have less ego strength than those who do. The danger posed by normative risk taking is that it is reinforcing; therefore, it is likely to be repeated. With repetition, of course, tolerance is developed; increased doses are needed thereafter to achieve the same desired effects. Without sufficiently competitive alternative methods to accomplish tension reduction, social acceptance, and so on, addiction and abuse and their attendant problems may follow.

Drug abuse (particularly among the young) and alcoholism (particularly among adults) are significant single factors for risk of suicide (see Chapter 15). Substance abusers are often also depressed and/or have significant personality disorders, commonly including conduct disorders and their symptomatic conflicts with the law. Acting-out and aggressive behaviors, impulsive behaviors, and recklessness are all more likely to occur in response to substance abuse. Involvement with the criminal justice and/or mental health system is a likely sequelae.

The alcoholic frequently has serious physical health problems and is more likely to have serious accidents, vehicular and otherwise, to suffer serious breakups in significant relationships, to have impaired occupational performance, and to die a premature death. The pathway toward death is littered with broken promises, lying, and failures. Underlying the alcoholic process are feelings of worthlessness, guilt, shame, and remorse. Further failure to break the cycle of abuse and bad feeling leads only to more abuse and bad feeling. In a sense, then, alcohol abuse as an ISDB may stem the pull of more directly self-destructive urges. The case of Juan T. (Case 18.1) well illustrates these dynamics.

CASE 18.1. The Case of Juan T.

Juan T., age 52, lived with his wife of 35 years and their nine children. He was known as a stable, hard-working, reliable employee (he had held the same job for 20 years) and a responsible family man. He also was a chronic alcoholic. He never sought help for his drinking problem, in spite of pleas from his family.

On the day of his death Juan T. drank as usual from the late afternoon into the early-morning hours. He fell asleep on top of his bed, fully clothed. Typically, when this happened, Juan T. would awake in the morning, make himself some instant coffee, and return to drink it in his bedroom. This morning, upon his return to the bedroom, he awoke his wife complaining of stomach pains; "I'm sick; there's something in my coffee. Take me to the hospital!," he said. He sounded frightened and desperate. His wife put her finger into the coffee and tasted a droplet. She reported that it "tasted very bitter."

Then, she realized he had mixed his coffee in one of three cups kept on the kitchen sinktop. This cup had been used the day before to pour a solution of drain cleaner to clear a blockage in the sink drain—and had not been washed out afterwards. With his coffee, Juan T. unknowingly had ingested a lethal amount of sulfuric acid. He died at the hospital 16 hours later.

CASE 18.2. The Case of Ralph V.

Ralph V., age 52, was found lying face down in a narrow hallway next to a closet containing three tanks of nitrous oxide in the dentist's office where he worked as an anesthetist. The regulator had been removed from one of the tanks and a tube had been taped to the open valve and extended to a mask held over Ralph V.'s face by his right hand. As is common to inhalers of nitrous oxide, Ralph V. appeared to have been in a sitting position when he lost consciousness. Usually, this position allowed for the hand holding the mask or tube to fall away, therefore allowing self-revival.

Ralph V. had no history of suicidal behavior. He had worked as a dental anesthetist for many years, serving two different practices on a permanent, part-time basis. His job was to administer nitrous oxide to patients. Recently, he had been promoted to a position as office manager for one of these dental practices.

In the other office, the one in which his body was found, there was some suspicion that he was using nitrous oxide recreationally. The dentist in this office had noticed that the nitrous oxide tanks were emptying at a faster than normal rate over the past few months. When Ralph was questioned, he maintained that there must be a leak in the tank. However, the tanks had recently been serviced and no leak was found. As a consequence, the dentist took the regulator off the tank, making it difficult for someone to abuse.

The night before Ralph was found dead, he drove to work and decided to spend the night due to inclement weather. His housemate reported that this was not unusual for him to do.

Drug-related deaths may occur as a direct (and intended or unintended) result of the injection, inhalation, or ingestion of a particular drug or as a result of medical complications (e.g., viral hepatitis). Among those who have died as a direct consequence of "accidental overdose" are some much publicized entertainers: Janis Joplin (age 27), Jim Morrison (age 27), Keith Moon (age 32), John Belushi (age 33), and Elvis Presley (age 42). The case of Ralph V. (see Case 18.2) is an example of an accidental overdose in a suspected chronic drug abuser.

In contrast, medical examiners often have some difficulty determining the manner of death in overdose cases in which, for example, the decedent was a drug abuser known to be self-medicating depression. The following case of Byron G. (see Case 18.3) was determined to be an accidental death but raises some questions regarding the decedent's lifestyle and possible motive for suicide.

UNPROTECTED SEXUAL BEHAVIOR

As U.S. views toward sex have liberalized, overt changes in sexual behavior have become noticeable. By the 1970s, in the United States, behavioral shifts in age of first intercourse (younger), array of sexual practices (wider), and number of premarital partners (more) were most obvious. A National Survey of Family Growth in 1970 found that 5% of women had premarital sex by the age of 15; in 1988 the proportion had risen to more than 25%

CASE 18.3. The Case of Byron G.

The victim was found dead on the floor of his bedroom. Cause of death was acute ethanol and codeine intoxication due to ingestion of overdose. Toxicological analyses revealed 0.17% ethanol, 2.64% codeine, and 0.08% morphine in the blood.

Byron G. was a 35-year-old man living with his wife and four children at the time of his death. In the past 12 years he had undergone several back and leg surgeries, the last of which only 6 months prior to his death resulted in the amputation of his left leg above the knee. During these years, the victim used Tylenol with codeine continually and in excessive amounts for control of pain and postoperative depression. Byron G. was open about his use of codeine and did not feel his excessive intake was a problem for him. In the past few days, observers reported he would take four pills at a time, then take two more as needed, often within only a couple of hours. In addition to abusing codeine, Byron G. abused alcohol. His pattern was to mix codeine with alcohol. He never expressed concern that he might overdose.

When Byron G. drank excessively, his wife slept in the living room. Byron, feeling overheated from the alcohol, often slept on the floor. Typically, he kept a large pitcher of water by the bed at night to handle the thirst resulting from excessive alcohol and drug use.

On the day of his death, Byron went out with his wife, brother, and sister-in-law. His mood was described as good, but he drank alcohol all day. When he returned home that night, he left to go to a neighborhood bar to play pool and drink some more. He returned home, quite drunk, around 11:30 P.M. To avoid an argument, his wife went to sleep in the living room. Byron G. stumbled into his bedroom, asked his son to bring him a pitcher of water, then closed the bedroom door. He was found dead the next morning.

On the nightstand were two vials of Tylenol with codeine #4; one was empty, the other, issued 12 days earlier, had 50 of 100 pills remaining.

(Berman, 1994). With sexual freedom, sexual activity also became more careless and reckless. Coitus often occurred without or with inconsistent use of effective contraception, in particular condoms.

In light of the well-publicized HIV epidemic and concerns for prevention, condom use increased among teenagers during first intercourse. However, thereafter, there has been a marked dropoff in condom use. Studies reported in the early 1990s reflect the following findings for young women: the younger the age at which sexual acts begin and the more sexual partners these women have had, the less likely their use of condoms (Byrne, Kelly, & Fisher, 1993). In a study of condom use in Canada, the percentage of men and women who used a condom was greater for women who had 1 partner than for women who had 10 partners; that is, those most at risk for sexually transmitted diseases (STDs) were least likely to use condoms (Berman, 1994)! One consequence of this neglect, of course, is unwanted pregnancy. Of greater concern with regard to our understanding of ISDB is the acquisition of STDs and, most profoundly, HIV infection.

Lesbian and bisexual women have a higher prevalence of HIV infection than do heterosexual women as a result of unprotected sex with women (e.g., sharing dildos) or with gay and bisexual men (Lemp et al., 1995). According to the Centers for Disease Control (1997), unprotected sexual activity between males accounts for one in three reported AIDS cases among adolescents and almost two-thirds of cases among young adult males (ages 20–24).

Given these risks, why would young sexual partners engage in unprotected sexual behavior? The reasons most often cited in the literature are (1) a low belief in self-efficacy (the skill to enact the preventive behavior), (2) a low intent to enact the preventive behavior, (3) perceived barriers to condom use (e.g., pleasure reduction or a pressure from a sex partner to participate in sex without a condom), (4) a desire for the negative outcome (e.g., to get pregnant or to contract AIDS), (5) substance abuse, and (6) personality traits, such as impulsiveness (Wulfert, Safren, Brown, & Wan, 1999).

Among gay men, unprotected anal intercourse is called barebacking. One particularly deviant and clear, yet indirect self-destructive variant of barebacking is *bug chasing*, in which HIV-negative gay men *seek to become infected* with the virus that causes AIDS. Gauthier and Forsyth (1999) reviewed these behaviors after surveying an availability sample through Internet chat rooms, personal ads, and so on. They found multiple motivations among gay male barebackers.

Bareback sex between two HIV positive men is often believed to be a nonissue ("For us, it's too late. So why shouldn't we party?"), even though it provides routes of transmission for other STDs, which can overburden the immune system and hasten death, and/or it risks infection with a more virulent strain of HIV, resulting in coinfection or recombination. Other views among practitioners spoke of a condom as a barrier to intimacy, thus any further risk was worth taking, and (illustrative of the theory of danger compensation) a belief that newer drug treatments that appeared would be able to check progression of the HIV infection, thereby giving greater freedom to risk.

Motivations for HIV-negative men to have unprotected sex with HIV-positive men (bug chasing) included the desire for intimacy and the belief that the infection was now medically manageable; a counterphobic desire to no longer live in fear of infection, thus to seek "relief" and less sexual inhibition by quickening the "inevitable" infection; the preference to experience sex filled with danger and excitement; and a desire to overcome feelings of isolation and loneliness by becoming members of the community, particularly one which gave status (as in membership in a selective club) and attained community sympathy.

A BRIEF NOTE ABOUT PROSTITUTION

Prostitutes are generally perceived as women at risk for STDs, including AIDS, for drug dependence and abuse, and/or for being physically abused. These are the "costs" of prostitution. Women who enter prostitution are disproportionately victimized by early sexual abuse or rape. Lacking cohesive family lives (they leave home at a young age also), they become sexually active (often unprotected) at an early age. The "benefits" of prostitution are perceived as outweighing the costs for these women, who find acceptance into and status within a peer group (a family of peers), the excitement and adventure of the "fast life," and economic rewards where once they felt devaluation (James, 1980; Viale-Val & Rattenbury, 1994).

RISK TAKING IN THE LAB

Most experimental studies of "risk-taking behavior" are laboratory-based examinations of game-playing styles and win–lose decision making. That is, they study influences on gambling behavior where earning money or succeeding are the goals and losing money or failure are the possible "risks." Understandably, any study with the possibility of physical loss (life or limb) or harm would probably not gain favor with a university's institutional review board, which considers the rights and safety of human subjects in research.

Nevertheless, a number of factors explaining the "risky bet" have been isolated and are helpful to our understanding of more dangerous risk taking decisions. To begin with, laboratory research on risk-taking can establish an *objective* measure of the *expected value* or outcome of any bet. When I toss a coin, for example, the probability of it landing on "heads" is pre-determined to be .50. The gaming industry is built on its knowledge of (and weighting of) probabilities.

However, human behavior is not that objective, although some potentially dangerous behaviors do have some measurable, albeit quite variable, outcomes. Safety records, for example, of various means of vehicular transportation are published annually by the federal government and consumer safety watchdog organizations. We daily "place our bets" regarding the likely outcomes of getting in a car or on a plane or a bike, with some knowledge that there is a low probability that death will result. In truth, most of us are ignorant of or naive to the true risk of these behaviors (can you state with any degree of accuracy the probability of your being killed as a result of commercial aircraft crashes?) and our decision to accept that risk is based on other variables, as described later (consider how prevalent the fear of flying is relative to its objective risk).

The only ISDB that has a clearly objective measure of outcome is Russian roulette (see later). In the typical example of Russian roulette, a six-chambered revolver is loaded with a single bullet, the chamber is spun and closed, and the gun is fired at the head. Thus, the probability of finding the bullet and probably dying as a consequence is 0.167 per try.

The expected value of a particular behavior is typically outweighed by its *expected utility*. Expected utility referes to the *subjective* value of risk. The more desirable the goal or the process, the greater incentive to the behavior's occurrence. Subjective value (probability) outweighs objective value. To test this, try to convince someone with a fear of flying with "rational facts" about the relative safety of airplane travel.

Motor vehicle accidents are the leading cause of accidental ("unintentional injury") death in the United States. In 1996, for example, 43,649 Americans lost their lives in an accidental crash of motor vehicles. But our reliance on these vehicles for myriad reasons makes these statistics meaningless to our daily decision making about driving. Moreover, with the advent of and statutory mandate to use safety belts and bags, we have been led to believe that death is even less likely. Keep in mind that those 43,649 individuals who lost their lives in 1996 also had these safety mechanisms available.

This leads us to the third major variable described by laboratory studies: *situational aspects*. Some outcomes of risk taking are strictly based on chance (e.g., Russian roulette). Others have a measure of skill involved (e.g., the vigilant and experienced automobile driver will have fewer accidents). Others yet involve a measure of skill and chance (e.g., smoking in bed or swimming far out from the ocean's shoreline).

The human mind, however, perceives situations and is capable of forming a belief that one can influence purely chance situations. Gamblers learn strategies (e.g., card counting) to gain a measure of control over the odds. This explains why the fear of driving is so far less prevalent than the fear of flying. Driving is considered to be under our personal control; flying is left in the hands of another (the pilot). But, for the most part, this belief is reinforced by our repetitive experiences of past successes or failures. The more we have succeeded (survived) at an activity, the less we perceive that activity as risky.

Several years ago, Berman (unpublished data) administered a questionnaire on risk-taking behaviors to a large sample of college age and adult subjects. When he compared males' level of "perceived risk" (i.e., danger to self) of experimenting with cocaine, those who admitted having tried cocaine gave a mean rating to this activity (on a scale from 0–100, with 0 being "no risk" and 100 being "great risk") of 20.7. In comparison, those who had not tried cocaine gave this activity a mean rating of 66.6.

Similarly, certain other high-frequency behaviors were perceived as low on perceived risk taking. These ranged from crossing the street in the middle of the block to driving a car 10 miles above the posted speed limit. Interestingly, the same finding resulted when asked about driving 20 miles above the posted speed limit, *except for adult women*. In contrast, other behaviors perceived to be at high risk were low in frequency of occurrence: taking a pill of unknown strength and purity or playing "chicken" with another car.

On one hand, these data suggest that experience decreases the perception of danger, therefore reinforcing its occurrence. Of course, it is equally possible that personality traits responsible for perceiving low or high risk in any activity (see later) determine the occurrence of the behavior to begin with.

This leads us to look at *individual aspects* of risk-taking bets. Needs for achievement, arousal, and success (to name but a few) might propel us to take greater chances. Fearful, inhibited, constricted persons most assuredly would bet conservatively, conserving resources and protecting themselves from real and perceived dangers. Great amounts of money have been made on Wall Street by risktakers. Of course, those who survived unscathed during the Great Depression would argue that the wiser bet was to not overplay the market.

Some have suggested that risk-taking behaviors are the result of a personality inclination or a situation-specific trait (Clark, Sommderfeldt, Schwarz, & Watel, 1990). Venturesomeness and impulsiveness are two such personality styles. Whereas venturesomeness refers to a conscious decision to risk or gamble, impulsiveness suggests "a complete failure to evaluate a situation as potentially dangerous" (Clark et al., 1990: 425) and both traits may be highly associated with alcohol and drug dependence and concomitant reckless behaviors and bad outcomes.

Finally, as there are individual propensities toward risk taking, there are also *group aspects*. Social psychological research has demonstrated that in choice situations, groups tend to move the individual toward the riskier of two choices. There also is a pressure toward group conformity. Moreover, there is a need to be approved of by and to attain status in some groups (e.g., gangs), whereby repetitive demonstrations of competence under conditions of danger define one as not cowardly.

Certain demographic findings might be of note here. Risk-taking behavior decreases with age and younger cohorts are more prone toward risk taking in general and drug experimentation in particular. Males are much more risk taking in their behaviors than are females. For example, in the sample noted previously, almost two out of three males (64%) stated that they had "driven a car above the speed limit on wet pavement" in contrast to only 37% of the females surveyed. Some behaviors are notably age and sex related. Table 18.3 shows the proportions of male versus female respondents who stated they had "driven a car while legally drunk." These data make clear why insurance premiums are so much higher for younger males.

TABLE 18.3. Percentage of Adult and College-Age Subjects Reporting Having Driven a Car While Legally Drunk

Gender	College age	Adult
Males	46%	22%
Females	24%	8%

Source: Berman (unpublished data). Used by permission of author.

TABLE 18.4. Percentage of Males among Unintentional Injuries, United States, 1996

Cause of death	Total number	% Male
Drowning/submersion	3,959	81%
Fall	11,292	54%
Residential fire/flames	3,375	58%
Firearms	1,134	89%
Motor vehicle	43,649	67%
Motorcyclist–traffic related	1,641	91%
Pedestrian	5,667	69%
Poisoning	9,510	74%
Suffocation	4,320	56%

Source: National Center for Health Statistics, Annual Mortality Data (1996).

Males are considerably more likely than females to die by unintentional injury by every means available. Table 18.5 reports 1996 mortality data by total numbers of decedents and percentage of males, as reported by the Centers for Disease Control and Prevention. Although it is probable that some unintentional deaths involve a greater proportion of male decedents because males engage the behavior in greater numbers than females (e.g., traffic-related motorcycling and firearms accidents), it is harder to make the same case for accidental poisonings, pedestrian-related accidents, or drownings.

RISK PERCEPTION AND MOTOR VEHICLE ACCIDENTS

As noted in Table 18.5, motor vehicle accidents (MVAs) result in more than 40,000 deaths annually in the United States and an additional 300,000 to 500,000 serious injuries. MVAs, in fact, are the number one cause of nonnatural death worldwide. Risk is inherent in driving. It varies as a function of roadway and weather conditions, vehicle condition, driver-related conditions (age, gender, attention, fatigue, scanning ability, sobriety, impairment, accident history, etc.), and the actions of others.

We have learned that risk taking is intimately tied to risk perception. Younger drivers, and especially younger male drivers, have riskier driving practices (e.g., speeding, tailgating, drinking and driving) and, consequently, higher accident rates. Younger drivers tend to report less perceived risk, particularly because they overestimate their personal immunity (see later) and the degree of control they have.

Personality factors are clearly associated with high-risk driving. Impulsivity, aggressiveness, psychopathology, stress, a generalized risk-taking propensity, and need for higher levels of arousal, for example, are all related to a greater involvement in accidents. Most profound is the influence of alcohol on visual perception, attention, reaction time, motor coordination, and so on, and, therefore on accidents. Alcohol, in turn, increases risk taking. What is of interest is that although most of us are aware of the risks of drinking and driving in general (and for others), our sense of personal immunity minimizes that perceived risk for ourselves.

One controversial theory in our attempt to understand risk perception is "danger compensation" or "risk homeostasis." These constructs have been used, for example, to explain why safety benefits lead to, and therefore may be offset (compensated for) by, *greater* risk taking. As an illustrative finding, drivers with studded tires have been observed to drive faster on curves on icy roads.

According to the theory for any given activity, such as driving, a person has some "target" of acceptable risk. Actions are adjusted accordingly to maintain this level (i.e., a homeostasis or equilibrium). If a perceived risk is higher than the target risk, behavioral changes (safer driving) will reduce the perceived risk; if a perceived risk is lower than one's target risk, behavioral changes (e.g., riskier driving) will occur to increase the perceived risk. This is akin to the dietary theory that posits that each of us has a "set point" with regard to our weight; we regain weight lost through a diet to achieve that set point. Drivers, therefore, drive faster as road conditions improve. One area of driving behavior in which this theory has not reflected research findings, however, is the wearing of seatbelts. Seatbelt users show less tendency to drive in a risky manner. Moreover, there is some evidence that the perceived risk increases, especially among younger drivers who wear seatbelts.

DRIVING AFTER ALCOHOL OR DRUG USE

A recent nationally representative study of almost 12,000 drivers 16 years and older estimated that, within a single year, 28% of all drivers in the United States had used alcohol, drugs, or both, within 2 hours of driving. As reported by the National Clearinghouse for Alcohol and Drug Information (see Figure 18.2), 23% of drivers used alcohol and 5% used

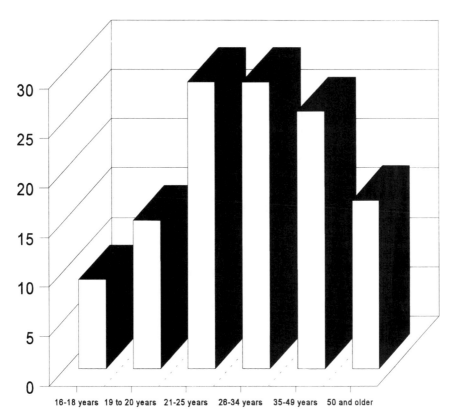

FIGURE 18.2. Percentage of drivers who drive 2 hours after alcohol use by age. *Source: SAMHSA News* (1999: 6).

a drug with or without alcohol and then operated a motor vehicle within 2 hours (National household survey on drug abuse, 1999).

Driving after drug use (most, 70%, used marijuana) was more common among very young drivers (ages 16–20), males, the never married, and the unemployed. Also, those with a recent history of arrest or current probation were more likely to drive soon after drug use. The majority of marijuana users did not believe that their ability to drive safely was affected. Driving after alcohol use was more common among those older than 20 (except for younger binge drinkers) and males.

Given this demographic profile of the at-risk driver, readers might wonder whether there is evidence for a more self-destructive drive (pun intended) among substance-using drivers. Some MVAs may, indeed, be directly self-destructive (i.e., suicides), although the proportion of such cases appears to be small (under 5%). In the earliest and most well-known study of single-car traffic fatalities, Tabachnick et al. (1973) reported that the great majority of these accidents occurred in the late evening or early morning, among drivers who had spent the evening drinking—a behavior that was part of their lifestyle.

RISK TAKING VERSUS INDIRECT SELF-DESTRUCTIVE BEHAVIOR

It is perhaps easier to distinguish direct from indirect self-destructive behaviors than to draw the line that clearly discriminates between normal, acceptable risk taking and excessive or pathological risk taking. Were probability estimates easily derived, perhaps we could agree on some level of risk (greater than 1%—3%—5%?) of loss of life or limb as the demarcation point between rational and excessive risk, although, as seen in the example of mountaineering on Mt. Everest below, this would be insufficient. On the other hand, maybe we should simply leave this determination to social attitudes; some behaviors are glorified by society, others condemned, and the rules for these attitudes are temporally and culturally determined.

In Farberow's (1980) classification presented at the start of this chapter, stress-seeking, risk-taking activities and occupations were incoporated into the overall definition of ISDB. At the same time, they were distinguished by their predominant motives—excitement, stimulation, challenge, and mastery. Consider the examples of mountaineering at its most prestigious level, ascending Mt. Everest, and Russian roulette, a life-threatening behavior.

THE ALLURE OF MT. EVEREST

When asked "Why climb Mt. Everest?," George Mallory responded with his infamous remark, "Because it's there!" Mallory died on the mountain in 1924. Everest was not conquered until 1953 by Sir Edmund Hillary and Tenzing Norgay. The peak was identified as the highest point above sea level in 1852. In the first century thereafter, two dozen deaths occurred among those attempting to reach its peak. Since then, more than 600 people have ascended to the summit of the mountain and more than 160 have died. These odds of survival (85.5% between 1970 and 1997) are not significantly better than than those posed by playing Russian roulette (83.3%). Interestingly, most of the deaths have occurred in the past two decades (15 people in 1996 alone), during which time significant advances in equipment and safety had occurred (recall our earlier discussion of *danger compensation*).

A study of seven Norwegian Everest climbers, all but one of whom reached the top of the mountain in a 1985 ascent, found them to score higher than comparison samples (including other elite Norwegian climbers) on all sensation-seeking subscales except that of Disinhibition. Thus, they were unusually high on boredom susceptibility, thrill and adventure seeking, experience seeking, and total score. They also were more extreme than, but had similar profiles to, other climbers in their freedom from worry and anxiety and showed less avoidance and more stability and maturity (Breivik, 1996).

With roughly equal odds of dying as those posed by playing Russian roulette, the motivation for climbing Mt. Everest has to be described as less a gamble than a calculated risk. Success in climbing depends partly on skill, on judgment, and on knowledge of one's equipment. Success at playing Russian roulette is totally left to chance.

RUSSIAN ROULETTE

Russian roulette is typically defined as a game. Clearly, it is a deadly game wherein the player challenges probability. Perhaps it is called a game because for some it is a diversion with rules—a means of proving one's courage, challenging an outcome beyond one's control, where the odds of losing are both fixed and high and the consequences permanent.

The first known description of Russian roulette occurs in the writings of Lord Byron, whose college roommate reportedly survived playing the as yet untitled game (Cutter, 1983). The Russian writer Mikhail Lermontoff wrote of the incident in a story called "The Fatalist" (1839). This description served as the protoype for the subsequent practice of Russian Army officers using a pistol in a gamble with death. Baechler (1979: 436) dates the origin of the game with these officers of the Czar.

"Winning" at Russian roulette, defined in process by the gun's hammer striking an empty chamber and in *outcome* by survival, involves none of the usual qualities of gamesmanship (skill, intelligence, courage, etc.). Rather, survival depends entirely on fate, to which the player willingly and passively submits. The outcome is a gamble with death; one exerts no control over this outcome. The spoils of victory are nothing more than what one began with—one's life!

Perhaps the goal of the game is to experience the rush of excitement in cheating fate. But where is the threshold between this type of arousal and a suicidal motivation to risk one's life for its gain. Moreover, that it is not that uncommon to find that a "player" has a past history of playing Russian roulette suggests more strongly that the ultimate motive in playing is to find the fatal bullet. Baechler (1975) claims that the sole purpose of playing Russian roulette is to play with one's life. Indeed, reports of depression, boredom, and both acute and chronic substance abuse often are found in the biographies of Russian roulette victims. The typical victim is an employed male who plays the game under the influence of alcohol or drugs in front of friends.

Baechler (1975) categorizes Russian roulette as an example of "ventured suicide"—conduct with a high probability of death but lacking the certainty of intended death. In contrast, Shneidman (1968) sees Russian roulette as an intentional death, categorizing a player as a "death darer," one who bets his continuation on a relatively low probability of survival (see Case 18.4).

Two studies reported in the literature suggest that Russian roulette is a death challenging form of exhibitionism, as it is frequently played in front of others. Fishbain, Fletcher, Aldrich, and Davis (1987) reported on 19 cases of male Russian roulette victims determined in Dade County, Florida between 1957 and 1985 and compared them to a control group of 95 randomly selected male firearm suicides. Russian roulette victims differed significantly from control subjects in race and ethnicity (more likely black, Latin, Catholic, and not a U.S. citizen), marital status (e.g., more likely single), greater alcohol use at time of act and

CASE 18.4. The Case of Alfred M.

On May 14, the victim died of a self-inflicted penetrating gunshot wound of the head while playing Russian roulette in front of friends.

Alfred M. was a 30-year-old man living with his family and his young son. His wife had left him and the boy 5 years earlier. Alfred had primary responsibility for parenting his son. He complained often of feeling burdened by this.

Alfred M. was always involved with guns and was knowledgable of their use and dangers. On occasion, however, he would carelessly point a gun at someone, although never at himself.

Alfred had enlisted in and saw combat in Vietnam. He enlisted in the service because he specifically wanted to be involved in warfare and gun play. Just prior to his death he tried to offer himself as a mercenary soldier in the Mideast, but was rejected because he had a history of heroin abuse. Although no longer a heroin abuser, he still frequently used marijuana and he drank beer daily. He had a high tolerance level for beer and was able to drink heavily, with the only effect being sleepiness.

Alfred was not known as someone who showed his feelings. Rather, he appeared almost detached in situations in which one might expect intense emotion. This was especially noticeable when he showed no overt response to the recent death of his mother.

When Alfred was 14 years old, he took his father's .38 revolver from the closet and played Russian roulette with his 6-year-old brother. The game included putting the muzzle of the gun against his brother's forehead above one eye and pulling the trigger. He then repeaeted the same actions by placing the gun to his own forehead. His brother did not know or recall whether or not there was a bullet in the gun. However, in retrospect, he commented how stupid he was and how lucky they both were not to have been hurt. This was the only time, prior to the death incident, that Alfred was known to play Russian roulette.

One month ago, after renting the movie *The Deerhunter*, Alfred began talking of wanting to play Russian roulette. [This film depicts American soldiers being forced to play Russian roulette as a form of torture, the captured soldiers alternating turns firing the gun until one found the loaded chamber]. Alfred could not find anyone interested in playing the game with him.

On May 14, Alfred worked on his construction job as usual. Work ended early, so he and a male friend decided to visit their girlfriends. While there, after drinking several beers, he again began talking of wanting to play Russian roulette. He told his friends how he had played the game one time as a youth with his brother. His friend had a gun and Alfred asked to hold it. The friend handed the gun to Alfred after emptying it of all its bullets. Alfred asked his friend for and was given one bullet. He loaded it in the gun's chamber, pulled the trigger, and died.

greater history of alcohol and drug abuse, and more likely to die in the presence of another. In fact, all the Russian roulette victims died in the presence of others. A similar study of 15 New York City male victims (Marzuk, Tardiff, Smyth, Stajic, & Leon, 1992c) found an overrepresentation of blacks and Hispanics and those single and unemployed. Alcohol or drugs were frequently present (78%) but were not statistically more present than in controls; except for the presence of cocaine, which was found almost twice as frequently (64% vs. 35%) among the Russian roulette victims. More than three-quarters of these deaths were witnessed by at least two or more other persons.

AUTOEROTIC ASPHYXIA: A SECOND LOOK

As noted in Chapter 5, sexual or *autoerotic* asphyxia is an arcane behavior that can lead to a self-inflicted, nonsuicidal death. When death occurs, it is the end result of a dangerous, habitual behavior that most likely has increased in complexity and potential lethality over the course of its practice.

Typically begun during adolescence or young adulthood and practiced almost exclusively by males (less than 4% of decedents are female [Burgess & Hazelwood, 1983]), practitioners of this secret behavior are often perceived outwardly to be happy and well-adjusted. Engaged in secret and in privacy, this behavior combines ritual with erotic gratification through fantasy. The autoerotic asphyxia practitioner typically ties a rope or ligature around the neck in an effort to produce and control voluntarily a constriction in the blood flow to the brain (anoxia). When orgasm is achieved through masturbation, the altered consciousness associated with anoxia heightens the intensity of orgasm. For some, the loss of control associated with ejaculation may carry the anoxia too far, causing the victim to black out and, if suspended, to die. Self-rescue mechanisms (slip knots, knives, etc.) often are found but either malfunctioned or could not be engaged quickly enough by the decedent to save the individual from hanging.

The typical autoerotic decedent is found partially or completely nude, in front of a mirror and/or attired in female clothing. Pornographic stimuli are often present as a fantasy aid. Sometimes, the body is elaborately and extensively restrained through the use of chains, belts, shackles, and so on, with protective padding placed between these bindings and the skin to prevent abrasion or discoloration. Rarely is the behavior accompanied by the use of alcohol or drugs.

A TYPOLOGY OF "SUBINTENTIONED DEATHS"

Shneidman (1968) classifies a death from autoerotic asphyxia as subintentioned and specifically as that of a "death chancer." In subintentioned deaths, decedents play a covert or unconscious role in hastening their own death. Evidence for this lies in their poor judgment, excessive risk-taking and recklessness, self-neglect, disregard of preventive advice, and abuse of alcohol and/or drugs. Implied in Shneidman's concept is a role of the unconscious in effecting a premature death. How else, he would argue, can we explain behaviors such as that of "victim-precipitated homicide," in which one person with some level of knowledge of lethal potential literally prods or goads another into killing him or her.

Among the types of subintentioned deaths, the *death chancer* leaves the outcome of his or her behavior entirely up to chance. They gamble with death, reflecting perhaps that the outcome of their behavior is entirely "in God's hands." Almost literally, these are the words of fundamentalist snake handlers, for example, who (as we saw earlier) regularly hold poi-

---

CASE 18.5. The Case of Samuel T.

According to a friend, Samuel T., a 44-year-old male, was a hard-working, industrious, and responsible man. However, in the past 3 months, since the death of his aunt who had raised him from birth and with whom he had lived, Samuel quit his job—refusing to return to work, began drinking heavily (after a lifetime of sobriety), and neither ate nor took care of himself. He died from a fall in his bedroom.

---

sonous snakes during religious services, believing that if bitten and should death result, it was meant to be.

The *death hastener* brings about a premature death by lifestyle and treatment noncompliance decisions. He or she unconsciously exacerbates a physical illness or disease by disregarding recommended medical treatment or safeguards (e.g., the diabetic who does not strictly follow insulin management or dietary instructions).

The *death experimenter* pursues a state of altered consciousness, increasingly risking and ultimately producing premature death. The person who copes with a pained life through chronic alcohol or drug abuse is an example of one who, perhaps unconsciously, chooses to cope by shortening that pained life. As drug tolerance increases, higher dosages are needed to produce the same effect; simultaneously, the risk of "accidental" overdose increases, as well.

Finally, the *death capitulator* appears to make an unconscious decision to simply "give up" or produce a premature death. This term might be used to explain "voodoo deaths," in which individuals, believing themselves cursed and expecting to die, act as if "frightened to death" and stop all measure of self-care and feeding. Consider the case of Samuel T. (Case 18.5), for example.

SUMMARY AND CONCLUSIONS

Imagine, if you will, the most dangerous thing you have ever done; and remind yourself what propelled you to attempt this particular activity. Were you young? Was this done on a dare, to prove your mettle, to gain some status among your peers? Did you do it for thrills and excitement or to undo some negative feeling such as boredom? Did you stop to think of possible consequences, of, perhaps, placing your life at risk? Was there a measure of skill and experience involved that you trusted would ensure your safety? Or was this pure recklessness, a mindless denial of the risk and your vulnerability?

Each of us has within us the potential to be both directly suicidal and indirectly self-destructive. Most of us have within our history examples of actions and choices that fit somewhere on the continuum that joins these polar opposites. In a sense, then, this chapter has attempted to delineate (to play on the words of Freud's pioneering work) the "suicidality of everyday life."

We have attempted to describe and discriminate the dynamics and intentions of this array of behaviors, to provide a theoretical framework for understanding, and to explicate a number of types of ISDB, their commonalities, and their idiosyncrasies. With time and more sophisticated research, as we come to understand better the suicidal mind and character, so will we come to differentiate the elusive threshold that differentially defines direct and indirect self-destructive behaviors.

To the extent that risk taking can be viewed as normative, constructive, and even necessary for achieving developmental tasks, we, as a society, should encourage experimentation and exploration. When health and life are potentially at stake, we have a further social responsibility, to ensure a protective frame within which our children can safely achieve these developmental goals. Similarly, we have a social responsibility to prevent those activities and behaviors that fall outside that protective frame and unnecessarily endanger our children and threaten either morbidity or premature mortality. This responsibility serves as the basis for all measure of prevention programs ranging from skills training and education to public awareness.

In Chapter 19 we move from ISDB to a consideration of the ethical, religious, and philosophical aspects of self-destructive behaviors.

FURTHER READING

Apter, M. J. (1992). *The dangerous edge: The psychology of excitement.* New York: Free Press. An insightful analysis and explication of the psychology of excitement and arousal states. Apter explores why we take unnecessary risks, why we enjoy putting our bodies under stress and expose ourselves to harm, the roles of boredom and panic, the protective frame that provides a zone of safety, and the conditions that lead to a misconceived confidence. This book is amply illustrated with real-life stories and examples.

DiClemente, R. J., Hausen, W. B., &Ponton, L. E. (1996). *Handbook of adolescent health risk behavior.* New York: Plenum. This volume covers the spectrum of behaviors that lead to excessive morbidity and premature mortality among adolescents. It covers epidemiological trends, preventive strategies, and the efficacy of treatment modalities.

Farberow, N. L. (Ed.). (1980). *The many faces of suicide: Indirect self-destructive behavior.* New York: McGraw-Hill. In his ground-breaking book Farberow brings together 28 authorities to examine the wide variety of behaviors examined in this chapter. The book is organized into seven sections ranging from theoretical understandings and classificatory schema to in-depth analyses of substance abuse behaviors, noncompliance with prescribed medical regimens, and high-risk sports. Several of the chapters in this volume remain two decades later as classic in our understanding of self-destructive behaviors.

Jessor, R. (Ed.). (1998). *New perspectives on adolescent risk-taking behavior.* Cambridge, UK: Cambridge University Press. An edited archive of a 3-day conference on the title's theme, held in Los Angeles in 1996. This is an excellent contemporary review of conceptual and research design issues, lifespan developmental perspectives, and new trends in the understanding of adolescent risk taking, with particular emphasis on the functional commonality of problem behaviors that compromise healthy development.

Plant, M., & Plant, M. (1992). *Risk-takers: Alcohol, drugs, sex, and youth.* London: Tavistock/Routledge. A short volume that overviews two areas of risk-taking behavior: the use (and misuse) of drugs and sexual risk taking by young people in England.

Zuckerman, M. (1979). *Sensation seeking: Beyond optimal level of arousal.* Hillsdale, NJ: Erlbaum. In this early compendium of his theory and research, Zuckerman explains sensation seeking as a personality trait and his prototypical models for measuring it. Readers are encouraged to trace the development of Zuckerman's work in this area by consulting his published research articles and book chapters over the two decades that followed this book.

19

Ethical, Religious, and Philosophical Issues in Suicide

Decide which day and at what time you intend to die, and let those know
who have agreed to be with you. Have your farewell note and other
documents (will, insurance policies) . . . beside you. An hour beforehand,
have an extremely light meal—perhaps tea and a piece of toast—so that the
stomach is nearly vacant, but not so empty as to feel nauseous or weak. . . .
Take three travel-sickness pills, such as Dramamine, to ward off nausea
caused by the excess of drugs taken later. Simultaneously, take four or five
beta- blocker tablets (such as Inderide, Lopressor, Corzide, or Tenoretic) to
slow down the heartbeat. . . . When about an hour has elapsed, take about
ten of your chosen tablets [e.g., Seconal or Nembutal] with as large a drink
of spirits or wine as you are comfortable with. . . . Have the remaining drugs
[perhaps a total of 60 × 100 mg; so about 50 more] already mixed into a
pudding, yogurt, or jam/preserves (whatever pleases you) and swallow all
this down as fast as possible. Throughout, keep plenty of alcoholic drink or
soda close by to wash all this down and also to help dilute the bitter taste.

—DEREK HUMPHRY

What's wrong with this quote? In his book, Humphry (1996) sidesteps crucial moral, ethical, religious, and philosophical issues that logically precede the mundane mechanics of suiciding. We consider just such issues in this chapter. Although no doubt many people lack
the practical wisdom or "tools" to suicide and end up alone and horribly botch even their
own deaths, surely a lot usually goes before, or should go before, concocting such lethal
recipes.

For example, a major *ethical* debate exists as to whether suicide is *ever* the right thing
to do. If it is, then for whom and under what circumstances? We might shudder to think of
our naive, vulnerable, depressed teenage sons or daughters reading the opening Humphry
quote. Humphry was once accused by an angry young woman of causing the suicide death
of her college roommate, who was found dead with an open copy of *Final Exit* in her lap.
Even in the state of Oregon (Humphry's home state and the only state allowing physician-
assisted suicide) one has to be certified by a medical doctor as terminally ill and within 6
months of death (plus other conditions) to be permitted to use physician-assisted suicide.
Here one has to be careful not to do a disservice to our friend, Derek Humphry. Humphry
is a sensitive, gentle, compassionate, bright man, attempting to confront extremely com-

plex, deeply ingrained, emotionally charged issues with a resolution that challenges fundamental human values.

Another issue we need to explore in this chapter is, Can suicide be *rational* or appropriate? Rene Diekstra once argued that Dutch suicidologist Nico Speijer's suicide was rational and specified eight conditions for a rational suicide (see Diekstra, 1986; cf. Werth, 1996). Some people contend that "rational suicide" is an oxymoron—in part because the depression, impulsivity, and other mental disorders present in the vast majority of suicides preclude rationality. But suicides can be rational (although most probably in fact are not). For example, Maris (1982a) devoted his presidential address to the American Association of Suicidology to the concept of rational suicide and argued for rational suicide in some circumstances. This important topic is explored in more detail later.

Still a third major subject in this chapter is, Should physicians help their patients die (many people don't realize that famous psychologist Sigmund Freud's death was probably a *physician-assisted suicide*)? Of course, doctors helped their patients die long before "Dr. Jack" (Kevorkian) appeared on the scene, under the guise of palliative care or pain control. What is new is legalized, active euthanasia, as we now see in Oregon and the Netherlands. Active killing, either in abortion or at the end of the lifespan with terminal patients, has always been highly controversial. After all, physicians take the Hippocratic oath, which (among other things) morally obligates them to "first do no harm." Kevorkian has gone so far in his iconoclastic zeal as to propose a new medical specialty named "obitiatry," devoted to physician-assisted suicide, which Kevorkian calls "medicide."

Most major world *religions* have ethically proscribed suicide as *hubris* (i.e., putting one's own individual will ahead of God's will) or as a violation of some scriptural commandment, such as "thou shalt not kill" (Deuteronomy 5:17). Religion concerns belief in and reverence for a supernatural power—a set of beliefs, values, and practices based on the teachings of a spiritual leader or leaders, usually embodied in a written text or texts. In this chapter we sketch the history of religious perspectives on suicide (cf. Chapter 4). There is little empirical data on the relationship between religion and suicide. However, Maris (1981a) did a sample survey in Chicago of suicide rates, religious affiliation, beliefs, and behaviors (e.g., church attendance) and some of these data are presented here. In this context, it would also be appropriate to consider suicidal religious cults (such as Jonestown and Heaven's Gate). Many religions seem to advocate leaving this world and going on to a better world in heaven. Some theologians have even argued that Jesus Christ was in effect a (sacrificial) suicide.

In the concluding section of this chapter we turn to more abstract, *philosophical* concerns. Ethics can be thought of as judgments of approval or disapproval, right or wrong, good or bad, virtue or vice, as sets of principles on right conduct or theories of moral values. *Philosophy* literally means "love of wisdom" and encompasses the study of metaphysics, ontology, epistemology, logic and language, ethics, aesthetics, and the history of philosophy. Philosophy can be thought of as a system of inquiry or demonstration, based on logical or mathematical reasoning rather than on empirical methods or physical science.

Peggy Battin is one of the preeminent suicidological philosophers. Early on Battin and Maris edited a smallish book, *Suicide and ethics* (1983; cf. Battin, 1996). In it they argued that there are two fundamental philosophical perspectives on suicide (the Kantian and the Utilitarian). Kant (cf. Rawls, 1971; Hill, 1983) might argue that suicide deviates from some ideal or duty, such as rationality. Utilitarian philosophers (such as Bentham or Narveson) might ask, Would suicide produce happiness or beneficial consequences and for whom? In this chapter we elaborate both the Kantian and Utilitarian perspectives on suicide. We also ask, "Whose life is the would-be suicide's?" Does our life belong to us, our family, our community or friends, the state? Can we do whatever we want to with our bodies? Finally, we ask, somewhat satirically, if you were suicidal would you want a philosopher as a psychotherapist?

ETHICAL ISSUES IN SUICIDE

Derek Humphry and Jack Kevorkian tend to focus on the "popular mechanics" and legal ramifications of assisted suicide, glossing over prior, crucial ethical issues in their rush to ghoulish gourmet recipes and the technical practicalities of death—ethical issues such as the following:

1. Whose life is it?
2. What is an "appropriate death"?
3. Do patients have the right to refuse life-saving treatment?
4. Are we morally obligated to suffer to please others?
5. How is active euthanasia any different from abortion?
6. We help loved ones—why not when they wish to die?

Is Suicide Ever or Never the Right Thing to Do?

In the introduction to this chapter we observed that some people believe that suicide is *never* justified. For example, far-right religious groups typically concede that even though all of us eventually have to die, none of us ever *has to* suicide. However, one has to question whether such dogmatic, rigid thinking is not overly simplistic and perhaps, because of that, irrational. At the other extreme, psychiatrist Thomas Szasz (see Box 19.1) argues that suicide is an inalienable right of individuals, and, in that sense, that suicide is *always* right.

To suggest that suicide may be right or ethical in certain circumstances raises the related topic of appropriate death and if suicide is ever an appropriate death. "Euthanasia" literally means "good death," which implies that there may also be "bad" or *in*appropriate death, or that some deaths (such as natural deaths) are more appropriate than others (such as suicides). For example, Avery Weisman (1984: 348) defines an "appropriate death" as a death that someone might choose, if he or she had a choice.

Any appropriate death includes several conditions being met. For example, (1) the dying person should be as free from pain as possible; (2) no unnecessary medical procedures should be performed; (3) the person should be allowed to die where and with whom he or she chooses; (4) interpersonal conflicts should be resolved, if possible; (5) preparations for one's death should have been made (including wills, good-byes, funeral plans, legal arrangements [such as a power of attorney], financial arrangements, etc.); (6) dying persons should yield control or share control of their dying to others they trust; (7) dying persons should have the degree of consciousness desired; and (8) the dying process should be the desired length of time (neither too long nor too short).

Something to keep in mind is that death is probably never appropriate when something short of death would have resolved the individual's life problems (many suicides are simply impatient, impulsive, and for whatever reason lack "staying power").

Of course, if the death is a *suicidal* death, several additional considerations for appropriateness may be required, because suicide has unique legal, medical, social, political, ethical, and religious implications. One way to explore the appropriateness of suicide is by taking a few minutes to read and discuss the case of Nico Speijer (see Case 19.1). So what do you think?

BOX 19.1. Libertarian Psychiatrist Thomas Szasz on Suicide Prevention

- If suicide is not an illness . . . but the act of a moral agent, then the only person ultimately responsible for it is the actor himself.

- . . . insofar as suicide is perceived as an undesirable act or event, people will insist on holding someone or something responsible for it.

- Psychiatrists now stigmatize suicide as much as priests did before them . . . psychiatrists patronize their patients and promise more than they can deliver . . . psychiatrists ally themselves with the police powers of the state.

- A person cannot be held responsible for something he does not control. . . . This is why persons who want to assume control over others typically claim to be responsible for them (called "paternalism").

- The physician is committed to saving lives. . . . He, thus, reacts . . . as if the patient had affronted, insulted, or attacked him.

- There is neither philosophical nor empirical support for viewing suicide as different, in principle, from other acts, such as getting married or divorced, working on the Sabbath, eating shrimp, or smoking tobacco.

- Insofar as suicide is a physical possibility, there can be no suicide prevention; insofar as suicide is a fundamental human right, there ought to be no such thing.

- . . . policies aimed at preventing suicide . . . imply a paternalistic attitude toward the "patient" and require giving certain privileges and powers to a special class of "protectors" vis-à-vis a special class of "victims."

- If the "patient" does not want such help and actively rejects it, the psychiatrist's duty ought to be to leave him alone.

Source: Szasz (1985). Reprinted by permission of the author.

Was Speijer right to suicide? He did have terminal cancer and could not find relief from his pain (in a PBS television program with Hugh Downs June 16, 1980, in New York City about the suicide of Jo Roman, about three-fourths of the viewing audience agreed that suicide was rational in the event of terminal cancer). Speijer had been ill for a long time and was in great pain from his intestinal cancer. He had thought a lot about his decision, discussed it with his wife, and did not act impulsively. He certainly was not mentally disordered, although he was understandably sad (just because one wishes to die does not mean *ipso facto* that one is clinically depressed).

Speijer had sought counsel from professional colleagues and, indeed, had written a book on assisted suicide with Professor Diekstra. In short, Nico Speijer met all eight of his own conditions for an appropriate suicide. So, was Speijer's suicide "rational"? In the next section we consider rational suicide, define it, and argue that although the vast majority of suicides are not rational, suicide in some circumstances certainly can be rational.

Rational Suicide

To many, "rational suicide" is an oxymoron; that is, all suicides are thought to be committed by people who are not thinking clearly, are depressed, are under the influence of some substance (especially, alcohol), are impulsive, are extremely stressed, are isolated from the

---

CASE 19.1. The Case of Nico Speijer

On September 25, 1981, the grand old man of suicidology and longtime champion of suicide prevention in the Netherlands himself committed suicide. He wrote this note to Rene Diekstra, who had been his pupil and friend:

> Dear Rene,
>
>   When you receive this letter, I will no longer be alive. As you know, I suffer from a carcinoma with a lot of metatases. Up to now I have been relatively capable of controlling the pain, but I cannot cope with it any longer and, therefore—as you yourself will very well understand—I have decided to put an end to my life. . . .
>
>   My wife has decided to go with me. After a marriage of forty years she prefers to die with me over having to stay behind all on her own. . . .

As Diekstra (1986) writes "How could it have happened that a man who had virtually all of his 76 years been a protagonist of suicide *prevention* committed suicide himself?

Actually in 1980 Speijer and Diekstra had published a book, *Aiding Suicide*, which gave some of the answers. Some of the conditions when suicide might *not* be prevented are:

- The choice of ending life by suicide is based on a free-will decision and is not made under pressure.
- The person is in unbearable physical or emotional pain with no improvement expected.
- The wish can be identified as an enduring one.
- At the time of decision the person is not mentally disturbed (*compos mentis*).
- No unnecessary and preventable harm is caused to others by the suicide.
- The helper should be a qualified health professional and an MD if lethal drugs are prescribed.
- The helper should seek professional consultation from colleagues.
- Every step should be fully documented and the documents given to the proper authorities.

---

checks and balances of other loving people, and so on. But is this true? Could one not be suicidal and rational?

"Rationality" can be defined as "exercising one's reason in a proper manner; having sound judgment, sensible, sane; not foolish, absurd, or extravagant; implying the ability to reason logically, as by drawing conclusions from inferences, and often connoting the absence of emotion" (*Webster's New World Dictionary*, 1966: 1207).

There are at least four fundamental ambiguities in the concept of rational suicide (for a more recent consideration of this topic, see Werth, 1996):

1. Having a *reason* versus a *right* to suicide.
2. Whether or not rational suicide *excludes* affect.
3. If suicides are not rational, are they *crazy*?
4. Whether suicides are *always* or *sometimes* irrational.

Maris (1982) discusses these four ambiguities.

1. It has been said (by Pavese) that "no one ever lacks a good *reason* to suicide"; nevertheless, suicide may still not be right, proper, or ethical. For example:

a. Suicide never just concerns the would-be suicide. Your suicide may resolve *your* problems but create severe lifelong problems for those who love you. That is, suicide can be a very selfish act—forgivable, but nonetheless, selfish. In short, what about the rights of *others* affected by suicide (parents, spouses, children, friends, etc.)?

b. If something short of suicide (taking antidepressant drugs or getting ECT, counseling, divorce, waiting a while, leaving home, changing jobs, getting a loan, prayer, etc.) would have had the same effect, then suicide is perhaps irrational (i.e., unnecessary or overkill).

c. What about God's rights? Does all life belong to God? Perhaps suffering has a purpose (for example, see the Judeo-Christian biblical story of Job). If all life belongs to God, we may not have a right to suicide, even though we have reasons to suicide.

d. Finally, suicide may be illegal or immoral, not an individual's right. Certainly, assisting suicide (as Dr. Kevorkian did) is illegal in most states. Although self-murder is no longer a crime (how could you punish the offender; take away his or her property or defile his or her dead body?), it does still threaten the state and is generally disapproved of in most circumstances, except perhaps in war.

2. It is hard to imagine rational suicide totally excluding *affect*. To be sure, affect can distort judgment, especially when one is in chronic, unremitting excruciating physical pain or in a psychotic or manic episode. In such circumstances one may be tempted to do *anything*, even commit suicide, just to stop the pain. On the other hand one can also be emotional *and* rational. All of us are at least thinking and feeling creatures. In fact, decisions can be rational because of emotion. For example, suicide may just not *feel* right in spite of an abundance of compelling reasons in favor of suicide. Finally, disemboweled, decathected reason or mind (the epitome of rationality) may be not be sufficient. Just think of all of the horrendous human actions justified in the name of unfeeling reason or a purely logical calculus.

3. Often suicide is taken as *prima facie* evidence for insanity or mental disorder. In surveying the Chicago Coroner's juries for suicides, Maris (1981) recounts being struck by how often Catholics were forgiven and given Christian burials in spite of their supposed mortal sin of suiciding, on the grounds that they were "temporarily insane." There are several subtleties here. For example, one can be not crazy and yet be irrational, or one can be mentally disordered and yet still capable of reasoning correctly.

Most people who suicide are sad, but they may not be clinically depressed. If an individual is acutely mentally disordered (and Kevorkian often did not check, test, or control for this), he or she probably should wait for several weeks and perhaps take some psychotropic drugs, then see later on whether he himself still has a persistent wish to suicide. Mentally disordered people often cannot consider their best alternative to suicide (i.e., cannot be rational). As one of our mentors, Edwin Shneidman, used to say: "Never kill yourself when you are depressed."

4. Most people who are against suicide argue that suicide is *always* irrational. Curiously, such people themselves tend not to be rational but, rather, are dogmatic and rigid (e.g., uncompromising pro-lifers). However, under most circumstances we are responsible for our *own* lives, both how and *if* they are lived (as opposed to largely paternalistic suicide interveners). Most of us would not like to see people cavalierly or whimsically killing anything—themselves, others, or animals (and usually there are laws against it). Nevertheless, we all have to die eventually. Sometimes death, even suicidal death, is "natural." In short, although suicide is often irrational, it is not *always* irrational.

Maris's presidential address to the American Association of Suicidology on the topic of rational suicide (see Box 19.2 and Maris, 1982a) opens with a quote from Edward Arlington Robinson's poem "Richard Cory." Cory seemed to outsiders to have everything anyone could imagine wanting, yet he suicided ("One calm summer's night he ... put a bullet through his head"). The point here is that suicide is a solution to the problem of life itself, under the best of circumstances (not just when life has gone awry).

Box 19.2 outlines the Maris argument for rational suicide. Under the *best* of circumstances, life is short, frequently painful (psychologically and physically), fickle and unpredictable, lonely, and anxiety generating. Thus, the human condition, not merely life gone astray, forms the basis for suicide. It is a wonder we are not all clinically depressed (instead of about 10% of us). Death and finitude are inevitable, even when we have a relatively "good life" (a "good enough" life, if you will). And, only in the oblivion or cessation of individual consciousness (i.e., only in death) is our psyche and body ever "at peace" (well, in death our psyche is likely annihilated).

The primordial human fear is fear of separation and death. All our psychological defenses are at best *distractions* from the fact that we all die and spend much of our living time essentially waiting to die and fearing it. Consciousness of our personal death is one of the curses of being a human being, and not (say) a cocker spaniel.

All the meaningful things in our lives (love, marriage, good friends, sexual euphoria, money, property, power, achievement, work success, art and music, religion, drugs, alcohol, travel to exotic places, play, etc.) are relatively ineffective defenses against death—cyn-

---

BOX 19.2. Maris on Rational Suicide

- Suicide is a solution to the problem of life itself, not some perverse response to a life gone awry. To understand suicide we must imagine abandoning life *at it best.*

- We have the regretable tendency to assume ... that if would-be suicides only "lived better," they would not *be* suicides.

- One reason we cannot understand and accept suicide is because suicide solves the life problem by abandoning life.

- Under the *best* of conditions life is short, periodically painful, fickle, often lonely, and anxiety generating.

- All human beings share the basic givens of life: a finite lifespan; periodic, unavoidable sickness, fatigue, and physical pain; a fickle and unpredictable life course; and the associated psychological burdens ... viz., anxiety, stress, and depression. ;

- Harshness has a complex relationship with suicide. People do not suicide simply because their lives are harsh.

- The vast majority of individuals and groups develop nonsuicidal solutions for adapting to the human condition across the entire spectrum of its harshness.

- Most individuals must ask themselves, would I prefer *something*, even a troubled and painful something, to nothing?

- Nevertheless ... nothing short of death can truly end the problems associated with being human. Does if follows then that suicide is rational? Have we been duped into living like eating spinach? Does it make sense to seek death and, if so, under what circumstances?

ically, they are merely postponements, deferrals, and distractions. The rational suicide argument contends that nothing short of death can truly end the life problems associated with being human (if there is no God, heaven, or hell).

Nevertheless, Maris argues that suicide is usually not the *best* alternative to resolve the human condition. For oneself, as well as for those who love us (suicide is selfish), death is a high price to pay for overcoming the tribulations of life. The suicidological resolution, in effect, is to end the world (which many religious cults in fact do for their entire cult). However, life does not seek death. Death is not the purpose of life. The goal of life is simply to live. All we need is a "good enough" life, not a perfect life, with no death ever. Just because all of us age and atrophy, it is not cause for despair. The process of loving, living, producing, and reproducing is not invalidated by the final product (i.e., our personal death).

One trait essential to life satisfaction is grace in the presence of necessity. Another is being lucky; for example, lucky not to be captured by irresistible, irreversible mental disorder or terminal physical illness early on. A third trait is resilience in the face of periodic bad luck and unavoidable insults to our life routines. Most suicides we have known have lost the ability to engage the world outside themselves and with it their reason, courage, and resources to be.

Euthanasia and Assisted Death

Well, then, should we help some people to die, and if so, who and under what circumstances? We *all* have to die, after all, so why not make dying as free from pain, as quick as desired, and not mutilating or lonely? One cannot help but think of what has happened to assisted death at the other end of the lifespan, when help has not been available (i.e., with abortion). Women often mutilate themselves and torture their fetuses by default. The same thing usually happens today with most suicides, when they shoot themselves in the head, in a drunken stupor, and in a lonely bedroom or hotel room. Clearly, many abortions and most suicides are not "good deaths."

Euthanasia itself is not one thing (Despelder & Strickland, 1996, Ch. 6). Euthanasia can be at least *active* or *passive*, *voluntary* or *involuntary*, and *direct* or *indirect*. A person could be against one type of euthanasia but in favor of another. "Active euthanasia" is an act that kills; "passive euthanasia" is the omission of act, which results in death. For example, passive or indirect euthanasia could be "no coding" a terminal cancer or heart patient, not resuscitating the patient or not doing CPR if the individual had a medical crisis.

"Voluntary euthanasia" is death in which the patient decides (perhaps by drafting a living will) versus "involuntary euthanasia," when someone other than the patient (e.g., if the patient is in a coma) decides (e.g., the patient's family, physician, or nurses).

"Direct euthanasia" is when death is the primary intended outcome, versus "indirect euthanasia," in which death is a by-product (e.g., administering narcotics to manage pain and secondarily causing respiratory failure).

All the types of euthanasia have associated problems. For example, active euthanasia is murder in most states. It also violates a physician's Hippocratic Oath (to first do no harm) and religious rules (does all life belong to God?) and has practical ambiguities (when is a patient truly hopeless?).

Passive euthanasia, on the other hand, is often slow, painful, and expensive. For example, comatose patient Karen Anne Quinlan (see DeSpelder & Strickland, 1996: 13–14, 221–232) lived for 10 years (even some time after her respirator was turned off) and seemed to grimace and gasp for breath. Her parents and their insurance company spent thousands of dollars on what proved to be a hopeless case. The U.S. Supreme Court ruled in *Cruzan* (1990) that hospitals cannot be forced to discontinue feeding comatose patients.

In the case (Case 19.2) of Elizabeth Bouvia, a quadriplegic cerebral palsy patient in California, sued to avoid being force-fed (as a noncomatose patient), her intention was to starve herself to death in the hospital (cf. Richard Dreyfuss in the movie *Whose Life Is It, Anyway?*). The California Supreme Court upheld Bouvia's right to refuse treatment, but others called the court's decision "legal suicide."

A celebrated spokesperson for euthanasia in the form of assisted suicide has been Derek Humphry, especially in his best-selling book, *Final Exit* (1996). As you can imagine, rational assisted suicide (Humphry assisted in his first wife's death [Jean] and in the death of his father-in-law), even for the terminally ill within 6 months of death, has proven highly controversial (particularly to Catholics and the religious right). Basically, Humphry has

---

CASE 19.2. The Case of Quadriplegic Elizabeth Bouvia

During the closing months of 1983 Elizabeth Bouvia, severely disabled by cerebral palsy (she was a quadriplegic), brought legal action in a Riverside county, California court, asking for custodial hospital care and simple treatment for pain, while she starved herself to death. Her case involved ethical issues of force-feeding a *noncomatose* patient and her right to refuse this treatment (see Despelder & Strickland, 1996: 232. Cf. Curzon, U.S. Supreme Court, 1990, for a decision about force-feeding of a *comatose* patient). Dr. Maris was an expert for the defense, opining as to whether or not Bouvia's request amounted to "legal suicide." The California Supreme Court upheld Bouvia's right to refuse treatment.

Elizabeth Bouvia's handicaps date from birth. She has no motor functions in her limbs or skeletal muscles except for extremely limited use of her right arm. She cannot change her own bodily position. This, together with pronounced spasticity and muscle contractions, aggravates the associated arthritis which she suffers from, and produces almost constant pain for which she requires medication.

Bouvia requires complete assistance in all matters of bodily hygiene, dressing, feeding, and other care functions. She is subject to multiple infections. However, she is able to speak quite well, to hold a cigarette in two fingers, to chew, and to operate her motorized wheelchair by means of a joystick.

She was able to complete a BA at San Diego State and started work on an MSW degree. In August 1982 she married Richard Bouvia, a machinist. After a year he left her and she filed for divorce. When Elizabeth was visiting her father in September 1983, she asked him to drive her to Riverside (California) General Hospital, where she requested that she be allowed to starve herself to death and filed suit.

Elizabeth said, "I know what's available to me out there and don't need or want it. My only outlet is talking or screaming. I'm trapped in a useless body. Unfortunately, I have a brain. It makes it all the worse [note: Many potential euthanasia patients are brain-dead or damaged]."

After checking out of the Riverside Hospital and into a hospital in Tijuana, Mexico, she hoped she would be allowed to starve herself (but she was not). She voluntarily decided to eat (on Easter morning, April, 1984) after checking out of the hospital and into a local motel.

written a "how-to" book on the practicalities of suicide for the terminally ill (see book reviews of *Final Exit* by Maris and others, Maris, 1992c).

His preferred rational suicide recipe (see the opening tease to this chapter) is four or five beta-blocker tablets, 40 to 60 100 mg tablets of a barbiturate (perhaps in pudding or Jell-O), taken with Dramamine (to settle the stomach), some Vodka (or favorite whiskey), and, finally, a plastic bag over the head, loosely fixed by a rubberband around the neck. Humphry recommends against guns (too messy), cyanide (too painful), hanging (too graphic), jumping (the individual could land on someone), and other mutilating, violent, painful, or uncertain methods.

One of the big questions about *Final Exit* seems to be its potential abuses (e.g., by people, especially those who are young, with treatable, reversible depressions; imagine a parent who lost a son or daughter because of Humphry's book). Having the lethal methods for suicide described in such vivid, explicit details worries many people that suicide will become too easy, and, thus, often will be clearly inappropriate (cf. Stone 1999, who tells readers how to make each one of several possible suicide methods lethal). Yet, Humphry is right that it is hard to get help with self-deliverance now, without fear of penalties. He argues that laws in states need to be changed to permit and specify procedures for physician-assisted suicide for the terminally ill, under highly controlled conditions.

A few states have undertaken just such reforms to permit legal assisted death. For example, Initiative 119 in the fall of 1991 in Washington (and Proposition 161 in the fall of 1992 in California) provided "aid in dying" for a person, if (1) two physicians certified the person to be within 6 months of (natural) death (i.e., to be terminally ill), (2) the person was conscious and competent, and (3) the person signed a voluntarily written request to die, witnessed by two impartial, unrelated adults. Both the Washington and the California referenda recently narrowly failed (by votes of about 45% in favor and 55% against).

Derek Humphry waged a similar legal battle in Oregon, first as president of the Hemlock Society (named after the famous suicide, Socrates, who drank hemlock in a kind of quasi-voluntary execution) and later as president of ERGO (Euthanasia Research and Guidance Organization) and the Oregon Right to Die organization (see Box 19.3). On November 4, 1994, Oregon became the first state in the United States to permit a doctor to prescribe lethal drugs expressly and explicitly to assist in a suicide (see Ballot Measure 16). The National Right to Life Committee effectively blocked the enactment of the Oregon assisted suicide law until 1997, when the measure passed overwhelmingly again. On March 25, 1998, an Oregon woman in her mid-80s stricken with cancer became the first known person to die in the United States under a doctor-assisted suicide law (most, if not all of Kevorkian's assisted suicides have probably been illegal).

Physician-assisted suicide has, however, been practiced for some time outside the United States, in the Netherlands. On February 10, 1993, the Dutch Parliament voted 91 to 45 to allow euthanasia. To be eligible for euthanasia or assisted-suicide in the Netherlands one must:

1. Act voluntarily.
2. Be mentally competent.
3. Have a hopeless disease without prospect for improvement.
4. Have a lasting longing (or persistent wish) for death.
5. Have the assisting MD consult at least one colleague.
6. Require the assisting MD to draw up a written report afterward.

The Dutch law opened the door for similar legislation in the United States, although the U.S. Supreme court seems to have slammed that door shut in Washington and New York

BOX 19.3. Oregon's Physician-Assisted Suicide Law

The electors of the state of Oregon made history on November 4, 1994, when they voted in favor of the Death with Dignity Act, which permits physician-assisted suicide under certain limited conditions. Known as a "prescribing bill," its sole task is to permit a doctor to legally and knowingly prescribe lethal drugs for suicide. The Oregon law does not permit injection of lethal substances in anybody. Actions by all parties must be voluntary–medical staff have a "conscience clause."

Ballot Measure 16 had been sponsored by Oregon Right to Die, an offshoot of the Hemlock Society, which was the measure's chief financial backer. But the day before it was to take effect, court proceedings brought by the National Right to Life Committee put the law on hold. In August 1995, a federal district judge declared the law unconstitutional on the grounds that it did not protect persons who were irrational from getting assistance in suicide.

The full text of Oregon's law is printed on pages 169 to 179 of the second edition of Derek Humphry's book, *Final Exit.*

On March 25, 1998, an elderly woman stricken with breast cancer became the first known person to die under the Oregon law. The Portland, Oregon woman in her mid-80s died about 30 minutes after taking a lethal dose of barbiturates mixed with syrup and washed down with a glass of brandy.

Oregon 's Death with Dignity Act, passed in 1994 and affirmed in 1995, allows doctors to prescribe lethal drugs at the request of terminally ill patients who have less than 6 months to live.

The law has been the focus of national debate since the first campaign in 1994, when voters passed it by a narrow margin, and in 1997, when it was put back on the ballot by the legislature and overwhelmingly passed again.

"This is a tragic and sad day for Oregon and the United States, " said Bob Castagna, a spokesman for the Oregon Catholic Catholic Conference. May God have mercy on all of us." But is it really a sad day? Now we are legally able to help those we love die without needless suffering and expense, like we have been able to do for our pets all along. What do YOU think?

on June 27, 1997. Box 19.4 discusses reviews of Dr. Herbert Hendin's book *Seduced by Death* (1997), which opposes physician-assisted death here in the U.S. and in the Netherlands. Although the idea of legal assisted suicide will remain highly controversial and divisive, quite likely bills similar to that of Oregon's Measure 16 will pass in other states in the next decade. A key issue in this legal reform will be safeguards against abuses (e.g., Hendin argues that physicians in the Netherlands have decided on their own in some cases to euthanize patients).

One of the most controversial, even radical, advocates of physician-assisted suicide ("medicide") has been Dr. Jack Kevorkian (see Kevorkian, 1991). Public awareness of assisted-suicide and whether or not it is rational has been focused largely on Kevorkian, the "suicide doctor." At last count (early in 1999) Kevorkian had assisted more than 100 suicides.

Initially, with Janet Adkins (see Case 19.3), Kevorkian used a suicide machine (which he dubbed a "mercitron"). This machine provided a motor-driven, timed release of three IV bottles; in succession they were (1) thiopental or sodium pentathal (an anesthetic producing rapid unconsciousness), (2) succinycholine (a muscle paralyzer like the curare used by African pygmies in poison darts to hunt monkeys), and (3) postassium chloride (KCl), which stopped the heart. The mercitron was turned on by the would-be suicide. Given some problems with malfunctions of the suicide machine, almost all of Kevorkian's suicides after Adkins were accomplished by a simple facial mask hooked up to a hose and a carbon monoxide canister, with the carbon monoxide flow being initiated by the suicides themselves. For most nonnarcotic users or addicts, 20 to 30 mgs of IV-injected morphine would also cause death.

All eight of Kevorkian's first clients were women (which is worth noting, given the usual excess male suicide rate) and mostly single, divorced, or widowed. Almost all of them were not terminally ill, or at least would likely not have died within 6 months. The toxicology reports at autopsy (by Frederick Rieders; these data were obtained from Dr. Dragovic, the Oakland County, Michigan, medical examiner) showed that only two of the eight assisted suicides had detectable levels of antidepressants in their blood at death. It could be concluded that Kevorkian's assisted suicides were, for the most part, not being treated for depressive disorder.

Given Kevorkian's obvious zealous pursuit of active euthanasia, one suspects that at least his early assisted suicides were not adequately screened or processed, for example, in accordance with the Dutch rules (discussed earlier) or other safeguards. Strikingly, Hugh Gale is reputed to have asked Kevorkian to take off the carbon monoxide mask and terminate the dying process and was perhaps ignored by Kevorkian.

BOX 19.4. The Dutch Case

[The following are excerpts from reviews of Dr. Herbert Hendin's book, *Seduced by Death: Doctors, Patients, and the Dutch Cure*. See *Suicide and Life-Threatening Behavior* (1998)]

On June 26, 1997, the United States Supreme Court handed down a unanimous decision on physician-assisted suicide. All nine justices concurred that both New York and Washington's state bans on the practice should stand.

The picture (Hendin paints in the Netherlands) is a frightening one of excessive reliance on the judgment of physicians, a consensual legal system that places support of the physician above individual patient rights in order to protect the euthanasia policy, the gradual extension of practice to include administration of euthanasia without consent in a substantial number of cases, and psychologically naive abuses of power in the doctor–patient relationship.

(For example:) "Many patients come into therapy with sometimes conscious but often more unconscious fantasies that cast the therapist in the role of executioner. . . . It may also play into the therapists illusion that if he cannot cure the patient, no one else can either" (Hendin, 1997: 57).

Samuel Klagsburn, MD, says of Hendin's argument: "He is wrong . . . suffering needs to be addressed as aggressively as possible in order to stop unnecessary suffering."

Hendin claims that in the Netherlands, "despite legal sanction, 60% of (physician-assisted suicide/death) cases are not reported, which makes regulation impossible."

Hendin goes on the argue that "a small but significant percentage of American doctors are now practicing assisted suicide, euthanasia, and the ending of patients' lives without their consent." But one also has to wonder: what about all those patients being forced to live and suffer without the patients' consent?

Dr. Hendin is, after all, the former executive director and current medical director of the American Foundation for Suicide Prevention. What would really be news is if Hendin came out in favor of physician-assisted death. Certainly, there are abuses of any policy. But is that enough of a reason to fail to assist fellow human beings in unremitting pain to die more easily? Death is one the most natural things there is and often is the only relief for some of us.

CASE 19.3. The First 15 Kevorkian-Assisted Suicides

Public awareness of assisted-suicides has been focused on the "suicide doctor," Jack Kevorkian. Initially, with Janet Adkins, Dr. Kevorkian used a *suicide machine* ("Mercitron" ... there is a computer-programmed machine now in Australia that involves an IV and the last question (really) is, "do you want to end your life"?, push "yes" or "no" (are you SURE you wish to delete?). The machine essentially was a motor-driven, timed release of 3 IV bottles: in order (1) *thiopental or sodium pentathal* (an anesthetic producing rapid unconsciousness), (2) *succinylcholine* (a muscle paralyzer like *curare*), and (3) *potassium chloride* (KCl; which stops the heart). The machine was activated by the would-be suicide. All of Kevorkian's later assisted-suicides (after Adkins) were by a simple facial mask hooked up to a carbon monoxide cannister; with the CO flow lever being tripped by the suicides themselves (20 to 30 mgs of IV-injected morphine would also work for most nonnarcotic users).

'Each Patient Is Unique'

Dr. Kevorkian has helped 15 people commit suicide in Michigan. Wrote one, Susan Williams, 52, "I'm happy to have his assistance, since I am unable to do this myself."

Janet Adkins, 54
June 4, 1990, Portland, Ore.
Alzheimer's disease
Kevorkian charged with murder; case dismissed.

Sherry Miller, 43
Oct. 23, 1991
Roseville, Mich.
Multiple sclerosis
Miller took a lethal dose of carbon monoxide. Again, murder charges were dismissed.

Marjorie Wantz, 58
Oct. 23, 1991, Sodus, Mich.
A pelvic disease
Wantz took a fatal injection, alongside Sherry Miller, in a secluded cabin.

Susan Williams, 52
May 15, 1992, Clawson, Mich.
Multiple sclerosis
Williams, who also suffered a skin disease, died in her home. No charges were filed against Kevorkian.

Lois Hawes, 52
Sept. 26, 1992
Warren, Mich.
Lung cancer
Hawes took a lethal dose of carbon monoxide.

Catherine Andreyev, 46
Nov. 23, 1992
Moon Twp., Pa.
Cancer
Andreyev died in the company of four friends, at a home in suburban Detroit.

Marcella Lawrence, 67
Dec. 15, 1992, Clinton Twp., Mich.
Heart disease, emphysema
"I wish [the lawmakers] could have [my pain] for one night," Lawrence once said.

Marguerite Tate, 70
Dec. 15, 1992, Auburn Hills, Mich.
Lou Gehrig's disease
Tate died after inhaling carbon monoxide, alongside Lawrence, at Tate's home.

Jack Miller, 53
Jan. 20, 1993
Huron Twp., Mich.
Bone cancer, emphysema
Miller, a former tree trimmer, was the first man to commit suicide with Kevorkian's aid.

Stanley Ball, 82
Feb. 4, 1993
Leland, Mich.
Pancreatic cancer
Kevorkian, who doesn't like to travel, drove to northern Michigan to aid Ball.

Mary Biernat, 73
Feb. 4, 1993, Crown Point, Ind.
Breast cancer
Biernat, whose cancer had spread to her chest, died at Stanley Ball's home.

Elaine Goldbaum, 47
Feb. 8, 1993, Southfield, Mich.
Multiple sclerosis
Goldbaum died in her apartment. Police confiscated the equipment she used but didn't arrest Kevorkian.

Hugh Gale, 70
Feb. 15, 1993
Roseville, Mich.
Emphysema, heart disease
Gale died in his living room, his wife by his side.

Jonathan Grenz, 44, Feb. 18, 1993, Costa Mesa, Calif. Cancer of the neck, lungs and chest
Grenz, a former real-estate agent, inhaled carbon monoxide in the home of a friend of Kevorkian.

Martha Ruwart, 41
Feb. 18, 1993
Cardiff-by-the-Sea, Calif.
Ovarian cancer
Ruwart, a former computer software engineer, had moved to Michigan last year to be near family.

It is difficult to be objective and clear-headed about assisted suicide, just as it is with abortion. Paradoxically, Jack Kevorkian may actually end up setting euthanasia and doctor-assisted suicide back several years. Not only has he lost (1991) his Michigan medical license (he was a pathologist) and in 1998 was charged again with murder (manslaughter) and convicted in 1999 (after videotaping the dying of an assisted suicide for the CBS television program *60 Minutes*), but Michigan and many other states (including South Carolina) have introduced bills to make previously legal assisted suicide a possible felony now, with concurrent fines and imprisonment.

These new laws may have a chilling effect on both active and passive euthanasia, even for legitimate pain control ("palliative care") previously offered to dying patients by physicians and nurses. For example, in Michigan it is now a felony to assist a suicide. People who wish self-deliverance from their final pain and suffering now will be more likely to mutilate themselves (the equivalent of coat hanger abortions), to die alone and disgraced, and to feel generally abandoned in their time of greatest need.

Jack Kevorkian needs to be separated from the issue of assisted suicide. He may be hot-headed, antiacademic, sensational, and publicity seeking, and may even see himself as messianic (much like an Old Testament prophet). He seems to be increasingly self-centered, dogmatic, insecure, and rigid. Readers are invited to read his book *Prescription Medicide* and make up their own minds. But, and this is important, the issue of physician-assisted suicide or death itself is not silly and transitory.

Finally, a few words about *pain control* are in order in this context. Of course, everyone has to die eventually, and many of us will suffer machine-prolonged debilitating illness and pain that diminishes the quality of our lives. Suicide and death, permanent annihilation of consciousness (if there is no afterlife), are effective means of pain control. We speak here primarily of physical pain, but, of course, psychological pain can be excruciating, too. Pain cannot always be controlled short of death. Most narcotics (like morphine drips) put users at a risk of respiratory death. Furthermore, narcotics often cause altered consciousness, nightmares, nausea, panic, long periods of disrupted consciousness and confusion, addiction, and so on.

To be sure, pain control technology is progressing rapidly (e.g., spinal implant morphine pumps). There are hospices which encourage classic pain-killing drinks, such as Cicely Saunder's "Bromptom's Cocktail" (a mixed drink of gin, Thorazine, cocaine, heroin, and sugar). It is also possible to block nerves or to use sophisticated polypharmacy to soften pain.

But some pain is relatively intractable (e.g., bone cancers, lung disease with pneumonia, congestive heart failure in which the patient chokes to death on his or her own fluids, gastrointestinal obstructions, and amputation stump pain). A few physicians have even made the ludicrous death-in-life proposal to give hopeless terminally ill patients a general anesthesia to control their pain! We do not always get well or feel better. Sometimes we just need to die, not to be kept alive to suffer pointlessly—and we deserve to be helped to die in such instances.

RELIGIOUS ASPECTS OF SUICIDE

Religion can be defined as " belief in and reverence for a supernatural power or powers as creator and governor of the universe" (*American Heritage College Dictionary*, 1993: 1153) or "a set of beliefs, values, and practices based on the teachings of a spiritual leader" (Jesus Christ, Moses, Allah, Krishna, Buddha, etc.).

Usually, being religious tends to protect people from suicide. For example, we saw in Chapters 3 (Table 3.5) and 7 (Figure 7.4) that predominantly Catholic or Muslim countries tend to have low suicide rates (e.g., Egypt, the Philippines, Iran, Mexico, Ireland). Later on in this chapter we present data that show that most religiously active *individuals* also tend to have lower suicide rates. Of course, suicide cults (e.g., Jonestown, David Koresh's Branch Davidians, the Solar Order, and Heaven's Gate) are exceptions to the rule that religion is a protective factor (see Maris, 1997).

Early on in the Judeo-Christian tradition suicide was not forbidden (see Chapter 4); in fact Jesus himself was a kind of sacrificial or altruistic suicide (he died "for our sins," the scriptures indicate). In the Christian Bible at least six or seven suicides are noted without disapproval. Conditions that the Bible implies justified suicide were (1) military defeat (Saul), (2) shame or justice (Judas), and (3) revenge (Sampson). It was not until St. Augustine's *City of God* (A.D. 412) and the Christian Council of Braga (A.D. 563) that the sixth commandment ("Thou shalt not kill") in the Book of Deuteronomy was interpreted to include suicide (self murder), as well as homicide. In fact, even homicide was all right if one was engaged in a "holy war" (cf. the Muslim *jihad*).

Most religions assert that we are not alone here on earth and that we are not fully in charge of our lives, that God has plans and purposes for us (although his or her will may be inscrutable). Religions tend to teach that our 70 to 80 years of life here on earth are not all there is. We may survive the death of our physical bodies and live on after death as spirits, souls, or disembodied minds. Hindus teach that we may be reborn in this world (the concept of transmigration of souls or samsara) and Buddhists argue that our physical bodies are not our true selves.

Most world religions contend that if we follow their scriptures, we will be rewarded (usually in heaven or a more perfect existence), but if we defy God and his or her teachings, we will suffer both in this life and in the afterlife (usually in hell or through forced rebirth). Judeo-Christian religions maintain that suffering and misfortune may actually be *good* for us (e.g., as in the *Book of Job*) and that God often tests us and our faith. Thus, suicide is an affront to God's will and can be seen as our all-too-human way out of his or her plans and purposes for our lives. As noted earlier, the real sin of suicide is hubris (the Greek word for "pride"), in which we selfishly put our own will ahead of God's will or simply drop out of life. Most religions contend that God would not give us more trials and tribulations than we could bear.

Typically, Protestants have higher suicide rates than do Catholics. This may be rooted in Martin Luther's idea of the "priesthood of all believers." That is, Protestants typically assume greater individual responsibility for their own salvation and for the resolution of their daily problems.

Catholics are more communal and protected by ritual (by the catechism, communion, saying the rosary, etc.) than Protestants are. Catholics tend to view the taking of life under most circumstances as solely the prerogative of God and, thus, tend to find suicide, abortion, euthanasia, capital punishment, and so on, all equally sinful and abhorrent. Jews tend to be a little less protected against suicide than Catholics are but a little more protected than Protestants.

Unfortunately, there are few empirical data on religion and suicide (see, e.g., McIntosh's [1996] review of doctoral dissertations on suicide, 1990–1995). The U.S. Census Bureau and Department of Vital Statistics are forbidden by the Constitution from surveying religious behaviors or opinions (Early's 1992 survey of the U.S. African American community is about all there is). In *Pathways to Suicide* (Maris, 1981) a sample survey about religion and suicide in Chicago was conducted, but there have not been other good, well-designed, empirical studies, with controls, concerning suicide and religion. As a result, we really do not know much about religion and suicide and tend to rely instead on theory and small ad hoc samples. We now turn to some of the Chicago data on religion and suicide.

Empirical Evidence on Religious Behavior and Suicide Rates

Well, does religion protect against suicide or not? What do the facts or data tell us (see Maris, 1981)? The short answer is that religion does tend to protect us from suicide, both individually and collectively, but it is not a simple causal connection. There are other variables or factors involved.

Much of our data is indirect and is "contaminated" by culture, ethnicity, and so on; such as in suicide rates by countries that are predominantly Catholic, Muslim, Protestant, Jewish, Buddhist, or Hindu (see Table 3.5 and Figure 7.4). Such data are inconclusive. For example, in Table 3.5 Hungary (with the second highest suicide rate) and Austria (with the fifth highest suicide rate) have some of the *highest* suicide rates in the world and are predominantly Catholic (68% and 90%, respectively). However, the Philippines (whose suicide rate is 65th) and Mexico (54th) have some of the *lowest* suicide rates in the world and are also predominantly Catholic (80 and 90%, respectively). Clearly, Catholic religion alone does not protect one against suicide; there must be other contributing factors involved.

We see a similar empirical pattern in predominantly Protestant countries. For example, Sweden and Finland are mainly Protestant countries (Lutheran) and have high suicide rates; whereas Norway, also predominantly Lutheran, has a relatively low suicide rate.

In countries with a Buddhist history, Japan has a high suicide rate (12th in the world), but Korea and China tend to have suicide rates in the middle range. Most Muslim countries (e.g., Iran and Egypt) tend to have low suicide rates. For comments on predominantly Hindu suicides in India, including *sati* or *suttee, karma,* and reincarnation, see Rao, in Farberow, 1975.

Glossing over the above subtleties, generally Protestants have the highest suicide rates, followed by Catholics (second), and Jews (third). However, when Maris examined Jewish suicides during World War II (Maris, 1981a: 246) buried in the only Jewish cemetery in Berlin (Weissensee), there was a dramatic increase in Jews suiciding as the war progressed (cf. Sonnefeld, 1998):

1940 = 59 suicides
1941 = 254
1942 = 811
1943 = 214
1944 = 34
1945 = 2

In the aforementioned Chicago sample survey of suicide, Maris (1981) was able to get direct information on religion and suicide, and to compare it with similar data in New York City. Table 19.1 reveals that overall in both Chicago and New York City Protestants have the highest suicide rates, followed by Catholics and Jews, in that order. Protestant and Catholic males (but not Jews) have suicide rates at least twice those of females, and in the oldest age group (age 65+) male suicide rates exceed female rates by a ratio of 3 to 1.

In data not presented here, Chicago Protestant and Catholic men preferred firearms and Protestant women preferred poisons as suicide methods (remember these data are from the 1960s and there probably have been changes). Catholic women preferred hanging in Chicago but poison in New York City. Jumping suicides were much more common in New York City across all religions and genders (Maltsberger, 1998, says that 40% of all suicides in New York City are by jumping). Note that Durkheim had predicted that suicide rates would have Protestants highest, Jews second, and Catholics third.

TABLE 19.1. Suicide Rate (per 100,000) by Religion, Age, and Sex, New York City, 1963–1967, and Cook County, Illinois, 1966–1968

Locality religion and race	≤24		25–44		45–64		≥65	
	M	F	M	F	M	F	M	F
Cook County[a]								
White Protestants	25	12	16	10	28	13	40	14
White Jews	22	—	15	—	28	—	26	—
White Catholics	13	7	11	8	16	6	24	8
New York City[a]								
White Protestants	47	19	46	17	42	22	62	20
White Jews	18	15	15	12	15	15	27	19
White Catholics	15	7	10	6	16	8	30	11

Source: Maris (1981: 248). Copyright 1981 by Johns Hopkins University Press. Reprinted by permission.
[a]Based on 1,056 white suicides in Cook County, Illinois, and on 2,975 white suicides in New York City. Percentages rounded off to nearest whole number.

Of course, religious preference or affiliation is not the same as religious activity or actual *behavior*. In data not shown here, nonfatal suicide attempters and suicide completers were less likely than natural deaths or a nonsuicidal national sample to attend church every week. Table 19.2 further shows that all suicides, regardless of their religious preference or gender, were much less likely to attend Christmas services than was the general nonsuicidal population. To sum up: Suicide completers and attempters are generally less involved in their religious communities and activities than is the general nonsuicidal population.

Thus, there is some modest empirical evidence that religion does protect against suicide. Protestant males have the highest suicide rates and were the least involved religiously. Catholic females had the lowest suicide rates and were the most involved religiously. Early (1992) and Nisbet (1995, 1998) provide similar data on African-American suicidal behaviors and ideation and the influence of religion.

Nevertheless, as we argue in the next section, if the norms, values, or objectives of a religion are in favor of suicide (as in the cults of Heaven's Gate, Branch Davidians, Order of the Solar Temple, or Jonestown), then clearly religion or social integration of a religious community does *not* protect one from suicide—quite the opposite.

TABLE 19.2. Church Attendance at Christmas by Sex, Suicide, and Nonsuicide (General) Samples, Cook County, Illinois (Whites)

Church services last Christmas	Protestant males[a]		Protestant females[b]		Catholic males[d]		Catholic females[d]	
	General	Suicide	General	Suicide	General	Suicide	General	Suicide
Did not attend	53	52	54	50	20	43	7	31
Attended	45	19	44	26	80	36	93	45
DK	2	29	2	24	0	21	0	24
Total	100%	100%	100%	100%	100%	100%	100%	100%
	(125)	(57)	(249)	(69)	(101)	(72)	(151)	(51)

Source: Maris (1981: 253). Copyright 1981 by Johns Hopkins University Press. Reprinted by permission.
[a]$Z = 2.1$, $p < .05$; [b]$Z = 1.0$, not significant; [c]$Z = 4.5$, $p < .001$; [d]$Z = 6.0$, $p < .001$.

Religious Cults and Concepts of Afterlife and Death

Religion as an institution typically concerns itself with death and the meaning or purpose of life. In many world religions the goal of life involves spiritual development, which transcends earthly flesh-and-blood existence. Christians, Buddhists, and Hindus all contend that the true self is not the physical body. In a sense, then, part of our "false self" has to die for us to be able to achieve spiritual maturity. The end of life in a sense is beyond earthly life—for example, in heaven, the afterlife, *nirvana*, or *moksha* (i.e., in spiritual enlightenment and fulfillment).

If we are evil, selfish, deluded, or accumulate bad *karma*, we cannot escape this world or we may go to hell or otherwise be punished. The bottom line is that many religions share with suicides the idea of escaping from pain and suffering of this world (see Maris, 1981: 258) and going to a better place or a different kind of existence, especially after death. Thus, it is not surprising that some religions are in effect "death cults" and may see suicide as a release from this "vale of tears" or even a graduation to a more perfect spiritual afterlife.

When Maris (1981) surveyed Chicago suicides, suicide completers were much more likely (82%) than natural deaths (51%) or nonfatal suicide attempters (68%) to conceive of death as "escape from pain and suffering" (Z test for death as escape, $p = .001$ for suicides vs. natural deaths). The second most common concept of death among all three groups (i.e., natural deaths, suicide completers, and nonfatal suicide attempters) was the belief that the death of our physical bodies was not the end of life but, rather, marked a transition to an "afterlife" of some kind (Maris, 1981: 258).

Perhaps the best way to illustrate how religious cults can become suicidal death cults is to consider briefly two examples: Jonestown and Heaven's Gate. Probably the most well known mass suicide in history took place November 18, 1978, when between 908 and 914 followers of Jim Jones drank cyanide and depressant-laced Kool-Aid (although a few members of the cult were shot to death—including Jones himself) in the jungle of Guyana, South America, at "Jonestown" (see Chidester, 1991).

Jones grew up in Indiana. His mother believed that her son eventually would become the messiah. Jones's father was a bigot, racist, and Klu Klux Klan member. Jones attended Butler University and was originally a Methodist minister. Later on Jones abandoned mainstream Christianity. He performed many evangelical faith-healing "miracles," which were really cheap tricks, such as producing chicken entrails while supposedly purging the ill of their cancers.

Many members of the People's Temple were poor, relatively uneducated African Americans, who signed over the deeds to their homes or life insurance policies to Jim Jones. In California (the Temple was in San Francisco before Guyana) family members began to protest to Congressman Leo Ryan about losing their estates property, money, and birthrights to Jones.

Partly to escape local ill will, Jones and his cult fled to Guyana, in north central South America. There he and the cult became even more isolated and extremist. For example, Jones came to believe that the world would be destroyed soon (the "apocalypse") by nuclear war. He grew increasingly paranoid, especially as some of his co-leaders (like Grace Stoen, with whom Jones had fathered a son; she later sued Jones for custody) defected.

The cult lived in crowded conditions in temperatures often exceeding 100 degrees Fahrenheit. Physical beatings, promiscuity (particularly by Jones), sexual abuse, and incest were commonplace in Jonestown (no wonder the cult called Jones "Father"!). Jones practiced a form of terrorism reminiscent of Orwell in which children and spouses spied on family members (who were often forbidden by Jones to have sex with their own spouses) and then told Jones, who chastised and/or severely punished (e.g., beat) the transgressors (cf. George Orwell's *1984*).

Preparing for the end of the world, which he thought was imminent, Jones held drills or practices (which he called white nights but were in fact "black nights") in which cult members drank Kool-Aid, not knowing whether or not it was poisoned—to prove their faith and loyalty to Jones. Note that in most cults it is the charismatic leader's intentions that are crucial. In effect, Jones himself decided that over 900 men, women, and children should commit suicide—not the cult members themselves.

A second example of a suicidal religious cult is Marshall Herff Applewhite and Bonnie Lu Nettles's Heaven's Gate (see Steiger & Hewes, 1997). On March 26, 1997, 38 members of the cult committed suicide in San Diego (Rancho Santa Fe), California.

Dressed all in black and wearing Nike sneakers, the cult members poisoned (using Humphry's methods described previously) their earthly bodies (which they called vehicles, containers, or shells) in an elaborate death ritual (including draping their bodies in shrouds and putting $5 in quarters in their pockets—for "long distance" calls?), hoping to get into a spaceship they thought was hidden in the tail of the Hale-Bopp comet.

The two leaders of the Heaven's Gate cult were originally from Houston, Texas. Applewhite was a former college music teacher (with an MA in music from the University of Colorado), opera singer, and choir director. He was the son of a Presbyterian minister. Bonnie Lu Nettles was an ex-nurse and astrologist, who died of cancer in 1985. They were know as "Bo" (Marshall) and "Peep" (Bonnie).

Taking their scriptural base mainly from the Book of Revelation, they believed in human individual metamorphosis (HIM). The idea was that a human being could metamorphize through ascetic discipline, hard work, and strict dieting and evolve to a higher kingdom. To prepare for the journey to this utopia one had to give up alcohol, tobacco, sex (even sometimes be castrated), work and regular jobs, and most material possessions. Salvation resulted from fasting and hard disciplined work.

Applewhite believed that if one prepared correctly, human beings could undergo "*chrysalis*" (i.e., become transformed like caterpillars into butterflies). He also thought that such perfected, enlightened beings could change their vibration rates, allowing them to disappear from sight, then reappear.

Applewhite contended that he had come to earth on a spaceship (a UFO) and only "woke up" to his real-life mission in his 30s. For the cult transformation was *bodily*, not just spiritual. The cult actually thought their perfected bodies were being transported to a higher level in a hidden spaceship.

The Heaven's Gate cult argued that when we leave this world we are "harvested." "Eschatology" refers to the science of the last days of the world as we know it—the close of this age. Marshall Applewhite believed the world was nearing a cataclysmic crisis and was about to be "recycled." Through suicide the Heaven's Gate cult members felt they escaped this world (a sinking ship, if you will) just in time.

In the next and concluding section of this chapter we examine the Kantian and Utilitarian philosophical perspectives on suicide.

PHILOSOPHICAL APPROACHES TO SUICIDE

We defined philosophy generally in the opening pages of this chapter as the love and pursuit of wisdom. Although philosophy subsumes ethics, it is more than ethics, and although religious people tend to be philosophical, they are also often irrational. Philosophy is distinct as a system of inquiry that is rigorously logical or mathematical. Often philosophers are seen as calm and rational, able to think clearly, unaffected by emotion, even as somewhat disembodied minds. Philosophy tends to be abstract and formal; a discipline many contend is focused more on method than on substance (see Plato, Aristotle, Kant, Hume, Russell, or Wittgenstein).

Some readers may be disturbed by philosophical discussions of suicide, in part because philosophy examines critically that which most of us take for granted: that life in almost all circumstances should be preserved. To suggest that suicide might make sense or be rational in some circumstances leaves many people dumbfounded, like the suggestion that there might not be a God or an afterlife. Unfortunately, many good religious people, well-intending suicide preventers, or compassionate clinicians seem to study philosophy (if at all) only to be able to defend their own dogma or biases. In fact, the study of philosophy can be disturbing. Whatever the truth is, we need to be prepared to go where it takes us.

The Kantian Perspective

There have been two basic philosophical perspectives in the study of suicide: the Kantian and the Utilitarian (see Battin & Maris, 1983; Battin, 1996). The ideal person, according to Immanuel Kant, is a rational agent with autonomy of will. Presumably, most suicidal behaviors compromise either the ideal of rationality or autonomy in some important way. Kant would argue that suicide is a violation of one's duty to oneself (see Kant, 1909: 80–116; cf. Rawls, 1971, on a Rawlsian value-free notion of rationality; rationality is taking the most effective means to a given end).

For example, Hill (1983) says that impulsive, apathetic, self-abasing, or hedonistic suicides deviate from an *ideal* (not from others' interests, values, or effect on others). Kant thought that suicide was *always* wrong, or nearly always wrong, because it throws away or degrades humanity in oneself. Hill's modified Kantian ideal would permit some suicides; for example, for persons facing the onset of permanent vegetative states, those in irremediable pain, or persons who act from strong moral convictions.

Kantians are nonconsequentialists. They believe that one ought to honor contracts and keep promises. Some Kantians assert formal moral rules reminiscent of Kant's so-called categorical imperative, such as the commandment in the book of Deuteronomy: "Thou shalt not kill."

The Utilitarian Perspective

Utilitarians, on the other hand, look at consequences. They might ask, What outcomes or consequences would my suicide have not just for me but for my family, for others, or for society in general? Utilitarians try to imagine what the results of a suicide might be. Bentham argued that we should "seek the greatest happiness for the greatest number" or the greatest balance of pleasure over pain.

Utilitarians argue that it is wrong to suicide if it will cause other persons anguish, sorrow, or emotional, social, legal or financial hardship.

However, Narveson (1983) contends that we own ourselves. He thinks that our bodies belong *to us* and ultimately we can do what we want to with them—as long as it does not clearly harm others. We do not have an obligation to "carry on" no matter how hard things are. We do not have to keep living just to satisfy the whims or capricious desires of remote others. Of course, we do not always *know* the consequences of our suicide in advance, so it is difficult to rationally assess them.

Most utilitarians argue that we are not just "private property." Suicide may solve the suicide's problems but cause immense damages to those who love or depend on the suicide.

Suicide is a selfish act most of the time. For example, many older white males tend to end their own pain without serious consideration of the consequences of their suicides for their children, spouses, colleagues, or friends (see Maris, 1982b).

Whose Life is It?

As we have seen, part of the philosophical issue in suicide is, Who owns our bodies? Narveson (1983: 240–253) contends that we are not the slaves of any other individual or of the community. That is, we own ourselves (see Box 19.5). As philosopher John Locke wrote: "Every man has a *property* in his own person," we own ourselves. It seems absurd to say: "It's your life, but you cannot do anything with it." The composer Brahms reputedly destroyed manuscripts of dozens of musical works which he thought were unworthy of publication. It may be our loss too and make us sad, but it was Brahms's property rights.

Narveson argues that surely we need not continue living just to satisfy someone else's values or interests. What if I and others value my life differently? Narveson would say I have the right to suicide if my suicide does not clearly harm others (but this criterion would seem to deter many suicides, would it not?).

BOX 19.5. Whose Life Is It, Anyway?

In a 1981 movie Richard Dreyfuss starred as a young sculptor, Ken Harrison, who was in a car wreck and overnight became a quadriplegic. After the accident Harrison becomes depressed and wants to starve himself to death in the hospital.

The central issue in the film is who decides life-and-death issues; power is a critical fact. Dr. Emerson (John Cassavetes) is Harrison's attending physician. Emerson forces Harrison to take 10-mg Valium injections and to undergo other treatments. When Harrison gets lawyer and a psychiatrist to sue the hospital to allow him to die (writ of *habeus corpus*), Emerson hires his own psychiatrist in an effort to have Harrison declared mentally incompetent.

The hospital argument is that if a patient is depressed, he or she cannot rationally decide to commit suicide or allow euthanasia. There is a "Catch-22" involved: If you want to suicide, you're crazy; if you were sane, you would never want to suicide. Thus, anyone wanting to suicide cannot make an informed decision, just because of the fact of his or her wanting to suicide alone.

The Harrison case is interesting because usually hospital euthanasia involves patients (such as Cruzan or Quinlan) who are brain dead or in coma. In Harrison's case only his brain was really alive; he felt nothing from the neck down.

At one point Harrison says: "If I were a dog or a cat that had been hit by a car, you would put me to sleep." Why should being a human being force individuals into expensive suffering just to please doctors, family, the state, the clergy, etc.?

Throughout the film Harrison uses humor as a psychological defense. As Freud argued, sometimes a sense of humor or resignation is all that keeps us going.

Another interesting aspect of the Harrison case was that he became sexually impotent after the paralysis. Is life worthwhile, if we cannot have sexual experiences? Harrison broke up with his fiancee but continued to flirt with a student nurse and a female doctor.

In the end Harrison is heard by a judge and is given the right to his own body. Still, it is not clear at movie's end if Harrison will now in fact decide to end his life. The real issue seemed to be getting the right to his own body, not the actual decision to exercise that right through suicide.

Pain is probably the most common reason given for a "rational" suicide. Empathy and love aside, no one else has to or *can* feel *my* pain. Early on in my career Maris wrote a master's thesis on Ludwig Wittgenstein's "private language argument" (see Wittgenstein, 1953; Maris, 1961). Wittgenstein inquires how we learn to use "sensation" (*Empfindung*) words such as "toothache." Because my mother never had my pain, how do I *know* that she taught me the correct word association for what I was sensing? Is there a private language of sensation, in which only I (or you) really know what my (your) pain words denote? The short answer is "no," language and words are public, not private; they connote common usage, not denote private experiences (says Wittgenstein).

In February 1985, Douglas Jacobs invited libertarian psychiatrist Thomas Szasz to speak on suicide prevention at the Harvard Medical School (Maris, 1986). Clearly, for Szasz, the individual's life belongs to him or her, not to God, the state, society, family, or friends. Szasz (1985) writes:

- "The only person ultimately responsible for suicide is the actor himself" (3).
- "Suicide prevention downgrades the individual's responsibility for the conduct of his own life and death" (19).
- "Psychiatrists should get out of the suicide business" (21).
- "We regard throwing away useless junk as quite reasonable, but we regard throwing away a useless life as a sign of mental illness" (Szasz, 1977, 111).

Of course, each of Szasz's points could be and was challenged (see Maris, 1986).

Would You Want a Philosopher as Your Psychotherapist?

When all is said and done and an individual is facing death, would he or she want a philosopher as a psychotherapist or death *confidant*? Imagine having Plato/Socrates, David Hume, Bertrand Russell, Ludwig Wittgenstein, or even Peggy Battin (who is a nice person) at your bedside. And if not, why not? Is it that most of us really do not want to take the responsibility for deciding to end our own lives—that we really want to be *told* (paternalism or maternalism) what to do, especially when it comes to suicide? More important, we suspect that most of us would like to be *talked out of* suicide, or at least hear some good arguments *for continuing to live*! Suicide or death is, after all, an irrevocable decision.

Another important consideration is that most of us do not want to be alone at the moment of our death. If suicide is our private right and our own individual decision, it can be a lonely event. Of course, our loved ones could support our decision to die and be there to the end. In any case in our experience people fear being alone more than they fear pain or death.

SUMMARY AND CONCLUSIONS

This chapter reviewed major ethical, religious, and philosophical issues in suicide. Among the key topics in the chapter were Derek Humphry's *Final Exit* and its fatal recipes, Dr. Jack Kevorkian's crusade for legalizing physician-assisted suicide, and Jim Jones and suicide cults.

We asked whether suicide is ever appropriate and, if so, under what circumstances? The chapter listed some conditions for possible rational suicides (like those of Nico Speijer) without really deciding the issue. Is "rational suicide" an oxymoron?—probably not. The chapter reviewed Maris's presidential address to the American Association of Suicidology and what could be meant by being "rational." Although suicide is usually not the best alternative to human pain (psychache), some suicides are more rational than others.

Another key current issue is whether we (especially physicians) should help terminally ill or emotionally hopeless patients die. If we do not, is that not abandonment or paternalism? We noted that euthanasia can be active or passive, voluntary or involuntary, and direct or indirect. We reviewed Derek Humphry's work and the various referenda (in Oregon, California, Washington, Michigan, etc.) for establishing assisted suicide laws. The guidelines for assisted suicide in the Netherlands were noted, along with strong objections by Dr. Herbert Hendin. Oregon's physician-assisted suicide law was considered in some detail.

Next we reviewed Dr. Jack Kevorkian's assisted suicides, starting with Janet Adkins in 1990 and continuing up to his 1999 manslaughter conviction for assisting a suicide on the CBS television program *60 Minutes*. To date, Jack Kevorkian has assisted over 100 suicides, most by carbon monoxide poisoning administered by the would-be suicides themselves. Although Dr. Kevorkian may be an iconoclastic zealot, the issue he addresses is important and will not go away. Some pain (physical and psychological) is intractable. Why do we give animals in such conditions deadly morphine injections but do not give such injections to human beings?

Most world religions proscribe suicide; for example, based on the Judeo-Christian scriptures, suicide may be considered a violation of the sixth commandment in the Book of Deuteronomy,

"Thou shalt not kill." Many religions regard our life and death as properly controlled by God, not by ourselves. Although religion tends to protect us, clearly other factors are at work, too (otherwise how could overwhelmingly Catholic Austria have one of the highest suicide rates in the world?). Some religious cults have actually become in effect suicide cults (such as Jonestown, Waco, Heaven's Gate, and the Solar Order).

Philosophy critically examines suicide in a logical and rational manner. The German philosopher Kant contended that suicide was *always* wrong; that is, it violated one's duty to oneself or the ideal of being human. On the other hand, utilitarians are consequentialists. For example, if our suicide would not do harm to others and would solve our problems, then utilitarians contend it might be rational. A key philosophical issue is, Whose life is it? Our own, our family and friend's, the state's, God's? Finally, we asked: Would you want a philosopher at the side of your deathbed or would you prefer some more affectually biased family member to be there, who loved you and did not want to let you "go"?

Chapter 20 turns from ethics, religion, and philosophy to explicit legal issues. What do U.S. courts say about suicide? What are the major types of suicides cases? Note the obvious: one's ethical, religious, or philosophical beliefs or arguments may be very different from what the law allows or sanctions.

FURTHER READING

Battin, M. P. (1996). *The death debate: Ethical issues in suicide*. Upper Saddle River, NJ: Prentice-Hall. A shortish academic treatise by a very bright and prolific philosopher, Margaret "Peggy" Battin, with a foreword by Dr. Timothy Quill. There are extensive notes for each of seven chapters. Battin surveys religious views for and against suicide, social arguments for and against suicide (including utilitarianism), Kant and the sanctity of human life arguments, paternalistic interventions, and suicide as a fundamental human right (whose life is it?) and concludes with a thorough consideration of physician-assisted suicide.

Early, K. E. (1992). *Religion and suicide in the African-American community*. Westport, CT: Greenwood Press. Does the African American church contribute to the low suicide rate of black

Americans, especially of black females? Early (in his sociology doctoral dissertation at the University of Florida) surveyed African pastors and 220 members of black churches. He concluded that the black church and family provide amelioration or buffering of social forces (alcoholism and substance abuse, depression, disrupted families and divorce, poverty, etc.) that would otherwise promote suicide. See similar work by Paul Nisbet in the psychiatry department at the University of Rochester Medical School. Such empirical studies of religion and suicide are rare.

Humphry, D. (1996). *Final exit: the practicalities of self-deliverance and assisted-suicide for the dying* (rev. 2nd ed.). New York: Bantam Doubleday Dell. First published in 1991 (see Maris, 1992: 514–516), *Final Exit* is subtitled "the practicalities of self-deliverance and assisted suicide for the dying." It is dedicated to helping the terminally ill have a "good death." Humphry addresses making the decision to die, getting a medical doctor to help, legal ramifications, the preferred methods or recipes for self-deliverance, life insurance, and social and psychological support. Much of the profits from *Final Exit* have gone to promote citizen initiatives (in Washington, California, and Oregon) legalizing physician-assisted suicide.

Kevorkian, J. (1991). *Prescription medicide: The goodness of planned death*. Buffalo, NY: Prometheus Books. Of course, all of us know something about the infamous "Dr. Death," Jack Kevorkian, a pathologist from Michigan, who, after his conviction (manslaughter) for a CBS *60 Minutes* episode on TV assisted suicide, had helped more than 100 people die. In *Prescription Medicide* we get a fascinating view of Kevorkian's iconoclastic personality, thirst for publicity, and his crusade against academia, U.S. prisons and courts, and the medical establishment. He advocates a new suicide machine ("mercitron"), a new medical specialty ("obiatry"), and a new form of euthanasia ("medicide") performed only by medical doctors.

Maris, R. W. (1981). The religious factor: Religion, culture, and concepts of death in suicide. In *Pathways to suicide: A survey of self-destructive behaviors* (Ch. 9). Baltimore, MD: Johns Hopkins University Press. One of the big problems in the study of religion and suicide is the conspicuous absence of empirical data. Maris was able to get a sample of Chicago suicides and the ask questions about the individual's religious attitudes and behaviors. Generally, he found that religious affiliation and activity tends to protect one against suicide (if the group's religious norms are against suicide). Of course, if one belongs to a death cult (such as Jonestown or Heaven's Gate), then religion is a risk factor, not a protective factor. Suicides were much more likely than controls to see death as an escape from pain and suffering.

Werth, J. L., Jr. (1996). *Rational suicide? Implications for mental health professionals*. Washington, DC: Taylor & Francis. Most people tend to assume that "rational suicide" is an oxymoron; that is, that all suicides are irrational (e.g., the products of mental disorder, impulse discontrol, stress, and anger). Werth counters that it is possible to make a rational decision to suicide. His book reviews the history of suicide, arguments against rational suicide, mental health professionals' attitudes toward rational suicide, criteria for rational suicide, ethical and legal implications, and future predictions. Werth concludes that there are no absolutes when working with suicidal individuals.

20

Suicide and the Law

Traditionally, society has felt that it was necessary to assign blame for every death, either to God (natural, accidental) or to man (homicide, suicide). If God was the responsible agent, nothing more needed to be done, but if man was to blame, there must be punishment for the guilty.

—ROBERT E. LITMAN

Perhaps one of the greatest paradoxes in modern attitudes toward suicide is that it is viewed not only as an intensely personal act of self-annihilation but also as an act for which others may be held to blame. Understanding this apparent contradiction requires us to have a historical perspective on social and cultural attitudes toward suicide.

A thorough review of this history is not within the scope of this chapter (however, see Chapter 4). But a brief iteration of sociocultural attitudes toward suicide, particularly with reference to issues of blameworthiness, sets the stage for our understanding modern Western views. In the Roman empire, suicides were often extolled as acts of civic duty and moral virtue, for example, when life was viewed as painful or purposeless. Suicides that affected the finances or security of the state were generally held to be dishonorable. Thus, a criminal facing death and the confiscation of his property for the commission of a felony could be charged with a second crime if he took his own life before trial (in an attempt to pass on his estate to his family). Slaves, who themselves, were their masters' property, were forbidden from "stealing" that property through their own suicide. Likewise, soldiers, as property of the state and necessary for the security of the state, were forbidden to "desert" through suicide. Good help was apparently hard to find and/or replace!

Between baptism and death, according to the Christian church, lay a lifetime of possible transgressions. Martyrdom guaranteed redemption, blissful immortality, and family income from the church. By teaching that life's purpose was to be free of sin in order to achieve the rewards of the hereafter, Christianity unintentionally promoted suicide as a means of providing a sort of "afterlifetime guarantee." This presented an embarrassing problem for the church. Accordingly, St. Augustine (A.D. 354–430) in *The City of God* vigorously expressed Christianity's unequivocal rejection of suicide as a violation of the sixth commandment: "Thou shalt not kill." Suicide was a mortal sin, the consequence of which was hell, not heaven.

As suicide now was considered a crime against God and ecclesiastical penalties resulted, later church writings added secular reasoning to bolster their objections to suicide. For example, St. Thomas Aquinas (1225–1274) concluded that a person killing himself both usurps God's power (to decide life and death) and injures the community of which he is a part.

The state soon echoed these arguments by providing civil mandates against suicide. A suicide in the Middle Ages was denied burial in consecrated ground (and, instead, was buried at the crossroads with a stake through the heart) and forfeited his goods to the state. The role of the coroner was established to rule on suicides, thereby enriching the royal coffers (if the suicide were a *felo de se*, a "felony against the self"). On the other hand, if the coroner's court decided that the perpetrator was deprived of reason due to madness, transient insanity, or young age, sanctions and penalties did not accrue. Thus, the link between suicide and pathology and society's concern for both the causes of suicide and its effects on survivors was established and recognized.

In the Massachusetts Bay Colony, Puritans continued to deny Christian burials to those who suicided but (choosing not to punish families) did not confiscate their goods (cf. Kushner, 1991: 21–27). By the mid-18th century, in both England and the United States, verdicts of insanity (*non compos mentis*) were increasingly common in cases of suicide, replacing almost entirely the earlier view of suicide as a felony. This transformation, from viewing suicide as a crime to one of disease, coincided with the development of modern U.S. psychiatry and the replacement of bloodletting by pharmacological intervention. Concepts of treatment and prevention replaced that of punishment, and the role of the caregiver began. Correspondingly, a shift in social attitudes to an enlightened view of mental illness shifted the concept of blameworthiness away from the individual, now seen as acting with diminished capacity, to society as custodial caretaker of the individual needing protection from himself (the concept of *parens patriae*).

However, society has not ceased to condemn suicide. The coroner, or medical examiner, continues to act as the representative of the state, assigning responsibility for each death to God (natural, and some accidental) or man (homicide, suicide, and some accidental). Surviving family members continue to feel stigmatized by suicide, sometimes pressuring coroners to change determinations to protect the family from a feared social condemnation. The suicide's survivors understandably may seek to externalize any self-blame by holding custodial caretakers responsible (blameworthy) for failing to protect their loved one from him- or herself.

Survivors also have reason to protect against the forfeiture of property, theirs as part of the suicide's estate. Life insurance policies, meant to compensate the family for the loss of a loved one and his or her future earning capacity, usually contain clauses excluding benefits for death due to suicide within 1 or 2 years of the date application was made. As it is assumed that in suicide the time of death is in the insured's control, insurance companies protect themselves against insureds having such an unfair advantage in their actuarial bet (i.e., of securing financial benefits for their decedents through a planned and premature death). A denial of insurance benefits often leads to contested manners of death, the determination of which may take place in the courtroom. The burden of the claimant in such cases is to prove that the death was an accident; it is the insurance company's burden to prove that the decedent intended to cause his or her own death (i.e., suicided).

Hence, we arrive at the foci for this chapter on *suicide and the law*. We first examine expectations of responsible caretaking (i.e., to prevent suicide) and cases in which it has been alleged that the caretaker failed to meet those expectations and, thus, may be held responsible for the consequences of that failure. Then, we turn our attention to cases of contested life insurance claims, examining decisions for assigning responsibility for a death, the consequence of which may amount to hundreds of thousands of dollars in benefits to the estate of the insured.

PARENS PATRIAE

In the contemporary United States, social custom and statutory regulation demand safe environments. These environments range from conditions of work—as enforced in child labor laws or toxic waste disposal regulations—to everyday settings and products (e.g., smoke-free buildings and child-proof safety caps on medications). Thus, businesses and individuals have a mandated responsibility to protect against possible and foreseeable harm to others.

When required public safety and protection are not afforded and the consequence of that negligence is harm or injury, the law allows those harmed to seek compensatory damages. For example, a slip and fall on an unsalted icy pavement in front of a store may lead to monetary damages for injuries sustained. A *tort* is a civil wrong alleged to have caused injury. In the common law, assault, battery, and false imprisonment comprise a set of torts in which intentional injury is charged. Negligence is another type of tort in which, if an injury was a proximate result, liability for failing to meet a standard of conduct may be held (see *Black's Law Dictionary*, 1979: 930–931).

With regard to suicide (the injury), those potentially held liable in a tort action are therapists, institutions, employers, and even product manufacturers (Berman, 1993). For example, take the case of an employer charged with maintaining a safe work environment. If, for reasons of negligence, unsafe working conditions exist and these, in turn, cause an injury to an employee, workmen's compensation laws provide for compensatory monies for any treatment costs, loss of income, and so on, that may result. However, if that now disabled employee becomes increasingly despondent and isolated, self-medicates his depression with alcohol, and ultimately suicides, the employer's negligence may now be linked to the

CASE 20.1. The Case of Jose Garcia

Jose Garcia was a 64-year-old railroad engineer, a 29-year employee with an exceptional work history. One morning, while unloading rails off a flatcar, Mr. Garcia slipped on some grease and fell, fracturing his wrist severely enough to require surgery. Expecting to fully recover and return to work, Mr. Garcia was frustrated at the pace of his rehabilitation. He continued to complain of swelling, numbness, and pain which made even mundane household chores unmanageable. After 5 months of medical leave (and hope for recovery), Garcia's injury was ruled a permanent disability by company physicians and he was forcibly retired from the job. Garcia felt abandoned and betrayed by his employer and his doctors.

Moreover, he was a defeated man. He prided himself on his loyalty to his employer and blamed himself for "cheating" by not completing the mandatory 30 years to retirement. He also blamed the railroad for causing his injury. He felt trapped by his injury, frustrated that he could not recover, and increasingly hopeless about his future. Lacking a focus for his free time, he became increasingly restless, agitated, and irritable. He spoke of feeling worthless and burdensome and displayed symptoms of a clinical depression. A lifelong history of heavy alcohol use now further potentiated his depression and increased his withdrawal from family supports. After drinking almost a dozen beers within a 3-hour period, he ended his life by a gunshot blast to the head.

suicide and that employer may be held responsible for causing a wrongful death. Consider the case of Jose Garcia (Berman, 1992; Case 20.1).

Like links on a chain, Garcia's suicide can be directly tied, retrospectively, first to his acute alcohol intoxication, later to his interpersonal withdrawal and isolation, and sequentially back to his depression, his hopelessness, his loss of job, his disability, his injury, and, ultimately, to the cause of the injury (i.e., the grease on which he slipped on the flatcar). As the railroad had the responsibility for maintaining a safe workplace and work conditions, the railroad may be held liable for not meeting its legal obligation, the *proximate cause* of Mr. Garcia's suicide.

The case of *Wade v. Transcontinental Railroad* (both names are fictitious) was filed as a wrongful death complaint by Ellen Wade, the widow of Steven. Compensatory damages were asked for "medical, funeral, and burial expenses, loss of financial support, love, companionship, comfort, affection, society, and solace." Transcontinental was charged with negligently owning, managing, and operating dangerous premises and for maliciously failing to guard or warn against dangerous conditions. (See Case 20.2.)

The railroad was known not to lock its exit doors; all were openable by a latch. No warning light or delay mechanism was installed as a safety device. A disoriented passenger or one with blurred vision might as well think this was a door to a bathroom as an exit from the train. Furthermore, a neurologist consulting for the plaintiff argued that the "strobing effect" of light and dark shadows through a train window could precipitate a seizure and altered consciousness in a predisposed individual. Most damning to the railroad's defense was the testimony of a retired investigator for the railroad who said that "management always treated unwitnessed events (such as Wade's) as suicides.

SUICIDE AND SCHOOLS

A failure to implement policies and procedures designed to protect and safeguard students places schools and school personnel in a position equally vulnerable to that of employers, if a death results. Consider, for example, the case of *Smith v Williams County School Board et al.* (names are fictional). (See Case 20.3.) By allegedly failing to fulfill its mandated responsibilities and policies, if it can be shown that they indeed were informed of Bobby's verbal communications and behavior, school personnel would be seen as breaching duties to protect and safeguard and to warn. That breach will then be tied directly to Bobby's death, as, it will be argued, his parents were deprived of an opportunity to intervene and seek help for him. This case was settled out of court for $350,000.

In the same state, teachers were required for their teaching certificate to "be able to recognize signs of emotional distress in students and to apply crisis intervention techniques with emphasis on suicide prevention." The parents of one 14-year-old male who killed himself with a .44 caliber handgun in a school bathroom stall subsequently charged their son's teachers and school administrators with "negligent failure to recognize signs of emotional distress, to refer him to a guidance counselor, and to notify them." It was shown that their son was assigned to keep a composition notebook for his seventh-grade English class, in which assignments would be written, to be periodically reviewed by his teacher. On the front cover of the spiral notebook were written the words "all that lives is born to die," "HATE," and "Diary of a Suicide."

Figure 20.1 presents an example of this youngster's writings contained within the notebook. The trial court in this case held that the school board was at fault for not notifying this boy's parents after school officials learned of his suicide attempt at school. Table 20.1 offers a listing of selected school-based suicide court cases.

CASE 20.2. The Case of *Wade v. Transcontinental Railroad*

Steven Wade, age 37, was traveling home by train after a weekend visit to his sister-in-law and nephew some 200 miles from home. Some 2 hours from arrival, with the train traveling at an estimated 40 miles an hour, he left the train through an openable door, landed on the rocky train track bed, and died instantly from multiple blunt-force trauma. His body was found some 40 yards from the point of impact. Two books that Wade had been seen carrying were found near his body. Transcontinental called Wade's death a suicide and produced a passenger who described a passenger fitting Wade's description exhibiting "some rather bizarre, agitated behavior." This witness further reported that the passenger "was twitching, wringing his hands together, talking to himself, uttering unintelligible words." The county coroner, a forensic pathologist, however, determined that the death was an accident.

At the age of 6 Steven Wade suffered a skull fracture in a biking accident. As a result, he had a craniotomy and a mild residual learning disorder. Subsequent to a second (car) accident while in the Marines, he developed a multiple seizure disorder ("trauma epilepsy"), characterized by tunnel vision and sense alteration (complex partial seizures), right-side clonic movement (Jacksonian seizures), and brief confusion and blackouts (absence seizures) in addition to headaches with visual blurring. These had been treated with medications, successfully enough to allow Steven to complete theology school. At the time of his death Steven was on 65% Veterans Administration disability and was prescribed Depakote, 500 mg, three times a day. He also had a diagnosis of diabetes for which he took daily medicine. Notably, he left all of his medicines at home before boarding the train for his sister-in-law's.

Steven was described by family and friends as in good spirits at the time of the trip and under no notable stress. He rarely drank but for a glass of wine with dinner and gave no history of labile mood or erratic behavior. He was reported to be frustrated by his disability but not self-pitying or depressed. He was a planful sort, curious and tenacious when he wanted to learn (thus the books found with him) and proud of his achievements in spite of his disability. He had never talked of suicide.

A retired railroad investigator testified in this case about his observations that a number of elderly passengers had literally walked off trains traveling as fast as 90 miles an hour, especially as the trains went up and down over mountainous elevations. In fact, he alleged, the railroad had assigned special agents to watch for passengers who showed signs of altitude sickness, disorientation, or violent behavior, and had actually installed physical restraints in each car for these occasions.

SUICIDE IN CORRECTIONAL FACILITIES

Suicide is the leading cause of death in correctional facilities. The typical jail suicide is that of a young intoxicated male recently arrested for a misdemeanor. Isolated and alone, humiliated and fearful, the young offender opts for an available method (usually hanging) to quickly end his problems within the first hours or days of incarceration. As patterns, methods, and risk factors of suicide in correctional facilities have been well researched (see

---

CASE 20.3. The Case of Smith v. Williams County School Board et al.

Bobby Smith was a 13-year-old, sixth-grade student at Van Dyke Middle School. On November 17, 1995, Smith went to the backyard of his family home, strung a rope over a branch of a large oak tree, fashioned a noose, and completed suicide by hanging. His family subsequently filed a wrongful death suit against the County School Board and a number of school personnel.

The complaint specifically alleged that the school had a duty to formulate and implement policies and procedures to provide adequate training and supervision regarding suicide prevention and intervention which, in turn required a duty to inform superiors and procedures to intervene after a suicide threat or attempt, and a duty to safeguard and protect students. At the heart of these alleged duties was a statute ("The Suicide Prevention Act") passed by the state 3 years earlier that required local school boards to develop and implement such policies and procedures. The County School Board had, indeed, complied with the mandate from the state and, at the time of Bobby's death, had trained school personnel to developed procedures in three separate countywide in-service trainings. Included among these intervention procedures for dealing with potential student suicide was the requirement for personnel to "notify the family or guardian immediately" in the event of a student's suicide threat or attempt.

At issue, then, in this case were the following allegations of fact: Two days before his suicide (November 15) Bobby Smith, as usual, rode home on the school bus but stayed on the bus to the end of the line because he wanted to talk to the driver, a woman who had befriended him after classmates had picked on Bobby. She reported that Bobby felt he had no one to talk to, that he seemed down but not overly depressed, and that he did not talk of suicide. The next day (November 16) Bobby spoke of suicide to at least two classmates, who minimized the significance of his communications. Later that night one of these classmates told her mother, who called the principal of the school the next morning (November 17).

Around 2:30 P.M. on the afternoon of the 16th, as students were leaving school to catch their bus rides, Bobby was observed to be "acting weird" by a classmate. When Bobby then went into a school rest room, the classmate soon followed. There he interrupted Bobby tying his football jersey to a railing above a toilet. The classmate then reported his observations to a schoolteacher as he ran to catch his bus. Neither the teacher nor the principal notified Bobby's parents of these alleged incidents or intervened directly to talk with Bobby.

Welch & Gunther, 1997, for a review; cf. issues of the newsletter *Jail Suicide Mental Health Update*), approaches to prevention of suicide in these facilities have also been frequently presented. Jails and prisons have custodial responsibilities toward their inmates; thus, the need for preventive measures to protect inmates from foreseeable self-harm is reasonably expected as a duty of these facilities (usually, the 8th and 14th Amendments to the U.S. Constitution are cited). Once again, when that duty to prevent is allegedly breached, when policies and procedures are either not followed or not written, the staff, administrators, and

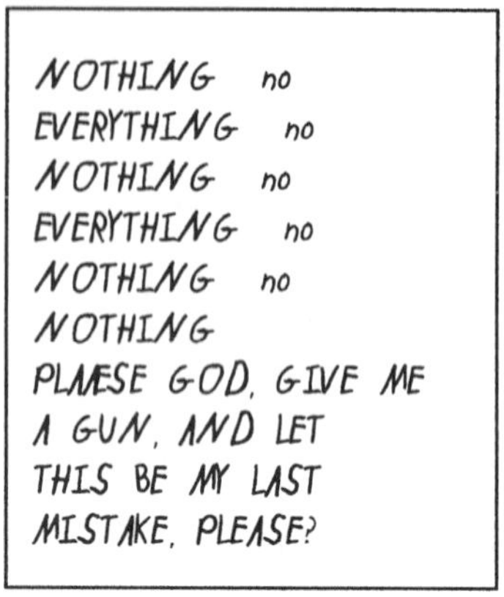

```
NOTHING  no
EVERYTHING  no
NOTHING  no
EVERYTHING  no
NOTHING  no
NOTHING
PLAESE GOD, GIVE ME
A GUN, AND LET
THIS BE MY LAST
MISTAKE. PLEASE?
```

FIGURE 20.1.   Notebook page from a 14-year-old's composition book.

elected officials responsible for these facilities are all subject to suit (see Maris, 1992b: 240–241).

The typical allegations in a complaint cite a lack of policies and procedures for screening and monitoring inmates, insufficient training of personnel to established policies and procedures, insufficient staffing to implement policies and procedures, and/or institutional conditions contributing to suicidal outcomes. Typically, as we shall see with malpractice cases, multiple complaints are lodged reflecting the interrelationship of these variables. The case of Cy Pope is illustrative of the above variables (Case 20.4).

MALPRACTICE

Of the approximately 31,000 suicides that occur annually in the United States, roughly one-half have had contact with the mental health system. Some fraction of those would have been in treatment or would have recently terminated treatment at the time of their suicide. It is not difficult to imagine how readily a bereaved family member might seek to exorcise feelings of pain, rage, and implied guilt by seeking to blame a caregiver for the family member's suicide (see Bongar et al., 1998).

Mental health professionals have well understood their duties with regard to patient care: simply put, they are to assess mental status and presenting problems, to diagnose, and

---

TABLE 20.1. Suicide and Schools: Selected Court Cases

Seattle, WA (1998): *Lewis v. Longview School District*

Valley View, IL (1997): *Grant v. Board of Trustees Valley View School District*

Polk County, FL (1997): *Wyke v. Polk County School Board*

Meridian, ID (1997): *Brooks v. Logan*

Milford, CT (1996): *Brown v. Board of Education*

Greece, NY (1996): *Shaner v. Greece Central School District*

Virginia, MN (1996): *Killen v. I.S.D.*

Cypress-Fairbanks, TX (1995): *Fowler v. Szostek*

Montgomery County, MD (1991): *Eisel v. Board of Education*

Springfield, OR (1985): *Kelson v. Springfield*

Source: American Association of Suicidology, Washington, DC.

CASE 20.4. The Jail Suicide of Cy Pope

Cy was a 24-year-old white male who suicided in a southern Georgia jail cell in 1994. The chronology of events of the case was as follows.

Cy saw an MD in October for "trouble sleeping" and was prescribed about 25 Dalmane. Cy had a prior diagnosis of "sociopathic personality." He had been in jail twice for a few months each for writing bad checks. Cy had an erratic work history, had gone AWOL while in the Army, and was a college dropout from Georgia Tech, where he played freshman football. Cy had just broken up with his girlfriend. He was on parole and was due to go to court for a hearing the day after he suicided in jail.

Cy had a poor, aggressive, even violent relationship with his father, who was a local football coach. His mother left his father and her four sons and moved to Texas. Cy had recently told his girlfriend and grandmother that he was thinking about killing himself.

Cy overdosed on the sleeping pills (Dalmane) he was given. He was found asleep by his grandmother (who was so upset she took the remaining Dalmane herself!) and taken to a local ER and then to a regional hospital. His diagnosis was "suicide attempt—overdose." The next day Dr. A discharged Cy, who went home and still sleepy drove his car into a school bus. Cy was arrested and taken to a local jail. At the jail Cy asked other inmates for razor blades to kill himself with.

After being released, Cy went home and got his father's pistol (which he stuck in his belt in the back of his pants) and rode off on his motorcycle. He was arrested a second time for driving erratically and booked again in the same jail on the same day he was first arrested. He was not searched, and Cy shot himself in the head as soon as he was placed in his cell.

Cy's family sued Dr. A (for medical malpractice) and the local jail for negligence and gross indifference. The jail had no policies, procedures, or training for managing suicidal inmates. The case was settled out of court.

---

to treat. One singular aspect of that duty of patient care involves protecting the patient from self-inflicted harm during the course of the patient's therapeutic work. The threat of suicide is the most frequently encountered mental health emergency for clinicians (Schein, 1976). Indeed, persons with diagnosed mental disorders have an increased probability of premature and nonnatural death, particularly because of the documented relationship between mental disorder and suicide. Moreover, surveys by Chemtob and his colleagues (Chemtob, Hamada, Bauer, Kinney, & Torigoe, 1988; Chemtob, Hamada, Bauer, Torigoe, & Kinney, 1988) have established midcareer probabilities of having a patient suicide in the range of 20–25% for psychologists and about 50% for psychiatrists.

Should the estate (family) of a patient who suicides allege that the patient's therapist violated a duty of care to their loved one and that that alleged violation proximately caused the suicide, a malpractice claim is likely to ensue. The therapist's behavior will now be scrutinized by attorneys and expert colleagues, and potentially by the court and a jury, to be evaluated relative to a loosely defined system of professional "shoulds" and "should nots," known as the *standard of care*. The standard of care is "that degree of care which a reasonably prudent person or professional should exercise in same or similar circumstances" (see

Black, 1979: 1260). If the caregiver is deemed to have acted below the standard of care, a breach in the duty of care through acts of either omission or commission, and the patient's suicide can be argued effectively to have directly and proximately resulted from that breach, that action can be considered malpractice (Black, 1979: 1103).

As we stated previously, the standard of care is defined legally as the duty to exercise that degree of skill and care ordinarily employed in similar circumstances by the average clinical practitioner. The operative words in defining that "average" practitioner speak to "reasonable and prudent" practice, although some courts have considered that connotation to be more stringent than that of "customary care and skill." Nevertheless, in practice the standard of care (and its possible breach) is opined by experts testifying for the plaintiff and defense who must bring their own figurative yardsticks to bear on the task of defining standard practices to the court. Thus, there is no universally agreed-on, uniform set of standards (however, see Bongar et al., 1998). Each expert must rely on his or her observations and knowledge of reasonable and expected clinical practices, prior court decisions establishing breaches of care, his or her own prior participation in malpractice actions that led to settlements prior to and in lieu of trial, and so on, to establish a convincing set of standards. Experts, however, are fallible and may, perhaps due to the self-aggrandizement involved in being an "expert," state ideal or optimal expectations as reasonable. Consider the following example:

> Both Dr. Smith, an expert for the plaintiff, and Dr. Jones, an expert for the defense, opined that in cases of observed suicidal risk the standard of care required that the caregiver be available and accessible to the patient. Dr. Smith, however, stated that this required the practitioner to carry a beeper on his or her person and that any other means of accessibility (e.g., an answering service or machine checked with reasonable frequency) was unacceptable relative to customary and expected behavior.

The duty to protect a patient is clearest when a patient is hospitalized. Indeed, evaluated acute risk for self-harm is one of the most common reasons for the hospitalization of a patient. The hospital setting is assumed to provide the maximum opportunity to monitor and safeguard a patient from self-destructive urges, to provide sanctuary from external sources of stress, to offer multiple hours of therapeutic interventions through different modalities (individual, group, and family therapy; milieu therapy; art therapy; etc.), to titrate pharmacological treatments to stabilize the patient's mood, thinking, and behavior, and so on. Once in the hospital, issues of safeguarding a patient's welfare range from providing policies and procedures regarding decisions for or against various levels of suicide watch status (such as constant observation or logged 15-minute checks and protocols for implementing these—see Table 20.2) to "suicide proofing" the unit (see Table 20.3), providing evaluated treatment plans, and providing discharge dispositions in favor of continuity of care and reflective of continued risk management.

For outpatient care, where the degree of control and oversight of a patient's mental status and behavior are considerably more limited, the foreseeability of a suicide governs the decision to, or not to, hospitalize a patient, voluntarily or involuntarily. Statutes for involuntary commitment (or emergency detention and protective custody) differ from one jurisdiction to another in their specificity but typically require evidence of suicide threat or attempt. For example, in Washington, DC, "the police or an M.D., with reason to believe a person is mentally ill, and because of that illness, is likely to injure himself [or others] if not immediately detained may, without a warrant, take the person into custody, transport, and make application for admission to a hospital for purposes of emergency observation and diagnosis" (Involuntary Commitment Statute, DC § 21:521). In contrast, in Oklahoma a peace officer or a licensed mental health professional who reasonably believes a person to

TABLE 20.2. Typical Levels of Suicide Watch Status in Inpatient Psychiatric Units

1:1 Constant observation

Staff member stays *within arm's length* of the patient 24 hours a day, so that physical contact can be immediate, if necessary. There are no exceptions to this rule, including visits by family, clergy, legal counsel, or bathroom use (door remains open). Patient is restricted to building. This is often referred to as to "special" a patient. Staff member in 1:1 role is often referred to as a "sitter."

Continuous eyesight (or "Line of Sight") observation

Staff member must have patient continuously in view 24 hours a day. There are no exceptions to this rule, including visits by family, clergy, legal counsel, or bathroom use.

Suicide precautions/close watch/close observation/checks

Staff member monitors patient every 15 minutes during both waking hours and sleep. Bathroom use is supervised with door closed. Patient may leave ward only for pressing medical reasons, as authorized by a physician, and must be escorted by two staff members

Open observation

Staff member monitors patient every 15 minutes during both waking hours and sleep. Bathroom supervision is optional. Patient reports to staff when changing geographical location.

Close supervision

Staff member monitors patient every 30 minutes and every 15 minutes when patient is asleep. No bathroom checks required. Patient reports to staff when changing geographical location.

Open supervision

Staff member monitors patient every 60 minutes during waking hours and every 30 minutes during sleep. Patient reports to staff when changing geographical location.

pose "a substantial risk of physical harm to the person himself as manifested by evidence of threats of, or attempts at, suicide or serious bodily harm" may call upon the police to take the person into protective custody and detention for up to 72 hours for purposes of an emergency examination (Oklahoma Mental Health Law § 5-206).

If a suicide were adjudged, retrospectively, to have been reasonably foreseeable, prospectively, then the duty to protect would suggest the need for constant or frequent ob-

TABLE 20.3. Recommendations for "Suicide Proofing" an Inpatient Psychiatric Unit

1. Supervise patients when it is necessary to use "sharps" (i.e., eating utensils). Count silverware and all other sharp objects before and after use by the patient. Use only electric razor.
2. Remove from patient any items that could be used in a suicide attempt (e.g., belts, neckties, shoelaces, matches, lighter, scissors, glass articles, jewelry).
3. Never place a patient who is on suicide precautions in seclusion. Do not allow patient to spend much time in room alone. Do not place patient in a private room.
4. Allow patients to take showers only, never a bath.
5. Install breakaway shower rods and recessed shower nozzles. Remove exposed pipes. Locate ventilation ducts at floor level.
6. Keep electrical cords to a minimum length.
7. Install windows of unbreakable glass with either tamper-proof screens or partitions too small to pass through. Keep all windows locked. Locate psychiatric unit on lower floor of hospital.
8. Lock all storage and supply closets, utility rooms, stairwells, and offices. Train all staff, both clinical and nonclinical (housekeepers, maintenance personnel) in security precautions.
9. Clear all gifts brought by visitors. Search patients after their return from passes
10. Train all new staff in policies and procedures and periodically update all current staff.

Sources: Benensohn & Resnick (1973) and various hospital Policy and Procedure Guidelines, courtesy of the American Association of Suicidology, Washington, DC.

servation and monitoring of that patient until a period of risk had passed. This can best be accomplished in a hospital setting. If the assessed foreseeable risk, however, was not sufficiently acute to warrant hospitalization or, especially, the implementation of involuntary committment procedures should the patient not comply with such a recommendation, then the duty to safeguard the patient is commensurately less. The scope of the duty to protect and safeguard a patient is always limited by the question of reasonableness. Practitioners reading this should consider whether they agree with the wife or with the court regarding the duty of the caregiver in Case 20.5.

With regard to the suicidal patient, the standard of care can generally be subsumed under three primary duties: to assess the patient's risk for suicide (foreseeability), to implement treatment designed to reduce the potential for suicide, and to safeguard the patient. The last duty requires the implementation of reasonable and proper precautions if necessary, against self-harm and oversight to ensure that a treatment plan is, indeed, carried out.

As should be evident, choices and judgments abound in the clinical relationship. The caregiver must make decisions in a context of risk (i.e., a suicide might result and cannot be guaranteed not to happen). The standard of care does not require perfect decision making; errors in judgment are human. Rather, it establishes the duty to make reasonable and appropriate decisions using sound clinical judgment. A documented (charted) rationale (with dates and times) for these decisions is always in the caregiver's best interest, given the possibility of a legal action should a suicide occur. Caregivers must not assume that if they said it, they need not write it in the chart.

The scope of clinical judgments and actions involved in the care of a suicidal patient is vast and beyond the purview of this chapter. We recommend that readers consult Bongar et al. (1998) for a thorough treatment of this subject. We would, however, like to briefly overview commonly alleged "failures" noted in malpractice actions, then illustrate the complexity and risk inherent in the clinical situation by some actual clinical vignettes.

Failures of Assessment

Patients presenting for treatment require consideration of potential suicide risk and therefore, an assessment of that risk (see Maris, Berman, Maltsberger, & Yufit, 1992). A reason-

---

CASE 20.5. The Case of *Farwell v. Un* (902 F.2d 282 [4th Cir. 1990])

The patient agreed to a voluntary hospitalization at a Veterans Administration hospital after an appointment and was sent home in the company of his wife to collect his belongings. Once home, he told his wife he would rather wait and admit himself the next day. In the morning he promised to go to the hospital that afternoon and sent his wife to work. When she returned, he was found dead, asphyxiated by hanging.

The estate (his widow) argued that when treating a patient with known or suspected suicidal tendencies, the psychiatrist had an "unbounded duty to take whatever other action is humanly possible" to ensure that the patient will voluntarily hospitalize himself. The court rejected this argument stressing that "such a stringent duty could only be discharged by . . . assuming actual physical custody of the patient or . . . mounting (constant) . . . close physical surveillance."

able assessment requires a clinical interview with direct and indirect questions about suicide ideation and/or behavior; relevant history taking and gathering of prior treatment records (including medication) and collateral information; a mental status evaluation of the patient's presenting behavior, mood, impulse control, insight, judgment, and so on; and establishing a specific diagnosis with a DSM code leading to a treatment plan.

Within the treatment planning lie other clinical assessments based on the assessed risk for suicide and diagnostic presentation (the need for inpatient vs. outpatient treatment, consideration of pharmacological interventions, the proper therapeutic modality and frequency, etc.). Within the hospital setting, levels of observation (constant, at 15, 30, or 60 minutes) must be determined and choice of unit (secluded, locked, with or without roommate, etc.), need for restraints, readiness for passes, and, ultimately, discharge all involve evaluations of the patient's current suicide risk.

Consider the following two case vignettes of adolescent patients (Cases 20.6 and 20.7) regarding the decision to admit to and discharge from the hospital. Readers should consider whether they believe the standard of care was violated.

Failures of Treatment

Decisions to medicate require adequate monitoring of medication benefit and side effects. Treatments must be designed and carried out appropriate to the patient's evaluated condition, must evidence awareness of the power of the therapeutic relationship and ethical standards, must be supervised effectively if administered by a team or by someone in training, and so on.

Case 20.7 illustrates an inadequately monitored psychopharmacological treatment. The lawsuit that resulted ended in a judgment against the defendant.

Hospital discharge decisions and outpatient terminations are difficult transitions to manage with regard to further disposition. One reason that suicides occur within 30 days of discharge from a hospital (Litman, 1992) is that inadequate attention is paid to the patient's need for further treatment and support to help deal with oftentimes the very same environmental stressors that prompted the need for hospitalization. Similarly, patients who form

---

CASE 20.6. The Case of Helen

Helen, age 14, was brought by her mother to an outpatient therapist. She was having nightmares, was not sleeping or eating, and had little energy to perform everyday tasks. In therapy she soon began recapturing memories of early sexual abuse by her father and emotional neglect by her mother. As these memories flooded into consciousness, she began acting out, staying out late, fighting with her mother, and punching holes in the apartment walls. The therapist increased Helen's sessions to three times a week and emergency appointments were scheduled whenever Helen threatened to kill either herself or her mother. Her therapist had Helen sign a "no suicide" contract and gave her home telephone number to Helen with instructions to call whenever the need arose. The therapist later argued that she only considered hospitalization when an actual suicide attempt had occurred. Unfortunately, Helen's first suicide attempt was her last—it was fatal.

CASE 20.7. The Case of John Powers

John Powers, age 19, had had behavior problems since the 10th grade. His first suicide attempt, a superficial wrist cut in his junior year in high school after being rebuffed by a girl, got him into psychotherapy and a diagnosis of conduct disorder. Later, after his first hospitalization, the diagnosis was changed to schizophrenia, paranoid type. Once discharged to aftercare, John became noncompliant with his prescribed medications. He began displaying problems in control and acted with suspicion toward everyone. He was referred to a local clinic that specialized in Prolixin, a drug that could be administered intramuscularly, thus enforcing compliance. He began treatments that, after a few months had to be increased in dosage because he showed signs of impulsivity and aggression.

Once again, after being rebuffed by a girl, he overdosed on 65 extra-strength Tylenol and was hospitalized. Once discharged he restarted his Prolixin treatments. However, he missed his second appointment, then canceled his next three appointments. One week later, again after a girl refused his advances, he killed himself with his father's shotgun on the front stoop of his home.

strong alliances with outpatient therapists may feel abandoned when therapy ends. The case of Barbara Baxter (Case 20.8) briefly illustrates how an inadvertent lack of attention to this dynamic can become proximately tied to a suicide months later.

Failure to Safeguard

Hospital units must be "suicide proofed," homes should be cleansed of available and accessible lethal weapons during periods of risk, and so forth. Inpatient units, also, should have well-defined policies and procedures for "suicide watch" and adequate staffing patterns to prevent self-harm behaviors on the unit. The case of Wanda Jones (Case 20.9) is typical of a hospital suicide that is likely to pose problems for the defense. It presents issues of alleged failure to safeguard (i.e., maintaining unsafe premises and dangerous substances within reach of the patient) and, possibly, failure to supervise (i.e., a questionable judgment regarding the level of watch [15 minutes vs. 1:1] given the level of suicidality and pathology at intake).

The typical lawsuit alleges a long list of "failures" in a petition for damages. Case 20.10, which was settled before trial, briefly illustrates how a plaintiff's attorney will position a case charging a caregiver with negligence.

Once filed, the *complaint* alleging acts of negligence must be defended. Each defendant's attorney or each defendant's liability insurance company's attorney will answer the complaint in writing asserting affirmative defenses that, if proven, will bar the plaintiff's claims. The defense also will often seek to have the court dismiss the complaint through a motion for summary judgment, arguing that the alleged facts do not demonstrate a violation of law. The formal investigatory phase of a lawsuit follows through a process known as *discovery*. Discovery entails such legal procedures as issuing subpoenas for documents (e.g., treatment records), hiring experts to review those records and express opinions regarding the plaintiff's allegations as breaches in the caregivers' duties to the patient (or to defend the caregivers' actions as within the standard of care), filing and answering

CASE 20.8. The Case of Barbara Baxter

Barbara Baxter, age 23, was a law student in her last year of law school when she entered outpatient therapy with a female therapist. She had complaints of depression and weight gain, transient suicidal ideation particularly when she felt unacceptable and became self-deprecating, and long-standing feelings of inadequacy stemming from her relationship with a critical father. She was diagnosed as having an adjustment disorder with depressed mood.

Treatment was provided weekly for 7 months, when her therapist learned that she would be moving out of town due to her husband's job transfer. Discussions regarding termination occured over the next 6 weeks until the end of therapy. Barbara's therapist strongly suggested that therapy continue—especially through the difficult postgraduation period of bar review, exam, and job search—and made one referral to a colleague.

Her therapist left town at the beginning of the summer and simply assumed that Barbara would follow through on the referral to continue her work. She made no effort to ensure that this transfer occurred and did not even call Barbara to reiterate the importance she placed on this work. Barbara simply felt abandoned and told fellow students she could not trust anyone to really care for her.

Five months later, after passing the bar exam but failing to be offered a job by the law firm at which she had spent the summer clerking, she killed herself with a gun she bought while awaiting the bar exam results. Her family sued, alleging her therapist abandoned Barbara by prematurely ending therapy and not making every effort to have therapy continue with a new therapist as deemed necessary by the therapist. Plaintiff's attorney linked Barbara's suicide to her not being offered a job which reactivated feelings of unworthiness and unlovability and her underlying depression, the ongoing treatment of which was both prematurely ended when her therapist abandoned her months earlier and exacerbated by the uncaring manner in which Barbara was left without further support.

CASE 20.9. The Case of Wanda Jones

Wanda Jones, age 23, had been hearing voices since her late teens. She also had become religiously delusional, believing that her only salvation—given a long list of unspecified sins—was to join Jesus in heaven. It was her attempt to hang herself to accomplish this end that got her hospitalized at Memorial Hospital. Diagnosed as schizophrenic, she was placed on suicide watch with 15-minute checks. The second day after her admission—within the 14 minutes between checks—she managed to find an open cleaning supply closet on the ward and ingest a toxic cleaning fluid. She died within minutes. Hospital standards requiring a locked closet made an evident breach an indefensible act of negligence.

CASE 20.10. The Case of Bobby Stewart

Bobby Stewart, age 14, was referred for inpatient hospitalization by his outpatient psychotherapist after receiving a phone call from Bobby's mother who had discovered blood on Bobby's pillow. When confronted, Bobby admitted to self-cutting his wrists with pieces of glass. Bobby was brought to the hosptial by his parents. Two days later they delivered to the attending psychiatrist copies of an undated journal and poems found in his room. These were replete with references to hating himself, to feeling worthless, to wishes to die, and to having a second chance (rebirth).

Bobby had a long history of violent temper outbursts, impulsive behavior, depression, and attention deficit problems. At the time of his admission he was on probation for arson and tampering with railroad tracks. He was on both Ritalin and Prozac and was awaiting a hearing for violating his probation for selling his precription medicines. He had significant problems with insomnia and readily admitted to suicidal thoughts.

Bobby was placed on an acute care ward with admitting Axis I diagnoses of dysthymic disorder, conduct disorder, and attention-deficit/hyperactivity disorder. His Axis V Global Assessment of Functioning was rated at 25. He was placed on 15-minute checks. His dosage of Prozac was increased and he started on Trazadone for his insomnia.

On the second day on the inpatient unit, Bobby's watch status was reduced to 30-minute checks. No self-damaging behaviors were noted; his affect, however, remained flat and his behavior was described as lethargic. On the fifth day on the unit Bobby refused to attend group therapy and ran from a family therapy session, slamming doors and hitting his fists against the hospital walls. He was placed in protective seclusion for 2 hours. On the same day he was found to be in possession of a straightened paper clip and he was caught eating a pencil. His Prozac was again increased in dosage. Nursing notes reflected that Bobby minimized his behaviors and denied the significance of his problems. Two days later he was discharged to the care of his parents (and against their objections) and referred to a partial hospitalization program which allowed him to be at home on evenings and weekends. Six days later, while at home, Bobby Stewart hung himself in his bedroom.

The plaintiff's Petition for Damages charged that at the time of Bobby's discharge from acute care, "it was reasonably foreseeable . . . that without twenty-four hour medical care, treatment, and supervision [Bobby] would engage in self-damaging and suicidal behavior." Specifically, the defendant inpatient psychiatrist was alleged to be "guilty of the following acts of negligence and carelessness by failing to measure up to the standards of due care, skill, and practice as required by members of his specialty" to wit: In negligently and carelessly:

1. Failing to accurately assess.
2. Failing to appropriately treat.
3. Failing to evaluate the efficacy of the care and treatment provided.
4. Ordering the discharge . . . from twenty-four hour in-patient care.
5. Discharging . . . when it was apparent that further care was needed.

CASE 20.10. (*cont.*)

6. Failing to advise [Bobby's parents] of his mental condition and the possibility of infliction of self harm.
7. Failing to accurately assess [Bobby's] failure to respond to care, treatment, and therapy during his hospitalization, including but not limited to medical treatment and individual and family therapies.
8. Failing to accurately assess and evaluate [Bobby] regarding self harm and suicidal iseation and plans.
9. Failing to provide the proper follow-up care after [Bobby] was discharged from . . . [the] acute care program.
10. Failing to properly evaluate and follow-up on [Bobby's] behavior that indicated desires for self-harm and suicide, including, but not limited to, written poems and attempts at hiding a sharp object during his in-patient hospitalization.
11. Keeping incomplete records and using inadequate charting methods during the course of treatmen; and
12. Abandoning [Bobby]!

Similarly, the hospital and other members of the inpatient treatment team were sued for an equivalent list of alleged acts of negligence.

---

interrogatories, and deposing all relevant parties to the case and each side's experts. Discovery is costly, time-consuming, and fraught with legal maneuvering. Ultimately, once filed a case is most likely to reach a settlement at some time before all parties reach the courthouse steps, as sending a case to a jury is risky to both sides. In some states mandated or voluntary arbitration is used to speed up disposition of cases, saving both time and money.

Suicidologists are often admitted as experts, given their specialized knowledge of the subject matter in dispute (see Maris, in Bongar, 1992: 241). The case of Norman Smith (Case 20.11) allows us an opportunity to follow the thinking of an expert called by the plaintiff. Readers should try to place themselves in the shoes of the expert for the defense and define what positions they might reasonably take to counter the plaintiff's allegations.

In spite of these opinions the burden on the plaintiff is to demonstrate a deviation from a duty and that that deviation directly caused the suicide of Mr. Smith. Even if a deviation from a duty of care can be demonstrated, if that negligence can be shown to not be a proximate cause of the suicide, then no liability can be found. Thus, for example, an expert for the defense in the case of Mr. Smith might well argue that in the 3 weeks after discharge, a number of *intervening acts*, both unforeseen and outside the control of the defendant, occured. Alternatively, the defense might pose that expecting the defendants to foresee a suicide over such a long period as 3 weeks was unreasonable; that there was no way to force Mr. Smith to seek outpatient treatment; that Mr. Smith had 4 days in the hospital with no self-destructive acts, including two day passes that were "uneventful" before discharge. Thus, as it could not be argued that he needed continued hospitalization, discharge was appropriate. Readers should consider whether they can think of other possible positions they might argue if they were to testify as experts for the defense?

CASE 20.11. The Case of Norman Smith

Norman Smith, a 37-year-old white male, died by a self-inflicted shotgun blast to the chest in the early morning of November 2. Mr. Smith's death followed a preceding late-night attack on his wife. Motivated by rage and despondency over her pending divorce from him, Smith attempted to strangle her, then hit her on the head with a hammer, before fleeing and killing himself with the gun he bought just the day before.

Struggling with marital problems Mr. Smith first attempted suicide on August 4 by running his car engine in the closed garage of his home. This nonfatal attempt resulted in outpatient counseling at City Hospital. Norman and his wife were seen sequentially by the therapist. During his wife's session, Norman listened to her conversation through the closed office door and got extremely agitated. He refused to enter into treatment, stating that he could not trust the therapist.

During the month of September Norman's behavior became more erratic and threatening. His wife moved out to her parents' house and filed divorce papers. The day after Norman was served with the papers he drank a quantity of alcohol, wrote a suicide note to his parents, and ingested a large number of over-the-counter sleeping pills. When he was observed by neighbors to be rolling around in the gravel outside his home, the police were called and he was transported to City Hospital's emergency room. His stomach was pumped. He was admitted first to a medical floor, then transferred to a psychiatric unit and admitted involuntarily on September 29.

Smith was placed on precautions with 15-minute checks as a suicide risk and remained so until October 9. During the intake assessment he was noted as angry, agitated, anxious, and guarded; he had ideas of reference, blamed his wife for all his problems, showed poor insight and judgment, and appeared paranoid. He was thought both homicidal and suicidal. He was diagnosed as a bipolar disorder (manic–depressive), mixed type, although paranoid schizophrenia could not be ruled out. Antipsychotic drugs were ordered in addition to lithium. A psychosocial history was ordered and completed. A psychological consultation was ordered to rule out psychosis. An interdisciplinary treatment team established a treatment plan that also included 1:1 supportive psychotherapy, group therapy, milieu and activity therapies. It was expected that he would be hospitalized for 3–4 weeks.

After coming off precautions Mr. Smith was allowed two day passes in the care of his mother. Both were uneventful. Two days later, on October 13, he was discharged with a 7-day supply of lithium carbonate (300 mg a day) and an outpatient referral to an aftercare facility "as needed." He never showed there for an appointment. Three weeks later he was dead.

Hospital records indicate that Mr. Smith's lithium—when his blood was last tested before discharge—was below therapeutic levels. The psychological consultation, a computer-scored MMPI, found no evidence to support psychosis, depression, or bipolar mood disorder. Rather it was seen as "marginally valid"and suggested the patient was "not suicidal now and unlikely to be suicidal in the near future," in spite of having the potential for impulsivity.

CASE 20.11. (*cont.*)

Experts for the plaintiff found the following:

Hospital charting, especially well-documented during the 9 days of 15-minute checks, failed to indicate Mr. Smith received any 1:1 individual psychotherapy during his inpatient stay. Neither the hospital psychiatrist nor the social worker had any notations, after intake, in Mr. Smith's medical chart.

The psychological evaluation was inadequate. The MMPI is insufficient to address the referral question, does not answer the question of suicide risk, and was questionably valid anyway.

No meeting with his wife or any family member was noted, particularly with regard to discharge planning and to provide a *Tarasof* warning. Moreover, there was no evidence of any evaluation of suicide risk at the time of discharge. The discharge medication, questionable given the lack of substantiation for a bipolar diagnosis, even if correct was not therapeutic at the time of discharge, was not connected to ongoing monitoring, and had no follow-up plan after 7 days.

Aftercare, *as needed*, for a patient as disturbed, guarded, and potentially impulsive as Mr. Smith was the equivalent of discharge without further need of intervention (i.e., abandonment).

CONTESTED LIFE INSURANCE

Suicide poses a special problem for life insurance contracts. Insurance companies consider that an applicant for insurance has a decided advantage in their actuarial bet regarding the applicant's expected lifespan, when the applicant is considering suicide at the time of application. To protect themselves, insurance companies typically use an exclusionary clause, such as the following, that denies benefits to the insured's estate if the death is by suicide within 2 years of the date the policy went into effect: "Suicide of the insured, while sane or insane, within two years of the issue date or the reinstatement date is not covered by this policy. If the insured does commit suicide, the only amount payable will be a return of the premiums paid for the policy less any indebtedness or partial surrender." The "sane or insane" phrase is intended to protect the insurance company from arguments that the suicide resulted from a mental disorder that prevented rational thought (i.e., the inability to form suicidal intent). Only a few courts have limited the meaning of this phrase (Nolan, 1988). On the other hand, family members have every reason to argue that their loved one's death was not a suicide; that is, that the decedent intended neither to suicide nor to defraud the insurance company at the time application for death benefits was made. If denied benefits, the estate of the insured may take the insurance company to court. There is a strong presumption of law that the decedent did not commit suicide. (In older British law, suicide used to be considered a crime. With possible criminal action the perpetrator was considered innocent until/unless proven guilty. Thus, the law presumed that suicide did *not* occur.) The insurance company, having denied benefits, has the burden to prove that the death was a suicide. Even if the coroner or medical examiner has determined the manner of death to be a suicide, this does not constitute legal proof that the death was a suicide. However, the medical examiner's determination usually would be introduced by the insurance company as one expert opinion among many regarding the decedent's manner of death. Even when the death is determined by the medical examiner or coroner to be an accident, the insurance company may seek a second opinion if it has reason to believe the medical examiner or coroner to be wrong. The life insurance company's denial of benefits then may be challenged in court. Such was the case in the death of Ron Peters (a pseudonym; see Case 20.12).

Death investigations are the work of the police and the coroner or medical examiner's office and their deputies. The determination of cause and manner of death ultimately is that of an informed opinion of the coroner or medical examiner. Should that opinion be in dispute, as when an insurance company or the decedent's estate questions a manner-of-death determination, litigation may ensue. Suicidologists often are called on by attorneys to help determine the manner of death, through the use of death investigations, including both the physical and "psychological autopsy" (see Clark, 1992). As the question of the decedent's intent most often has to be reconstructed (the decedent of course is no longer available to inform us of his or her "state of mind"), interviews with family, friends, and colleagues; analyses of archival documents and records (e.g., school, employment, criminal, and military); and site investigation all serve to establish the character, lifestyle, coping patterns, and possible precipitating motives (or lack thereof) of the decedent. In legal cases, the typical question being addressed is whether the death was a suicide, accident, or homicide. Correspondingly, opposing sides attempt to present evidence for or against suicide intent (and/or motive). In the case of Mr. Peters (Case 20.12), lawyers for the estate would argue that Mr. Peters was a chronic user of drugs and had habitually used Isoflurane to cope with

---

CASE 20.12. The Case of Ron Peters

Ron Peters was a 49-year-old white male found dead at approximately 11:00 P.M. in his locked room at the Drop Inn Motor Hotel. Mr. Peters was found face down in his bed on a hand towel which had been soaked with approximately half a bottle of isoflurane. Isoflurane is a volatile anesthetic agent, resulting in complete incapacitation within 10 minutes of inhalation. Toxicological analyses found a .06 blood alcohol level.

Mr. Peters was a registered nurse anesthesist with approximately 15 years' experience in the field. Recently, he had complained frequently of insomnia and other symptoms of depression. He had numerous problems that gave rise to his depression, including a recent divorce, a more recent loss of employment because of mood swings, suspected drug (Valium) and alcohol abuse, failure to show up for or appear on time for work, and a consequent termination of his license to practice. He had severe financial difficulties including bankruptcy and federal tax liens.

The County Coroner determined Mr. Peters's death to be an accident. The insurance company contested the determination, arguing that the effects of lying face down on a cloth soaked with isoflurane were well-known to Mr. Peters and that he had intent to suicide. The case was settled out of court.

---

his insomnia. Moreover, evidence that he had been drinking suggested he was unaware how much anesthetic he had poured on the hand towel.

Self-inflicted deaths under circumstances that suggest a lack of capacity for intention (e.g., under the influence of alcohol or psychosis) are threshold cases, the final determination of which in court often depends on the strength of either side's expert testimony. Consider, for example, the case of comedian Freddie Prinze (Litman, 1988) presented in Box 20.1.

Some deaths pose extremely difficult manner-of-death determinations (e.g., unwitnessed drownings, falls from heights, and single-car accidents). These, in particular, demand the skills of a trained suicidologist to conduct a death investigation to assess whether or not the death was a suicide. Berman (1993) has provided two such cases in depth with reference to unwitnessed asphyxiation by drowning. The psychological autopsy attempts to establish the decedent's intent at the time of death (see Chapter 3). Some states only permit an insurer to deny a claim on the basis of suicide if it can be proven that the insured had suicide intent at the time the insurance policy was applied for.

The case of John Davenport (Case 20.13) is a most unusual example in that it first raises the interesting question of whether a suicide is a suicide if, by law, it was a homicide; then whether the insurance policy was fraudulently obtained, given evidence of suicidal intent at the time of application.

An intensive investigation of both site and character often is necessary for the suicidologist to offer to the court a considered opinion as to the manner of death. Even then, experts on opposing sides of a case may view data selectively and with a perhaps unconsciously prejudiced eye. The unusual case of Bob Charles (Case 20.14) illustrates how both plaintiff and defense experts can develop plausible opinions and conclusions, based on their

---

BOX 20.1. The Case of Freddie Prinze

Freddie Prinze was a 22-year-old comedy star who shot himself in the temple one night in the presence of his manager after calling a number of people, including his mother and his estranged wife, and telling them, "I'm going to do it." He also wrote a suicide note, which declared, among other things, that "no one else is responsible." At various periods, in the 2 years before his death, Mr. Prinze had taken out substantial amounts of life insurance with different beneficiaries. The total exceeded $1 million. At the trial, the focus was on intention.

The argument for accident hinged on two elements in Freddie Prinze's lifestyle. First, he was a habitual user and abuser of cocaine and methaqualone. In fact, during the 24 hours before his death, he had ingested 10 to 15 tablets of methaqualone. There was question about how much methaqualone it would take to produce impaired intention in an habitual user. Second, Mr. Prinze often played with his gun. Friends explained that it was a symbol to him of power and control. He was known to have put a gun to his head several times when the safety was on, or when it was not loaded, and mimic (rehearse?) shooting himself. The plaintiff presented the scenario that Mr. Prinze had been putting on an act of pretending to shoot himself and the discharge of a loaded gun had been a great mistake from his point of view. By this view, he had not intended to die, even though he told everybody he was going to shoot himself and the circumstances of his life were extremely stressful. The jury accepted this point of view, but in a decsion worthy of Solomon, decided that only a small portion of the insurance money was payable, because Mr. Prinze had not answered questions on the insurance application forms truthfully, which asked whether the person used drugs and alcohol.

CASE 20.13. The Case of John Davenport

John Davenport was a highly successful businessman, a risk-taking entre-preneur who bought and sold a number of small ventures on his way to amassing a fortune. His last venture, however, was a gamble that failed. Seeking to replicate an earlier success, Davenport bought a coal mine and secured a lucrative contract with the state power company to supply coal. To accomplish the purchase and to support the expensive start-up costs to open up the mine, Davenport secured millions in business loans with per-sonal credit. This was a "no-lose proposition" he told friends. He also bought $5 million in life insurance, as required by his creditors. "If [he] failed," he also told friends, "his family would be taken care of."

Within 2 months the mine delivered its first shipment of coal. How-ever, the production was under the anticipated and promised tonnage and it was of inferior quality. The power company threatened that it would cancel its contract if the sulfur content of the next shipment was not sig-nificantly lessened.

Davenport, an experienced coal man, knew that to possibly reach veins of higher-grade coal he would have to dig much deeper in the mine. This was inordinately expensive and was confounded by the collapse of a retaining wall, the repair of which would delay the effort for months. He was ruined and talked of suicide to over a dozen friends and colleagues, with special emphasis on "taking care of [his] family."

Knowing that the insurance policy would not pay if he were to sui-cide, Davenport turned to his right-hand man, Smee, with his plan. Smee had worked for Davenport for more than 15 years and was known to be in-tensely loyal. He would do anything for Davenport, a man he idolized and called a friend. Davenport, known as an engaging, controlling, persuasive, sometimes intimidating man, convinced Smee that he was a ruined man and that Smee alone could save his family from going down with him. Tearfully and pleading, he asked Smee if he would kill him (i.e., assist in his suicide). Smee ultimately acquiesced and agreed to Davenport's plan to "make it look like a homicide during an act of burglary at the mine."

Early one night when no one was around Smee and Davenport met at the mine office, arranged the scene to look like a break-in had oc-curred, and accomplished the plan. Davenport was killed with three bul-lets from a revolver Smee borrowed that day. Ruled a homicide, the insur-ance company paid Davenport's widow $5 million.

Smee was the last person to be suspected of the homicide, but after a protracted investigation and much happenstance and luck, Smee was charged with Davenport's murder. When faced with the threat of life im-prisonment, Smee told of Davenports's plan. Given his reputation for honesty and integrity in the community, and backed by many reporters who spoke of Davenport's suicidality over the last several months, Smee's confession was accepted and a plea bargain of "assisting a suicide" was entered with and agreed to by the court. The insurance company sued Davenport's estate for the return of the insurance monies.

Further psychological investigation revealed that Davenport did not disclose on his application for the insurance any medical history of note. He gave a fictitious address for a nonexistent family doctor and otherwise listed his dentist. Not revealed was a 30-year trail of manic behavior and treatment and prior suicidal behavior much earlier in his life.

CASE 20.14. Ain't No Bull . . . the Case of Bob Charles

Bob Charles, age 47, worked for 18 years as a farmer and dairyman. When the government offered to buy out his dairy herd, he sold off his stock and took a job with the Artifical Breeding Service of the state university. His new job was as a field representative and salesman of bull semen and artifical insemination products. For this work he drove a pickup truck from farm to farm disseminating bull semen from a 600-gallon liquid nitrogen tank (used to freeze the bull semen) housed in a camper shell covering the truck bed. At the time of his death he had worked at this job for 3 years.

On a sweltering Monday after Father's Day (the temperature reached 102°), Mr. Charles ran some errands, then began his route. Before noon he had made 5 of 14 scheduled deliveries. Observers along the highway noted that the camper doors were flapping open. He was last observed crossing a bridge around 12:15 P.M. From 2:30 P.M. on, his truck was observed by several witnesses to be parked by the banks of the river near the bridge under a tree. At 2:00 A.M. the next morning, the truck was observed in the same location by a state police officer. Investigating more closely, the officer found the frozen body of Mr. Charles in a seated position behind the closed doors of the camper shell. His face was in almost direct contact with the outflow tract of the nitrogen gas. Two valves were observed to be opened, thus releasing the liquid nitrogen almost directly to Mr. Charles's face. Mr. Charles had died almost instantaneously from a flash-freezing of his larynx caused by the escaping gas. There was no evidence of foul play. The county coroner ruled Mr. Charles's death to be a suicide. The insurance company refused to pay his heirs $200,000 in death benefits and an additional $200,000 in accidental benefits on a policy obtained by Mr. Charles 9 months before his death. Litigation ensued over the question of whether his death was an accident or a suicide.

Arguing that Mr. Charles's death was an accident, the expert for his estate observed:

1. Neither Mr. Charles nor any member of his biological family was known to have a history of suicide, suicide attempt, depression, or other mental disorder. His physical health was good.

2. Mr. Charles did not abuse alcohol or drugs.

3. His family described him as happy and stable; there were no known marital problems; family members described the family as "close." Allegations that he was upset over his older son being homosexual were unfounded.

4. Though typically a note writer, he left no suicide note.

5. The last person on his route to see him alive described no behavior "out of the ordinary."

6. His children reported he was "careless around machinery."

7. He had described plans to plant a crop later in the week and was looking forward to a good harvest in the near future.

8. The night of his death, he had plans to meet his wife for a once postponed anniversary dinner and overnight. Though suffering from life-threatening breast cancer, she reported that her husband was supportive.

(cont.)

CASE 20.14. (*cont.*)

9. Although one of his sons said that his father was "depressed over finances," he had sufficient assets to acquire various loans and had a steady income.

10. The coroner who conducted the autopsy was inexperienced in evaluating liquid nitrogen asphyxial deaths.

This expert concluded: "Because of the 102° weather, Mr. Charles entered the camper with the intent to do paperwork and turned the valves slightly open to drip behind him and cool him. The evaporating liquid nitrogen cooled him, but simultaneously replaced and deprived him of needed oxygen. He became dizzy, sat down, and was further overcome. Because of his hypoxia, he was unable to rescue himself. The wind closed the doors and he was effectively entombed in a very cold refrigeration unit."

In contrast, the expert for the defense (as expected) strongly supported the coroner's determination of a suicidal death based on the following observations of both site and person:

1. There is no compelling reason for Mr. Charles to have been in the camper with the doors shut. It is possible that Mr. Charles pulled off the road to close the doors to the refrigeration unit, but there would be no reason for him to have entered the camper. Even if he had reason, the doors could not have accidentally slammed shut and there would be no reason for him to manually shut the doors behind him.

2. Given the extreme heat of the day, if he had wished to cool down, he would have stayed in the cab of the truck which had a fully operating and functional air-conditioning system. He had no reason to enter the camper to cool down.

3. Mr. Charles's body position in the camper gave no evidence of an accidental fall or trip. His glasses were appropriately positioned on his face. He was found in a sitting position, not sprawled.

4. His body was found "as close as possible to the outflow tract of gasses," the equivalent of a contact gunshot wound. If the gas had already been flowing, he would have known of its danger and would have kept greater distance.

5. For the gas to be flowing, two valves had to be manually turned on. Both had been observed to be off at his last delivery stop. They were now turned on inside a closed camper by someone with knowledge, familiarity, and experience to know not to.

6. Mr. Charles was not known to readily display affect. He reportedly showed no response upon learning of his son's homosexuality, was known not to fight openly with his wife, and was described by one informant as one who "nothing ever bothered." This was not a man who readily communicated pain. Thus, it is consistent that few reporters knew of any problems he might have been having.

7. Yet, his sons told the police that he was "depressed over finances." A friend reported that, upon the sale of his dairy herd Mr. Charles was "depressed, tearful, and regretful." Indeed, one of the loans recently acquired by Mr. Charles (which also placed him in greater "financial straits," as reported by a colleague) was taken to finance a repurchase of cows.

CASE 20.14. (*cont.*)

8. Considerable evidence has been found to suggest Mr. Charles was seriously concerned about his finances. Several notes and payments were coming due in the next several months. His net worth at the time of his death was the lowest it had ever been since receiving the buyout of his herd. He had called his banker the Friday preceding his death to "discuss finances." Found in the cab of his truck, near his checkbook and some bills, were "Post-it" notes with writing stating, "How am I going to pay this back?"

9. He had reason to fear losing his wife. Diagnosed with breast cancer in March, she had a bilateral modified mastectomy in April. On the afternoon of his death she had a scheduled chemotherapy appointment. A friend reported that Mr. Charles was despondent over his wife's cancer and had "reacted strongly" upon learning of a woman friend's recent death.

10. The delayed, belated anniversary dinner scheduled the night of his death was to be at a motel at which he actually made (incorrectly) a reservation for the next evening. Something was likely interfering with his thought processes. Also, he was already behind in his planned route and delivery schedule for the day, threatening once again a postponement of the anniversary date. One report suggested that Mr. and Ms. Charles had fought over the weekend and that she did not intend to meet him for the planned anniversary dinner and overnight.

11. Other signs of anxiety and confusion appear in his records from the morning's route. Uncharacteristically, he made a calculation error on one bill and, on another invoice, miswrote a well-known customer's name. Furthermore, there is a noticable hand tremor evident on the invoices from the late morning.

This expert concluded: "Bob Charles was emotionally inhibited; problems and feelings generally were not known by others. In spite of this, we see signs of anxiety regarding his finances, regrets over the loss of his dairy herd, and anxiety over his wife's deteriorating health. All these weighed heavily on him and led to some seepage of otherwise overcontrolled emotions. Little evidence of a "close family" was presented. There may well have been marital problems, Mr. Charles was not happy, and his stability was threatened by very real and difficult stressors. This man longed to reconnect to an earlier life as a dairyman, but financial problems and his relationship with his wife placed that in jeopardy. With knowledge, familiarity, experience, and opportunity Mr. Charles had an immediate and available end to the pressures mounting within. He was able to effect his death instantaneously by means of a self-inflicted blast from an available supply of liquid nitrogen in the back of his truck."

own intensive investigations and possible ideological biases. As is evident from their respective observations, these cases are equivocal because the information derived is complicated and may support either viewpoint (i.e., figuratively, there is no "smoking gun").

The final determination, as it should be, is up to the court or jury to decide. As with our earlier discussion regarding malpractice, the adversarial system in this setting rests the final determination on the skills of the attorneys and the believability of an expert's responses to the attorney's questions. Case 20.14, presented earlier as Case 12.1, presents the opinions of two opposing experts. Readers might find each to be convincing in their rationales.

It has been attributed to Harvard Medical School psychiatrist and forensic expert Thomas Gutheil that for a bereaved plaintiff "a *tort action* is the oldest antidepressant." A suicide is usually a bad outcome that leaves bad feelings. Almost every suicide leaves survivors who are acutely bereaved and looking to blame someone or something for those bad feelings. Their loved one is dead and someone has to be to blame!

Attorneys make their living in an adversarial arena. They serve as gladiators—either for angry and pained plaintiffs seeking recompense for their grief allegedly caused by another's negligent caretaking of for that other who will feel unjustly accused for being something less than perfect, omniscient, and able to predict the future. As parents feel unjustly blamed for their children's problems, when most parents try to their very best, so do defendants struggle to prove their intent and practice to have been reasonable and prudent. Litigation of the sort reviewed in this chapter ultimately is the only test of who has what responsibility when we form fragile alliances with lives held in the balance.

SUMMARY AND CONCLUSIONS

In this chapter we primarily emphasized two areas of interface between the law and suicide: equivocal deaths and negligence cases. In equivocal deaths the suicidologist acts as death investigator, bringing to bear skills and expertise in ascertaining behavioral factors and observations common to site and method that describe the intent of the decedent and, thus, the manner of death. The opinions derived from the expert suicidologist's investigation may affect the payout of millions of dollars in life insurance proceeds.

Similarly, in negligence cases, millions of dollars may be involved. However, more important is the involvement of the caretaker potentially held responsible for not protecting the life of the decedent. When the caretaker is a clinician, a finding of negligence is a finding of malpractice. A finding of malpractice can be both personally and professionally devastating.

Clinical work with suicidal patients is hard enough. It is even made even more difficult by the threat of "failure," as perceived and evidenced by the intentioned death of a patient, and, yet again, by the threat of a malpractice action. Clinicians, like others responsible for the protection and caretaking of those they serve and treat or for whom they have custodial duties, must practice with these possibilities as figurative "background noise" to their everyday observations, judgments, decisions, and actions. This reality "comes with the territory" and frames the clinical paradigm (see Chapter 21).

One upside of this reality is that an awareness of one's potential for malpractice may force a clinician to sharpen his or her focus on what constitutes good treatment of the suicidal patient. It is to this theme that we now turn in the next chapter.

FURTHER READING

Applebaum, P. S., & Gutheil, T. G. (1991). *Clinical handbook of psychiatry and the law.* Baltimore: Williams & Wilkins. An award-winning contribution to the forensic literature, each chapter of this book presents case summaries, a review and interpretation of legal stautes, an outline of the clinical issues involved, obstacles to good patient care, and an "action guide" to reference appropriate responses to clinicolegal dilemmas.

Berman, A. L. (1993). Forensic suicidology and the psychological autopsy. In A. A. Leenaars, A. L. Berman, P. Cantor, R. L. Litman, & R. W. Maris (Eds.), *Suicidology: Essays in honor of Edwin S. Shneidman* (pp. 248–266). Northvale, NJ: Aronson. Illustrated with a focus on two cases of equivocal death by unwitnessed drowning, this chapter outlines the use of the psychological autopsy in questions of negligence by custodial caretakers.

Bongar, B. (1991). *The suicidal patient: Clinical and legal standards of care.* Washington, DC: American Psychological Association. Bongar combines clinical expertise with case law examples to support this didactic text regarding the management of suicidal patients. Included are a number of specific suggestions and recommendations for optimizing clinical practice.

Bongar, B., Berman, A. L., Maris, R. W., Silverman, M. M., Harris, E. A., & Packman, W. L. (Eds.). (1998). *Risk management with suicidal patients.* New York: Guilford Press. Written by an interdisciplinary team of behavioral scientists and legal experts, this book presents guidelines and recommendations for the care and treatment of the suicidal patient in both outpatient and inpatient settings, including psychopharmacological treatments.

Nolan, J. L. (Ed.). (1988). *The suicide case: Investigation and trial of insurance claims.* Chicago: American Bar Association. A short volume of collected papers authored by plaintiff's and defense attorneys, a psychiatric expert, and a medical examiner relative to legal cases involving possible suicides and insurance contracts with exclusion clauses relating to suicide.

Simon, R. I. (1992). *Clinical psychiatry and the law.* Washington, DC: American Psychiatric Press. This book is an excellent guide to the clinical management of legal issues potentially faced by mental health practitioners. Each chapter (Chapter 12 is on the "Clinical Risk Management of the Suicidal Patient") begins with a clinical case and is followed by a series of pertinent questions answered from a perspective toward recommending practical guidelines and considerations.

PART V

TREATMENT AND PREVENTION

21

Treatment and Prevention of Suicide

> As to how to help the suicidal individual, it is best to look upon a suicidal act as an effort to stop unbearable anguish or intolerable pain by "doing something." Knowing this usually guides us as to what treatment should be.
> —Edwin S. Shneidman

By virtue of a symptom, set of symptoms, a complaint(s), or problem(s), an individual seeks or is referred, taken (e.g., by parents), or commanded (e.g., by the court) to seek help from a person with specialized skills, licensed to observe and evaluate, refer to or offer treatment, and then treat, successfully it is hoped, the presenting issues. This is the *clinical paradigm*. It defines roles of patient and caregiver and simply outlines the patient–caregiver relationship and the help-giving process. But, with the suicidal patient, these are anything but simple.

In this chapter, we outline the complexities of working with the suicidal patient with an intent to integrate principles of good clinical intervention with those of suicide prevention. In this regard, and as we shall discuss here, mental health intervention is within the spectrum of prevention. The distinction between treatment and prevention is essentially one of timing: in prevention we attempt to intervene *before* the onset of a problem; clinical treatment begins once a problem has developed and, too often, well after optimal points of intervention have passed.

Moreover, as Vlasak (1975) has noted, certain features, typically present with the suicidal patient, are incongruous with a "good patient's" role and obligations. For example, the patient who intentionally has injured him- or herself is both the perpetrator and victim of his or her action, in contrast to being the innocent victim of an undesirable disease or injury. Moreover, not all suicidal patients share their caregiver's belief that they should be provided with life-sustaining treatment; some may maintain a persistent wish to die. Treatment compliance and the attainment of a reciprocal, collaborative relationship are often difficult.

High-risk patients have a number of character traits, skill deficits, and attachment difficulties that both explain their suicidality and negatively affect *treatment alliance*. Among these are significant psychopathology, limited impulse control (act first, think later), alcohol and/or drug abuse, and poor relational, communication, emotional regulation, and problem-solving skills. Among suicidal adolescents, in particular (but, perhaps, common to all life stages), stage-specific developmental characteristics further make the forming of a therapeutic alliance difficult—for example, idealism and absolutism (black and white thinking), externalizing attributions, and so on. Attachment patterns common to suicidal adolescents

509

have been described as "unresolved/disorganized" (Adam, Sheldon-Keller, & West, 1996) and further combine to interfere with working alliances. Thus, treatment dropout rates are high. As the quality of the therapeutic alliance is the greatest single factor affecting treatment outcome, recognizing these issues is critical to developing a treatment plan with any chance of successful implementation.

Compliance with treatment, both medication and psychotherapy, is a significant treatment problem when dealing with suicidal patients. Children and adolescents, even after treatment in a hospital emergency room for a suicide attempt, have low rates of compliance with recommended outpatient follow-up appointments (see Litt, Cuskey, & Rudd, 1983). Suicidal adolescents may not comply for a variety of reasons, including a desire to maintain drug or alcohol use, nihilistic attitudes, or a fear of being labeled as crazy (see Trautman, Stewart, & Morishima, 1993). Suicidal children, whose referrals for follow-up are most often governed by their parents, often do not comply because of parental denial, embarrassment, or pathology (see Box 21.1). Antisocial and paranoid patients are simply difficult to engage and align with in treatment.

With regard to medication, patients with bipolar disorders object to the blunting of the high of their manic cycling and, thus, often do not maintain themselves on lithium (see Case 21.1). Uncomfortable side effects often lead others to discontinue medication treatments. Geriatric patients may forget to take prescribed medications or mis-take dosages. Making compliance a focus for treatment increases the likelihood that it will be attained. This can

---

BOX 21.1. Some Common Reasons for Noncompliance

Patient
Denial of problem/pathology; minimization of pathology
Behavior has secondary gain (e.g., control of other's attention)
Reluctance to relinquish "sick" role
Familial reinforcement to maintain "sick" role ("identified patient")
Nihilism/negative expectancy set
Autonomy/control (refusal to seek/accept help); ambivalence/fear of dependency
Psychopathology (personality disorder, e.g., antisocial or psychosis); paranoia
Avoidance of affect (e.g., anger, rage, hopelessness)
Fear of exposure/humiliation (being seen as "sick"; announcing sexual orientation . . .)
Antimedication attitudes
Religious attitudes
Prior therapeutic failures

Parent (in regard to child patient)
Denial of severity of child's problems/pathology; minimization
     Pollyanish beliefs (the crisis has passed, the problem is resolved)
Ignorance; moralism (e.g., bad child labeling)
Fear of exposure/humiliation (of own pathology,);
     Implication of poor parenting/communication
     Protection of family secrets
Refusal to face parental issues (e.g., marital discord/conflict; parental substance abuse)
Guilt (possible genetic transmission of mental disorder)
Refusal to face own hostility, detachment . . .
Financial limitations; managed care/insurance limitations

CASE 21.1. The Case of Nick Traina

"I will never forget the sheer beauty of him. . . ," wrote Danielle Steele (1998) of her son, Nick Traina's, birth in her loving memoir *His Bright Light*. But within a year "all hell broke loose." Nick "exploded into life," doing things he was not supposed to do, saying things no child his age said. He also did not sleep—an early sign of the trouble that was to come. By the time he was 2 he was enchanting all whom came into contact with him; but, at home, he was a terror, uncontrolled and often uncontrollable. Soon after a sister was born Nick, now 4, became rageful. He wet his bed every night; at times, he defecated in the bathtub. His drawings were black and angry. He destroyed toys. Control was not in his behavioral vocabulary. "Being with him was like trying to harness a tornado," Steel observed.

By the time Nick was 11, his mother was constantly worried about him. Everything he did was more extreme—brighter, faster, louder, harder, meaner. There were signs he was self-medicating with whatever he found in the bathroom—Tylenol, Sudafed. By age 12 it was clear he was seriously experimenting with drugs—alcohol, pot, LSD; later yet, he would try mushrooms, speed, ecstacy, and cocaine. He began isolating himself. His journals spoke of his sadness, fear, loneliness, and depression. Soon, he wrote of his thoughts of suicide and of an attempt to kill himself by suffocation with a plastic bag; thwarted by a change of mind. But he still felt hateful and hated. Prophetically, he wondered whether he was manic–depressive.

It took 3 more years before he was correctly diagnosed. In between ages 12 and 15, he was in and out of boarding schools and psychiatrists' offices. He had no impulse control; he could not abide by others' rules; he could not comply with treatment. It was as if he was controlled by demons; all the time more hostile, more depressed, more isolated, more bizarre. There followed a series of hospitalizations, short- and longer-term stays. And finally a psychological evaluation that mentioned for the first time "a variant of bipolar disorder." Prozac was first ordered and seemed to help, but only for a while; a year later he was prescribed lithium and finally he appeared balanced, good-humored, calm. He was able to get heavy into his music, a band he formed, performing, and gaining some success.

Turning 18, Nick declared his independence, "I'm 18 now, you can't make me!" Four months later he decided he was cured, that he did not need to take his lithium. Within weeks he was again manic, and soon therafter made his first and nearly lethal suicide attempt by heroin and an unknown assortment of drugs. Miraculously, he recovered; his lithium was restarted. Ten days later, while on an inpatient psychiatry ward, he made a second attempt, overdosing on some drugs brought in by friends. Again, he bounced back, stabilized, and soon seemed to be once again happy and passionate about his music. But with the music scene came the lure of alcohol and drugs, the stress of performing, the inevitable conflicts with fellow band members, and noncompliance with his lithium . . . and a year later his suicide by morphine overdose.

only be accomplished with an empathic acknowledgment and understanding of the patient's reported reasons for noncompliance (a past history of unpleasant experiences on medications, concerns for addiction, loss of control, etc.); moreover, acknowledging that all medications of consequence have side effects of consequence but that these hopefully will be minimized. With this as a groundwork, approaches to destigmatizing and normalizing psychopharmacological interventions can be made. These might include analogizing to physical conditions for which the patient willingly takes medication, describing a variety of common biochemical deficiencies commonly regulated by medication, providing bibliographic material written by or about celebrities who have been helped by medication, cognitively reinforcing the patient's freedom to choose to be well or ill, and noting by history the patient's relapsing or symptom exacerbation when prior medications were discontinued relative to improved functioning when on medication.

COUNTERTRANSFERENCE

Suicidal communications, in the form of behaviors (e.g., nonfatal attempts), threats, and verbalized ideation, are common to a number of mental disorders (e.g., schizophrenia and alcohol abuse). Conversely, a number of mental disorders have suicidal behavior as one of several symptom criteria, a proportion of which define the disorder (e.g., major depression and borderline personality disorder). Thus, suicidal behaviors are commonly observed in the clinical paradigm.

In fact, suicidal behaviors are the most frequent mental health problems presenting to hospital emergency departments and that result in inpatient admissions. This is particularly true among children and adolescent inpatient psychiatric admissions.

Given our difficulty in accurately predicting when and if any at-risk patient might attempt suicide, the potential for a patient acting on suicidal urges (and consequently causing lethal medical damage) is a constancy in the clinical situation and is anxiety provoking to the clinician. Surveys of clinicians consistently report that suicidal behaviors and communications are among the most stressful of all patient behaviors encountered (Deutsch, 1984; Farber, 1983) and the threat of an actual suicide of a patient is the greatest practice-related fear (Menninger, 1990; Pope & Tabachnick, 1993). Consequently, and perhaps not surprisingly, some therapists simply refuse to treat suicidal patients (Bernstein, Feldberg, & Brown, 1991; Jobes, 1995; Jobes & Berman, 1993).

Berman (1986a) estimated that one in six individuals who complete suicide is actively engaged in psychotherapy at the time of their deaths and that one-half of completers have had experience with the mental health system at some time. It is of interest, then, to consider whether these suicides might be considered *prima facie* evidence of treatment failures. Moreover, it is of interest to consider whether these suicides were consequent to some *iatrogenic effect*. Iatrogenesis is defined as a caregiver-induced negative effect (or illness caused by health care), such as hopelessness engendered by a lack of response to sequentially prescribed antidepressants or the anger and distrust induced and reinforced by involuntary hospitalization.

Perhaps, the most significant contributor to iatrogenesis is *negative countertransference*. In its most contemporary usage, negative countertransference is defined by a range of aversive reactions (thoughts, feelings, behaviors) that are manifested in clinicians in reaction to working with their psychotherapy patients. These reactions range from anger to hopelessness to dislike. In the traditional meaning of the term, these reactions are unconscious and stem from the therapist's relationships in childhood (e.g., to parents). Often, however, these responses are conscious and directly related to a difficult-to-treat patient.

As noted previously, suicidal patients readily engender fears and anxieties in clinicians. They present complicated and often chronic histories, maintain a high level of anticipatory threat, impose strong transferential feelings and behaviors stemming from conflictual relationships with their primary caregivers (parents), pose potential emergency situations (such as the need for hospitalization or for intervention should they act out suicidally) and potential malpractice litigation, should they complete suicide during the therapist's watch. Each and every one of these anxieties must be successfully managed by the clinician in order to maintain an effective and helpful therapeutic position. This is no small task.

Pioneering theoretical work in this area was presented by Maltsberger and Buie (1974) who described the most common and dangerous form of countertransference evoked by the suicidal patient as "countertransference hate." Countertransference hate, they proposed, consists of both aversion—a strong dislike leading to rejection and possible abandonment—and malice—a sadistic desire to tease or harm.

There is little doubt that suicidal patients harbor much rage, can be manipulative or help rejecting, and engage in a number of interpersonally alienating behaviors. Suicidal patients who have diagnoses of schizophrenia, schizophrenic spectrum disorders, or borderline personality disorder are, indeed, difficult to treat. These patients may experience extreme distress at having to tolerate aloneness, may be terrified at anticipated abandonments, and may have diffuse boundaries—any or all of which test the most experienced of therapists' skills at maintaining appropriate therapeutic positions. Moreover, a patient who threatens suicide is, at once, rejecting the offered help and efforts of the therapist.

Maltsberger and Buie posit that countertransferential acting out, the result of a therapist's unconscious murderous impulses, can lead to suicidal behavior. Bloom (1967) was among the first to provide evidence of therapists who denied or repressed their hostility toward their patients in six cases of suicide. More recently, Judd, Jobes, Arnkoff, and Fenton (1999) tested these observations empirically on a sample of 23 discharged, suicidal inpatients matched to a sample of nonsuicidal inpatients from a long-term psychoanalytic treatment facility. Verbatim transcripts of case presentations by the patients' treating therapists, made between 3 and 12 months of admission, were coded and analyzed blindly for 14 categories of negative countertransference (described instances of inattention during a session, self-blame, angry and hopeless attitudes, etc.). Indeed, significant differences between groups were found on both total and covert countertransference variables.

Negative therapist attitudes toward suicidal patients are also observable in the pejorative labeling attributed to difficult-to-treat patients. Suicidal patients are often seen, for example, as "manipulative," suggesting that they are devious and indirect in attempting to control others and/or outcomes, rather than more simply deficient in skills to be in better control. As few people like to be manipulated, perhaps especially therapists whose job it is to manipulate, protective distancing is likely to result from perceived manipulators. This is the antithesis of what is needed to change a patient's interpersonal behavior and to teach more effective skills.

Similarly, therapists are wont to label help-rejecting patients "resistive." Rather than seeing this as an obstacle of therapy, resistance needs to be reframed as one of the reasons this patient needs therapy; that is "resistance" is a protective device, probably learned in childhood, that has gained functional autonomy with age. Patients need to be helped to analyze the defense and to learn to risk trusting behaviors in the context of the therapeutic relationship.

Finally, suicidal persons challenge caregivers to examine their own issues regarding life and death, to keep clear the boundary between personal beliefs and professional ethics, and to examine carefully their attitudes toward involuntary detention and treatment. Readers should consider, for example, the following scenario proposed by Tanney (1995b) in determining their response to an acutely suicidal person:

> *Would you lie?* You approach a person-at-risk (PAR) standing on the railing of a bridge clearly threatening to jump. You are the only potential interventionist. You approach cautiously, calmly engage the PAR in dialogue, establish rapport, and invite the PAR to come down off the bridge abutment and accompany you back to your office. The PAR agrees, but on one condition; that is, if after giving you a reasonable opportunity to intervene, that if the PAR decided to return to the bridge and complete the intended suicide, that you would do nothing to stop the PAR. How would you respond?

FROM ASSESSMENT TO DISPOSITION

Risk assessment initiates treatment by first addressing the appropriate setting. If a patient is evaluated as at high risk for imminent suicidal behavior, immediate action is called for to protect the patient from him- or herself. Psychiatric hospitalization is generally thought to provide the most secure environment and best opportunity to provide sanctuary, to manage and observe behavior, and to initiate treatments. Thus a rationale or cost-benefit analysis for inpatient hospitalization is the first consideration for an acutely suicidal patient.

The decision to hospitalize is based on a number of criteria reflective of the patient's acute psychopathology, observed ability to regulate self, alternative sources of support and monitoring, and so on, that determine danger-to-self evaluations. Among the variables to consider are the following:

- Axis I psychopathology that describes symptoms of dyscontrol or impending decompensation such as disorientation, dissociation, and impulsive behavior; high levels of perturbation (agitation); thought disorder (e.g., hallucinations and delusions); and/or high levels of rage, panic, or uncontrolled violent behavior.
- Axis III medical problems consequent to a suicide attempt placing the patient in danger of losing life, if untreated.
- Axis IV stress at high and unresolvable levels.
- Axis V GAF (Global Assessment of Functioning Scale) score of 20 or lower.
- Attachment problems such as the absence of a supportive family or surrogate system to monitor and prevent isolation or the presence of an abusive, rejecting, or psychiatrically impaired interpersonal system; the absence of a therapeutic alliance; or the absence of other attachments of personal value and efficacy, such as employment, function and so on.
- Highly death intentioned suicidal thinking or behavior indirectly suggesting high intent, such as an attempt made by a male under conditions of low rescuability (e.g., made in a locked hotel room).
- Evaluated acute risk in the context of a family history of suicide.

The case of Helen (Case 20.6) is a tragic example of a therapist setting the bar too high in determining criteria for when her patient could benefit from a more stabilizing environment.

There are clear *benefits* to the stabilization and sanctuary that hospitalization provides: The patient is removed from sources of stress; an immediate change in (pathological) system dynamics is effected; 24-hour support and monitoring are available that counteract isolation and loneliness and encourage activity and interpersonal involvement; maximum control over suicidal and aggressive urges is available; hope and mastery are instilled through stepwise goal attainment programs; medical consequences and/or complications from self-injurious behavior can be treated and monitored; and medications may be reconsidered and titrated to therapeutic levels. For some, hospitalization is an aversive experience and is, thus, a contingent reinforcer to sufficient self-regulation to deter future rehospitalization.

There also are clear *costs*: hospitalization interrupts the consistency and alliance building of an outpatient contract; reinforces regression and, for some, fosters an institutional dependency; and removes the patient from the *in vivo* context in which coping and mastery skills need to be applied and reinforced. Furthermore, the hospitalized patient loses some degree of autonomy and may feel stigmatized. These pose significant problems to outpatient alliances (problems of trust, for example) and reentry, for example, for an adolescent who must now return to school and peers.

It should therefore be of no surprise that therapist variables also enter into the decision to hospitalize a patient. For example, therapists differ in their capacity to tolerate stress and uncertainty. Therapist variables, such as those just discussed, underlie research findings that describe disagreements among clinicians' disposition recommendations in the same case scenario. A recently reported analogue study found relatively low levels of agreement among eight senior attending psychiatrists who viewed videotaped emergency service assessment interviews on both the evaluation of danger to self and decisions to admit to (vs. release from) hospital treatment (Way, Allen, Mumpower, Stewart, & Banks, 1998). Engelman, Jobes, Berman, and Langbein (1998) reported that decisions to detain were highly variable among emergency service personnel, depending on prior experience (e.g., individuals with different patterns—high frequency vs. low frequency—of detaining patients) and perceived bed availability.

One point should be made eminently clear: Hospitalization does not necessarily *prevent* suicide. Suicides can occur in hospitals, although policy and procedural safeguards typically deter such outcomes, on passes and via elopement from an inpatient unit, and quite soon after discharge, suggesting that this is a particularly crucial treatment decision point. Also, the decision to hospitalize is best considered when the patient voluntarily consents to this treatment setting. Involuntary hospitalization is mandated by state statute under conditions (with regard to suicide) of evaluated imminent danger to self.

The case of PR (Case 21.2) presents such a consideration. Readers should place themselves in the shoes of the psychiatric resident or the attending psychiatrist and make a determination whether they would decide to detain this patient for further observation. For this decision, readers should further assume that state statutes allow them to detain this patient for further observation for up to 72 hours before discharging him or her or seeking a court-ordered involuntary hospitalization.

INPATIENT TREATMENT

The immediate treatment goal of inpatient hospitalization is the absence of current suicidal ideation and intent. Within the typical parameters of managed care, this goal must be met rapidly; economic pressures are now added to the matrix of considerations in determining discharge decisions. Clearly, when the patient is still considered to be unsafe from his or her own self-destructive urges, a well-documented appeal for extended treatment should allow sufficient additional time to stabilize most patients.

At the most acute phase of risk, an imminently suicidal patient is immediately confronted with a treatment environment in most psychiatric inpatient units that promotes protection, safety, and connectedness. The patient is denied access to immediately accessible

CASE 21.2. The Case of PR

PR, a 22-year-old single male, is brought to the emergency room on a Saturday morning by the police on a "certificate of evaluation" after failing to show up for his outpatient psychiatric appointment. His psychiatrist expressed concern regarding PR's increasing hopelessness and suicidality. PR allegedly told a cousin (who relayed the message to the psychiatrist) that "his meds weren't helping and had never helped." He told his cousin that he was going to be evicted from his apartment, if he didn't have rent money by Sunday and stated, "This was his last weekend . . . that he would not be around on Sunday." He claimed that he heard voices telling him to cut himself or cause a gas explosion. He said he planned to kill himself by a gas explosion and that "It's going to be a messy scene." When his cousin asked how he felt, should others get harmed in the explosion, he said, "I'll be dead; I don't care."

PR's first hospital admission was at the age of 12. Diagnosed as having a major depression, he was admitted with a history of school vandalism and stealing, enuresis (once or twice a week), and morbid obesity; he furthermore admitted to increasing suicide ideation. He was hospitalized for 7 months with major treatment foci being his body image, anxiety and anger management, and social withdrawal.

His second hospitalization occurred at the age of 20. Brought to the hospital by his mother for episodes of angry outbursts, paranoia (he feared he was being watched through holes in their apartment wall), self-cutting ("X's" on arms "in honor of those who had turned against him"), and symptoms of visual hallucinations, he was involuntarily admitted. After four days he was discharged with an Axis I diagnosis—adjustment disorder with mixed disturbances of emotions and conduct—and an Axis II diagnosis—borderline personality disorder.

PR had been unemployed for 6 months and had given up looking for work. He reportedly ran out of marijuana 3 days ago and said he was "going crazy." During his high school years he reportedly dealt drugs and was dependent on amphetamines. He currently was taking Depakote (250 mg twice a day) and Zoloft (100 mg orally every day).

Upon intake at the hospital, PR stated to the on-call psychiatric resident, "I worried a lot of people today," that he did not want to harm himself, that he was just frustrated about his situation. He was calm and cooperative, oriented to time, person, and place, and organized and goal directed in his thinking. His mood was appropriate; he denied having audio or visual hallucinations and delusional thinking. He did admit to some paranoid thoughts regarding "people standing behind me." He stated that he had threatened to cause a gas explosion to get attention—"to rile [his family] up," that he needed and wanted to look for work. Offered hospitalization, he declined because he "would not do be able to seek work if [he] were hospitalized." He wanted to spend Sunday searching the paper's classifieds. He stated that his rent had been extended by Goodwill.

After consulting with the attending psychiatrist by phone, the psychiatric resident released PR with a follow-up outpatient appointment scheduled on Monday with his outpatient psychiatrist.

means to suicide—for example, sharp objects are confiscated at admission—and units are reasonably suicide-proofed in their design; for example, breakaway shower rods are used and windows are barred or effectively screened internally. Watch procedures and monitoring protocols are established ranging from one-to-one constant observation to various levels (e.g., 15 minutes) of logged checks. No unit, however, can be totally suicide proofed and in-hospital suicides do occur. In addition, it should be kept in mind that a suicidal act can lead to death in less than 5 minutes; thus, any level of surveillance other than that of close observation, one-to-one or group, is insufficient to prevent suicide. The case of Wanda Jones (Case 20.9) illustrates the inadequacy of typical watch procedures with a severely disturbed patient and an indefensible act of negligence by the hospital.

Multidisciplinary Treatment Plan Goals

A typical initial treatment plan will evolve at admission or after a few days' observation. Figure 21.1 illustrates how this might be written for a patient admitted after a suicide attempt. Secondary treatment goals, of course, would be established for assessed underlying problems (for depressed mood, social skills, self-esteem, etc.).

Genral Principles of Inpatient Management

Inpatient care usually involves a screening evaluation and team-developed treatment plan, treatment according to that plan, followed by discharge planning and implementation. As indicated by the initial and follow-up evaluations of suicide risk, affirmative precautions are instituted—with an ever present awareness that suicides can occur in the best of inpatient units. Unit policies and procedures should define steps to safeguard the environment and protect the patient, in addition to staff responsibilities, roles, and so on.

No-Suicide Contracts

"No suicide safety contracts" are commonly employed in inpatient psychiatry units. These written and signed documents reflect an understanding (in truth, no "contractual" exchange actually occurs) between hospital staff and the suicidal patient. The hospital promises to provide the patient safety, a responsibility it already has, while the patient commits to not act in a suicidal manner and to inform the staff should suicidal urges become overwhelming.

The no-suicide contract actually is a clinical tool used to assess the therapeutic alliance and to identify explicitly a treatment goal. A patient's refusal to sign represents his or her lack of alliance or oppositionalism to the primary treatment goal (i.e., life vs. death). On the

Date	Problem	Long- and Short-Term Goals	Intervention
12/28/__	Potential for violence—self and others. Shot self and fired gun in mother's home without warning.	Patient will be free from harm and will not harm others during this hospitalization.	• Provide safe environment/15-minute checks. • Administer medications as per MD order as necessary. • Encourage time-outs to decrease stimulation as necessary. • Patient to sign no-self-harm contract.

FIGURE 21.1. Sample inpatient treatment plan.

other hand, his or her acceptance of the contract's terms (typically documented in the chart simply as "patient contracted for safety") should not delude caregivers into a false sense of security. Patients deceive; patients may not have sufficiently developed defenses to resist unpredictable and episodic suicidal urges (after all, this is, in part, why patients are hospitalized); patients who have been wounded in prior exchanges with caretakers (e.g., parents) simply cannot be trusted to invest long-term meaning in such transient promises. Moreover, the danger exists that the contract will replace staff attention to a careful assessment of other signs of increased risk for suicidal behavior, as in the case of Alicia (see Case 21.3).

CASE 21.3. Case of Alicia

Alicia, age 18, was admitted to the hospital with comorbid diagnoses of major depressive disorder, single episode; dysthymic disorder; and post-traumatic stress disorder. Her mother had been murdered when Alicia was 2. Alicia believed her father was the murderer. Until the age of 11, she was physically and sexually abused by both her father and one brother. After informing a teacher of the abuse, Alicia was removed to a series of foster families throughout her teen years. When she learned that she would be expected to testify against her father and brother, Alicia got depressed. She reported sleep difficulties, flashbacks of the abuse, difficulty concentrating with a consequent drop in grades, and thoughts of suicide by choking herself with a sweater or taking poison. She also began self-mutilative wrist scratching "to let out the pain."

On the inpatient unit she was hypomanic and sexually inappropriate. She was put on suicide precautions and was closely observed for over a month as she continued to voice suicidal plans. She told a nurse, " I've always thought of killing myself since the day I was born . . . I know I'll commit suicide some day; it's just too much pressure." In spite of this statement, she signed a safety contract, promising to inform staff if she felt like harming herself and before she would do anything to hurt herself. Her mood and behavior on the unit continued to be unpredictable and labile. By month 3 of her hospitalization, she had been removed from constant observation, graduating to "frequent observation," then "frequent awareness" levels. After 3 months she began to discuss and consider discharge disposition with the treatment team. She interviewed for a group living facility but was rejected. Given a second opportunity to interview, she excitedly began rehearsing her interview style; but she again did poorly when evaluated, and was rejected a second time. Returning to the ward, she was sullen, rude, and demanding; she blamed the group home director for not accepting her. However, by the next day, her mood and behavior were described as "softer, less complaining, claims not to be sad." She denied suicidal intent. There was no thought to reinstitute any level of suicide observation; the staff considered her safety contract to still be in effect.

When awakened the next morning, she was observed to be dawdling in her room. Encouraged to prepare for breakfast, she went to the bathroom. Ten minutes later, nursing staff noticed a knotted sheet over her closed bathroom door. When the door was opened, Alicia's lifeless body fell to the floor. She was blue, not breathing, and pulseless. A code was called and CPR instituted, but she could not be resuscitated.

Discharge Procedures

The frequency of suicides that occur shortly after hospitalization is disturbing. Several implications need to be considered: Did the assessment of suicide risk at the time of discharge inadequately consider the toxic effect of the external social milieu or the loss of constant support provided by hospital care? Was the patient sufficiently advised of the need for continued compliance with the treatment plan and referral for outpatient care? Did the patient intentionally deceive/mislead the treatment team in appearing well-enough for discharge? Was follow-up outpatient care not sufficiently accessed? Was the patient's family or significant other insufficiently aligned with follow-up care needs or with the continued need for surveillance and reporting?

The case of Norman Smith (Case 20.11) exemplifies a discharge with inadequate attention to assessment of risk, aftercare planning, treatment compliance, and medication monitoring.

OUTPATIENT TREATMENT

Outpatient treatment begins with the assessment of suicide risk and the decision not to hospitalize (cf. Bongar et al., 1998). If the risk for suicidal behavior is high but not sufficiently imminent to demand hospitalization, the need for monitoring may still be present through the period of perturbation or crisis. A person close to the patient and capable of providing both vigilance and relief from aloneness should be considered and may be necessary. Home environments should be suicide proofed, as much as possible, particularly as they pertain to available and accessible firearms and medications. Frequent contact with the primary caregiver is important through either increased session visits and/or telephone communication. Pharmacological interventions should be considered for assessed diagnoses (see the section "Psychopharmacotherapy" below). With these immediate supports established, treatment planning ensues.

TREATMENT PLANNING

Treatment planning involves designing interventions that aim first at reducing the risk of suicidal behavior and second at reducing the predisposition to being suicidal (dealing with the underlying mental disorder, etc.). It is a truism that the better the assessment, particularly in understanding the suicidal person's vulnerabilities and pathologies, aims or goals of suicidal behavior, and resources (protective factors), the easier the treatment planning. In addition to deciding structural issues such as the site of treatment (inpatient vs. outpatient), treatment planning speaks to the sequencing of treatment, for example, with dual-diagnosis patients; the particular type(s) of psychosocial intervention; the need for biological interventions, such as medication or electroconvulsive therapy; the frequency and duration of interventions; the measurable goals of interventions, the accomplishment of which leads to termination from treatment and follow-up planning; and environmental manipulations and enhancements to support treatment goals.

Treatment planning further specifies particular symptom remission related goals (the reduction in frequency, intensity, duration, or specificity of suicidal ideation; decreased hopelessness; improved access to supports, etc.). Specific throughout the treatment planning should be considerations of ongoing risk assessment and the need for collateral consultations.

In this regard, Jobes et al. (1998) have introduced a creative, collaborative model for outpatient treatment planning dictated by specific risk assesment. The Collaborative Assessment and Management of Suicidality (CAMS) is intended to facilitate building a therapeutic alliance through a working partnership between therapist and patient to understand the patient's suicidality. By identifying key constructs that underlie the patient's suicidal state, treatment goals and interventions are targeted and shaped.

Built on a multitheoretical model, the CAMS model asks both patient and clinician to complete a Suicide Status Form (see Figure 21.1) and, then, to build specific treatment goals

Suicide Status Form
(patient)

Patient name: _____   Clinician: _____
ID # _____   Date: _____

1) RATE PSYCHOLOGICAL PAIN: The cause of my pain is: _____	Little pain: 1 2 3 4 5 :Intolerable Pain
2) RATE EXTERNAL PRESSURES: (STRESSORS): My biggest stressor is: _____	Low external pressures: 1 2 3 4 5 :High external pressures
3) RATE AGITATION: (EMOTIONAL UPSETNESS): What upsets me most is: _____	Low agitation: 1 2 3 4 5 :High agitation
4) RATE HOPELESSNESS: The reason I am hopeless is: _____	Absolutely hopeful: 1 2 3 4 5 :Absolutely hopeless
5) RATE SELF-REGARD: The best description of my self is: _____	Extremely positive: 1 2 3 4 5 :Extremely negative
6) RATE IMPULSIVENESS: The reason I am impulsive is: _____	Low impulsiveness: 1 2 3 4 5 :High impulsiveness
7) RATE COPING ABILITY: The best description of my coping ability is: _____	Completely able to cope: 1 2 3 4 5 :Completely unable to cope
8) RATE OVERALL RISK OF SUICIDE:	Extremely low risk: 1 2 3 4 5 :Extremely high risk (will <u>not</u> kill self) (will kill self)

1) How much is being suicidal related to thoughts and feelings about <u>yourself</u>?
   Not at all: 1   2   3   4   5 : completely
2) How much is being suicidal related to thoughts and feelings about <u>others</u>?
   Not at all: 1   2   3   4   5 : completely

In order of importance, list your top five reasons for wanting to live and your top five reasons for wanting to die

REASONS FOR LIVING	REASONS FOR DYING
1)	1)
2)	2)
3)	3)
4)	4)
5)	5)

The one thing that would help me no longer feel suicidal would be: _____
_____

I agree to maintain my safety between outpatient sessions: YES ___ NO ____
Patient signature: _____

FIGURE 21.2. CAMS Suicide Status Form, patient version, initial session (Jobes et al., 1998).

to reduce or alleviate intrusive symptoms (see top of form) or strengthen attachments noted in reasons for living (see bottom of form). For example, were a patient to have rated a high level of hopelessness (item 4) about his marriage, a treatment goal might be to improve marital relations. Interventions to achieve this goal might include cognitive therapy to address distorted thinking or couple therapy to improve communications.

TREATMENT APPROACHES

Crisis Intervention

Crisis intervention and management approaches to the suicidal patient are designed to ensure the patient's safety and life until the precipitant crisis situation can be resolved and a precrisis equilibrium restored. The "steps" of crisis intervention might involve (1) restricting access to lethal means (e.g., removal of available and accessible weapons); (2) decreasing personal isolation (e.g., monitoring activities and behavior through constant interpersonal watch); (3) decreasing anxiety, agitation, or insomnia (e.g., through medication or relaxation training procedures); (4) increasing accessibility (e.g., through telephone availability) and frequency of contact; (5) establishing a collaborative, problem-solving focus to treatment and fostering the patient's problem-solving skills; (6) removal from stressful or toxic environments (e.g., through hospitalization); (7) system interventions to shift immediate (e.g., family) dynamics; and (8) negotiating safety considerations and developing contingency plans.

Common Errors of Suicide Interventionists

Niemeyer and Pfeffer (1994) analyzed intervention responses of 215 crisis interventionists, medical residents and master's level counselors who had frequent contact with suicidal people. Based on responses to a self-report instrument involving hypothetical scenarios, they identified the following 10 recurring themes that summarized inadequate responses:

1. *Superficial reassurance.* A tendency to emphasize the more optimistic or positive aspects of a situation risks alienating the person in distress, implicitly rejects and contradicts a communication of anguish or hopelessness, and deepens feelings of isolation. Prematurely offering prepackaged meaning for expressed difficulties, as in a religious or secular philosophy, also discounts the depth of pain often felt by the person in distress. *Example:* "But, you have so much to live for." "God works in mysterious ways." "Things can't be all that bad."

2. *Avoidance of strong feelings.* A retreat into intellectualization or premature advice-giving concurrently avoids empathic understanding and models the containment of strong emotions. *Example:* "Your tears suggest that you're depressed. Maybe we should consider some medication."

3. *Professionalism.* Similarly, caregivers might insulate or protect themselves from the exhausting task of empathic pairing by seeking refuge in the boundaries afforded by their role. This may overly distance and detach the caregiver and convey disinterest. Most important, it does not build upon the relationship. *Example:* "You can tell me, I'm a professional and have been trained to be objective about these things."

4. *Inadequate assessment of suicidal intent.* Often, veiled, indirect communications of suicide risk may be met with reassurance while more direct statements are ignored or even contradicted. *Example:* "You sound [say you are] suicidal, but what is really bothering you."

5. *Failure to identify the precipitating event.* It is important to recognize the context of, and specific triggers for, suicidal behaviors. A focus on precipitating events allows for the development of action plans later in the intervention. Patients need their pain (and its context) understood before being ready to move on. *Example:* "What do you think your [deceased] wife would want from you? . . . Don't you think she'd want you to be more productive, to get on with your life."

6. *Passivity.* Interventions at times of crisis need to be active, engaging, focused, and structuring. Passive responses tend not to join the person at risk to a more collaborative alliance. *Example:* "I'm here to listen . . ." vs. "It must be very hard to talk about what's bothering you."

7. *Insufficient directiveness.* Similarly, crises require directive management. Sometimes empathic listening needs to shift to the negotiation of safe structures for further work. *Example:* "Why don't you put the gun down?" vs. "I know holding the gun in your hand makes you feel more in control. But it also makes me feel anxious, and I don't want my anxiety to get in the way of my helping you. I want you to put the gun down, so we can just talk, OK?"

8. *Advice giving.* Problem solving must follow a thorough assessment of the problem and the establishment of a working alliance. Collaborative work, particularly designed to shape the person at risk's problem-solving skills, will lead to better resolutions than will premature advice. *Example:* "You're not thinking rationally. We need to identify an alternative way to interpret what happened . . ."

9. *Stereotypical responses.* The press of a crisis may force shortcuts in the form of unwarranted, stereotypical assumptions based on demographic profiles, typologies, and so on. rather than paying sufficient attention to the individuality of each person in distress. *Example:* "Most men have this sort of difficulty."

10. *Defensiveness.* Difficult-to-treat persons in distress may display characterological patterns of anger, help rejection, provocative communications, interpersonal distrust, and so on. They may attack the caregiver's competence, understanding, and/or caring. Responses to these communications must be nondefensive and noncontradictory; rather, they must reflect empathy and open discussion to how these beliefs affect a working alliance. *Example:* "Well, no, I have never been suicidal myself, but I can still help you." or "Sure I've had thoughts of suicide myself, but I've always found better solutions to my problems."

Brief Therapy

Brief therapy is a time-limited intervention that, especially in the era of managed care, attempts to focus on maximizing change, accomplishing goals and need fulfillment, and problem-solving. One example of this interventive approach is *solution-focused brief therapy* (SFBT). As described by Fiske (1997), SFBT transfers the treatment focus from problems and pathology to solutions and competencies. This shift in focus is toward the future—doing more of what works and something different if something is not working. The model emphasizes exceptions to the problem ("nothing occurs always!"), using the patient's strengths, competencies, resources, and successes; helping patients define their goals; and effecting small changes that generate yet larger, more profound, and pervasive changes.

Cognitive-Behavioral Therapy

Cognitive-behavioral therapy (CBT) is also structured and problem focused. In a time-limited approach, CBT aims to identify and change dysfunctional cognitions (thoughts, beliefs, schemas, etc.) and behaviors. Problems are conceptualized as having interacting dysfunctional thoughts, moods, and behaviors. By identifying and changing any one component, problem solving can occur.

The basis for a cognitive approach is rooted in a substantial body of research linking cognition and suicidality (cf. Ellis & Newman, 1996). Hopelessness, problem-solving deficits, perfectionism, and a variety of dysfunctional attitudes and irrational beliefs have been found to be characteristic of suicidal individuals. Teaching problem-solving thinking, reattaching to reasons for living, and defusing black-and-white thinking, then, become tools for correcting maladaptive thinking.

For adults, the typical point of attack is on the patient's cognitive distortions and automatic negative thoughts that underlie a depressive mood state, or even more malignant states of hopelessness (cf. Berchick & Wright, 1992). For children and adolescents, behaviors are easier to observe and monitor, therefore modify (Trautman, 1995). For both adult and adolescent patients, the CBT therapist is active and assertive, providing explanations and positive feedback with frequency.

Above all, the CBT model is collaborative. Therapist and patient (and, perhaps, the patient's family) identify the patient's problems, strengths, and previous attempts at problem solving. By viewing the world through the patient's eyes, the therapist is able to identify and label the patient's errors in thinking, automatic thoughts such as overgeneralization ("Other people can do this; I can't; I'm a loser."), jumping to conclusions ("Hurting myself is the only way to feel better"), and dysfunctional attributions ("My parents fight because of me; I should never have been born") and to help the patient develop alternative explanations, interpretations, and beliefs. In particular, a primary target of treatment is to change the patient's view of suicide as the most desirable (or only) alternative to the present, pained experience of living. Problem-solving thinking and skills are developed and practiced (homework is often assigned). A significant goal of treatment is to increase the frequency of pleasant and rewarding thoughts and experiences (activities).

Dialectical Behavior Therapy

Dialectical behavior therapy (DBT) was developed by Linehan (1993) specifically to treat the chronic suicidal patient who lives a suicidal career high in suicidal ideation, frequent in suicide talk and/or threat, and high in repetitive suicide attempts of varying degrees of lethality. DBT differs from traditional cognitive-behavioral approaches to treatment in that it is based on making behavioral techniques more compatible with psychodynamic models (see below). The model posits that the chronic suicidal individual (1) lacks and must acquire self-regulation (of emotion and behavior) and distress tolerance skills and (2) must be motivated to strengthen and generalize skills to out-of-therapy situations.

DBT utilizes a problem-solving strategy, addressing patient behaviors through a collaborative behavioral analysis and hypothesis formulation. Possible changes (behavioral solutions) are then generated to be tested and evaluated. Dialectical strategies balance and attempt to synthesize coexisting opposites and tensions, helping the patient accept reality as ambiguous and constantly changing. The therapist validates the patient's view of life (and death) while implementing alternative problem-solving analyses and responses. Detailed chain analyses of environmental and behavioral events linked to suicidal behavior are conducted to elicit patterns (i.e., regularities in precipitants and consequences) and to identify alternative solutions. The patient's capacity (skills) to modify problematic precipitating events or conditions that inhibit or interfere with the use of existing skills must then be understood. Skills, then, are either taught or inhibiting forces reduced. A commitment to learning nonsuicidal behavioral responses while tolerating negative affect is a significant target of DBT treatment.

Psychoanalytic/Psychodynamic Approaches

Psychoanalytic/psychodynamic approaches to treating the suicidal patient assume that suicidal behavior is an expression of unconscious conflict (behavioral approaches do not interpret unconscious factors). The goal of treatment is to gain insight (making the unconscious conscious) in order to resolve the intrapsychic pain, self-hatred, and so on. The classic psychoanalytic approach, or Freudian model, theorized that suicidal urges were expressions of a turning inward of aggressive/hostile impulses—an attack against the ambivalently held, internalized love object. Writing in *Mourning and Melancholia*, Freud (1917/1963) noted that "self-reproaches are reproaches against a loved object which have been shifted away from it onto the patient's own ego" (248). Libido invested in another ("object libido") is withdrawn and directed back into the self and an identification takes place between the ego and the lost object. The ego could only kill itself, Freud argued, "if it can treat itself as an object." This concept of "retroflexed rage" was described by Shneidman (1980b) as "murder in the 180th degree."

Karl Menninger (1938) elaborated on this perspective of hostility, extending the concept of the death instinct to explain suicidal drives as a combination of three motivations—the wish to kill (aggression), the wish to die (guilt), and the wish to be killed (escape)—with one of these predominating in each suicide.

More modern analytical approaches define the core conflict in different terms, each then posing a different "cause" for suicidality to be understood and resolved. *Object relations* theory emphasizes that suicidality represents a failure in the task of separation–individuation. The suicide act is an attempt to rid the self of the bad internal objects and to reunite with idealized omnipotent love objects. Research on attachment styles among suicidal teens and adults supports this model, finding many more "insecure" styles of attachment, ranging from avoidant to enmeshed and clinging. Alternatively, suicide is seen as a resolution to problems of separation and individuation through a regressive wish to return to a state of symbiosis.

Self psychology theorists argue that suicide vulnerability arises from threats of being overwhelmed/fragmented by negative self-judgments (e.g., worthlessness and guilt) in the context of an intolerably intense experience of aloneness or unsoothable isolation. Soothing security can be derived from having soothing self-objects (introjects) and/or from having available external holding resources. Lacking these internal resources and absent external resources for soothing, there is a profound and intolerable state of aloneness. Suicide avoids the experience of a crumbling self.

Suicide, in turn, may avoid having to accept a changed sense of self (Smith, 1985). Individuals maintain an internalized view of self—an unconscious, life-guiding abstraction that is rigidly held. When threatened (e.g., by undeniable assault from others) intrapsychic control is maintained. The suicides of Vincent W. Foster, Jr. (see Chapter 11) and Admiral Jeremy Boorda illustrate these types who choose death rather than dishonor and seek to preserve a preferred sense of self under unendurable threats from without to their persona/character.

These psychodynamic formulations inform psychodynamic interventions, such as the analysis of transference, exploration of intrapsychic pain and negative early life events, identification of painful affect states, interpretation of defenses and the motives that maintain self-devaluation, attention to issues of individuation and self-soothing, and so on. Central to the treatment is the role of the therapeutic relationship. The psychodynamic therapist plays the role of "good enough parent," establishes self–object transferences that convey acceptance and confirmation ("mirroring"), protects against feared disintegration/annihilation from painful affect, models soothing and nurturing, interprets transferential impulses that seek to punish a hated parent or seek rescue while supporting ego functioning, perseveres in the face of suicide ideation or through assaults on his or her competence, and so on.

Psychopharmacotherapy

Psychopharmacotherapy does not target suicidal behavior per se. There simply is no antisuicide pill. Rather, pharmacological strategies are diagnosis-specific treatments that aim to regulate the biochemistry associated with predisposing, suicidogenic pathologies. There is, for example, persuasive research evidence (see Chapter 16) linking diminished serotonin (5-HT) metabolism and depression, thus suggesting that the administration of selective serotonin reuptake inhibitors (SSRIs) should effect a reduction in suicidality (cf. Goldblatt, Silverman, & Schatzberg, 1998).

Antidepressant medications (see Chapter 16), particularly the less toxic SSRIs, and lithium and carbamazepine for bipolar disorders are core considerations for pharmacological intervention in suicidal patients. These medications also may reduce episodic impulsive and aggressive behavior. Neuroleptics and antipsychotics are to be considered to manage chronic schizophrenia, as might the short-term use of a benzodiazepine for acute anxiety states.

The effectiveness of psychopharmacological interventions has been widely debated in the literature, with particular questions raised regarding the quality of the research (transparent double-blind studies, use of inactive placebos, high rates of dropout, etc.; cf. Fisher & Greenberg, 1989). Randomized clinical trial pharmacotherapy studies targeting depression typically exclude individuals at high risk for suicide (Linehan, 1998) and have high rates of subjects dropping out of research studies (Sommers-Flannagan & Sommers-Flannagan, 1996). In addition, there has been little to no scientific evidence to date demonstrating that antidepressants are more therapeutic for treating depression in children and adolescents than are placebos (Fisher & Fisher, 1996; Sommers-Flannagan & Sommers-Flannagan, 1996).

Even the newer antidepressants (SSRIs) show little gain in effectiveness relative to imipramine, developed almost a half century ago. Their clear benefit is in the diminution of significant side effects. Concurrently, there are side effects (e.g., irritability and insomnia) and adverse, often paradoxical reactions (e.g., rage and excitation) and case reports of emergent suicide ideation while on these medications (Teicher, Glod, & Cole, 1990).

Perhaps the most persuasive research on the effectiveness of medication is with lithium maintenance treatment in mood disorders. Tondo, Jamison, and Baldessarini (1998) reviewed 28 relevant reports on lithium treatment published between 1974 and 1996. Noting many methodological limitations, they specifically observed that all 12 studies that observed suicide rates with and without lithium maintenance treatment consistently found suicide rates to be lower during maintenance treatment.

Table 21.1 outlines a sequence of psychopharmacotherapeutic interventions for suicidal behaviors. This sequence is not exhaustive; rather, it suggests a way of proceeding that should keep the patient and caregivers aware of and involved in the interventions as they unfold within the total treatment plan.

Electroconvulsive Therapy

Electroconvulsive therapy (ECT), in its modern form, is generally considered safe and effective in the treatment of major depression and mania and should be considered for suicidal patients whose disorders are refractory to psychopharmacological interventions. However, perhaps because there is a paucity of randomized controlled studies to document its

TABLE 21.1. Psychopharmacotherapeutic Intervention Sequence for Suicidal Behavior

Consider potential value of trial medication.
Discuss pros and cons of various medications with patient.
Obtain informed consent.
Slowly initiate medication trial; monitor side effects and adverse symptoms.
Request, if available, blood levels of active metabolites.
Document justifications for discontinuing, decreasing, or increasing dosages beyond
    recommended/accepted levels.
Establish end points (goals of symptom reduction are clarified).
Document justifications for adjunctive somatic therapies (additions of other
    psychoactive medications).
Undertake adequate trials (time frames match or exceed recommendations).
Document alternative approaches, if reevaluation of medication regimen is warranted.

Source: Adapted from Silverman (1998). Copyright 1998 by The Guilford Press. Adapted by permission.

effectiveness—or because of negative public perceptions, fueled by such popular books/films as *One Flew Over the Cuckoo's Nest*—it has not gained widespread use or acceptance. Moreover, its position on the hierarchy of interventions is often one "of last resort," only for those difficult-to-treat patients, thus, suggesting frustrated caregivers wishing for "magic bullets." This latter perspective is fueled by the fact that the mechanism of its action remains shrouded in mystery, although it is believed that ECT affects serotonin function (Metzger, 1998).

SOCIAL SYSTEM INTERVENTIONS

Family Therapy

Family therapy seeks to alter system dynamics when suicidal behavior is viewed as an expression of family dysfunction and transactional difficulties. For suicidal children and adolescents, in particular, it is considered a most significant intervention, paralleling the child's need for individual therapy, as family problems often precipitate suicidal behavior among youth. Among early trauma frequently linked to later suicidal behaviors are early family loss (e.g., through death or divorce), physical and sexual abuse, and parental psychopathology.

The goal of family therapy is to improve family functioning. This may be accomplished in a number of ways designed to reduce enmeshment and support greater individuation, increase tolerance and flexibility, identify and resolve communication problems, clarify dysfunctional alliances, reveal and accept previously held secrets, increase mutually rewarding behaviors among family members, decrease punitive interactions among family members, and so on. Moreover, family members might be educated about, taught to understand triggers for, and to monitor suicide risk in a suicidal member.

Group Therapy

Group therapy seeks to help suicidal patients acquire and maintain a social support network. Concurrently it affords a safe haven in which social skill deficits may be observed and social skill development may occur. Interpersonal learning and support are developed through the sharing of problems, perceived commonalities among group members, and reinforcing feedback among members and by therapists. In particular, the impact of one's behavior on others can be observed and understood. Among the skills that may develop in group are those of listening and empathy, an understanding of group qua family dynamics, and the containment and regulation of impulses (e.g., of aggression). Group leaders/therapists model good parents and teaching specific skills while exploring pathological defenses, cognitive distortions, and so on.

A NOTE ABOUT TREATING OLDER ADULTS

The treatment of geriatric patients requires a flexible treatment plan that takes into account the ego weakening, social, and developmental factors common to both later years and the individual case. Richman (1994) emphasizes the recognition and treatment of both mental and physical illnesses, alcoholism, and depression; social isolation and marginalization (being treated by family members as if no longer an integral and functioning participant in life issues, shared information, etc.); and coping with multiple losses common to aging. Social isolation is, also, a key factor in DeLeo's outreach model (DeLeo, Carollo, & Dello Buono, 1995). These caregiver–researchers make proactive use of the telephone to reach out to isolated (76% lived alone), at-risk elders and have shown a promising reduction in suicidal behaviors among this population.

TREATMENT EFFECTIVENESS

Research on treatment effectiveness is both difficult and rare. Linehan (1998) decried the overall quality of this research, finding only 20 published studies, using randomized clinical trials (RCTs), the only research model allowing for causal inferences regarding the effectiveness of treatment. Of these 20 studies, only slightly more than one-half (55%) operationally defined "suicidal behaviors," only 2 studies (10%) used standardized assessments, and only 3 studies (15%) used blind assessment. Moreover, almost one-half of published RCTs targeting suicidal behavior (45%) excluded high-risk patients; this percentage increased to 88% when examining pharmacotherapy studies targeting depression. Of those few RCT studies that included high-risk patients, findings have demonstrated the effectiveness of telephone follow-up and home visits in reducing likelihood of repeated attempts, short-term ([6 months] but not longer-term [18 months]) benefits to cognitive–behavioral interventions, DBT (through 24 months), and efforts to improve ease of access to emergency room treatment.

Hawton et al. (1998) similarly reported that there was some promise shown for brief problem-solving treatment approaches (CBT) delaying the onset of repetitive suicide attempts, that home-based treatment and treatment compliance efforts (the provision of a card to allow patients to make emergency contact with services) similarly affected repetition, and that treatment effects appeared most profound in women. Overall, however, a meta-analysis of 20 RCTs involving more than 2,600 patients did not detect statistically significant treatment effects.

Rudd and Joiner (1998) added to this list the observed utility of psychoeducational approaches but concluded, "We simply do not know what patients (e.g., diagnostic subgroups, comorbid problems, severity of risk, age groups) are best suited for specific treatment approaches (i.e., hospitalization vs. a range of outpatient alternatives)" (145).

Discouraging as the empirical data appear, readers should be reminded that outcome studies focusing on suicidal behaviors are difficult to accomplish given the low base rate of these behaviors and, therefore, the large number of subjects needed. Furthermore, factors such as the influence of insitutional review boards that are skittish about potential liability should adverse outcomes result, and the necessity for establishing adequate surveillance (other than patient report) of behaviors to be measured (see Chapter 3), make these studies difficult to accomplish. Finally, it should be noted that treatment outcome studies require standardized treatments, often conducted with "how to" manuals, that may not mirror treatment (as usual) as practiced in caregivers' offices. Given this, laboratory-based treatments may not reflect real world practice.

THE PREVENTION PARADIGM

In 1987, a 2½-year-old toddler named Jessica McClure made front-page headlines across the United States. Trapped for more than 2 days 22 feet down a backyard well into which she had fallen, Jessica was helpless; her survival was impossible without emergency intervention. A massive rescue effort was, indeed, instituted, at great financial expense, and Jessica was rescued to the universal relief of the riveted public. Now, years later, she is a healthy and thriving teen.

Jessica's rescue examplifies the clinical paradigm—built on roles of patient and caregiver and models of treatment that are initiated by the early detection and identification of acutely at-risk conditions/individuals (evidencing signs and symptoms of distress) and ranging to the long-term maintenance and protection of those with chronic conditions threatening to relapse or give up under the cumulative burden of symptoms, demands for coping and adaptation, and unachieved goals. Treatment focuses on the individual at risk and aims to reduce or reverse pathology and suicidal vulnerability

Imagine, instead, a model of intervention that had been instituted before Jessica's unfortunate entrapment—perhaps, a legally mandated locked well cover; or construction code requirements allowing secondary and easy access routes to remove objects (and children) from backyard wells; or intensive parent education programs regarding safety and risk. These strategies reflect a different paradigm of intervention, one that incorporates the clinical model into a broader perspective strategically linked to target populations at risk for the development of specific disorders and dysfunctions (i.e., *prevention*). As shown on the Institute of Medicine's (1994) intervention spectrum (Figure 21.3), prevention attempts to intervene before the initial onset of the target problem versus treatment which begins once a case has been identified.

Similar to the treatment paradigm, prevention encompasses the concepts of risk reduction (disease prevention) and resiliency (health promotion). Thus, suicide prevention can proceed toward reducing the prevalence of known risks or vulnerabilities or increasing protective, immunizing factors. But whereas the clinical paradigm rests primarily on a mental health model (observe, find, treat) and too often involves tertiary prevention (*after* a pathological process has developed), the prevention paradigm rests on a public health model and primary prevention (observe [surveillance], understand etiology and pathways, and interrupt/intervene *before* process develops).

Conceptually, the field of prevention has evolved from simple tripartite models to complex, multifactorial systems that recognize the complexity of self-destructive behaviors and individuals. Moreover, in recent years suicide prevention has come to embrace a melding of mental health and public health thinking, as traditional paradigms have been insufficient in addressing these complexities. Clinical models (e.g., the medical model) assumed that suicide is a behavioral manifestation of underlying pathology, and therefore one treats the underlying disorder (e.g., depression). A more complex variation of this model understands

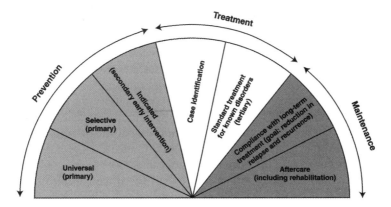

FIGURE 21.3. The mental health intervention spectrum. *Source:* Institute of Medicine (1994). Copyright 1994 by National Academy Press. Reprinted by permission.

that suicidal behavior is consequent to both distal and proximal antecedent conditions—that is, predisposing and precipitating conditions (e.g., depression in males who then increase acute alcohol intoxication leading to relationship conflicts and loss). The more complex public health variation of this approach is to understand the more universal mechanisms and processes that lead to these negative outcomes, then designing preventive interventions to reduce long-term vulnerabilities.

As can be seen, the public health approach moves our thinking toward interventions earlier along the pathway, ideally before the disorder develops (*primary prevention*). The public health approach also forces our interventions "out of the box" of focusing just on the individual at risk (host) and into the realm of the environment and the agents of self-destruction. Thus, early interventions might be designed to increase coping skills in children (host), restrict access to available means such as firearms (agent), and/or increase community/parent education toward the importance of safe gun storage behaviors (environment).

Gordon's (1983) operational model further shifts our thinking "outside the box." This model identifies target groups for such interventions, ranging from the broad-based, *universal* interventions to those more *selective*, to the yet more *indicated* (see Figure 21.3). Universal interventions are directed toward the entire population, incorporating specific subgroups at risk. Improving easy access toward health care for all or promoting risk awareness training in schools as part of general health education courses are examples of universal approaches. Selective interventions specifically target those at greater risk for being/becoming suicidal, for example, children of depressed or substance-abusing parents. Indicated interventions target a yet more focused at-risk group that already manifests a risk factor or condition placing group members at increasingly high risk for suicide (e.g., those who have made a suicide attempt). This last target, again, merges the more preventive, larger-scale, public health focus into more secondary/tertiary (after risk develops) prevention, with its more narrow, clinical–mental health focus.

Beginning with its inclusion of agents and the environment in its preventive focus, public health models have incorporated injury control strategies into suicide prevention approaches. In fact, the Centers for Disease Control and Prevention has subsumed suicide into its public health agenda by bifurcating injuries into those that are unintentional (e.g., accidents), and those that are intentional (e.g., suicides). With evidence that reducing the availability of popular and readily available means of committing suicide can lower suicide rates

(Kreitman, 1976), application of accident prevention findings to suicide prevention becomes both possible and promising. Adapting and expanding on Haddon and Baker's (1981) model, Silverman and Maris (1995) presented an outline of preventive interventions specifically linked to measurable outcomes at particular phases of prevention (see Table 21.2).

This approach to prevention, to alter the external environment to protect the individual at risk, contrasts with more traditional public health approaches that rely on education or legislation to persuade or mandate behavioral change. The difficulty with the educational approach is that it requires a long-term commitment (duration of message), multiple booster "shots" (frequency of message), and attention to and reduction of powerful countervailing messages (e.g., glamorization through media portrayals of unhealthy lifestyles). Consider the time, effort, and cost of mounting successful smoking reduction or AIDS prevention programs. The difficulty with the legislative process is that few public health professionals have mastered the art of lobbying and persistence of effort to gain sufficient support for social engineering programs to benefit the public good.

Moreover, suicide prevention efforts must compete with an ever-shifting landscape of

---

TABLE 21.2. Adaptations of Haddon and Baker's Injury Control Strategies to Suicide Prevention

Primary prevention

   1. Prevent initial creation of hazard.
     • Do not manufacture handguns for nonsecurity civilian use.
     • Improve social support systems.
   2. Reduce amount of hazard created.
     • Control distribution (sales) of firearms.
   3. Prevent release of already existing hazard.
     • Set standards for purchasing of firearms.
     • Limit access to alcohol (amount, frequency, timing).

Secondary prevention

   4. Modify rate of release or spatial distribution of hazard from its source.
     • Package medications as individual tablets to prevent rapid consumption of large quantities.
   5. Separate, in time and space, hazard from person.
     • Legislate to prevent access to firearms by severely mentally ill persons.
     • Separate ammunition from firearms.
   6. Interpose a barrier between hazard and person.
     • Place barriers on high bridges and buildings.
     • Promote "safe guns," e.g., requiring palm print identification for use.
   7. Modify contact surfaces to reduce injury.
     • Prevent access to bridges and to building rooftops.
   8. Strengthen resistance of persons who might be injured.
     • Offer school-based health promotion programs.
     • Train parent–firearms owners in safe firearm storage methods and necessity.

Tertiary prevention

   9. Rapidly detect and limit damage that has occurred.
     • Improve professional education to assess and treat suicidal individuals.
  10. Initiate immediate and long-term reparative actions.
     • Improve follow-up treatment for and compliance behaviors among attempters.

Source: Adapted from Haddon & Baker (1981). Copyright 1981 by Lippincott Williams & Wilkins. Adapted by permission.

other societal/public health problems requiring preventive relief (AIDS, homelessness, etc.), stigmatic and ambivalent attitudes that limit understanding of suicides as preventable deaths, social forces promoting suicide (e.g., physician-assisted deaths), and disagreement among suicide preventionists regarding the most effective approach (where legislators could be convinced they would get the "most bang for the buck"). In truth, to date we know little about what works; this, then makes for a hard sell for large-scale, government-sponsored programs. It does suggest, however, the need for large-scale pilot programs with evaluation research defining promising "best practices."

Prevention programming also requires clearly delineated, empirically sound answers to several basic questions that underlie the development of preventive interventions (cf. Silverman & Maris, 1995). Consider the following, partial list of questions and decision points in focusing suicidal behavior as a target for preventive effort. These are offered to help guide prevention programming decisions rather than to provide definitive answers.

- *What is the target of our effort?* Do we hope to reduce the rate of suicide (a low-frequency event to begin with), suicide attempts (a more difficult to measure, higher-frequency event), suicide ideation (perhaps common to one-fourth of the adolescent population in any year, but by itself usually transient and not life-threatening), or predisposing vulnerabilities to being suicidal (depression, alcohol abuse, psychosis, etc.)? Alternatively, should we attempt to build competencies, enhance wellness, strengthen coping skills, and increase protective factors?

- *Who is at risk for the target behavior?* Is there a well-defined population at risk for completing suicide or attempting suicide? Do we know enough about pathogenesis and etiology to establish, for example, who among the population of depressed adolescents is likely to engage suicidal behaviors, or when an adult male alcoholic is at increased risk?

- *How should we identify who is at greatest risk?* In what setting—schools, primary care physicians' offices, clinical caregivers' offices, hospital emergency departments, and so on—might we best reach the population at risk? With what methods/procedures should we identify risk: screening questionnaires, computer interviews, specially trained interviewers? What questions are most effective at screening those most at risk? Can we be assured that what we are asking is being interpreted by the patient in the same way as the interviewer interpreted it (cf. Velting, Rathus, & Asnis, 1998)?

- *When is someone most at risk? When and where should we intervene?* Are there particular precipitating events that increase risk among those predisposed to suicidal behavior? Are these moments (e.g., relationship breakups among adult alcoholics) accessible to intervention? Should we intervene at other points in the causal chain, perhaps ones more vulnerable to intervention? Are there particular settings, contexts, environments, situations, and so on, that increase risk and are accessible to intervention?

- *What interventions are effective at lowering risk?* Should the approach be educational, legislative, or environmentally manipulative (cf. Brent & Perper, 1995)? Do we have sufficient program evaluation studies to document an effective intervention? What interventions will result in immediate versus longer-term reduction of risk? What interventions are most feasible, most likely to be adopted by the targeted community? What interventions are cost-effective? Should the chosen approach be universal (e.g., communitywide), selective (e.g., people with signs of depression), or indicated (people who have already engaged self-destructive behavior)?

- *What interventions are effective in protecting against risk?* Should we teach elementary school children depression awareness and management skills? Should we enhance high school environments promoting social connectedness, relationship skills, and so on? Should we reduce the accessibilty and availability of firearms? Should we decrease the toxicity of medications? Should we reach out and provide social supports for elderly persons at risk to combat social isolation and loneliness?

With regard to youth suicide, the first generation of prevention programs relied primarily on just two conceptual strategies: (1) recognition and referral of at-risk youth and (2) reduction of risk factors. As critically reviewed by the Centers for Disease Control (1992), these programs too often were seen as stand-alone models, inadequately linking together other community resources and risk-prevention programs; rarely focused on means-reduction efforts that had at least some empirical support; and, in general, rarely measured desired outcomes and potential iatrogenic effects. Moreover, they rarely had a primary prevention focus. Table 21.3 outlines these programs.

These preventive efforts have yet to commit resources to promoting protective factors among younger children, targeting developing resiliency in later (i.e., teen) years. To this end, Berman and Jobes (1995) have outlined a conceptual model of primary prevention interventions that focus on decreasing the individual child's potential for later suicidality. These include skill-based approaches to manage depression, anger and aggression, or loneliness and to enhance competencies such as decision making, social skills, and problem-solving skills. These approaches are educational, thus school-based; manualized, thus teachable without extensive training of trainers; and time-limited (e.g., eight sessions), but requiring booster shoots over subsequent years of development.

With regard to elderly suicide, Conwell (1998) has reviewed public health preventive interventions in late-life populations. Among universal models he describes means-restriction approaches (e.g., gun control legislation and restricting access to drugs with high

TABLE 21.3. First-Generation Youth Suicide Prevention Programs

Prevention program	Summary description
School gatekeeper training	Education of school personnel (counselors, teachers, coaches, etc.) to identify and refer at-risk students to mental health caregivers.
Community gatekeeper training	Education of the nonschool community in contact with youth (clergy, pediatricians, police, etc.) to identify and refer at-risk students to mental health caregivers.
General suicide education	Classroom centered, knowledge-based training of students to increase self-awareness and peer observation of risk and help-seeking/referral skills.
Screening programs	School-based administration of a screening questionnaire to all students with follow-up triage of identified at-risk students.
Peer support programs	School- or community-based support groups aimed to foster social and coping competencies, peer relationships, and networking among at-risk youth.
Crisis centers and hotlines	24-hour anonymous telephone support systems offering nonjudgmental listening, problem solving, and crisis intervention to callers.
Means restriction	Delaying or thwarting access to available and accessible means for self-harm, particularly firearms.
Postvention/cluster prevention	School and community interventions to reduce potential imitative ("copycat") suicides after an index suicide.

Source: Berman & Jobes (1995). Copyright 1995 by The Guilford Press. Reprinted by permission.

BOX 21.2. Does Training Primary Care Physicians to Assess Depression Prevent Suicide?

Yes: Rutz, von Knorring, and Walinder (1989).

No: Rutz, von Knorring, and Walinder (1992).

Issue Summary: Physicians generally have difficulty detecting mental disorders; therefore they undertreat them. This observation led to an experimental educational program to train all general practitioners on the Swedish island of Gotland (pop. 56,000). The primary goal of this intervention was to increase knowledge about the diagnosis and treatment of patients with affective disorders. The year after the 2-day training program, attended by 90% of the island's general practitioners, it was found that significantly more patients with depressive disorder were identified and adequately treated than in the prior year. There was a reduction in sick leave for depressive disorders, fewer inpatient care days recorded for depression, and increased numbers of prescriptions for antidepressant medications. Most profoundly, the suicide rate on Gotland dropped significantly, relative to the rates for both Gotland and Sweden as a whole before the initiation of the training program.

In a follow-up study 3 years after the project ended, it was found that the pronounced positive effect initially observed had not lasted and that its principal influence was on depressed women, not men. Gotland's suicide rate had returned to near baseline levels. The study's relatively small sample size and limited time frame suggested that the early results might have been an artifact of temporal fluctuations in suicide rates.

---

lethality) and those that decrease functional disability and social isolation. Among selective models dealing with high-risk elderly persons he describes community outreach approaches and interventions in primary-care settings designed to improve recognition and treatment of depressed and suicidal older patients. One example of this latter approach is known as the Gotland study (see Box 21.2).

Spearheaded by parent survivors of suicide, Jerry and Elsie Weyrauch, cofounders of the Suicide Prevention Advocacy Network (SPAN), a unique collaborative (public and private sector) conference of experts met in Reno, Nevada in late 1998 to review and evaluate "best practices" in suicide prevention. Based on a growing belief that the time was ripe and good-enough answers existed to the questions posed earlier to establish a national strategy for suicide prevention, the outcome of this meeting was a list of 81 recommendations for preventing suicide. These, then, were passed to the U.S. Surgeon General, reformulated into a tighter blueprint for addressing suicide prevention as part of the nation's Year 2010 health objectives, and presented to the public on July 28, 1999, as the *Surgeon General's Call to Action*. This essential step toward establishing a national strategy also embraces suicide prevention fully within public health. Moreover, the United States joins other countries in the world community, notably Norway and Finland, that have adopted a national plan to prevent suicide.

The recommended strategies, subsumed under the acronym *AIM* (assessment, intervention, methodology) includes 15 key recommendations. Although, as noted with regard to treatment interventions, we lack clear and convincing evidence, based on controlled research studies, of the effectiveness of specific interventions, these recommendations best express state-of-the-art thinking regarding suicide prevention. The need exists to demonstrate

TABLE 21.4. The U. S. Surgeon General's Call to Action Recommendations

Awareness: Appropriately broaden the public's awareness of suicide and its risk factors.
- Promote public awareness that suicide is a major public health problem and, as such, many suicides are preventable.
- Expand awareness of and enhance resources in communities for suicide prevention programs and mental and substance abuse disorder assessment and treatment.
- Develop and implement strategies to reduce the stigma associated with mental illness, substance abuse, and suicidal behavior and with seeking help for such problems.

Intervention: Enhance services and programs, both population-based and clinical care.
- Extend collaboration with and among public and private sectors to complete a National Strategy for Suicide Prevention.
- Improve the ability of primary-care providers to recognize and treat depression, substance abuse, and other major mental illnesses associated with suicide risk. Increase the referral to specialty care when appropriate.
- Eliminate barriers in public and private insurance programs for provision of quality mental and substance abuse disorder treatments and create incentives to treat patients with coexisting mental and substance abuse disorders.
- Institute training for all health, mental health, substance abuse, and human service professionals (including clergy, teachers, correctional workers, and social workers) concerning suicide risk assessment and recognition, treatment, management, and aftercare interventions.
- Develop and implement effective training programs for family members of those at risk and for natural community helpers (e.g., coaches, hairdressers, and faith leaders) on how to recognize, respond to, and refer people showing signs of suicide risk and associated mental and substance abuse disorders.
- Enhance community care resources by increasing the use of schools and workplaces as access and referral points for mental and physical health services and substance abuse treatment programs and provide for support for persons who survive the suicide of someone close to them.
- Promote public/private collaboration with the media to ensure that entertainment and news coverage represent balanced and informed portrayals of suicide and its associated risk factors including mental illness and substance abuse disorders and approaches to prevention and treatment.

Methodology: Advance the science of suicide prevention.
- Enhance research to understand risk and protective factors related to suicide, their interaction, and their effects on suicide and suicidal behaviors. In addition, increase research on effective suicide prevention programs, clinical treatments for suicidal individuals, and culture-specific interventions.
- Develop additional scientific strategies for evaluating suicide prevention interventions and ensure that evaluation components are included in all suicide prevention programs.
- Establish mechanisms for federal, regional, and state interagency public health collaboration toward improving, monitoring systems for suicide and suicidal behaviors and develop and promote standard terminology in these systems.
- Encourage the development and evaluation of new prevention technologies, including firearm safety measures, to reduce easy access to lethal means of suicide.

Source: U.S. Public Health Service (1999).

their efficacy, but, more important, the humanitarian demand is to proceed with or without such evidence, until sufficient trials with sufficient samples can be measured for desired changes. With this in mind, and to provide a template for future understanding, Table 21.4 presents these recomendations.

SUMMARY AND CONCLUSIONS

The effective prevention of suicide and suicidal behaviors is in the best interest of all communities. Prevention efforts communicate that life is valued. It should make no difference whether that message is given to those suffering with cancer, with AIDS, with alcoholism, or with suicidal despair. Prevention efforts might actually save lives, provide years of productive life, and, in so doing, enhance protective factors that generalize across the sepctrum of potential mental and public health problems.

We have emphasized in this chapter the spectrum of preventive interventions that incorporates both individual clinical treatment approaches and population-based prevention models. We have also emphasized that, to date, we lack sufficient empirical support for the effectiveness of these interventions. However, even if we accomplish a more scientific basis for these efforts, we are not naive enough to believe that we can prevent all suicides. And with each of these suicides, there will be many survivors. In the next chapter we turn our attention to these secondary vicitms of suicide, family members, friends, associates, and others who are affected by the suicide of a loved one. With this focus, we come full circle in our consideration of prevention—that is, postvention, interventions to assist the grief work of those bereaved by a suicide.

FURTHER READING

Chiles, J. A., & Strosahl, K. D. (1995). *The suicidal patient: Principles of assessment, treatment, and case management.* Washington, DC: American Psychiatric Press. As a treatment protocol collaboratively developed by a psychiatrist and a psychologist, this volume articulates a problem-solving and learning-based model of acute care and case management of patients making nonfatal suicide attempts and with suicide ideation.

Kleespies, P. M. (Ed.). (1998). *Emergencies in mental health practice.* New York: Guilford Press. A well-edited series of chapters focusing on crisis theory and emergency intervention in crises ranging from acute suicidality to self-injurious behavior, alcohol and drug-related episodes; and medical conditions precipitating psychological emergencies.

Leenaars, A. A., Maltsberger, J. T., & Niemeyer, R. A. (Eds.). (1994). *Treatment of suicidal people.* Washington, DC: Taylor & Francis. Chapters cover the range of interventions with at-risk people from crisis intervention to: family therapy, adolescent therapy, geriatric therapy, psychopharmacotherapy, hospitalization, and so on.

Linehan, M. M. (1993). *Cognitive-behavioral therapy of borderline personality disorder.* New York: Guilford Press. With its accompanying skills manual this pioneering text establishes Linehan's dialectic behavior therapy approach. Although developed to treat females with borderline personality disorder, it has wide application to suicidal patients. It is most helpful in its focus on the skills of emotional regulation and distress tolerance.

Silverman, M. M., & Maris, R. W. (Eds.). (1995). Suicide prevention: Toward the year 2000. *Suicide and Life-Threatening Behavior, 25* (1). The special issue of this journal integrates a vast body of literature and presents a systematic discussion of prevention theory and practice. Models of risk reduction, theoretical and conceptual foundations to suicide prevention, and practical recommendations are presented throughout the 16 articles, including setting specific and population specific perspectives.

Zimmerman, J. K. (Ed.). (1995). *Treatment approaches with suicidal adolescents.* New York: Wiley. Similarly focused on the range of treatments applicable to working with at-risk adolescents (psychoanalytic and cognitive treatments, group therapy, psychopharmacotherapy, etc.) and, in particular, helpful techniques for enhancing outpatient treatment compliance.

22

In the Wake of Suicide:
Survivorship and Postvention

David A. Jobes, Jason B. Luoma,
Lisa Anne T. Hustead, and Rachel E. Mann

A person's death is not only an ending: it is also a beginning—for the survivors. Indeed, in the case of suicide the largest public health problem is neither the prevention of suicide, nor the management of attempts, but the alleviation of the effects of stress in the survivor-victims of suicidal deaths, whose lives are forever changed. . . .

—Edwin S. Shneidman

On a cool crisp day in November, Joan Smith came home from work early with plans to make a special dinner for her son, Jimmy—his favorite, tacos and enchiladas. Upon first entering the house, she had a strange feeling. Hearing music playing from the basement recreation room, she was relieved to know that Jimmy was home from school, probably playing a video game downstairs. As she walked down the basement stairs to say a quick hello, she was struck dumb by the sight she beheld. Jimmy's body was sprawled on the carpet, blood everywhere, and her husband's handgun (which he kept under their bed for protection) was next to his body. Jimmy was dead. He died from a self-inflicted gunshot wound to the right temple. A five-page suicide note was neatly folded in his breast pocket. The note described his feelings of depression and despair, particularly since the breakup with his girlfriend, Julie. There were song lyrics and apologies to his parents, sister, friends, and girlfriend. He asserted that in the long run, they would be better off without him; he knew he was disappointing all who loved him and alienating anyone who tried to care.

What had happened to Jimmy? Jimmy had been a precocious but troubled, 14-year-old eighth-grader. His parents, Bill and Joan Smith, had a good marriage and had always worked hard to provide Jimmy and his older sister, Tammy, a happy and comfortable home life. For the first 12 years of his life, Jimmy seemed to have it all; both family and friends often referred to Jimmy as the "golden boy." Both handsome and bright, Jimmy seemed to excel in whatever he chose to pursue. Successful in academics and sports, Jimmy was popular among his peers, especially the girls.

During seventh grade, however, Jimmy's life began to change. Over the course of that year, he seemed to become increasingly withdrawn and depressed. More and more of his time was spent alone at home watching MTV or playing computer games. According to his parents, when he did leave the house, he would spend time with "troublemakers." Tom and Nate were the so-called troublemakers; both boys came from broken homes, did poorly in school, listened to heavy metal rock music, and were reputed to be "druggies."

No one in the Smith household could understand the sudden change in Jimmy or why he was spending more and more time with Tom and Nate. Teachers and coaches expressed their concerns to Jimmy's parents and there were a handful of meetings at school about what was happening to Jimmy. Over the summer before his eighth-grade year, Jimmy changed his appearance dramatically, he wore beat-up, wornout clothes and let his hair grow long, dying it green. There were increasing fights with his parents. One major fight centered on his refusal to play baseball that summer, a sport in which he had previously excelled as a pitcher. Bill and Joan Smith increasingly felt like they were losing the son they had known and loved; Tammy had said she could not relate to her brother at all.

When the eighth grade school year started, Jimmy announced that he was dropping out of school. Shocked and dismayed by this bold announcement, and by his general behavior, Jimmy's parents sent him to a psychologist for help. Family sessions were combative and unproductive and Jimmy reported that he hated seeing the "shrink" in individual meetings. About a month into the school year things seemed to improve somewhat, when Jimmy became involved with a girl named Julie. Even though she was a "Deadhead" and seemed somewhat depressed and spacey, Jimmy's parents thought the relationship had a positive stabilizing influence on Jimmy. However, after going together for a month, Julie suddenly broke off the relationship with Jimmy. In turn, Jimmy was completely devastated by the breakup and he spoke to no one, not even Tom and Nate. He refused to meet with his therapist, and his parents began to wonder whether he needed more specialized treatment or perhaps even hospitalization. Three days later, Jimmy was found dead by suicide.

What will happen now to the survivors of Jimmy's suicide? Suicides rarely occur in an interpersonal vacuum; in the wake of most suicides there are often "survivors" who may be deeply affected by the death. Typically, survivors are family, friends, and coworkers of the deceased. Nevertheless, others who may not have even known the deceased personally can also be profoundly affected by a suicide. As we discuss further on, the aftermath of suicide poses distinct challenges for suicide survivors and even puts some individuals at risk who may be especially affected by the suicide of another person.

The goal of this chapter is to take a journey through the experience of surviving a suicide and all the personal, professional, research, and public health implications thereof. The first portion of this journey examines different aspects of the suicide survivor's experience. The second part examines how the reporting of a suicide either on television or in the newspaper may cause certain vulnerable individuals to imitate the reported suicidal act. Finally, this journey involves an examination of "postvention," a term that broadly refers to a range of professional and paraprofessional efforts directed to those in need after a tragedy. For our purposes, we focus on postvention efforts that are uniquely tailored for the particular needs of bereaved suicide survivors.

WHO ARE SURVIVORS?

Edwin S. Shneidman (cited in McIntosh, 1996) has estimated that each suicide intimately affects at least six other people. Based on the number of suicides since 1972 (through 1995), it is estimated that the number of survivors of suicide in the United States is 4.06 million. That would amount to about 1 in every 64 Americans in the mid-1990s. Critically, the number of suicide survivors is estimated to grow by 180,000 each year. But who are these legions of survivors (see Exercise 22.1)?

Let us return to the case of Jimmy. Following a tragedy like the suicide of Jimmy, there are inevitably countless questions that can never be answered. But one question worth trying to answer is who the survivors of Jimmy's suicide are. Perhaps most obviously, Jimmy's parents and sister, as family, would typically be seen as survivors. With regard to time spent with and proximity to Jimmy, Tom, Nate, and Julie are also potential survivors.

But what of Jimmy's sixth-grade girlfriend, someone he has not even spoken to in over a year? What about Jimmy's teachers and coaches, from grade school on? Is the bus driver who pulls up to Jimmy's house the next day and waits patiently (because Jimmy is always late) a survivor of his suicide? Is the psychologist who Jimmy refused to see for over a month a survivor? Are peers who never met Jimmy, or neighbors who saw him deliver papers a few years back, survivors of Jimmy's tragic suicidal death?

In our view, no one can externally or arbitrarily define who is a survivor and who is not a survivor; there can be no rigid or strict definition of the term. Indeed, for hundreds of years much pain and anguish have resulted from the negative social labeling to which suicide survivors are often subjected. In this regard, a common assumption about survivors of suicide is that they are somehow explicitly or implicitly to blame for the death. The survivor is often perceived to have either directly caused the person to kill him- or herself or alternatively as having done nothing to prevent the death. Such social perceptions are unfair and

---

EXERCISE 22.1. How Many Survivors Are There in an Average Suicide?

Determining the number of survivors of a suicide is largely a subjective decision. Many people would include only the nuclear family when determining who should be called a survivor. But what about close friends? What about girlfriends or boyfriends? How about the case of a middle-age man? What about his parents, in-laws, brothers, sisters? It is apparent that the number of survivors varies widely depending on the breadth of the definition applied. What is your definition of a suicide survivor? This exercise will help you to look at your own definition of what a suicide survivor is and how this may relate to other peoples' definitions.

Exercise: Consider a typical adolescent male (like Jimmy Smith) who completes suicide. Write in the number of people in each of the following categories you think might be impacted by this suicide.

Category:	No. of people
Parents:	_____
Siblings:	_____
Friends (and girlfriends):	_____
Grandparents:	_____
Teachers and coaches:	_____
Classmates:	_____
Total:	_____

What is your total? Does it agree with the most commonly cited average of six survivors (Shneidman, as cited in McIntosh, 1996)? Why do you think your average was higher or lower? Might you have been more or less inclusive in your definition? Why did you choose to include the people you did?

deeply wounding and can potentially generate tremendously destructive shame in people who are already deeply grieved and guilt-ridden. Although there are situations in which family, friends, and lovers contribute to the suicide through abuse, neglect, and hatred, the focus in this chapter centers on the nonabusive/loving survivors, who are often shocked and bereaved by the loved one's death.

Some neighbors and teachers at school blamed Jimmy's parents. Yet the Smiths referred their son to a professional and met with teachers and school personnel, but still he died. In the eyes of many, Bill and Joan Smith failed their beloved son, Jimmy. Is his death Julie's fault? According to his suicide note, it was Julie's breakup with him that was the principal reason for his suicide. Might Nate and Tom be blamed because of their negative influences, that led Jimmy into a more destructive and depressive lifestyle? In a sense, no one deserves to be blamed for something that cannot ultimately be controlled—the volition and acts of another autonomous human being. Given this perspective, we would advocate moving from a socially stigmatizing and blaming sense of who is a survivor to a more explanatory and healing definition. Simply stated, survivors of suicide are self-defined. They are any and all people, both close and distant, who experience the pain of a suicidal death and who acknowledge that this loss has affected them in painful and sometimes profound ways. Suicide survivorship is not an elite club, no one wants to join it. But suicide, and survivorship, is truly a democratic phenomena. Anyone can be affected; anyone can suddenly become a survivor of another's suicidal death.

The contemporary suicide survivor movement has done much to educate and combat social stigma and stereotypes connected to losing someone to suicide. But ignorance and stigmatization still surround suicide survivorship. We should perhaps not be surprised; the stigma of surviving suicide has a distinct and extensive cross-cultural history that is critical to our understanding of this topic.

Historical Perspective

As Colt (1987) has discussed vividly, there is a lengthy history to the social stigma that has often been connected to suicide. A litany of disturbing acts and rituals have been practiced throughout the world in response to the perceived shamefulness of suicide. Often these acts were directed toward the suicide attempter or were performed on the body of the deceased. Moreover, in certain cultures, additional action was sometimes taken against the surviving loved ones of the deceased.

For many centuries throughout Europe, Asia, and Africa, custom or law often required that the corpse of a suicide be subjected to various acts of abuse. Much of this treatment of the suicide's body was meant to prevent the deceased's ghost from wandering about causing famine, drought, and disease. Moreover, desecration of the corpse had the added effect of being a potential deterrent to others who may be contemplating the shameful act of suicide or punishment for the suicide on their family. Ritual acts performed on the corpse of a suicide included decapitation, burying the body outside tribal territories or city limits, cutting off the hands of the deceased and burying them separately, beating the body with chains, throwing the body to wild beasts, public burning of the corpse, and burying the corpse at a crossroads with a stake through the heart (Cain, 1972).

Primitive rituals and taboos against suicide were increasingly adopted into organized religion throughout medieval Europe (Colt, 1987). Civil law and attitudes propagated by the church ultimately led to penalizing the survivors of the suicide. Because the suicide had perpetrated a sinful act against God (and the crown) in taking his or her own life, someone had to be punished. However, given that the deceased was literally beyond the reach of civil authority, penalties could only be exacted from the next of kin. Essentially, survivors were treated as accessories to the criminal act of suicide. Accordingly, in England the goods of the deceased were forfeited to the feudal lord; while in France goods of the deceased as well as the property of the surviving widow were surrendered. Sometimes the surviving widow was even forced to pay a fine to the deceased's in-laws in compensation for the shame brought on the family by the suicide (Colt, 1987).

Given this state of affairs, it is understandable that survivors of suicide in this era were encouraged to disguise suicide deaths. Bodies were quickly buried, suicide notes were destroyed, and valuables were smuggled out of the house. Over time, however, desecration of the corpse and the automatic forfeiture of property to the crown began to be replaced by a crude form of investigation into the cause of death. In turn, direct blame and civil punishment of surviving family members gradually began to decline over time as suicide was increasingly linked to madness and insanity.

In 18th-century England, trials in the Coroner's Court were held posthumously, to determine whether the deceased had been insane and, therefore, innocent of a crime (*non compos mentis*) or has in fact been guilty as a criminal against him- or herself (*felo de se*) and thereby subject to punishment which may have included forfeiture of property and desecration of the corpse (Colt, 1987). During the Enlightenment of the 18th century, punishment of innocent survivors increasingly began to be challenged by the more educated. Ultimately, changes in law and attitude led to important changes in the stigma associated with suicide. Even though survivors were no longer directly punished by civil authority, a whole new social stigma began to be connected to survivors of suicide. This new form of stigma was intimately wrapped up in prevailing fears, superstitions, and prejudices connected to madness and insanity.

The evolution of suicide being associated with mental illness, rather than a sin or a crime, became clearly established in the 19th century. In this era, the prevailing medical view and research of the day closely linked insanity to heredity. Indeed, as discussed by Colt (1987), there was a flood of publications among 19th-century medical scholars that examined insanity and suicide within successive generations of certain family trees. However, much of this scholarship, which was also spurred on by the eugenics movement, was largely anecdotal and the published cases often were not accurately studied. Importantly, according to this view, a survivor who shared the genes of the deceased also was potentially doomed to similar mental illness and even suicide. Fortunately, by the mid-20th century, these theories of heredity and suicide were tempered, when more rigorous empirical work was conducted (however, see Maris, 1997).

Nevertheless, the Victorian era of respectability ushered in yet another form of stigma which in many ways still lingers to the present day. Even though suicide survivors were no longer formally punished, they were still informally punished by the judgments of society—the looks, the whispers, the avoidance by friends, extended family, and neighbors. Some of the roots of contemporary social stigma toward survivors can be traced to the era when a suicide within one's family was a source of distinct social shame. Family reputations were tainted, property values were lowered, funerals were hastily conducted, and information about the death was kept from children. Suicide was the family secret, the source of gossip, a reason to blame and shun the survivors of the deceased. Suicide survivors were thus doomed to an internal prison of their own private shame, trapped with feelings of guilt, hurt, loss, and anger.

It is remarkable to note that even though suicide has been studied for many years by sociologists and mental health scholars, little direct attention was paid to suicide survivorship until the early 1960s. In this regard, the "discovery" of the survivor phenomena was largely an indirect result of psychological autopsy work undertaken by members of the Los Angeles Suicide Prevention Center. As a tool to help determine the medicolegal manner of death (see Chapter 3), the psychological autopsy work of Litman, Curphey, Shneidman, Farberow, and Tabachnik (1963) led to an increasing awareness that survivors of suicide had a tremendous need to talk about their pain, grief, guilt, and anger. This discovery prompted Shneidman (1967) to coin the term "postvention," broadly referring to posttraumatic crisis interventions that are specifically tailored to assist the grieving survivors of suicide. The contemporary survivor movement was launched in the 1960s and a steady march toward destigmatization, increased understanding, empathy, and healing for survivors of suicide was undertaken.

Contemporary Perspective

Much has changed for suicide survivors over the past 30 years. Even while stigma and stereotypes continue to linger, awareness about the suicide survivor's experience has greatly increased among suicidologists as well as the general public. Since the late 1970s, mental health professionals, public health officials, crisis center personnel, and scholars/researchers have begun to pay a great deal more attention to survivors of suicide—their issues, concerns, needs, and contributions. The increased attention paid to suicide survivors over the past 20 to 30 years is fundamentally connected to the grass-roots development and proliferation of survivor-of-suicide support groups. A recent listing of the number of support groups in the United States and Canada puts the number at over 300 (American Association of Suicidology, 1996).

Some initial attempts to bring suicide survivors together for support can be traced back to the late 1960s, but these groups began to take firm hold in the late 1970s. As discussed by Appel and Wrobleski (1987), the rapid growth of suicide-survivor support groups appears to be inextricably linked to the general self-help movement born in the 1960s and the growth of bereavement groups which occurred in the late 1960s and early 1970s. The initial bereavement self-help groups were not specific to suicidal deaths. The organization Compassionate Friends, for example, was developed for bereaved parents who lost children through all manners of death. But even among the bereaved, many suicide survivors still felt the sting of stigma—in contrast to a mother who loses a child to cancer, the mother of a child who commits suicide *could* be seen as having missed a chance to prevent her child's death. Such perceptions ultimately led survivors of suicide to seek out each other and find support in their common experience through support groups that were specifically for suicide survivors. (See Box 22.1.)

The 1970s was also a critical period of growth for the field of suicidology. Interestingly, the evolution of the survivor movement mirrors the evolution of the larger field of suicidology as a confluence of forces came together to significantly raise public awareness about the problem of suicide. A tremendous amount of media attention and public awareness was directed toward the "epidemic" of adolescent suicide during the 1970s (Maris, 1985; McIntosh, 1987). Indeed, the federal government responded at the national level, through the Department of Health and Human Services, by launching the Secretary's task force on Youth Suicide. The task force was made up of leading suicidologists throughout the United States with the charge of comprehensively addressing concerns about adolescent suicide with the aim of decreasing the adolescent suicide rate (U.S. Department of Health and Human Services, 1989).

The net result of the increasing public and professional awareness about suicide led to a growing appreciation of the survivor experience as well as the long-ignored needs of survivors of suicide (Appel & Wrobleski, 1987). In turn, clinicians, scholars, and researchers began increasingly to study and write about survivors of suicide. Albert Cain's (1972) book, among the first examinations of the topic, was soon followed by a flood of publications on

BOX 22.1. A Brief Chronology of the Survivor Movement

The evolution of the survivor movement is one of the most remarkable developments within contemporary suicidology. Beginning in the late 1970s, an inexorable process began that continues to the present day which has helped move survivors of suicide from the shadows of shame and blame into the forefront of suicidology and suicide prevention. The following is a chronology of key events:

- **1977–1980:** There is the formation of the first suicide-specific survivor support groups. These early efforts include "Ray of Hope," founded by Elizabeth ("Betsy") Ross in Iowa City; "Survivors of Suicide," founded by Iris Bolton in Atlanta; "Heartbeat/Survivors After Suicide," founded by LaRita Archibald; and a co-led (survivor and professional) survivor support group at the Los Angeles Suicide Prevention Center.

- **Spring 1980:** Iris Bolton makes first survivor-oriented presentation at the Annual Conference of the American Association of Suicidology (AAS) held in Alburqueque. At same conference, Adina Wrobleski chairs several sessions on surviving suicide.

- **Spring 1983:** At AAS Annual Conference in Dallas, survivors convened and began plans for developing a "Survivors Committee" within AAS. The purpose of this committee was to identify and assert needs of survivors within the Association and to the Board of AAS.

- **1984:** Persistent advocacy and work of survivors Bolton, Wrobleski, Archibald, Stephanie Weber-Harding, Edward Dunne, and Karen Dunne-Maxim led to AAS Board formally recognizing the Survivor Committee as the official postvention arm of AAS.

- **1989:** First AAS-sponsored "Healing After Suicide" conference held in Denver (chaired by LaRita Archibald). Iris Bolton was elected to AAS Board of Directors. Celebrity survivors (e.g., Marriet Hartley, Joan Rivers, and Judy Collins) began to speak out publicly about surviving suicide and become involved in the field. The American Suicide Foundation, later renamed the American Foundation of Suicide Prevention (AFSP), began to mobilize survivor support for generating funding for suicide-related research.

- **1993:** AAS publishes first issue of *Surviving*, as a survivor-specific newsletter.

- **1994:** Survivor Committee becomes Survivor Division within AAS.

- **1996:** SPAN (the Suicide Prevention Advocacy Network) is founded by the Weyrauch family as a survivor-based grass roots advocacy group promoting suicide prevention.

- **1998:** SPAN (with support of CDC and SAMSHA) convened first National Suicide Prevention Conference in Reno, NV to develop a national suicide prevention strategy which ws accepted as a guiding plan by Surgeon General, Dr. David Satcher. SPAN's letter writing campaign and grass-roots lobbying efforts on Capital Hill led to resolutions in both Houses of Congress in support of suicide prevention. Survivor Karen Dunne-Maxim was elected President of AAS.

Source: Interviews and recollections of Edwin S. Shneidman, Iris Bolton, LaRita Archibald, Edward Dunne, Karen Dunne-Maxim, Sam Heilig, Jerry and Elsie Weyrauch, and Norman Farberow.

the topic of suicide survivorship. Much of the initial work in this area was largely conceptual and anecdotal, but as time passed, research relating to the survivor experience gradually began to accumulate.

Research Perspective

There have been many theories postulated about the reputed course of "normal" bereavement. Theorists such as Kübler-Ross (1969) and Bowlby (1980) have described bereavement as a linear process. Bereavement is typically depicted as a process beginning with shock and numbness, followed by yearning, protest, and disorganization, ultimately ending with reorganization (Rudestam, 1992). Many of the so-called stage models of bereavement discuss similar processes with some variation. According to this perspective, an individual whose grief process follows the linear progression of these models is experiencing "normal" grief. However, when a person deviates from this progression, or experiences grief in longer duration, or does not experience certain emotions, it is hypothesized that the person is experiencing a form of "pathological grief." In contrast, as empirical research has progressed in this area, the difficulty of predicting the process and length of time in which an individual will grieve has become increasingly apparent (Bonanno, Keltner, Holen, & Horowitz, 1995). In fact, researchers and clinicians alike are increasingly discarding the notion of "normal" grief. Clearly, there are many common emotions experienced when coping with death, but the order and duration of these emotions are often different from one individual to the next.

One area of research has examined the possible differences in bereavement resulting from different modes of death. A recent review by McIntosh (1993) looked only at studies that compared groups of suicide survivors to various other control groups. After reviewing results from 16 studies, McIntosh (1993: 158) suggested several generalizations that could me made regarding bereavement from suicide:

> (1) There are many more similarities than differences between suicide survivors and other bereaved groups, particularly other sudden death survivors such as by accidental death, (2) there are possibly a small number of grief reactions or aspects of grieving that may be differ for suicide survivors, but the precise differences are not yet entirely clear or consistent, (3) the course of suicide survivorship may differ from that of other suicide survivors over time, but (4) by some time after the second year differences in grief seem minimal or indistinguishable across survivor groups.

Cleiren, Diekstra, Kerkhoff, and van der Wal (1994) conducted a longitudinal study investigating the recovery process of first-degree family members of victims of a suicide, traffic accident, or illness at 4 and 14 months after the death. These investigators found that suicide survivors experienced a greater sense of guilt at the loss than did survivors of accidents or illnesses. In contrast, feelings of depression and suicidal ideation were felt with similar frequency and intensity across all three groups. Another longitudinal study (Farberow, Gallagher, Gilewski, & Thompson, 1987; Farberow, Gallagher-Thompson, Gilewski, & Thompson, 1992a, 1992b) found that grief took a longer time to subside among suicide survivors when compared to natural death survivors but that differences in grief became insignificant by 2½ years postloss.

One in-depth investigation of the recovery process of survivors by Van Dongen (1993) found somewhat different results from other past research. Thirty-five adult survivors participated in a lengthy, detailed interview in which they were asked questions pertaining to experiences and relationships since the death of their loved one. The purpose of the study was to develop a thorough and precise description of suicide survivors' experiences within the first year of bereavement. Often survivors showed a desire to learn why their loved one had committed suicide. Communication between the family members at this time was described as intense while they tried to retrace the steps of the victim in an attempt to find answers to the question, "Why?" Most survivors in this sample reported that the funerals were helpful but upsetting experiences. Survivors reported that the most helpful funeral experiences were those in which the clergy provided an appropriate service, many people attended, and the survivors were able to fully cry and express their intense grief (Van Dongen, 1993).

Survivors' reactions to suicide also seem to depend to some extent on the kinship ties to the deceased. In general, adult children of suicides tend to show less grief than do either spouses or parents (Owen, Fulson, & Markuson, 1982; Sanders, 1980). In addition, a recent study suggests that higher levels of attachment may be related to increased guilt, shame, shock, and mental preoccupation for suicide as well as survivors of accidental deaths (Reed & Greenwald, 1992).

One important area of research that has distinct implications for suicide survivorship pertains to the importance of social support in the bereavement process. Research has shown that, in general, individuals who report adequate levels of social support have a more positive outcome than those who feel socially isolated (Range & Niss, 1990; Reed, 1993, 1998). Why might suicide survivors feel that they have lower levels of social support? As discussed earlier, throughout history, suicide has often resulted in negative consequences for survivors. Recently a number of studies have in fact found that between 62% and 80% of suicide survivors report high rates of hurtful comments made by persons who are potentially in the position to be supportive (Davidowitz & Myrick, 1984; Lehman, Ellard, & Wortman, 1986; Range & Niss, 1990).

Van Dongen (1993) found that 69% of the suicide survivors in their study perceived themselves as receiving strong social support. However, despite the high rate of social support, 26% of survivors still reported at least some negative stigmatization that tended to appear in more subtle forms. For instance, one survivor in Van Dongen's study perceived another individual's discomfort with him or her.

Research further suggests that people may tend to have different attitudes toward survivors of suicide than survivors of other types of death (see Exercise 22.2). In this regard, research about attitudes toward suicide might provide some insight into attitudes toward survivors. Wellman and Wellman (1986) found that 50–70% of respondents from two surveys (both men and women) believed that no one should ever be allowed to commit suicide. Using four national surveys conducted between 1977 and 1983, Singh, Williams, and Ryther (1986) studied the acceptability of suicide under a variety of circumstances (i.e., an incurable disease, financial problems, disapproval of the family, and being tired of living). They consistently found that suicide was the most acceptable when the suicide victim had an incurable disease (such as terminal cancer).

EXERCISE 22.2. How Do You See Suicide Survivors?

- How do you personally view the survivors of Jimmy's suicide (see previous pages)? Do you think they are to blame for his suicide?
- How do you think they would be doing a year after Jimmy's death? What about 5 years?
- How might their reactions be different if Jimmy had died of cancer? How might you view the survivors differently?

Several other experimental studies have examined the potential impact of numerous variables on attitudes toward suicide and/or survivors of suicide (e.g., age of the deceased). One study conducted by Range and Goggin (1990) examined community attitudes toward the suicide of persons ages 10, 18, 30, and 65. For each of the specified age groups, participants were randomly presented with fictitious newspaper articles about a death by either suicide or a viral illness. Participants were then asked about their perceptions of the victim and the victim's family. The researchers found that participants' attitudes were more negative toward victim and family members in the death by suicide scenario than in the viral illness scenario. They also found that subjects believed the families of the 18- and 30-year-olds would grieve longer than families of 10- and 65-year-olds. The authors suggest that a possible explanation for this finding is that people view the deaths of young and old people as having less of an impact on the family and community than the middle-age groups. In a related study, Range, Bright, and Ginn (1985) discovered that subjects perceived suicidal adolescents as more psychologically disturbed and placed more blame on these parents than on those with suicidal children.

From a somewhat different perspective, Reynolds and Cimbolic (1988) looked at how the survivor's relationship to the deceased moderated the way in which the survivor was perceived. In this analog study, students were presented three fictional case histories that described a child's suicide, a spouse's suicide, or a parent's suicide. Participants were then asked to provide ratings of their attitudes toward the survivor. Though the subjects generally perceived all suicide survivors negatively, the researchers found that the child survivors were perceived significantly less negatively than parent and spouse survivors. Based on these results, Reynolds and Cimbolic suggested that a survivor's relationship to the victim might affect the type and amount of social support that is received.

It is clear from past research that many suicide survivors experience a great deal of pain during the recovery process. Most report a great variety of emotions, ranging from anger and guilt to disbelief and shame. Research has suggested that, in many ways, bereavement from suicide is similar to bereavement from other forms of death. Bereavement by suicide may differ in course, but by 2 years or so, survivors of suicide appear to be adjusting about as well as survivors of other types of death. Research has also supported the important role that social support may play in the course of bereavement. Related findings suggest that those people in the position to provide social support (e.g., family members, friends, and colleagues) may tend to have more negative attitudes toward the survivors of suicide than do survivors of other forms of death. Research in this area underscores the need for further education about suicide and suicide survivorship in order to combat stigmatization and increase possible social support that seems so critical in the suicide survivor's healing process.

HELPING SUICIDE SURVIVORS

Having a general sense of the history of survivorship and the empirical research related to being a suicide survivor are critical components to our understanding of the topic. But what about actually helping survivors of suicide deal with these deaths (see Box 22.2)? Interventions and responses to suicide survivors may range from clinical interventions to more informal types of healing and support. As Dunne (1987) has noted, many people who have experienced the loss of a loved one to suicide often do not seek professional assistance for a variety of reasons. One reason may be distrust of professionals who are seen as having failed to save their loved one. Survivors may also fear that even a professional help giver may blame the survivor for the death of the loved one. Indeed, when survivors do seek the

BOX 22.2. Responding to the Child as a Survivor

The death of a parent or other close relative can be a very difficult experience for any child. Often adults have difficulty knowing how to approach child survivors of suicide. This box outlines some guidelines that may be helpful in responding to the grief and pain of a child survivor of suicide.

Grief reaction	Adult response
Shock and numbness: Often serves as a cushion against the full impact of the tragedy.	Provide an atmosphere which encourages the open expression of all initial reactions to the event, even unusual ones, such as laughing.
Denial: Blatant denial is not an unusual reaction, especially among younger children.	Communicate all facets in a clear, concise way and avoid a power struggle about the truth. Don't be unduly concerned if denial seems to wax and wane.
Sadness: Tearfulness and sadness are common reactions among grieving children.	Encourage children to talk about these feelings and validate them as appropriate. Initiate conversations about the deceased.
Anger: Anger may be directed at the deceased, event, or other adults.	Accept the anger and allow children to express it. You may want to encourage physical activities as a way to relieve tension.
Anxiety: Children may experience fears of abandonment or that the other parent may die. If a sibling is lost, children often fear for their own safety.	Reassure children that arrangements have been made for their caretaking. Encourage children to resume routine activities. Encourage them to take part in rituals for the deceased which provide social support.
Shame: Children may be ashamed of being seen as grieving, different from peers.	Encourage normal peer activities as soon as possible, especially recreation with other peers.
Guilt: Children may often believe they were the cause of the tragedy or worry about negative interactions with the deceased They may also feel guilt that they are not as "sad" as the rest of the family about the loss.	Help children to see the causative factors were not related to their behavior. Explain that every relationship has negative and positive aspects but our feelings cannot cause another's death. Clearly, give children permission to go on enjoying living.
Physical problems: Frequent illnesses and somatic complaints are common in children who are grieving.	Create an atmosphere where children have permission to verbalize their physical concerns. For example, tolerate frequent visits to the nurse, if necessary.
Academic problems: Confusion, concentration difficulties, memory lapses, and preoccupation with deceased.	Provide additional help or tutoring for children of all ages. Older children may benefit from a temporary reduction in their academic load.

Source: Adapted from Parkin & Dunne-Maxim (1995). Copyright 1995 by American Foundation for Suicide Prevention. Adapted by permission.

help of mental health professionals, they may sometimes encounter a clinician who is not familiar with the unique aspects of suicide bereavement. This may result in the well-meaning but perhaps naive clinician inadvertently stigmatizing or wounding the grieving suicide survivor.

From a clinical perspective, Dunne (1987) offers some parameters for conducting individual psychotherapy with a suicide survivor. These parameters include considerations that pertain to the clinician, the client, the timing of the psychotherapy, and the nature of the psychotherapy itself. For many clinicians, the topic of suicide has the potential to evoke strong negative countertransference and may bring out the worst in a clinician. Due to the difficulty of working with the issue of suicide, even seasoned clinicians may make clinical errors (Jobes & Maltsberger, 1995). Clinicians' concerns about malpractice liability, fears about losing a patient to suicide (and thereby becoming a survivor), and even their own potential death anxiety may interfere with sound clinical work.

Psychotherapy is not necessarily required for every survivor of suicide. However, individual psychotherapy, sometimes in combination with other modalities such as couple or family therapy, can be quite helpful. Typically, therapy is most appropriate for those survivors who become unable to function because of their grief. Basically, when grief becomes profoundly debilitating in either professional or personal spheres, some form of psychotherapy may be warranted. Although client motivation, timing, and the specific type of psychotherapy are always important considerations, it is probably best for survivors to find a supportive and flexible form of treatment that enables them to define what is best for them in the course of their grieving process. Dunne (1987) suggests that an involved, humanistic, and compassionate approach is preferable to overly directive or passive/inactive approaches (refer to Dunne, 1987).

In addition to a suicide's blood relatives, who may need and benefit from the help of a professional, other survivors of the deceased, who are not relatives, may have also special professional needs. As discussed by Berman, Jacobs, and Jobes (1993), there is sometimes an obvious need to respond to a group of survivors who are not family (e.g., coworkers, class mates, even casual acquaintances). Indeed, Zinner's (1985) notion of "group survivorship" conceptualizes many groups as extended families that may need to mourn the loss of a member.

Certain groups, such as an office staff that loses staff member to suicide, may benefit from the intervention of an outside consultant to facilitate a process of understanding, support, and healing. In such situations, interventions may involve both individual and group meetings that provide the opportunity to (1) disseminate accurate factual information about the death, (2) assess the needs of individuals and the group to guide further interventions, and (3) begin a process of healing by using the group system as a vehicle of support and comfort (Berman, Jacobs, & Jobes, 1993).

In general, effective formal or informal help for suicide survivors involves some form of learning about the specific suicide (and perhaps about suicide in general), acknowledging the range of feelings about the suicide to supportive others (e.g., grief, loss, guilt, and anger), and ultimately reframing the event by finding an acceptable understanding of the suicide within the framework of their own life (refer to Schuyler, 1979).

In other words, to successfully resolve the tragedy of a suicide, each survivor must develop his or her own unique interpretation of the act as well as develop an understanding of the consequences of the act for them (Zinner, 1990). In that spirit, a survivor can begin to deal with the misperception, "I could have (should have) done something to prevent this death." Fundamentally, dealing with this common perception is central to successful survivorship. Indeed, as Jobes and colleagues have asserted (Berman et al., 1993):

Ultimately suicide survivors (not by their own choosing) must face some difficult realities inherent in living and dying. In the face of a suicide death, perhaps no reality is more difficult to reconcile than the realization that none of us can be truly responsible for anyone's life, or death. Paradoxically, in that insight, we may experience the terror of our limits to influence and simultaneously find courage and relief from the pain of surviving another's suicide. (272)

CLINICIANS AS SURVIVORS

Suicide is the most commonly encountered clinical emergency (Bongar, 1992; Schein, 1976). Recent surveys suggest that about half of psychiatrists and one-quarter of psychologists will lose a patient to suicide during the course of their career (Jobes & Berman, 1993). Additional data suggest that about one in six people who complete suicide (about 5,000 patients/year) are currently in therapy (Berman, 1986a). Although patient suicide is relatively commonly encountered, it has been little researched and few clear findings have emerged.

The loss of a patient to suicide is often a difficult event for therapists. Kleespies, Penk, and Forsyth (1993) surveyed 292 clinical psychology predoctoral interns about experiences relating to losing a patient to suicide. Those who had lost a patient to suicide exhibited high levels of intrusive thoughts relating to patient suicide as well as avoidance of situations that might remind them of the suicide. Another study suggested that clinician survivors often have stress levels equaling those of bereaved patients (Kleespies, Smith, & Becker, 1990). Often therapists have high levels of self-blame and guilt about their role in the patient's suicide, along with fears of losing standing with professional colleagues (Tanney, 1995). Many therapists lose confidence in their professional competence and may fear relatives' reactions and the possibility of malpractice suits (Valente, 1994). Some clinicians may refuse to treat suicidal patients in the future, whereas others may improve their suicide prevention skills (Kleespies et al., 1993). Many clinicians begin to take patient's suicidal ideas or threats more seriously and become more cautious, accepting more responsibility for monitoring suicidal patients.

In the difficult days following a patient's suicide, social and collegial support for the clinician survivor is important (Tanney, 1995). Often clinician survivors can benefit from attending support groups composed of clinicians who have experienced a completed suicide. Consultation is also important for clinician survivors, especially when working with patients who are currently at risk for suicide (see Case 22.1). When the bereaved family and the clinician choose to meet, both parties may feel vulnerable and need support (Valente, 1994). The presence of another therapist on such occasions can allow the primary clinician to experience personal feelings without having the responsibility to provide counseling to the family.

SUICIDE MODELING AND IMITATION

There is another aspect left behind after a suicide—the potential for others to imitate the deceased. Indeed, central to the idea of *surviving* suicide is the notion that survivors do not pursue the same death as the deceased.

Marilyn Monroe was 36 years old at the time of her death. She had starred in 22 films and was an internationally renowned movie star. A controversial public figure throughout her career, Monroe was both beloved by devoted fans (who sent her up to 5,000 letters per day) and widely criticized as a no-talent blond bombshell. Since her death, Marilyn Monroe

CASE 22.1. The Case of a Therapist Survivor

Jane is 28-year-old clinical psychologist, working in private practice with three other colleagues. Jane began to see Helen, a 24-year-old physical therapist who worked in a children's rehabilitation hospital. Helen had severe bulimia—she was bingeing and purging three to four times per day and exercising 2–4 hours daily. Helen told of her parents and their divorce when she was quite young, her alcoholic father, and her mother who had been depressed for many years since the divorce. She also told of being sexually abused by her neighbor over a period of 4 years (from the ages of 14 to 18). Helen ultimately escaped the abusive relationship when she went to college. This was when her obsessive exercising and bingeing and purging began.

Treatment with Helen progressed well. She regularly attended checkups with her physician to monitor her medical status and behavioral management did much to reduce instances of bingeing and purging. In this context, Jane was stunned when Helen suddenly and precipitously descended into a deep depressive state. She became even more concerned about Helen's increased use of alcohol and marijuana. During this period, Helen began talking about some of her suicidal thoughts and fantasies. She stated that she was tired and just wanted to finally end the pain. Helen's decent into suicidal despair was alarmingly rapid. Jane considered hospitalizing Helen as the risk increased. The consulting psychiatrist increased the antidepressant medication and they began to meet twice per week. Helen only seemed to deteriorate.

On an overcast Saturday afternoon, Helen called Jane at home. Helen was drunk and had apparently injected herself with some Demerol that she had stolen from a nursing station at the hospital. Her speech was slurred and she was sobbing uncontrollably. She revealed to Jane that she was standing on her 11th-story apartment balcony and was thinking about jumping. In the midst of Jane's pleading for her to step back inside the apartment, Helen jumped to her death.

With Helen's tragic death, Jane was plunged into a personal and professional nightmare. She immediately called her supervisor who was supportive but did not know exactly what Jane should do. Jane remembers that he seemed particularly worried about the "potential for legal issues." Jane decided to attend the funeral, which was very awkward. She felt as if the family treated her with disdain. Jane perceived that they blamed her for Helen's death; she had failed to save Helen from herself. Colleagues seemed to keep their distance. She perceived that they too felt that she had somehow failed. Jane's crisis deepened and was intensified when an attorney hired by Helen's family called to inform her that she was being sued for malpractice. This litigation was especially agonizing. After almost 2½ years, the case was dismissed.

Jane entered therapy, cut back on her practice, and even questioned whether she should stay in the field. She read literature on being a "survivor" of suicide but found that very little was written about being a clinician who survives the death of a patient. As a clinician survivor, she felt as if she was left to make her own sense of Helen's tragic death. However, she did find remarkable support from other clinicians who had lost patients to suicide. Four years later, Jane is doing much better, and increasingly has renewed energy for clinical work. But some nights when she lies awake in bed she still plays through her mind the fateful days leading up to that Saturday afternoon. If only she had . . .

has become a cultural icon; dozens of books, movies, and various retrospectives continue to examine and reexamine her life and sudden suicidal death.

Monroe was notably depressed and despondent in the months preceding her death. Toward the end of her life, Monroe had developed a reputation of being a troubled, temperamental, pampered star, who was impossible to work with. Monroe actively sought psychoanalytic treatment in an effort to address her various emotional problems. After a string of highly publicized divorces and the financial failures of her last two movies, Monroe's personal life was in disarray and her movie career was in limbo.

In her final weeks and days, Monroe largely lived in isolation. She spent most of her time in the simple two-bedroom Brentwood bungalow, where she died on the evening of August 5, 1962. She was last seen alive by her housekeeper, Mrs. Murray, who discovered her lifeless body at 8:00 P.M. As discussed by Litman (1996; Litman did the psychological autopsy on Monroe for Los Angeles Medical Examiner Theodore Curphey), Monroe had made previously foiled suicide attempts. Interestingly, on the night of her fatal overdose she made phone calls to friends and her analyst, who apparently failed to intervene. When Mrs. Murray discovered Monroe's body, she called Monroe's analyst who came to the house and determined that she had died of an overdose of sleeping pills. Empty pill bottles were found at her bedside; no suicide note was found at the death scene.

The news of Monroe's sudden death spread like wildfire, both nationally and internationally. In retrospect, her death would become known as the prototypical "celebrity suicide." As a widely recognized national–international movie star, Marilyn Monroe's suicide was widely reported throughout the news media. Years later, sociologist David Phillips began his seminal research studying possible effects of newsprint reporting of celebrity suicides on national suicide rates in the months immediately following the printing of such stories. Phillips (1974) found a 12% increase in the U.S. national suicide rate in the month following Monroe's suicide (the highest increase following any celebrity suicide that Phillips studied). Using an approach that investigated expected versus observed suicides, Phillips found an excess of 303 suicides following newspaper coverage of Monroe's suicide. The systematic, and sometimes controversial, empirical study of suicide imitation effects had been launched.

The Werther Effect

In his original 1974 paper, Phillips coined the term "Werther effect" to describe the potential impact of a celebrity suicide to inspire others to similarly end their lives. The term was based on the reported effect among young European romantics to commit suicide after a fictional hero depicted in Goethe's 1774 novel, *The Sorrows of Young Werther*. In recent years, other terms for the Werther effect have appeared in the literature, such as suicide "contagion" or "copycat" suicides; groupings of youthful suicides are commonly referred to as suicide clusters. Whatever the name, studying the potential imitative modeling effects in suicidal behavior has become an important (and sometimes contentious) line of research in suicidology.

With important implications for First Amendment rights, much controversy has surrounded research examining media effects on possible imitative suicidal behavior. At this time, many suicidologists believe that the reporting of a suicide either on television or in the newspaper may cause certain vulnerable individuals to imitate the reported suicidal act. This general view is based on a line of research that has specifically focused on whether newspaper articles, television reports, and fictional stories on suicide appear to correlate with statistically significant increases in suicide rates (Motto, 1967, 1970; Phillips, 1974, 1979; Wasserman, 1984).

However, although many studies have suggested that media reports of suicide may spark copycat suicidal behaviors, much of this research has been plagued with methodological problems as well as some inconclusive findings. In an attempt to clarify some to the controversies and contradictions in this research, we examine the historical background on the Werther effect and review the empirical research on the potential effect of media coverage on suicidal behavior (with an emphasis on newspaper articles, television reports, and fictional television stories; cf. Chapter 10).

Historical Perspective

As noted, the term "Werther effect" was derived from a popular novel written by the German author Goethe more than 200 years ago (Phillips, 1974). In this story, the hero (Werther) dramatically commits suicide by a pistol shot to the head after a failed love affair. Although no definitive evidence is available, it was widely perceived throughout Europe that many young men in the late 18th century imitated Werther—his apparel, his romantic persona, and particularly his method of suicide (Alvarez, 1975). As a result of the novel's reputed effect, it was banned in several European countries (e.g., Italy) and cities (e.g., Leipzig and Copenhagen). Some hundred years later, Durkheim (1897/1951) reexamined the research linking imitation and suicidal behavior. In his review, Durkheim found no evidence of imitative effects and proclaimed that "'suicide exposes a state which is the true generating cause of the act and which probably would have produced its effect even had imitation not intervened'" (quoted in Barraclough, Shepherd, & Jennings, 1977: 528). Although Durkheim did acknowledge that imitation and suggestion may be important, he thought they influenced only a small proportion of the population and had relatively little effect on the national suicide rate.

Following Durkheim's work, nearly 60 years passed before the relationship between suicide and imitation was revisited. At that time, several studies were conducted, but the results were inconsistent and at times contradictory (Motto, 1967; Seiden, 1968). Regardless of these problems, the research continued to develop and methodological design improve. As is discussed, the research originally focused on the effects of newspaper suicide stories and later examined the influence of television reports and fictional movies on the national suicide rate.

Effect of Newspaper Coverage

Since the early late 1960s–early 1970s, researchers have focused on whether newspaper stories about suicide can influence the national suicide rate. In one of the first studies examining the effect of newspaper stories on suicide, Motto (1967) examined the incidence of suicide in seven cities that had lost newspaper coverage for a certain period due to strikes. He compared the suicide rate for the month without newspaper coverage with the incidence in the same month of the previous 5 years. Motto had thought that the suicide rate would decrease during the newspaper strikes. However, he did not find support for his hypothesis or for the Werther effect. In a subsequent study, Motto (1970) used a similar study design and found that the suspension of a newspaper publication did result in a substantially lower suicide rate. A particularly interesting finding from this study was that the suicide rate for women decreased by more than 60%, whereas the rate for men tended to rise. Although no specific pattern was revealed, Motto's results provide some support for the hypothesis that sensational newspaper reporting may cause imitative suicidal behavior. Overall, however, these studies provide inconsistent results and fail to provide strong evidence for the Werther effect.

Following Motto's (1967, 1970) studies, researchers developed an alternative research design that proved to be more useful and provided a more direct estimate of the impact of newspaper suicide stories. These studies tended to examine all suicide stories reported in a newspaper for a designated period. Normally, researchers focused on front-page articles because they tended to be more visible to the newspaper audience.

In addition, suicide statistics were compiled from the time before and after the suicide articles to determine whether or not the suicide rate increased or decreased. As discussed earlier, one of the first studies using this design was conducted by Phillips (1974) who found that suicide rates between 1946 and 1968 rose significantly 7 to 10 days after front-page suicide stories and that rates stayed elevated (up about 3%) for up to 10 days following the article. This effect on suicide rates appeared to be about twice as strong among adolescents as among adults. Phillips (1979) also examined the number of motor vehicle fatalities following a newspaper suicide article and found that single-vehicle crashes tended to increase after suicide articles, with a greater increase in vehicle accidents occurring after a highly publicized article.

In a subsequent study, Wasserman (1984) expanded Phillips's study and examined the front-page suicide stories from 1946 to 1977. In contrast to Phillips, Wasserman found that an increase in suicide rates only occurred after a celebrity suicide. Following Wasserman's article, other researchers criticized previous work on newspaper stories that combined all types of suicide stories. As a result, researchers began focusing on the significance of specific type of suicides, especially publicized celebrity suicides. For instance, Stack (1987) found that suicide stories on U.S. political and entertainment celebrities were related to the most significant rise in suicide rates. It is possible that this increase in suicides following a celebrity suicide may be due to the large amount of publicity given to these articles versus other suicide stories.

Effect of Television Coverage

A much smaller body of research has examined the effect of television suicide stories (see Box 22.3). These studies have focused on heavily publicized stories or on television series that have depicted suicides. Bollen and Phillips (1982), in an attempt to replicate Phillips's (1974) newsprint findings, found a significant rise in suicides in the week following TV news reports during 1972–1976. In addition, they provided evidence that the rise in suicides occurred after and not before the TV news story. They also replicated Phillips's earlier finding that the effect of the suicide story appeared to last up to 10 days following the program.

Schmidtke and Hafner (1988) examined the effect of a six-episode television film, *Death of a Student*, on the suicide rate in Germany. In this study, the investigators were specifically interested in the age and sex effects on imitative behavior. Their results indicated that the suicide rate rose immediately after the television film for those individuals whose age and sex were most similar to the model. This finding illustrated the importance of similarities between the model and the imitator. In contrast to previous findings, they also found that the imitation effect probably lasted for longer than a 10-day period following the broadcast.

Two recent studies of a potential Werther effect related to the suicide of rock star Kurt Cobain have provided additional data that failed to support the notion of celebrity suicide copy-cat effects (Jobes, Berman, O'Carroll, Eastgard, & Knickmeyer, 1996; Martin & Koo, 1996). Jobes et al. (1996) conducted a quasi-interrupted time-series analysis of suicide mortality data obtained from the King County Medical Examiners Office in Seattle, Washington (Cobain's hometown and site of his death). These investigators used 7-week surveillance periods of completed suicides that occurred both before and after Cobain's death in

---

BOX 22.3. Do Television Stories Cause Suicide? Evidence from Two Contradictory Studies

Yes: Philips and Carstensen (1986) analyzed the relationship between 38 nationally televised stories about suicide from 1973 to 1979 and the fluctuation of the rate of suicide among U.S. teenagers before and after these stories. They found that the number of teenage suicides increased for up to 7 days after a TV story and that increases in suicide were highly correlated with the amount of coverage of the story. In addition, rates of suicide appeared to increase as much after general-information stories as feature stories about a particular suicide. They also controlled for six alternative explanations and for fluctuations in suicide due to the effects of specific day of the week, month, holiday, and yearly trends. They concluded that the best explanation of their results was that television stories tend to trigger additional suicides among adolescents.

No: Kessler, Downey, Milavsky, and Stripp (1988), in response to the article just cited, performed a study that critically evaluated their results. They improved on the above study through using more years of data (1973–1984), more comprehensive information on news stories about suicide, a more exact measure of the number of teenagers exposed to each suicide, and more refined statistical analyses. Kessler et al. replicated Philip and Carstensen's (1986) findings about increased rates of suicide following television stories during the years of 1973–1979. However, during the years of 1981-1984, this trend actually reversed itself—lower rates of suicide tended to follow television stories on suicide. Kessler et al. suggested that this reversal in rates of suicide might be due to changing perceptions of suicide beginning in 1980. Several results also contradicted the idea that increased rates of suicide following TV programs during 1973–1979 were due to imitative effects. Additional analyses also showed that the number of teenagers exposed to stories about suicide was unrelated to rates of suicide. Finally, evidence showed that news stories specifically about youth suicide (hypothesized to be more likely to be imitated) were unrelated to rates of teenage suicide.

1994. Data for the same surveillance periods pertaining to suicides for 1993 and 1995 (adjusted for day of the week) were obtained as equivalent comparison-control years. As shown in Figure 22.1, there was no notable increase in suicides following Cobain's death in 1994. In addition, overall suicide rates for 1994 (even after Cobain's death) were consistently lower than overall rates seen in the 1993 and 1995 comparison control years. This unexpected finding suggested that Cobain's death did not apparently inspire Seattle youth to take their lives as would be expected by the Werther effect.

As a follow-up to this initial analysis of completed suicides, Jobes et al. (1996) applied a similar quasi-interrupted time-series methodology for suicide crisis calls to the Seattle Crisis Clinic for the years 1993, 1994, and 1995 during the exact same surveillance time periods. Data from this analysis provided some striking results. As shown in Figure 22.2, suicide crisis calls markedly increased after Cobain's suicide, especially when compared to the 1993 and 1995 control years for the same time periods. This so-called Cobain effect, speaks implicitly to the possibility that Cobain's death actually inspired young people to reach out for help rather than imitate his fatal behavior. The authors suggest that unique aspects pertaining to Cobain's death may account for these results. For example, there is some evidence that the news media did a fairly responsible job of reporting the death. Various interventions within the Seattle community may have also had a positive impact. Finally, the particularly grisly method of death (a shotgun wound to the head) may have created a no-

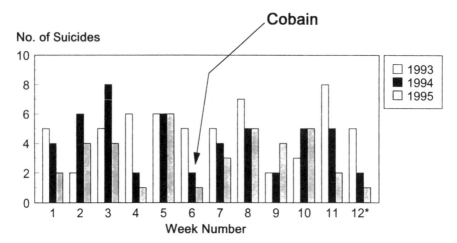

FIGURE 22.1. Suicides in King County, Washington, by week, late February to mid-May, several years. *Partial week. *Source:* Medical Examiner's Office, King County, Washington.

tably different image of the suicidal act, particularly in comparison to a Marilyn Monroe "sleeping beauty" overdose image of suicide.

Similar to the Jobes et al. (1996) findings, Martin and Koo (1996) found no evidence of a Cobain effect in a controlled-comparison national study of Australian youth. As Cobain was also popular in Australia, these researchers had expected an increase in suicide completion rates (especially among youth) in the days following Cobain's death. Yet, such was not the case. Even though his suicide was widely reported throughout the Australian media, there were increases in neither general suicide completions nor the method of his death (firearm) in the days following his suicide. The suicide rates for 1994 after Cobain's death were actually lower than rates for the preceding 5 years during the same time periods.

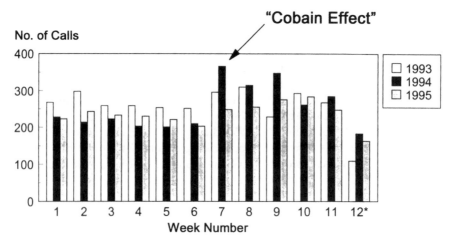

FIGURE 22.2. Suicides crisis calls to the Seattle Crisis Clinic by week, late February to mid-May, several years. *Partial week. *Source:* Seattle Crisis Clinic.

Effect of Fictional Suicide Stories

In addition to the research on nonfiction newspaper and television stories, a growing body of research has concentrated on the impact of fictional suicide stories on imitative behavior. Prior to the early 1980s, this research was primarily based on laboratory studies (Phillips, 1982). Although this research was useful, Phillips developed a naturalistic methodology to examine the effect of soap opera suicides. Specifically, he focused on the suicide rate 1 week prior to the soap opera episode and 1 week following the program. He found that there was a significant increase in the suicide rate in the week following the soap opera suicide. Furthermore, Phillips found that the number of motor vehicle deaths from single-car motor fatalities increased following a soap opera suicide.

In a subsequent study, Kessler and Stripp (1984) attacked Phillips's (1982) methodology and invalidated his results. Unlike Phillips, who only knew the month of the soap opera suicide, Kessler and Stripp were able to determine the specific day of the episode. They also found several more soap opera suicides that were ignored by Phillips. As a result, Kessler and Stripp did not find a significant relationship between soap opera suicides and subsequent suicides and motor vehicle fatalities.

Gould and Shaffer (1986) examined four television movies focusing on suicide and its effect on the suicide rate in New York City. They found that there was a significant rise in the youth suicide rate following these films. In addition, a significant increase in the number of attempted suicides in area hospitals was reported. In an effort to generalize these findings, Gould, Shaffer, and Kleinman (1988) examined the suicide rate following these four movies in three other U.S. cities: Cleveland, Dallas, and Los Angeles. From their analyses, they found a significant rise in the suicide rate in New York and Cleveland but not in Dallas or Los Angeles. It seems that these differences may be due to the fact that geographic areas provided different education programs on suicide prevention following the television movie.

These studies have sparked a flourishing interest in the effects of other television movies on adolescent suicide. Berman (1988) attempted to replicate the Gould and Shaffer (1986) study. In contrast, Berman found that suicidal behavior by fictional characters was unrelated to rates of suicide by adolescent viewers. In the course of his investigation, Berman found that suicide rates actually decreased following televised suicide movies. In his conclusion, however, Berman discussed the potential importance of imitation effects and argued for further research exploring whether the interaction of several factors such as characteristics of the viewer, the stimulus, and the suicidal method used in the story influenced subsequent suicidal behavior.

Summary of Suicide Imitation Effects

In 1845, Amariah Brigham, the founder and editor of the *American Journal of Insanity*, wrote:

> "No fact is better established in science than that suicide is often committed from imitation. A single paragraph may suggest suicide to 20 persons. Some particulars of the act, or expressions, seize the imagination, and the disposition to repeat it, in a moment of morbid excitement, proves irresistible." (quoted in Motto, 1967: 156)

For several years, researchers have attempted to provide empirical evidence for Brigham's statement. Although many of the findings suggest that media coverage on suicides may cause imitative suicidal behavior, the evidence still remains inconclusive (Gould & Shaffer, 1988; Motto, 1967, 1970; Phillips, 1974, 1979).

To determine the primary effect of media coverage, more research is necessary. Future research should focus not only on the effect of newspaper and television programs, but also on the effect of the Internet on the suicide rate. In addition, more research is needed on the effect of suicide stories on the number of attempted suicides (Phillips, Lesyna, & Paight, 1994). Until now, the vast majority of research has focused solely on completed suicides. Moreover, it would be interesting to examine whether advertisements for suicide prevention centers influence the suicide rate. By expanding the current research on the Werther effect and exploring these suggested research areas, a better understanding of the factors that influence suicide contagion may be provided.

SUICIDE POSTVENTION

Shneidman (1971) coined "postvention" as a term that describes appropriate and helpful acts that come after a dire event. As discussed by Shneidman (1980), "Postvention, then, consists of activities that reduce the aftereffects of a traumatic event in the lives of the survivors. Its purpose is to help survivors live longer, more productively, and less stressfully than they are likely to do otherwise" (234).

Whereas Shneidman's original use of the term was broad-based and inclusive of any traumatic event, "postvention" has increasingly been linked to suicide-specific intervention efforts designed to prevent suicide imitation effects as well as to considerations of overall immediate postsuicide care for survivors of suicide. We organize major suicide postvention efforts by examining programs and initiatives that come from public health perspectives as well as school-based (community-based) postvention initiatives.

Public Health Perspective

In recent years, the importance of suicide postvention following suicide attempts and completed suicides has been increasingly recognized by the Centers for Disease Control and Prevention (CDC), crisis intervention centers, school districts across the country, and the public at large (Celotta, 1995; Kalafat & Underwood, 1989; Lamb & Dunne-Maxim, 1987; Mauk, Gibson, & Rodgers, 1994). Many organizations and groups have developed literally hundreds of specific suicide postvention guidelines to help civic leaders, crisis workers, mental health professionals, school faculty, students, and the general community deal with suicidal events. Because it is impossible to thoroughly review the range of different suicide postvention approaches, we initially focus our attention on federal (CDC) efforts before considering two typical approaches to school-based suicide postvention programs.

In the aftermath of a completed suicide, there is an obvious need for a coordinated effort in the community to decrease the risk of copycat suicidal behaviors or even a potential cluster of suicides. In the wake of a suicide, community leaders are often confronted with sometimes competing needs to prevent further suicides while helping a community cope with the loss that has occurred. To further complicate an already difficult situation, media interest in a community suicide is often present and can potentially raise the risk for further copycat suicidal behaviors. How does the community cope? How can suicide prevention and healing be linked? How can the "news" of a community suicide be appropriately reported without fanning the flames of further suicide risk?

From the mid-1980s through the 1990s, the CDC has provided notable leadership in its attempts to answer the difficult questions of suicide postvention. By using identifying problem issues, using various resources, and bringing experts together, the CDC has developed excellent postvention guidelines that have fundamentally defined and shaped our contemporary suicide postvention efforts. Two sets of guidelines are particularly noteworthy. The first set of guidelines provides specific suicide postvention guidelines for use in the general community environment (Centers for Disease Control, 1988), the second set of guidelines provides specific suggestions that pertain to media coverage of suicide events (Centers for Disease Control and Prevention [CDC], 1994).

The 1988 CDC Postvention Guidelines outline general steps of a coordinated community-based crisis intervention response after a suicide within the community. The principal purpose of these guidelines is to prevent further suicidal behavior and contain potential suicide clusters. In addition, these guidelines also make suggestions as to how to best facilitate healing after the suicidal death. The guidelines specifically suggest that postvention initiatives be implemented by leaders in the community that have an involvement in public health, mental health services, and education. Oftentimes this might not just represent individuals within the community but community-based agencies as well. The first step in implementing a crisis response is for the appropriate people and agencies to identify and create a coordinating committee that will manage the day-to-day response within the community. This committee should be an ongoing entity that is developed and maintained *before* a crisis response is needed so that appropriate postvention action can be taken in a planful and decisive manner. The guidelines recommend that one agency be selected to act as the "host" agency to function as the postvention control center, to coordinate, implement, and monitor all suicide prevention and postvention activities undertaken by the coordinating committee. (See Box 22.4.)

BOX 22.4. Guidelines for the Reporting of Suicide

- When information is provided to the media, it should be given in an efficient and accurate manner.

- "No comment" or a general refusal to speak to the media is often not a useful response for the public official to make. These responses may create an adversarial relationship with the media that prevent the chance to influence and shape the information that is made known to the public.

- Professionals should take time to explain the scientific basis for the concerns about suicide contagion and assist the media in finding ways of reporting the information to avoid such risks.

- The suicide event should not be explained as the result of one single precipitating factor but as the result of many events.

- Sensationalizing the suicide through ongoing and excessive reporting should be avoided.

- Excessive details on the method used by the individual should be avoided.

- The suicide should not be portrayed as a successful means to an end or a viable option for uncomfortable circumstances; for example, reporting a suicide as a way of "getting back" at strict parents or as a result of a breakup with a boyfriend or girlfriend.

- Reports of public expressions of grief (e.g., public eulogies and remembrance pages in a yearbook) should be minimized so as not to glorify the deceased person.

- Glorification can be avoided by providing a balanced account of the deceased person's positive qualities as well as the problematic characteristics that are associated with the suicidal behavior.

Source: Centers for Disease Control and Prevention (1994).

Once a host agency has been identified and the coordinating committee has been established, key personnel who are potentially in a position to intervene and directly make contacts with friends and classmates of a potential suicide victim should be identified and appropriately trained. These intervenors need to be contacted and in place *before* a potential crisis so that they can be properly prepared to handle the crisis situation (e.g., how to announce the death and provide support to youth). These intervenors would also be responsible for identifying youth who may be particularly at risk for suicidality and most in need of support and care. In the midst of a crisis it is critical that individuals such as family members, friends, girlfriends, boyfriends, and past attempters can be identified and attended to, as these individuals may be at a potentially higher risk for self-destructive behaviors. Sometimes a mental health evaluation and referral to professional services are warranted for these at-risk survivors.

As discussed by O'Carroll (in Jobes et al., 1996), a workshop sponsored by the Association of State and Territorial Health Officials, the New Jersey Department of Health, and the CDC was convened to bring together suicidologists, public health officials, researchers, and news media professionals from around the country. The workshop was designed to share concerns and perspectives on the questions related to suicide contagion and media coverage and explore ways in which reporting of suicide could minimize potential contagion without compromising the independence or integrity of news media professionals. A tangible product of this meeting was a set of recommendation guidelines that were ultimately endorsed by the CDC (1994). These recommendations generally suggest that a suicide should be handled in such a way as to not glorify the victim or the act. When information is provided to the news media, it should be given in an accurate and efficient manner. Further recommendations are made for how a spokesperson can best cooperate with and provide accurate, but responsible information to the news media. For example, it is suggested that "no comment" or a general refusal to speak with the media is often not a useful response for the public official to make. The guidelines acknowledge the appropriate role of the media, and that media coverage of a suicide does not necessarily create an automatic danger for contagion; it is the way in which such information is portrayed that matters. Therefore, uncooperative responses sometimes create an adversarial relationship with the media that does not necessarily prevent further suicides and potentially misses the positive opportunity to influence and shape the information that is made known to the public. When the media consults professionals, time should be taken to explain the scientific basis for the concerns about suicide contagion and assist the media personnel in finding ways of reporting the information to avoid such risks.

The CDC recommendations further suggest several ways in which the media can report a suicide to thwart suicide contagion.

First, the suicide event should not be explained as the result of one single precipitating factor but as the result of many events. Second, sensationalizing the suicide by ongoing and excessive reporting of the suicide maintains a preoccupation with suicide in at-risk individuals. Sensationalism also occurs through the inclusion of detailed reports of the morbid facts including photographs and videos of such things as the funeral or the site of the suicide. Excessive details on the method used by the individual should also be avoided. Third, the suicide should not be portrayed as a successful means to an end or a viable option for uncomfortable circumstances (e.g., reporting a suicide as a way of "getting back" at strict parents or as a result of a breakup with a boyfriend or girlfriend). Reports of public expressions of grief (e.g., public eulogies, flags flown at half-mast, or remembrance pages in a yearbook) should be minimized so as not to glorify the deceased person. Glorification can also be avoided by providing a balanced account of the deceased person's positive qualities as well as the problematic characteristics that are associated with the suicidal behavior (CDC, 1994).

School-Based Postvention

The potential role of schools in youth suicide prevention has been argued for decades. Indeed, Freud and the members of the Vienna Psychoanalytic Society discussed the pivotal role that educational systems can play to prevent and intervene in youthful suicidal behavior (Berman, 1986a). In a more contemporary sense, the call for school-based prevention programming has grown since the late 1970s, when dramatic rises in adolescent suicide rates brought increased attention to the issue. Over recent years the idea of school-based suicide prevention has been hotly debated. As discussed by Berman and Jobes (1991), the initial explosion of school-based suicide prevention programs over the past decades may be said to reflect more our humanitarian spirit than a reasoned approach to suicide prevention. The initial flurry of programs was followed by call for more research and a more methodological approach to school-based programs. One controversial study by Shaffer, Garland, Gould, Fisher, and Trautman (1990), which indicated the possibility of negative effects of such programs for at-risk suicidal youth, caused many in the field to pause and reconsider otherwise well-intended school-based initiatives. Further reflection among leaders in the field as well as ongoing empirical work has led to a general consensus that schools can play an appropriate and important role in youth suicide prevention and postvention (Berman & Jobes, 1991; CDC, 1991; Celotta, 1995; Kalafat & Underwood, 1989; Lamb & Dunne-Maxim; Mauk et al., 1994). In recent years, more measured approaches to school-based programs have been developed which embrace the spirit of CDC guidelines and perspectives gained from experience and research.

The Suicide Prevention Project (SPP), developed by Lamb and Dunne-Maxim (1987), represents one thoughtful approach to school-based postvention programming. Central to the SPP model is the importance of postvention policy and structuring a *process* for successful suicide postvention. The guiding principles of this model emphasize the following: (1) the suicide should not be dramatized or glamorized, (2) doing nothing can be as dangerous as doing too much, and (3) students cannot be helped until faculty are helped. Further suggestions are made on the development of policy pertaining to dealing with school survivors, contact with the victim's parents, and interactions with the news media (Lamb & Dunne-Maxim, 1987). With regard to the postvention process, these authors believe that it is best to engage an expert consultant to help facilitate a school's suicide postvention plan. Phase one of the process of postvention in this model involves meetings facilitated by the consultant with administrators and faculty. These meetings involve a working-through of feelings, issues, specific decisions, and the imparting of factual information about suicide and suicide prevention. In phase two of the model, faculty and staff help the students with their grief and facilitate appropriate referrals for those who appear to be most at risk. This can be facilitated by faculty-led discussion groups, drop-in hours for students to talk to staff and faculty, and a general message that faculty and staff are available to help and provide support.

Another approach has been developed by Kalafat and Underwood (1989). Similar to the SPP model, this approach emphasizes the importance of identifying a list of students who were particularly close to the adolescent so that these individuals can meet with the school psychologist at a selected time. It is further recommended that students be allowed to leave class if they are in need of emotional support regarding the suicide. In addition, specific sites throughout the school are set up so that students may see a mental health professional either individually or in a group setting. Kalafat and Underwood also provide recommendations for how the school should respond to the media following suggestions of the CDC. The model emphasizes the importance of using a single spokesperson who meets with the media as quickly as possible to provide a written, factual, nonsensational statement pertaining to the death and the school's response to the crisis.

SUMMARY AND CONCLUSIONS

Suicide usually creates tragic circumstances for those left behind—the survivors of a loved one's suicide. However, it is promising to note that after centuries of stigmatization, shame, and devastation linked to surviving suicide, recent developments of the last 20 years have created an important evolution of thinking about suicide survivorship. Indeed, spurred on by a courageous group of ground-breaking survivors and leading suicidologists, we have witnessed the extraordinary evolution of contemporary suicide postvention. Along with our evolving understanding, there are now whole new avenues for personal support and healing after a suicide. Survivors are making their presence known to other survivors in the bond created by their shared tragedy and therein finding strength, support, and the courage to go on. Moreover, survivors are making their presence know to nonsurvivors as well. In recent years we have seen the astonishing power of survivor advocacy for mobilizing the media, politicians, and professionals alike to further improve our efforts to educate, study, and prevent suicide.

In many ways, increased attention to the plight of survivors of suicide has sparked a flurry of research into suicide bereavement and suicide contagion/imitation effects. In turn, this research has increased public and professional awareness and has spurred work in postvention. Our increasing knowledge about postvention now helps shape postsuicide responses to prevent further suicides and speed healing of those left behind.

It is encouraging to note that modern-day survivors of suicide are increasingly able to step out of the shadows of shame and guilt to claim the healing and respect they have always deserved but have rarely received throughout history. Given this legacy, it is even more poignant to note that survivors of suicide are now helping to shape the nation's contemporary suicide prevention agenda. In the wake of suicide, there is the reality of personal loss beyond comprehension, but there is also the promise of courage, support, and healing insights that are helping to advance ongoing efforts to understand and prevent future suicides and the suffering that almost always follows these tragic deaths.

FURTHER READING

Dunne, E. J., McIntosh, J. L., & Dunne-Maxim, K. (Eds.). (1987). *Suicide and its aftermath: Understanding and counseling the survivors* (pp. 245–260). New York: Norton. A good overview of multiple issues related the impact of suicide on survivors. Several chapters are very relevant to survivors, including chapters by Colt on the history of the suicide survivor, Dunne on the needs of suicide survivors in therapy, and Lamb and Dunne-Maxim on postvention in schools.

Jobes, D. A., Berman, A. L., O'Carroll, P. W., Eastgard, S., & Knickmeyer, S. (1996). The Kurt Cobain suicide crisis. *Suicide and Life-Threatening Behavior, 26,* 260–271. A recent study of using modern statistical techniques to analyze data on the "Werther effect." Good for those interested in the Werther effect, the effect of suicide in the media, or interested in the suicide of Kurt Cobain

Kalafat, J., & Underwood, M. (1989). Responding to at-risk students' attempts and completions. In J. Kalafat & M. Underwood (Eds.), *LIFELINES: A school based adolescent suicide response pro-*

gram (pp. 3–19). Dubuque, IA: Kendall/Hunt. An excellent examination of school-based prevention programs.

Litman, R. E. (1996). Sigmund Freud on suicide. In J. T. Maltsberger & M. J. Goldblatt (Eds.), *Essential papers on suicide. Essential papers in psychoanalysis* (pp. 200–220). New York: New York University Press. An eloquent analysis of the Freudian perspective and suicide.

McIntosh, J. L. (1993). Control group studies of suicide survivors: A review and critique. *Suicide and Life-Threatening Behavior, 23,* 146–161. A thorough review of some of the best research on bereavement by suicide and grief.

Tanney, B. (1995). After a suicide: A helper's handbook. In B. L. Mishara (Ed.), *The impact of suicide.* New York: Springer. A practical guide to assisting those professionals who become suicide survivors.

References

Abbar, M., Amadeo, S., Malafosse, A., et al. (1992). An association study between suicidal behavior and tryptophan hydroxylase markers. *Clinical Pharmacology, 15*(1), 299.

Abbar, M., Courtet, P., Amadeo, S., et al. (1995). Suicidal behaviors and the tryptophan hydroxylase gene and suicidality. *Archives of General Psychiatry, 52*, 846–849.

Abel, E. L., & Zeidenberg, P. (1985). Age, alcohol, and violent death: A post-mortem Study. *Journal of the Study of Alcohol, 46*, 228–231.

Åber-Wistedt, A., Wistedt, B., & Bertilsson, L. (1985). Higher CSF levels of HVA and 5-HIAA in delusional compared to nondelusional depression. *Archives of General Psychiatry, 42*, 925–926.

Abram, H. S., Moore, G. L., & Westervelt, F. B. (1971). Suicidal behavior in chronic dialysis patients. *American Journal of Psychiatry, 127*, 1199–1204.

Achté, K. A., & Lönnqvist, J. (1975). Suicide in Finnish culture. In N. L. Farberow (Ed.), *Suicide in different cultures*. Baltimore: University Park Press.

Adam, K. S. (1990). Environmental Psychosocial and Psychoanalytic Aspects of Suicidal Behavior. In S. J. Blumenthal & D. J. Kupfer (Eds.), *Suicide over the life-cycle*. Washington, DC: American Psychiatric Press.

Adam, K. S., Bouckoms, A., & Streiner, D. (1982). Parental loss and family stability in attempted suicide. *Archives of General Psychiatry, 39*, 1081–1085.

Adam, K. S., Sheldon-Keller, A. E., & West, M. (1996). Attachment organization and history of suicidal behavior in clinical adolescents. *Journal of Consulting and Clinical Psychology, 64*, 264–272.

Addington, D. E., & Addington, J. M. (1992). Attempted suicide and depression in schizophrenia. *Acta Psychiatrica Scandinavica, 85*, 288–291.

Addy, C. L. (1992). Statistical concepts of prediction. In R. W. Maris, A. L. Berman, J. T. Maltsberger, & R. I. Yufit (Eds.), *Assessment and prediction of suicide*. New York: Guilford Press.

Adelson, L. (1974). *The pathology of homicide*.

Ägren, H. (1983). Life at risk. *Psychiatric Development, 1*, 87–103.

Ägren, H., & Terenins, L. (1985). Hallucinations in patients with major depression: Interactions between CSF monoaminergic and endophinergic indices. *Journal of Affective Disorders, 9*, 25–34.

Ahlburg, D., & Schapiro, O. (1984). Socio-economic ramifications of changing cohort size: An analysis of U.S. postwar suicide rates by age and sex. *Demography, 21*, 97–105.

Allebeck, P., & Bolund, C. (1991). Suicides and suicide attempts in cancer patients. *Psychological Medicine, 21*, 979–984.

Allebeck, P., Allgulander, C., & Fisher, L. D. (1988). Predictors of completed suicide in a cohort of 50,465 young men. *British Medical Journal, 297*, 176–178.

Allebeck, P., Bolund, C., & Ringback, G. (1989). Increased suicide rate in cancer patients: A cohort study based on the Swedish cancer-environment register. *Journal of Clinical Epidemiology, 42,* 611–616.

Allen, J., & Haccoun, D. (1976). Sex differences in emotionality: A multidimensional approach. *Human Relations, 8,* 711–722.

Allen, N. H. (1983). Homicide followed by suicide: Los Angeles, 1970–1979. *Suicide and Life-Threatening Behavior, 9,* 15–23.

Allgulander, C. (1994). Suicide and mortality patterns in anxiety neurosis and depressive neurosis. *Archives of General Psychiatry, 51,* 708–712.

Allgulander, C., & Lavori, P. W. (1991). Excess mortality among 3302 patients with "pure" anxiety neurosis. *Archives of General Psychiatry, 48,* 599–602.

Allgulander, C., Allebeck, P., Przybeck, T. R., & Rice, J. (1992). Risk of suicide by psychiatric diagnosis in Stockholm County. *European Archives of Psychiatry, 241,* 323–326.

Alston, M. (1986). Occupation and suicide among women. *Issues in Mental Health Nursing, 8,* 109–119.

Altman, H., Sletten, I. W., Eaton, M. E., & Ulett, G. A. (1971). Demographic and mentalstatus profiles. Patients with homicidal, assaultive, suicidal, persecutory and homosexual ideation. The Missouri Automated Standard System of Psychiatry. *Psychiatric Quarterly, 45,* 57–64.

Alvarez, A. (1970). *The savage god.* New York: Random House.

Alvarez, A. (1975). Literature in the nineteenth and twentieth centuries. In S. Perlin (Ed.), *A handbook for the study of suicide.* New York: Oxford University Press.

Amador, X. F., Friedman, J. H., Kasapis, C., Yale, S. A., Flaum, M., & Gorman, J. M. (1996). Suicidal behavior in schizophrenia and its relationship to awareness of illness. *American Journal of Psychiatry, 153,* 1185–1188.

Amchin, J., Wettstein, R. M., & Roth, L. H. (1990). Suicide, ethics, and the law. In S. J. Blumenthal & D. J. Kupfer (Eds.), *Suicide over the life-cycle.* Washington, DC: American Psychiatric Press.

American Association of Suicidology. (1996). *Directory of suicide survivor support groups.* Washington, DC: Author.

American Heritage College Dictionary. (1993). Boston: Houghton Mifflin.

American Psychiatric Association. (1987). *Diagonostic and statistical manual of mental disorders* (3rd ed., rev.). Washington, DC: Author.

American Psychiatric Association. (1994). *Diagnostic and statistical manual of mental disorders* (4th ed.). Washington, DC: Author.

Andreasen, N. C. (1987). Creativity and mental illness: Prevalence rates in writers and their first degree relatives. *American Journal of Psychiatry, 144,* 1288–1292.

Andreasen, N. C., & Black, D. W. (1995). *Introductory textbook of psychiatry.* Washington, DC: American Psychiatric Press.

Andreasen, N. C., & Noyes, R. (1975). Suicide attempted by self-immolation. *American Journal of Psychiatry, 132,* 554–556.

Andrews, J. A, & Lewinsohn, P. M. (1992). Suicidal attempts among older adolescents: prevalence and co-occurrence with psychiatric disorders. *Journal of the American Academy of Child and Adolescent Psychiatry, 31,* 655–662.

Anthony, J. C., & Petronis, K. R. (1991). Panic attacks and suicide attempts. *Archives of General Psychiatry, 48,* 11–14.

Appel, C. P., & Wrobleski, A. (1987). Self-help and support groups: Mutual aid for survivors. In E. J. Dunne, J. L. McIntosh, & K. Dunne-Maxim (Eds.), *Suicide and its aftermath: Understanding and counseling the survivors.* New York: Norton.

Appleby, L. (1994). Panic and suicidal behavior. *British Journal of Psychiatry, 164,* 719–721.

Appleby, L., Mortensen, P. B., & Faragher, E. B. (1998). Suicide and other causes of mortality after post-partum psychiatric admission. *British Journal of Psychiatry, 173,* 209–211.

Apter, A., Gothelf, D., Orbach, I., & Weizman, R. (1995). Correlation of suicide and violent behavior in different diagnostic categories in hospitalized adolescent patients. *Journal of the American Academy of Child and Adolescent Psychiatry, 34,* 912–918.

Apter, A., Kotler, M., Sevy, S., Plutchik, Brown, S., Foster, H., Hillbrand, M., R., Korn, M., & van Praag, H. M. (1991). Correlates of risk of suicide in violent and nonviolent psychiatric patients. *American Journal of Psychiatry, 148,* 853–887.

Apter, A., Plutchik, R., Sevy, S., Korn, M., & van Praag, H. M. (1989). Defense mechanisms in risk of suicide and risk of violence. *American Journal of Psychiatry, 146,* 1027–1031.

Apter, A., van Praag, H. M., Plutchik, R., Sevy, S., Korn, M., & Brown S. (1990). Interrelationships among anxiety, aggression, impulsivity and mood.: A. serontonergically linked cluster? *Psychiatry Research, 148,* 191–199.

Apter, M. J. (1992). *The dangerous edge: The psychology of excitement.* New York: Free Press.

Arbeit, S. A., & Blatt, S. J. (1973). Differentiation of simulated and genuine suicide notes. *Psychological Reports, 33,* 283–297.

Arieli, A., Gilat, I., & Aychek, S. (1996). Suicide among Ethiopian Jews: A survey conducted by means of a psychological autopsy. *Journal of Nervous and Mental Disease, 184,* 317–319.

Aries, P. (1962). *Centuries of childhood.* New York: Vintage Press.

Arnetz, B. B., Horte, L. G., Hedberg, A., Theorell T., Allander, E., & Maker, H. (1987). Suicide patterns among physicians related to other academics as well as to the general population. *Acta Psychiatrica Scandinavia, 75,* 139–143.

Asarnow, J. R. (1992). Suicidal ideation and attempts during middle childhood: Associations with perceived family stress and depression among child psychiatric inpatients. *Journal of Clinical Child Psychology, 21,* 35–40.

Åsberg, M. (1980). Biochemical abnormalities in depressive illness. In G. Curzon (Ed.), *The biochemistry of psychiatric disturbance.* New York: Wiley.

Åsberg, M. (1986). Biochemical aspects of suicide. *Clinical Neuropharmacology, 9*(4), 374–376.

Åsberg, M., Bertilsson, L., & Martensson, B. (1984). CSF monoamine: metabolites, depression, and suicide. In E. Usdin et al. (Eds.), *Frontiers in biochemical and pharmacological research in depression.* New York: Raven Press.

Åsberg, M., Cronholm, B., Sjoquist, F., et al. (1971). Relationship between plasma level and therapeutic effect of nortriptyline. *British Medical Journal, 7,* 331–334.

Åsberg, M., Eriksson, B., Matensson, B., et al. (1986a). Therapeutic effects of serontonin uptake inhibitors in depression. *Journal of Clinical Psychiatry, 40*(4), 3–35.

Åsberg, M., Nordstrom, P., & Träskman-Bendz, L. (1986b). Biological factors in suicide. In A. Roy (Ed.), *Suicide.* Baltimore: Williams & Wilkins.

Åsberg, M., Nordstrom, P., & Träskman-Bendz, L. (1990). Cerebrospinal fluid studies in suicide: An overview. *Annals of the New York Academy of Sciences, 487,* 243–255.

Åsberg, M., Träskman, L., & Thorén, P. (1976). 5-HIAA in the cerebrospinal fluid: A biochemical suicide predictor? *Archives of General Psychiatry, 136,* 559–562.

Åsberg, M., Thorén, P., & Träskman, L. (1976). Serotonin depression—biochemical subgroup within the affective disorders? *Science, 191,* 478–480.

Asch, S. (1955, November). Opinions and social pressure. *Scientific American,* pp. 31–35.

Asnis, G. M., Friedman, T. A., Sanderson, W. C., Kaplan, M. L., van Praag, H. M., & Harkavy-Friedman, J. M. (1993). Suicidal behaviors in adult psychiatric outpatients, I: Description and prevalence. *American Journal of Psychiatry, 150,* 108–112.

Atkinson, J. M. (1978). *Discovering suicide: Studies in the social organization of sudden death.* London: Macmillan.

Avery, D., & Winokur G. (1977). The efficacy of electroconvulsive therapy and antidepressants in depression. *Biological Psychiatry, 12,* 507–523.

Avery, D., & Winokur, G. (1978). Suicide, attempted suicide, and relapse rates in depression. *Archives of General Psychiatry, 35,* 749–753.

Axelsson, R., & Lagerkvist-Briggs, M. (1992). Factors predicting suicide in psychotic patients. *European Archives of Psychiatry and Clinical Neurosciences, 241,* 259–266.

Babbie, E. (1996). *The practice of social research.* Belmont, CA: Wadsworth.

Baechler, J. (1975). *Suicides.* New York: Basic Books.

Baldessarini, R. J., & Jamison, K. R. (1999). Summary and conclusions: Effects of medical interventions in suicidal behavior. *Journal of Clinical Psychiatry, 60*(suppl. 2), 117–122.

Bancroft, J., Hawton, K., Simkin, S., Kingston, B., Cumming, C., & Whitwell, D. (1979). The reasons people give for taking overdoses: A further inquiry. *British Journal of Medical Psychology, 52,* 353–365.

Banki, C., & Arato, M. (1983). Amine metabolites and neuroendocrine responses related to depression and suicide. *Journal of Affective Disorders, 5*, 223–232.

Barnes, F. C., & Helson, R. A. (1974). An empirical study of gunpowder residue patterns. *Journal of Forensic Sciences, 19*, 448–462.

Barraclough, B. (1972). Suicide prevention, recurrent affective disorder, and lithium. *British Journal of Psychiatry, 121*, 391–392.

Barraclough, B., & Hughes, J. (1987). *Suicide: Clinical and epidemiological studies.* London: Croom Helm.

Barraclough, B., & Shepard, D. M. (1994). A necessary neologism: The origin and uses of suicide. *Suicide and Life-Threatening Behavior, 24*, 113–126.

Barraclough, B., Bunch, J., Nelson, B., & Sainsbury, P. (1974). A hundred cases of suicide. *British Journal of Psychiatry, 125*, 355–373.

Barraclough, B., Shepherd, D., & Jennings, C. (1977). Do newspaper reports of coroners' inquest incite people to commit suicide? *British Journal of Psychiatry, 131*, 528–532.

Bartels, S. J., Drake, R. E., & McHugo, G. J. (1992). Alcohol abuse, depression, and suicidal behavior in schizophrenia. *American Journal of Psychiatry, 149*, 394–395.

Battin, M. P. (1991). *Crisis, 12*, 73–79.

Battin, M. P. (1996). *The death debate: Ethical issue in suicide.* Upper Saddle River, NJ: Prentice Hall.

Battin, M. P., & Maris, R. W. (1983). *Suicide and ethics.* New York: Human Sciences Press.

Baumrind, D. (1987). A developmental perspective on adolescent risk-taking in contemporary America. In C. E. Irwin (Ed.), *Adolescent social behavior and health: New directions for child development.* San Francisco: Jossey-Bass.

Beardslee, W., Bemporad, J., Keller, M., & Klerman, G. (1983). Children of parents with major affective disorder: A review. *American Journal of Psychiatry, 140*, 825–832.

Beasley, C. M., Dornself, B. E., Bosomworth, J. C., et al. (1991). Fluoxetine and suicide: A meta-analysis of controlled trials of treatment for depression. *British Medical Journal, 303*, 685–692.

Beasley, C. M., Potvin, J., Masica, D. N., et al. (1992). Fluoxetine: No assocation with suicidality in obsessive–compulsive disorder. *Journal of Affective Disorder, 24*, 1–10.

Beautrais, A. L., Joyce, P. R., Mulder, R. T., Fergusson, D. M., Deavoll, B. J., & Nightingale, S. K. (1996). Prevalence and comorbidity of mental disorders in persons making serious suicide attempts: A case-control study. *American Journal of Psychiatry, 153*, 1009–1014.

Beck, A. T. (1986). Hopelessness as a predictor of eventual suicide. *Annals of the New York Academy of Sciences, 487*, 90–96.

Beck, A. T. (1990). Suicide Intent Scale. In S. J. Blumenthal & D. J. Kupfer (Eds.), *Suicide over the life cycle.* Washington, DC: American Psychiatric Press.

Beck, A. T., Brown, G. K., Steer, R. A., Dahlsgaard, K. K., & Grisham, J. R. (1999). Suicide ideation at its worst point: A predictor of eventual suicide in psychiatric outpatients. *Suicide and Life-Threatening Behavior, 29*, 1–9.

Beck, A. T., Davis, J. H., Frederick, C. J., Perlin, S., Pokorny, A. D., Schulman, R. E., Seiden, R. H., & Wittlin, B. J. (1973). Classification and nomenclature. In H. L. P. Resnik & B. C. Hathorne (Eds.), *Suicide prevention in the seventies.* Washington, DC: U.S. Government Printing Office.

Beck, A. T., Kovacs, M., & Weisman, A. (1979). Assessment of suicidal intention: The Scale for Suicidal Ideation. *Journal of Consulting and Clinical Psychology, 47*, 343–352.

Beck, A. T., & Steer, R. A. (1989). Clinical predictors of eventual suicide. *Journal of Affective Disorders, 17*, 203–209.

Beck, A. T., Steer, R. A., & Brown. G. (1993). Dysfunctional attitudes and suicidal ideation in psychiatric outpatients. *Suicide and Life-Threatening Behavior, 23*, 11–20.

Beck, A. T., Steer, R. A., Kovacs, M., & Garrison, B. (1985). Hopelessness and eventual suicide: A 10-year prospective study of patients hospitalized with suicidal ideation. *American Journal of Psychiatry, 142*, 559–563.

Beck, A. T., Steer, R. A., Sanderson, W. C., & Skeie, T. M. (1991). Panic disorder and suicidal ideation and behavior: Discrepant findings in psychiatric outpatients. *American Journal of Psychiatry, 148*, 1991–1995.

Beck, A. T., Weisman, A., Lester, D., & Trexler, L. (1974). The measurement of pessimism: The Hopelessness Scale. *Journal of Consulting and Clinical Psychology, 42,* 861–865.

Beck, R. W., Morris, J., & Lester, D. (1974). Suicide notes and risk of future suicide. *Journal of the American Medical Association, 228,* 495–496.

Becker, B. J. (1986). Influence again: An examination of gender differences in social influence. In J. S. Hyde & M. C. Linn (Eds.), *The psychology of gender: Advances through metaanalysis.* Baltimore: John Hopkins University Press.

Becker, E. (1973). *The denial of death.* New York: Macmillan.

Bedeian, A. (1982). Suicide and occupation: A review. *Journal of Vocational Behavior, 21,* 206–223.

Bell, A. P., & Weinberg, M. S. (1978). *Homosexualities.* New York: Simon & Schuster.

Benensohn, H., & Resnick, H. L. R. (1973). Guidelines for "suicide proofing" a psychiatric unit. *American Journal of Psychotherapy, 26,* 204–211.

Berchick, R. J., & Wright, F. D. (1992). Guidelines for handling the suicidal patient: A cognitive perspective. In B. Bongar (Ed.), *Suicide: Guidelines for assessment, management, and treatment.* New York: Oxford University Press.

Berglund, M. (1986). Suicide in male alcoholics with peptic ulcers. *Alcoholism, 10,* 631–634.

Berglund, M., & Nilsson, K. Mortality in severe depression. *Acta Psychiatrica Scandinavica, 76,* 372–380.

Bergman, B., & Brismar, B. (1994). Hormone levels and personality traits in abusive and suicidal male alcoholoics. *Alcoholism: Clinical and Experimental Research, 18,* 31–316.

Berkowitz, L. (1962). *Aggression: A social–psychological analysis.* New York: McGraw-Hill.

Berman, A. L. (1978, April). *Sex roles and attribution of suicidality.* Paper presented at the 11th annual meeting of the American Association of Suicidology, New Orleans.

Berman, A. L. (1979). Dyadic death: Murder-suicide. *Suicide and Life-Threatening Behavior, 9,* 15–23.

Berman, A. L. (1986a). Notes on turning 18 (and 75): A critical look at our adolescence. *Suicide and Life-Threatening Behavior, 16,* 1–12.

Berman, A. L. (1986b, November). *Interventions in the media and entertainment sectors to prevent suicide.* Paper presented at the USDHHS Task Force Conference on Strategies for the Prevention of Youth Suicide, Bethesda, MD.

Berman, A. L. (1987). Suicide and the mass media. In R. Yufit (Ed.), *Combined proceedings of the 20th annual meeting of the American Association of Suicidology and the 19th International Congress of the International Association of Suicide Prevention.* Denver, CO: American Association of Suicidology.

Berman A. L. (1988). Fictional depiction of suicide in television films and imitation effects. *American Journal of Psychiatry, 145,* 982–986.

Berman, A. L. (1992). Five potential suicide cases. In R. W. Maris, A. L. Berman, J. T. Maltsberger, & R. I. Yufit (Eds.), *Assessment and prediction of suicide.* New York: Guilford Press.

Berman, A. L. (1993). Forensic suicidology and the psychological autopsy. In A. A. Leenaars, A. L. Berman, P. Cantor, R. L. Litman, & R. W. Maris (Eds.), *Suicidology: Essays in honor of Edwin S. Shneidman.* Northvale, NJ: Jason Aronson.

Berman, A. L. (1996). Dyadic death: A typology. *Suicide and Life-Threatening Behavior, 26,* 342–350.

Berman, A. L., & Jobes, D. A. (1991). *Adolescent suicide: Assessment and intervention.* Washington, DC: American Psychological Association.

Berman, A. L., & Jobes, D. A. (1995). Suicide prevention in adolescents (age 12–18). Suicide prevention: Toward the year 2000. In M. M. Silverman, & R. W. Maris (Eds.), *Suicide and Life-Threatenting Behavior, 25,* 143–154.

Berman, A. L., & Samuel, L. (1990). Suicide among multiple sclerosis patients. *Proceedings of the 23rd Annual Meeting of the American Association of Suicidology, USA* (pp. 267–268). Washington, DC: American Association of Suicidology.

Berman, A. L., Jacobs, D. G., & Jobes, D. A. (1993). Case consultation: Tillie. *Suicide and Life-Threatening Behavior, 23,* 268–272.

Berman, A. L., Leenaars, A. A., McIntosh, J., & Richman, J. (1992). Case consultation: Mary Catherine. *Suicide and Life-Threatening Behavior, 22,* 142–149.

Berman, S. (1994, June). *STDs and adolescence: Synergy between behavior and vulnerability.* Paper presented at the national conference on Risk-Taking among Children and Adolescents, Arlington, VA.

Bernstein, R. M., Feldberg, C., & Brown, R. (1991). After-hours coverage in psychology training clinics. *Professional Psychology: Research and Practice, 20,* 204–208.

Beskow, J., Runeson, B., & Asgard, U. (1990). Psychological autopsies: Methods and ethics. *Suicide and Life-Threatening Behavior, 20,* 307–323.

Bettelheim, B. (1943). Individual and mass behavior in extreme situations. *Journal of Abnormal Psychology, 38,* 417–452.

Black, D. W., & Winokur, G. (1990). Suicide and psychiatric diagnosis. In S. J. Blumenthal & D. J. Kupfer (Eds.), *Suicide over the life-cycle.* Washington, DC: American Psychiatric Press.

Black, D. W., Winokur, G., & Nasrallah, A. (1987). Suicide in subtypes of major affective disorder: A comparison with general population suicide mortality. *Archives of General Psychiatry, 44,* 878–880.

Black, H. C. (1979). *Black's law dictionary.* St. Paul, MN: West.

Black, S. T. (1989). *Gender differences in the content of genuine and simulated suicide notes.* Paper presented at the annual meeting of the American Association of Suicidology, Denver, CO.

Blair-West, G. W., Mellsop, G. W., & Eyeson-Annan, M. L. (1997). Down-rating lifetime suicide risk in major depression. *Acta Psychiatrica Scandinavica, 95,* 259–263.

Blalock, H. M., Jr. (1979). *Social statistics.* New York: McGraw-Hill.

Blalock, H. M., Jr. (1985). *Causal models in the social sciences.* New York: Aldine.

Blanchard, B. C., & Blanchard, R. J. (1984). Affect and aggression: An animal model applied to human behavior. In R.J. Blanchard & D.C. Blanchard (Eds.), *Advances in the study of aggression* (vol. 1). New York: Academic Press.

Bland, R. C., Newman, S. C., & Orn, H. (1997). Help-seeking for psychiatric disorders. *Canadian Journal of Psychiatry, 42,* 935–942.

Bland, R. C., Newman, S. C., Orn, H., & Stebelsky, G. (1993). Epidemiology of pathological gambling in Edmonton. *Canadian Journal of Psychiatry, 38*(2), 108–112.

Blau, P. M. (1977). *Inequality and heterogeneity.* New York: Free Press.

Blau, T. H. (1980). The lure of the deep. In N. L. Farberow (Ed.), *The many faces of suicide: Indirect self-destructive behavior.* New York: McGraw Hill.

Bloom, V. (1967). An analysis of suicide at a training center. *American Journal of Psychotherapy, 123*(8), 918–925.

Blumenthal, S. J. (1990). An overview and synopsis of risk factors, assessment, and treatment of suicidal patients over the life cycle. In S. J. Blumenthal & D. J. Kupfer (Eds.), *Suicide over the life cycle: Risk factors, assessment, and treatment of suicidal patients.* Washington, DC: American Psychiatric Press.

Blumenthal, S. J., & Kupfer, D. J. (1986). Generalizable treatment strategies for suicidal behavior. *Annals of the New York Academy of Sciences, 487,* 327–340.

Blumenthal, S. J., & Kupfer, D. J. (1988). Overview of early detection and treatment strategies for suicidal behavior in young people. *Journal of Youth and Adolescence, 17,* 1–23.

Blumenthal, S. J., & Kupfer, D. J. (Eds.). (1990). *Suicide over the life cycle: Risk factors, assessment, and treatment of suicidal patients.* Washington, DC: American Psychiatric Press.

Blumer, H. (1969). *Symbolic interactionism.* Englewood Cliffs, NJ: Prentice Hall.

Bohannan, P. (Ed.). (1960). *African homicide and suicide.* Princeton, NJ: Princeton University Press.

Boland, C. (1985a). Suicide and cancer: I. Demographic and social characteristics of cancer patients who committed suicide in Sweden 1973–1976. *Journal of Psychosocial Oncology, 3,* 17–30.

Boland, C. (1985b). Suicide and cancer: II. Medical and care factors in suicides by cancer patients in Sweden, 1973–1976. *Journal of Psychosocial Oncology, 3,* 31–52.

Bollen, K. A., & Phillips, D. P. (1982). Imitative suicides: A national study of the effects of television news stories. *American Sociological Review, 47,* 802–809.

Bonanno, G. A., Keltner, D. A., Holen, A., & Horowitz, M. J. (1995). When avoiding unpleasant emotions might not be such a bad thing: Verbal-autonomic response dissociation and midlife conjugal bereavement. *Journal of Personality and Social Psychology, 69,* 975–989.

Bongar, B. (1991). *The suicidal patient: Clinical and legal standards of care.* Washington, DC: American Psychological Association.

Bongar, B. (Ed.). (1992). *Suicide: Guidelines for assessment, management, and treatment.* New York: Oxford University Press.

Bongar, B., Berman, A. L., Maris, R. W., Silverman, M. M., Harris, E. A., & Packman, W. (Eds.). (1998). *Risk management with suicidal patients.* New York: Guilford Press.

Bonner, R., & Rich, A. (1987). Toward a predictive model of suicidal ideation and behavior. Some preliminary data in college students. *Suicide and Life-Threatening Behavior, 17,* 50–63.

Booth, R. E., & Zhang, Y. (1996). Severe aggression and related conduct problems among runaway and homeless adolescents. *Psychiatric Services, 47,* 75–80.

Borg, S. E., & Stahl, M. (1982). A prospective study of suicides and controls among psychiatric patients. *Acta Psychiatrica Scandinavica, 65,* 221–232.

Botsis, A. J., Plutchik, R., Kotler, M., & van Praag, M. H. (1995). Parental loss and family violence as correlates of suicide and violence risk. *Suicide and Life Threatening Behavior, 25,* 253–260.

Bowen. (1982). Hanging—A review. *Forensic Science International, 20,* 247–248.

Bowlby, J. (1973). *Separation.* New York: Basic Books.

Bowlby, J. (1980). *Attachment and loss: Vol. 3. Loss: Sadness and depression.* New York: Basic Books.

Boxer, P., Burnett, C., & Swanson, N. (1995). Suicide and occupation: A review of the literature. *Journal of Occupational and Environmental Medicine, 37,* 442–452.

Boyd, J. Y. (1983). The increasing rate of suicide by firearms. *New England Journal of Medicine, 308,* 872–874.

Boyd, J. Y., & Moscicki, E. K. (1986). Firearms and youth suicide. *American Journal of Public Health, 308,* 872–874.

Boyer, B. (1975). Meanings of a bizarre suicidal attempt by an adolescent. *Adolescent Psychiatry, 4,* 371–381.

Boyer, R., Lesage, A. D., Grunberg, F., Moisette, R., Vanier, C., Butear-Menard, C., & Loyer, M. (1992). Mental illness and suicide. In D. Lester (Ed.), *Suicide '92.* Denver: American Association of Suicidology.

Brandt, R. B. (1975). The morality and rationality of suicide. In S. Perlin (Ed.), *A handbook for the study of suicide.* New York: Oxford University Press.

Braunig, P., Rao, M. L., & Fimmers, R. (1989). Blood serotonin levels in suicidal schizopherenic patients. *Acta Psychiatrica Scandinavica, 79,* 206–209.

Breault, K. D. (1986). Suicide in America: A test of durkheim's theory of religious and family integration, 1933–1980. *American Journal of Sociology, 92,* 628–656.

Breault, K. D. (1988). Beyond the quick and dirty: Reply to Girard. *American Journal of Sociology, 93,* 1479–1486.

Breed, W. (1963). Occupational mobility and suicide among white males. *American Sociological Review, 28,* 179–188.

Breed, W., & Huffine, C. L. (1979). Sex differences in suicide among older white Americans: A role of developmental approach. In C. J. Kaplan (Ed.), *Psychopathology of aging.* New York: Academic Press.

Breier, A., & Astrachan, B. M. (1984). Characterization of schizophrenic patients who commit suicide. *American Journal of Psychiatry, 141,* 206–209.

Breivik, G. (1996). Personality, sensation seeking and risk-taking among Everest climbers. *International Journal of Sport Psychology, 27,* 208–320.

Brent, D. A., Bridge, J., Johnson, B. A., & Connolly, J. (1998). Suicidal behavior runs in families: A controlled family study of adolescent suicide victims. In R. J. Kosky, H.S. Eskkevari, & S. Hadi (Eds.), *Suicide prevention: The global context.* New York: Plenum.

Brent, D. A., Johnson, B. A., Perper, J., & Connolly, J. (1994). Personality disorder, personality traits, impulsive violence, and completed suicide in adolescents. *Journal of the American Academy of Child and Adolescent Psychiatry, 33,* 1080–1086.

Brent, D. A., Johnson, B. A., Perper, J., Connolly, J., Bridge, J., Bartle, S., & Rather, C. (1994). Personality disorder, personality traits, impulsive violence, and completed suicide in adolescents. Journal of the American Academy of Child and Adolescent Psychiatry, 33, 1080–1086.

Brent, D. A., Kalas, R., & Edelbrock, C. (1986). Psychopathology and its relationship to suicidal ideation in childhood and adolescence. *Journal of American Academy of Child Psychiatry, 25,* 666–673.

Brent, D. A., & Kolko, D. J. (1990). The assessment and treatment of children and adolescents at risk for suicide. In S. J. Blumenthal & D. J. Kupfer (Eds.), *Suicide over the life-cycle.* Washington, DC: American Psychiatric Press.

Brent, D. A., & Perper, J. A. (1995). Research in adolescent suicide: Implications for training, service delivery, and public policy. *Suicide and Life-Threatening Behavior, 25,* 222–230.

Brent, D. A., Perper, J. A., & Allman, C. (1987). Alcohol, firearms, and suicide among youth: Temporal trends in Allegheny County, Pennslyvania, 1960–1983. *Journal of the American Medical Association, 257,* 3369–3372.

Brent, D. A., Perper, J. A., Goldstein, C. E., Kolko, D. J., Allan, M. J., Allman, C. J., & Zelenak, J. P. (1988). Risk factors for adolescent suicide: A comparison of adolescent suicide victims with suicidal inpatients. *Archives of General Psychiatry, 45,* 581–588.

Brent, D. A., Perper, J. A., Moritz, G., Allman, C., Friend, A., Roth, C., Schweers, J., Balach, L., & Baugher, M. (1993). Psychiatric risk factors for adolescent suicide: A case-control study. *Journal of the American Academy of Child and Adolescent Psychiatry, 32,* 521–529.

Brent, D. A., Perper, J. A., Moritz, G., Baugher, M., Roth, C., Balach, L., & Schweers, J. (1993). Stressful life events, psychopathology, and adolescent suicide: A case control study. *Suicide and Life-Threatening Behavior, 23,* 179–187.

Brent, D. A., Perper, J. A., Moritz, G., Baugher, M., Schweers, J., & Roth, C. (1994). Suicide in affectively ill adolescents: A case-control study. *Journal of Affective Disorders, 31,* 193–202.

Briere, J., & Runtz, M. (1986). Suicidal thoughts and behaviors in former sexual abuse victims. *Journal of Behavioral Sciences, 18,* 413–423.

Bronisch, T., & Wittchen, H. U. (1994). Suicidal ideation and suicide attempts: Comorbidity with depression, anxiety disorders, and substance abuse disorders. *European Archives of Psychiatry and Clinical Neurosciences, 244,* 93–98.

Brown, G., Ebert, M., Goyer, P., Jimerson, O., Klein, W., Brunner, W., & Goodwin, F. (1982). Aggression, suicide and serotonin relationship to CSF amine metabolites. *American Journal of Psychiatry, 139,* 741–746.

Brown, G., & Goodwin, F. (1986). Human Aggression and Suicide. *Suicide and Life-Threatening Behavior, 16,* 223–243.

Brown, G., Linnoila, M., & Goodwin, F. (1992). Impulsivity, aggression, and associated affects: Relationship to self-destructive behavior and suicide. In R. W. Maris, A. L. Berman, J. T. Maltsberger, & R. Yufit (Eds.), *Assessment and prediction of suicide.* New York: Guilford Press.

Brown, J. H., Henteleff, P., Barakat, S., & Rowe, C. J. (1986). Is it normal for terminally ill patients to desire death? *American Journal of Psychiatry, 143,* 208–211.

Brown, N. O. (1959). *Life against death.* New York: Viking Books.

Brown, R. (1990). Life events and their effect on suicide: The case of physicians. *Advances in Medical Sociology, 1,* 178–188.

Brown, W., & Pisetsky, J. E. (1960). Suicidal behavior in a general hospital. *American Journal of Medicine, 29,* 307–315.

Buchholtz-Hansen, P. E., Wang, A. G., & Danish University Antidepressant Group. (1993). Mortality in major affective disorder: Relationship to subtype of depression. *Acta Psychiatrica Scandinavica, 87,* 329–335.

Buda, M., & Tsuang, M. T. (1990). The epidemiology of suicide: Implications for clinical practice. In S. J. Blumenthal & D. J. Kupfer (Eds.), *Suicide over the Life Cycle* (pp. 17–38). Washington, DC: American Psychiatric Press.

Buie, D. H., & Maltsberger, J. T. (1983). *The practical formulation of suicide risk.* Cambridge, MA: Firefly Press.

Bulik, C. M., Carpenter, L. L., Kupfer, D. J., & Frank, E. (1990). Features associated with suicide attempts in recurrent major depression. *Journal of Affective Disorders, 18,* 29–37.

Bunney, W. E., Jr., & Fawcett, J. A. (1965). Possibility of a biochemical test for suicidal potential. *Archives of General Psychiatry, 13,* 232–239.

Burgess, A. W., & Hazelwood, R. R. (1983). Autoerotic asphyxial deaths and social network response. *American Journal of Orthopsychiatry, 53,* 166–170.

Burnett, C., Boxer, P., & Swanson, N. (1992). *Suicide and occupation: Is there a relationship?* Cincinnati, OH: National Institute for Occupational Safety and Health.

Burnley, I. (1994). Differential spatial aspects of suicide morality in New South Wales and Sydney, 1980–1991. *Australian Journal of Public Health, 18,* 293–304.

Burnley, I. (1995). Socio-economic and spatial differences in morality and means of committing suicide in New South Wales, Australia, 1985–1991. *Social Science and Medicine, 41,* 687–698.

Burr, J., McCall, P., & Powell-Griner, E. (1994). Catholic religion and suicide. *Social Science Quarterly, 75,* 300–318.

Busch, K. A., Clark, D. C., Fawcett, J. A., & Kravitz, H. M. (1993). Clinical features of inpatient suicide. *Psychiatric Annals, 23,* 256–262.

Byrne, D., Kelly, K., & Fisher, W. (1993). Unwanted teenage pregnancies: Incidence, interpretation, and intervention. *Applied and Preventive Psychology, 2,* 101–113.

Caesar, J. (1955). *Alexandrian, African, and Spanish Wars* (A. G. Way, Trans.). [Loeb Classical Library]. Cambridge, MA: Harvard University Press.

Cain, A. C. (Ed.). (1972). *Survivors of suicide.* Springfield, IL: Thomas.

Caine, E. (1978). Two contemporary tragedies: Adolescent suicide/adolescent alcoholism. *National Association of Private Psychiatric Hospitals Journal, 9,* 4–11.

Cairns, R. B., Patterson, G., & Neckerman, H. J. (1988). Suicidal behavior in aggressive adolescents. *Journal of Clinical Child Psychology, 17,* 298–309.

Caldwell, C., & Gottesman, I. I. (1992). Schizophrenia high risk factor for suicide: clues to risk reduction. *Suicide and Life-Threatening Behavior, 22,* 479–493.

Campbell, P. C. (1966). Suicide among cancer patients. *Connecticut Health Bulletin, 80,* 207–212.

Camps, F. E. (Ed.). (1976). *Gradwohl's legal medicine.* Chicago: Yearbook Medical Publications.

Camus, A. (1945). *The myth of Sisyphus.* (J. O'Brien, Trans.). London: Harris Hamilon.

Canetto, S. S. (1992). Gender and suicide in the elderly. *Suicide and Life-Threatening Behavior, 22,* 80–97.

Cantor, C. H., Tyman, R., & Slater, P. J. (1995). A historical survey of police suicide in Queensland, Australia, 1843–1992. *Suicide and Life-Threatening Behavior, 25,* 499–507.

Cantor, C., Hill, M., & McLachlan, E. (1989). Suicide and related behavior from river bridges: A clinical perspective. *British Journal of Psychiatry, 155,* 829–835.

Caplehorn, J. R., Dalton, M. S., Haldar, F., Petrenas, A. M., & Nisbet, J. G. (1996). Methadone maintenance and addicts' risk of fatal heroin overdose. *Substance Use and Misuse, 31,* 177–196.

Capstick, A. (1960). Recognition of emotional disturbance and the prevention of suicide. *British Medical Journal, 1,* 179.

Card, J. J. (1974). Lethality of suicidal methods and suicide risk: Two distant concepts. *Omega, 5,* 37–45.

Carey, G., & Goldman, D. (1997). The genetics of antisocial behavior. D.M. Stoff, J. Breiling & J.D. Maser (Eds.), *Handbook of antisocial behavior.* New York: Wiley.

Carlson, G. A., & Cantwell, D. P. (1982). Suicidal behavior and depression in children and adolescents. *Journal of American Academy of Child Psychiatry, 21,* 361–368.

Carmen, E., Rieker, P. P., & Mills, T. (1984). Victims of violence and psychiatric illness. *American Journal of Psychiatry, 141,* 378–383.

Cassell, E. J. (1979). Reactions to physical illness and hospitalizations. In G. Usdin & J. M. Lewis (Eds.), *Psychiatry in general medical practice.* New York: McGraw-Hill.

Catalano, R., Hawkins, D., Krenz, C., Gilmore, M., Morrison, D., Wells, E., & Abbott, R. (1993). Using research to guide culturally appropriate drug abuse prevention. *Journal of Consulting and Clinical Psychology, 61,* 804–811.

Celotta, B. (1995). The aftermath of suicide: Postvention in a school setting. *Journal of Mental Health Counseling, 17,* 397–412.

Centers for Disease Control. (1988). CDC recommendations for a community plan for the prevention and containment of suicide clusters. *Morbidity and Mortality Weekly Report, 37,* 1–12.

Centers for Disease Control. (1991). Attempted suicide among high school students—United States, 1990. *Morbidity and Mortality Weekly Report, 40,* 633–635.

Centers for Disease Control. (1992). *Youth suicide prevention programs: A resource guide.* Atlanta: Author.

Centers for Disease Control and Prevention. (1994). Suicide contagion and the reporting of suicide: Recommendations from a national workshop. *Morbidity and Mortality Weekly Report, 42,* 13–18.

Centers for Disease Control and Prevention. (1996, April 21). *Morbidity and Mortality Weekly Report, 44*(15) 289–291.

Centers for Disease Control and Prevention. (1997). *HIV/AIDS Surveillance Report, 9,* 1–37.

Centers for Disease Control and Prevention. (1998). *HIV/AIDS Surveillance reports.* Atlanta: Author.

Chandy, J. M., Blum, R. W., & Resnick, M. D. (1996). Female adolescents with a history of sexual abuse. *Journal of Interpersonal Violence, 11,* 502–518.

Charlifue, S. W., & Gerhart, K. A. (1991). Behavioral and demographic predictors of suicide after traumatic spinal cord injury. *Archives of Physical and Medical Rehabilatation, 72,* 488–492.

Charlton, J. (1995). Trends and patterns in suicide in England and Wales. *International Journal of Epidemiology, 24,* S45–S52.

Chemtob, C. M., Hamada, R. S., Bauer, G., Kinney, B., & Torigoe, R. Y. (1988). Patients' suicides: Frequency and impact on psychiatrists. *American Journal of Psychiatry, 145,* 224–228.

Cheng, A. T. A. (1995). Mental illness and suicide: A case-control study in East Taiwan. *Archives of General Psychiatry, 52,* 594–603.

Chessick, R. D. (1992). The death instinct revisited. *Journal of the American Academy of Psychoanalysis, 20,* 3–28.

Chidester, D. (1991). *Salvation and suicide: An interpretation of Jim Jones, the Peoples Temple, and Jonestown.* Bloomington: Indiana University Press.

Chynoweth, R., Tonge, J. I., & Armstrong, J. (1980). Suicide in Brisbane: A retrospective psychosocial study. *Australia and New Zealand Journal of Psychiatry, 14,* 37–45.

Clark, D. (1991, January 28). *Suicide among the elderly.* Final report to the AARP Andrus Foundation.

Clark, D. (1992, December). Suicide risk and persons with AIDS. *Suicide Research Digest, 6,* 12–13.

Clark, D. C., & Fawcett, J. (1992). An empirically based model of suicide risk assessment for patients with affective disorder. In D. Jacobs (Ed.), *Suicide and clinical practice* (pp. 55–73). Washington, DC: American Psychiatric Press.

Clark, D. C., & Fawcett, J. A. (1992). Review of empirical risk factors for evaluation of the suicidal patient. In B. Bongar (Ed.), *Suicide: Guidelines for Assessment, Management and Treatment.* New York: Oxford University Press.

Clark, D. C., & Horton-Deutsch, S. L. (1992). Assessment in absential: The value of the psychological autopsy method for studying antecedents of suicide and predicting future suicides. In R. W. Maris, A. L. Berman, J. T. Maltsberger, & R. I. Yufit (Eds.), *The Assessment and prediction of suicide* (pp. 144–182). New York: Guilford Press.

Clark, D. C., & Kerkhof A. J. (1993). Panic disorders and suicidal behavior. *Crisis, 14,* 2–5.

Clark, D. C., Gibbons, R. D., Fawcett, J., & Scheftner, W. A. (1989). What is the mechanism by which suicide attempts predispose to later suicide attempts? A mathematical model. *Journal of Abnormal Psychology, 95*(1), 42–49.

Clark, D. C., Sommderfeldt, L., Schwarz, M., & Watel, L. (1990). Physical recklessness in adolescence and its relationship to suicidal tendencies. *Journal of Nervous and Mental Disease, 178,* 423–433.

Clarke, R. V., & Lester, D. (1987). Toxicity of car exhaust and opportunity for suicide. *Journal of Epidemiology and Community Health, 41,* 114–120.

Clarke, R. V., & Lester, D. (1989). *Suicide: Closing the exits.* New York: Springer-Verlag.

Clarke, R. V., & Lester, D. (1991, April). *Explaining choice of method for suicide.* Paper presented at the annual meeting of the American Association of Suicidology, Boston.

Clarke, R. V., & Mayhew, P. (1989). Crime as opportunity: A note on domestic gas suicide in Britain and The Netherlands. *British Journal of Criminology, 29,* 35–46.

Cleiren, M. R. H. D., Diekstra, R. F. W., Kerkhof, A. J. F. M., & van der Wal, J. (1994). Mode of death and kinship in bereavement: Focusing on "who" rather than "how." *Crisis, 15,* 22–36.

Cobb, N., & Etzel, R. A. (1991). Unintentional carbon monoxide related deaths in the United States, 1979–1988. *Journal of the American Medical Association, 266,* 659–663.

Cohen, A. S., Vance, V. K., & Runyan, J. W. Jr., et al. (1960). Diabetic acidosis: An evaluation of the cause, course and therapy of 73 cases. *Annals of Internal Medicine, 52,* 55–86.

Cohen, L. J., Test, M. A., & Brown, R. L. (1990). Suicide and schizophrenia: Data from a prospective community treatment study. *American Journal of Psychiatry, 147,* 602–607.

Cohen, L. S., Winchel, R. M., & Stanley, M. (1988). Biochemical markers of suicide risk and adolescent suicide. *Clinical Neuropharmacology, 2,* 423–435.

Cohen, S. L., & Fiedler, J. E. (1974). Content analysis of multiple messages in suicide notes. *Life-Threatening Behavior, 4,* 75–95.

Cohen-Sandler, R., Berman, A. L., & King, R. A. (1982a). A follow-up study of hospitalized suicidal children. *Journal of the American Academy of Child Psychiatry, 21,* 398–403.

Cohen-Sandler, R., Berman, A. L., & King, R. A. (1982b). Life stress and symptomatology: Determinants of suicidal behavior in children. *Journal of the American Academy of Child Psychiatry, 21,* 178–186.

Coleman, J. S. (1962). *Centuries of childhood.* New York: Vintage Press.

Coleman, L. (1987). *Suicide clusters.* Boston: Faber & Faber.

Colt, G. H. (1987). The history of the suicide survivor: The mark of Cain. In E. J. Dunne, J. L. McIntosh, & K. Dunne-Maxim (Eds.), *Suicide and its aftermath: Understanding and counseling the survivors.* New York: Norton.

Colt, G. H. (1991). *The enigma of suicide.* New York: Summit Books.

Colton, M. E., & Marsh, J. C. (1984). A sex-roles perspective on drug and alcohol use by women. In C. Widom (Ed.), *Sex Roles and Psychopathology.* New York: Plenum.

Colton, P. G., Drake, R. E., & Gates, C. (1985). Critical treatment issues in suicide among schizophrenics. *Hospital and Community Psychiatry, 36,* 534–536.

Connelly, J. F., Cullen, A., & McTigue, O. (1995). Single road traffic deaths-Accident or suicide? *Crisis, 16,* 85–89.

Conroy, R. M. (1993). Low cholesterol and violent death: The evidence, the gaps, the theory and the practical implications. *Irish Journal of Psychological Medicine, 10,* 67–70.

Convit, A. J., Jaeger, S. P., Lin, M., Meisner, J., & Volavka, J. (1988). Predicting assaultiveness in psychiatric inpatients: A pilot study. *Hospital and Community Psychiatry, 39,* 429–434.

Conway, J. V. P. (1960). The investigation of suicide notes. *Journal of Forensic Sciences, 5,* 48–71.

Conwell, Y. C., Caine, E. D., & Olsen, K. (1990). Suicide and cancer in late life. *Hospital and Community Psychiatry, 41,* 1334–1339.

Conwell, Y. C., Duberstein, P. R., Cox, C., Hermann, J. H., Forbes, N. T., & Caine, E. D. (1996). Relationships of age and Axis I diagnoses in victims of completed sucides: A psychological autopsy study. *American Journal of Psychiatry, 153,* 1001–1008.

Cooper, J. E. (Ed.). (1994). *WHO pocket guide to the ICD–10 classification of mental and behavioral disorders.* Washington, DC: American Psychiatric Press.

Cooper, P. (1973). *The medical detectives.* New York: McKay.

Copi, I. (1994). *Introduction to logic.* New York: Macmillan.

Corbitt, E. M., Malone, K.M., Haas, G. L., & Mann, J. J. (1996). Suicidal behavior in patients with major depression and comorbid personality disorders. *Journal of Affective Disorders, 39,* 61–72.

Coren, S., & Hewitt, P. L. (1998). Is anorexia nervosa associated with elevated rates of suicide? *American Journal of Public Health, 88,* 1206–1207.

Cormier, H., & Klerman, G. (1985). Unemployment and male–female labor force participation as determinants of changing suicide rates of males and females in Quebec. *Social Psychiatry, 20,* 109–114.

Cornelius, J. R., Salloum, I. M., Day, N. L., Thase, M. E., & Mann, J. J. (1996). Patterns of suicidality and alcohol use in alcoholics with major depression. *Alcoholism: Clinical and Experimental Research, 20,* 1451–1455.

Cornelius, J. R., Salloum, I. M., Mezzich, J., Cornelius, Jr., M. D., Fabrega, H., Ehler, J. G., Ulrich, R. F., Thase, M. E., & Mann, J. J. (1995). Disproportionate suicidality in patients with comorbid major depression and alcoholism. *American Journal of Psychiatry, 152,* 358–364.

Coryell, W. (1988). Panic disoders and mortality. *Psychiatric Clinics of North America, 11,* 433–440.

Coryell, W., & Tsuang, M. (1982). Primary unipolar depression and the prognostic importance of delusions. *Archives of General Psychiatry, 39,* 1181–1184.

Coryell, W., Noyes, R., & Clancy, J. (1982). Excess mortality in panic disorder. A comparison with primary unipolar depression. *Archives of General Psychiatry, 39,* 701–703.

Cote, T. R., Bigger, R. J., & Dannenberg, A. L. (1992). Risk of suicide among persons with AIDS: A national assessment. *Journal of the American Medical Association, 268,* 2066–2068.

Council on Scientific Affairs. (1987). Results and implications of the AMA–APA Physician Mortality Project. Stage II. *Journal of the American Medical Association, 257,* 2949–2953.

Cowdry, R. W., Gardner, D. C. (1988). Pharmacotherapy of borderline personality disorder: Alprazolom, carbamazebine, trifluoperazine, and tranylcypromine. *Archives of General Psychiatry, 45,* 111–119.

Cox, B. J., Direnfeld, D. M., Swinson, R. P., & Norton, G.R.(1994). Suicidal ideation and suicide attempts in panic disorder and social phobia. *American Journal of Psychiatry, 151,* 882–887.

Cox, V. C., Paulus, P. B., & McCain, G. (1984). Prison crowding research: The relevance for prison housing standards and a general approach regarding crowding phenomena. *American Psychologist, 39,* 1148–1160.

Crosby, K., Rhee, J., & Holland, J. (1973). Suicide by fire: A contemporary method of political protest. *International Journal of Social Psychiatry, 23,* 60–69.

Cull, J. G., & Gill, W. S. (1982). *Suicide Probability Scale (SPS).* Los Angeles: Western Psychological Services.

Cumming, E., & Lazar, C. (1981). Kinship structure and suicide: A theoretical link. *Canadian Review of Sociology and Anthropology, 18,* 271–281.

Curren, W. J., McGarry, A. L., & Petty, C. S. (Eds.). (1980). *Modern legal medicine, psychiatry, and forensic science.* Philadelphia: F. A. Davis.

Custer, R. L. (1984). Profile of the pathological gambler. *Journal of Clinical Psychiatry, 45,* 35–38.

Cutter, F. (1983). *Art and the wish to die.* Chicago: Nelson-Hall.

Darbonne, A. R. (1969). Study of psychological content in the communications of suicidal individuals. *Journal of Consulting and Clinical Psychology, 33,* 590–596.

Davidowitz, M., & Myrick, R. (1984). Responding to the bereaved: An analysis of helping statements. *Death Education, 8,* 1–10.

Davidson, L., & Gould, M. S. (1989). Contagion as risk factor for youth suicide. *Report of the Secretary: Task Force on Youth Suicide.* Washington, DC: U.S. Government Printing Office.

Davidson, L., & Linnoila, M. (1990). *Risk factors for youth suicide.* New York: Hemisphere.

Davis, R. (1978). Dimensions of black suicide: A theoretical model. *Suicide and life-threatening behavior, 8*(3), 161–173.

Davis, R. (1980a). Black suicide and the relational system. *Research on Race and Ethnic Relations, 2,* 43–71.

Davis, R. (1980b). Suicide among young blacks: Trends and perspectives. *Phylon, 41,* 223–229.

Davis, R. (1981). Female labor force participation, status intergration, and suicide, 1950–1969. *Suicide and Life-Threatening Behavior, 11,* 111–123.

de Catanzaro, D. (1986). A mathematical model of evolutionary pressures and reflecting self-preservation and self-destruction. *Suicide and Life-Threatening Behavior, 16,* 84–99.

de Catanzaro, D. (1992). Prediction of self-preservation failures on the basis of quantitative evolutionary biology. In R. W. Maris, A. L. Berman, J. T. Maltsberger, & R. I. Yufit (Eds.), *Assessment and prediction of suicide.* New York: Guilford Press.

De Vane C. L. (1994). Pharmacogentics and drug metabolism of newer antidepressant agents. *Journal of Clinical Psychiatry, 55,* 38–45.

Dean, P. J., Range, L. M., & Goggin, W. C. (1996). An escape theory of suicide in college students:

Testing a model that includes perfectionism. *Suicide and Life-Threatening Behavior, 26,* 181–186.

DeLeo, D., & Marazziti, D. (1988). Biological predication of suicide: The role of serotonin. *Crisis, 9,* 1009–1018.

DeLeo, D., Carollo, G., & Dello Buono, M. L. (1995). Lower suicide rates associated with a Tele-Help/Tele-Check service for elderly at home. *American Journal of Psychiatry, 152,* 632–634.

Delk, J. L. (1980). High-risk sports as indirect self-destructive behavior. In N. L. Farberow (Ed.), *The many faces of suicide: indirect self-destructive behavior.* New York: McGraw Hill.

Denny, K. M. (1995). Russian roulette: A case of questions not asked? *Journal of the American Academy of Child and Adolescent Psychiatry, 34,* 1682–1683.

Department of Health and Human Services. (1989). Alcohol, drug abuse, and mental health administration. *Report of the Secretary's Task Force on Youth Suicide. Vol. 1: Overview and recommendations* (DHHS Publication No. ADM 89–1621). Washington, DC: U.S. Government Printing Office.

Derogatis, L. R., Morrow, G. R., Fetting, J., Penman, D., Piasetsky, S., Schmale, A. M., Henrichs, M., & Carnicks, C. L. (1983). The prevalence of psychiatric disorders among cancer patients. *Journal of the American Medical Association, 29,* 751–757.

Despelder, L. A., & Strickland, A. L. (1998). *The last dance: Encountering death and dying* (5th ed.). Mountain View, CA: Mayfield.

Deutsh, C. J. (1984). Self-reported sources of stress among psychotherapists. *Professional Psychology, 15,* 833–845.

Deykin, E. Y., Alpert, J. J., & McNamarra, J. J. (1985). A pilot study of the effect of exposure to child abuse or neglect on adolescent suicial behavior. *American Journal of Psychiatry, 142,* 1299–1303.

Deykin, E. Y., Buka, S. L., & Zeena, T. H. (1992). Depressive illness among chemically dependent adolescents. *American Journal of Psychiatry, 149,* 1341–1347.

DiBiance, J. T. (1979). The hemodialysis patient. In L. D. Hankoff & B. Einsidler (Eds.), *Suicide theory and clinical aspects.* Littleton, MA: PSG.

Diekstra, R. F. W. (1986). The significance of Nico Speijer's suicide: How and when should suicide be prevented? *Suicide and Life-Threatening Behavior, 16,* 13–15.

Diekstra, R. F. W. (1990). An international perspective on the epidemiology and prevention of suicide. In S. J. Blumenthal & D. J. Kupfer (Eds.), *Suicide over the life-cycle.* Washington, DC: American Psychiatric Press.

Diekstra, R. F. W., Maris, R. W., Platt, S., Schmidtke, A., & Sonneck, G. (Eds.). (1989). *Suicide and its prevention: The role of attitude and imitation.* Leiden: E. J. Brill.

DiMaio, V. J. M. (1999). *Gunshot wounds: Practical aspects of firearms, ballistics, and forensic techniques.* Boca Raton, FL: CRC Press.

Dinwiddie, S. H., Reich, T., & Cloninger, C. R. (1992). Psychiatric comorbidity and suicidality among intravenous drug users. *Journal of Clinical Psychiatry, 53,* 364–369.

Dishion, T. J., & Patterson, G. R. (1997). The timing and severity of antisocial behavior: Three hypotheses within an ecological framework. In D.M. Stoff, J. Breiling & J. D. Maser (Eds.) *Handbook of antisocial behavior.* New York: Wiley.

Dollard, J., Doob, L., Miller, N., Mowrer, O., & Sears, R. (1939). *Frustration and aggression.* New Haven: Yale University Press.

Dorpat, T. L., & Ripley, H. (1960). A study of suicide in the Seattle area. *Comprehensive Psychiatry, 1,* 349–359.

Dorpat, T. L., Anderson, W. F., & Ripley, H. S. (1968). The relationship of physical illness to suicide. In H. P. L. Resnick (Ed.), *Suicidal behaviors: Diagnosis and management.* Boston: Little, Brown.

Douglas, J. D. (1967). *The social meanings of suicide.* Princeton, NJ: Princeton University Press.

Douglas, J. D. (Ed.). (1970). *Understanding everyday life.* Chicago: Aldine.

Doyle, B. B. (1990). Crisis management of the suicidal patient. In S. J. Blumenthal & D. J. Kupfer (Eds.), *Suicide over the life-cycle.* Washington, DC: American Psychiatric Press.

Doyle, J. A. (1989). *The male experience.* Dubuque, IA: William C. Brown.

Dublin, L. L. (1963). *Suicide: A sociological and statistical study.* New York: Ronald Press.

Ducharme, S. H., & Freed, M. M. (1980). The role of self-destruction in spinal cord injury mortality. *Science Digest, 2,* 29–38.

Dugan, T. F., & Belfer, M. L. (1989). Suicide in children: Diagnosis, management, and treatment. In D. Jacobs & H. N. Brown (Eds.), *Suicide: Understanding and responding.* Madison: International Universities Press.

Duggan, C. F., Sham, P., Lee, A. S., & Murray, R. M. (1991). Can future suicidal behaviour in depressed patients be predicted? *Journal of Affective Disorders, 22,* 111–118.

Duncan, C. E., & Edland, J. F. (1974). Suicide notes. *Legal Medical Annual,* pp. 113–120.

Dunne, E. J. (1987). Special needs of suicide survivors in therapy. In E. J. Dunne, J. L. McIntosh, & K. Dunne-Maxim (Eds.), *Suicide and its aftermath: Understanding and counseling the survivors.* New York: Norton.

Dunne, E. J., McIntosh, J. L., & Dunne-Maxim, K. (Eds.). (1987). *Suicide and its aftermath: Understanding and counseling the survivors.* New York: Norton.

DuRant, R. H., Krowchuk, D. P., Sinal, S. H. (1998). Victimization, use of violence, and drug use at school among male adolescents who engage in same-sex sexual behavior. *Journal of Pediatrics, 132,* 113–118.

Durkheim, E. (1951). *Suicide: A study in sociology.* New York: Free Press. (Original work published 1897)

Durkheim, E. (1966). *Suicide.* New York: Free Press.

Dwivedi, K. N., Brayne, E., & Lovett, S. (1992). Group work with sexually abused adolescent girls. *Group Anaylsis, 25,* 477–489.

Dyck, R. J., Bland, R., & Newman, S. (1999, April). *The examination of life history and parasuicidal behavior: suicide in Alberta.* Paper presented at the 16th research symposium, Edmonton, Alberta, Canada.

Eagly, A. H. (1987). *Sex differences in social behavior: A social role interpretation.* Hillsdale, NJ: Erlbaum.

Earls, F., Escobar, J. I., & Manson, S. M. (1990). Suicide in minority groups: Epidemiologic and cultural perspectives. In S. J. Blumenthal & D. J. Kupfer (Eds.), *Suicide over the life-cycle.* Washington, DC: American Psychiatric Press.

Early, K. E. (1992). *Religion and suicide in the African-American community.* Westport, CT: Greenwood Press.

Easterlin, R. A. (1987a). *Birth and fortune: The impact of numbers on personal welfare.* New York: Basic Books.

Easterlin, R. A. (1987b). Easterlin hypothesis. In J. Eatwell & P. Newman (Eds.), *The new Palgrave: A Dictionary of economics,* New York: Stockton.

Eaton, W. W., & Kessler, L. G. (1985). *Epidemiologic field methods in psychiatry: The NIMH Epidemiologic Catchment Area program.* New York: Academic Press.

Echohawk, M. (1997). Suicide: The scourge of Native American people. *Suicide and Life-Threatening Behavior, 27,* 66–67.

Edland, J. F., & Duncan, C. E. (1973). Suicide notes in Monroe County: A 23 year look (1950–1972). *Journal of Forensic Sciences, 18,* 364–369.

Egeland, J., & Sussex, J. (1985). Suicide and family loading for affective disorders. *Journal of the American Medical Association, 254,* 915–918.

Ehrlich, M. (1991). *Les mutations sexuelles.* Paris: Presses Universitaires de France.

Eichelman, B., & Hartwig, A. (1993). The clinical psychopharmacology of violence. *Psychopharmacology Bulletin, 29,* 57–63.

Eisele, J. W., Reay, D. J., & Cook, A. (1981). Sites of suicidal gunshot wounds. *Journal of Forensic Sciences, 26,* 480–485.

Eisenberg, L. (1980). Adolescent suicide: On taking arms against a sea of trouble. *Pediatrics, 66,* 315–320.

Eisler, R. M., & Blalock, J. A. (1991). Masculine gender role stress: Implications for the assessment of men. *Clinical Psychology Review, 11,* 45–60.

Ellis, T. E. (1988). Classification of suicidal behavior: A review and step toward integration. *Suicide and Life-Threatening Behavior, 18,* 358–371.

Ellis, T. E., & Newman, C. F. (1996). *Choosing to live: How to defeat suicidal behavior through cognitive therapy.* Oakland, CA: New Harbinger.

Emerson, B., & Cantor, C. (1993). Traon suicides in Brisbane, Australia, 1980–1986. *Crisis, 14,* 90–94.

Engelman, J. E., Hessol, N. A., Lifson, A. R., Lemp, G. F., Mata, A., Rutherford, G. W., Goldblum, P., Bott, C., & Stephens, B. (1988). *Suicide patterns and AIDS in San Francisco.* Paper presented at the 4th International Conference on AIDS.

Engelman, N. B., Jobes, D. A., Berman, A. L., Langbein, L. I. (1998). Clinician's decision making about involuntary commitment. *Psychiatric Services, 49*(7) 941–945.

Entmacher, P. S., Krall, L. P., & Kranczer, S. N. (1985). Diabetes mortality from vital statistics. In A. Marble, L. P. Krall, & R. F. Bradley (Eds.), *Joslin's diabetes mellitus.* Philadelphia: Lea & Febiger.

Erikson, E. H. (1950). *Childhood and society.* New York: Norton.

Evans, G., & Farberow, N. L. (1988). *The encyclopedia of suicide.* New York: Facts on File.

Evenson, R. C., Sletten, I. W., Altman, H., & Brown, M. L. (1974). Disturbing behavior: A. study of incidence reports. *Psychiatric Quarterly, 48,* 266–275.

Eyman, J. R., & Eyman, S. K. (1992). Personality assessment in suicide prediction. In R. W. Maris, A. L. Berman, J. T. Maltsberger, & R. I. Yufit (Eds.), *Assessment and prediction of suicide.* New York: Guilford Press.

Famularo, R., Stone, K., & Popper, C. (1985). Preadolescent alcohol abuse and dependence. *American Journal of Psychiatry, 142,* 1187–1189.

Farber, B. A. (1983). Psychotherapists' perceptions of stressful behavior. *Professional Psychology: Research and Practice, 14,* 697–705.

Farber, M. L. (1968). *Theory of suicide.* New York: Funk & Wagnalls.

Farberow, N. L. (1969). *Bibliography on suicide and suicide prevention.* (DHHS Public Health Service Publication No. 1979). Washington, DC: United States Government Printing Office.

Farberow, N. L. (Ed.). (1975). *Suicide in different cultures.* Baltimore: University Park Press.

Farberow, N. L. (Ed.). (1980). *The many faces of suicide: Indirect self-destructive behavior.* New York: McGraw Hill.

Farberow, N. L., & Shneidman, E. S. (1957). Suicide and age. In E. S. Shneidman & N. L. Farberow (Eds.), *Clues to suicide.* New York: McGraw-Hill.

Farberow, N. L., & Shneidman, E. S. (Eds.). (1961). *The cry for help.* New York: McGraw-Hill.

Farberow, N. L., & Simon, M. D. (1975). Suicide in Los Angeles and Vienna. In N. L. Farberow (Ed.), *Suicide in different cultures.* Baltimore: University Park Press.

Farberow, N. L., Gallagher, D. E., Gilewski, M. J., & Thompson, L. W. (1987). An examination of the early impact of bereavement on psychological distress in survivors of suicide. *Gerontologist, 27,* 592–598.

Farberow, N. L., Gallagher-Thompson, D. E., Gilewski, M. J., & Thompson, L. W. (1992a). The role of social supports in the bereavement process of surviving spouses of suicide and natural death. *Suicide and Life-Threatening Behavior, 22,* 107–124.

Farberow, N. L., Gallagher-Thompson, D. E., Gilewski, M. J., & Thompson, L. W. (1992b). Changes in grief and mental health of bereaved spouses of older suicides. *Journal of Gerontology: Psychological Sciences, 47,* 357–366.

Farberow, N. L., Litman, R. E., & Nelson, F. L. (1988). A survey of youth suicide in California. In R. Yufit (Ed.), *Proceedings of the 21st annual meeting of the American Assocation of Suicidology.* Denver: American Association of Suicidology.

Farberow, N. L., Shneidman, E. S., & Leonard, C. V. (1963). *Medical bulletin 9: Suicide among general medical and surgical hospital patients with malignant neoplasms.* Washington, DC: Department of Medicine and Surgery, Veterans Administration.

Farley, F. (1986, May). The big T in personality. *Psychology Today, 20.*

Farmer, R., & Rohde, J. (1980). Effect of availability and acceptability of lethal instruments on suicide mortality: An analysis of some international data. *Acta Psychiatrica Scandanavia, 66,* 436–446.

Farrell, M. P., & Rosenberg, S. D. (1981). *Men at midlife.* Boston: Auburn.

Farrell, W. (1988). *Why men are the way they are.* New York: Berkeley.

Faulkner, A. H., & Cranston, K. (1998). Correlates of same-sex behavior in a random sample of Massachusetts high school students. *American Journal of Public Health, 8* 262–266.

Faupel, C. E., Kowalski, G. S., & Starr, P. D. (1987). Sociology's one law: Religion and suicide in the urban context. *Journal for the Scientific Study of Religion, 26,* 523–534.

Fava, G. A., Grandi, S., & Savron, G. (1992). Panic disorder and suicidal ideation. *American Journal of Psychiatry 149,* 1412–1412.

Fava, M., & Rosenbaum, J. F. (1992). Suicidality and fluoxetine: Is there a relationship? *Journal of Clinical Psychiatry, 53,* 103.

Favazza, A. R. (1989). Why patients mutilate themselves. *Hospital and Community Psychiatry, 40,* 137–145.

Favazza, A. R. (1996). *Bodies under siege.* Baltimore: Johns Hopkins University Press.

Favazza, A. R., & Conterio, K. (1989). Female habitual self-mutilators. *Acta Psychiatrica Scandinavica, 79,* 283–289.

Favazza, A. R., & Rosenthal R. J. (1993). Diagnostic issues in self-mutilation. *Hospital and Community Psychiatry, 44,* 134–139.

Fawcett, J. (1993). The morbidity and mortality of clinical depression. *International Clinical Psychopharmacology, 8,* 217–220.

Fawcett, J. A. (1992). Suicide risk factors in depressive disorders and in panic disorder. *Journal of Clinical Psychiatry, 53,* 9–13.

Fawcett, J. A., Clark, D. C., & Busch, K. A. (1993). Assessing and treating the patient at risk for suicide. *Psychiatric Annals, 23,* 244–255.

Fawcett, J. A., Scheftner, W. A., Fogg, L., et al. (1987, May). Acute versus long-term clinical predictors of suicide. In *CME syllabus and proceedings summary* (pp. 206–207), 140th annual meeting of the American Psychiatric Association, Chicago, Illinois.

Fawcett, J., Busch, K., Jacobs, D., Kravitz, H., &. Fogg, L. F. (1997). Suicide: A four-pathway clinical biochemical model. In D. Stoff & J. J. Mann (Eds.), *The neurology of suicide—From the bench to the clinic* (pp. 288–301). New York: New York Academy of Sciences.

Fawcett, J., Scheftner, W. A., Fogg, L., & Clark, D. C. (1990). Time-related predictors of suicide in major affective disorder. *American Journal of Psychiatry, 147,* 1189–1194.

Fawcett, J., Scheftner, W., Clark, D., Hedeker, D., Gibbons, R., & Coryell, W. (1987). Clinical Predictors of suicide in patients with major affective disorders: A controlled prospective study. *American Journal of Psychiatry, 144,* 35–40.

Feinstein, R., & Plutchik, R. (1990). Violence and suicide risk assessment in the psychiatric emergency room. *Comprehensive Psychiatry, 31,* 337–343.

Felix, O. M., Munoz, R., & Newcomb, M. D. (1994). The role of emotional distress in drug use among Latino adolescents. *Journal of Child and Adolescent Substance Abuse, 3,* 1–22.

Felner, R. D., & Silverman, M. M. (1995). In M. M. Silverman & R. W. Maris (Eds.), *Suicide prevention: Toward the year 2000.* New York: Guilford Press.

Felts, W. M., Chenier, T., & Barnes, R. (1992). Drug use and suicide ideation and behavior among North Carolina public school students. *American Journal of Public Health, 82,* 870–872.

Fenton, W. S., McGlashan, T. H., Victor, B. J., & Blyler, C. R. (1997). Symptoms, subtype, and suicidality in patients with schizophrenia spectrum disorders. *American Journal of Psychiatry, 154,* 199–204.

Ferris, C. F., & deVries, G. J. (1997). Ethological models for examining the neurobiology of aggressive and affiliative behaviors. In D.M. Stoff, J. Breiling & J.D. Maser (Eds.), *Handbook of antisocial behavior.* New York: Wiley.

Fifield, L. (1975). *On my way to nowhere: Alienated, isolated, drunk.* Los Angeles: The Gay Community Services Center.

First 15 Kevorkian-assisted suicides. (1993, March 8). *Newsweek,* p. 46.

Firth, R. (1961). Suicide and risk-taking in Tikopia society. *Psychiatry, 24,* 1–17.

Fishbain, D. A., D'Achille, L., Barsky, S., & Aldrich, T. (1984). A controlled study of suicide pacts. *Journal of Clinical Psychiatry, 45,* 154–157.

Fishbain, D. A., Fletcher, J. R., Aldrich, T. E., & Davis, J. H. (1987). Relationship between Russian roulette deaths and risk-taking behavior: A controlled study. *American Journal of Psychiatry,* *144*, 563–566.

Fisher, R. L., & Fisher, S. F. (1996). Antidepressants for children: Is scientific support necessary? *Journal of Nervous and Mental Disease, 184*, 99–102.

Fisher, S., Greenberg, R. P. (Eds.). (1989). *The limits of biological treatments for psychological distress.* Hillsdale, NJ: Erlbaum.

Fiske, H. (1997). Solution-focused brief therapy in suicide prevention. In J. L. McIntosh (Ed.), *Proceedings of the 30th Annual Conference of the American Association of Suicidology.* Washington, DC: American Association of Suicidology.

Flavin, D. K., Franklin, J. E., & Frances, R. J. (1986). The acquired immune deficiency syndrome (AIDS) and suicidal behavior in alcohol-dependent homosexual men. *American Journal of Psychiatry, 143*, 1440–1442.

Folstein, M. F., Folstein, S. E., & McHugh, P. R. (1975). "Mini-mental state": A practical method for grading the cognitive state of patients for the clinician. *Journal of Psychiatric Research, 12*(3), 189–198.

Fox, B. H., Stanek, E. J., Boyd, S. C., & Flannerty, J. T. (1982). Suicide rates among cancer patients in Connecticut. *Journal of Chronic Disease, 35*, 89–100.

Frances, A., & Pfeffer, C. R. (1987). Reducing environmental stress for a suicidal ten-year-old. *Hospital and Community Psychiatry, 38*, 22–24.

Frances, R. J., Wikstrom, T., & Alcena, V. (1985). Contracting AIDS as a means of committing suicide. *American Journal of Psychiatry, 142*, 656.

Franklin, C. W. (1988). *Men and society.* Chicago: Nelson-Hall.

Frederick, C. J. (1969). An investigation of the handwriting of suicide persons through suicide notes. *Journal of Abnormal Psychology, 73*, 263–267.

Freemantle, N., House, A., & Song, F. (1994). Prescribing selective serotonin reuptake inhibitors as a strategy for prevention of suicide. *British Medical Journal, 309*, 249–253.

Freud, S. (1955). Beyond the pleasure principle. In J. Strachey (Ed. and Trans.), *The Standard edition of the complete psychological works of Sigmund Freud* (vol. 18). London: Hogarth Press. (Original work published 1920)

Freud, S. (1963). Mourning and Melancholia. In J. Strachey (Ed. and Trans.), *The standard edition of the complete psychological works of Sigmund Freud* (vol. 14). London: Hogarth Press. (Original work published 1917)

Friedman, P. (1967). Suicide among police: A study of 93 suicides among New York City policemen, 1934–1940. In E. S. Shneidman (Ed.), *Essays on self-destruction.* New York: Science House.

Friedman, R. C., Aronoff, M. S., Clarkin, J. F., Corn, R., & Hurt, S. W. (1983). History of suicidal behavior in depressed borderline inpatients. *American Journal of Psychiatry, 145*, 1023–1026.

Friedman, S., Jones, J. C., Chernen, L., & Barlow, D. H. (1992). Suicidal ideation and suicide attempts among patients with panic disorder: A survey of two outpatient clinics. *American Journal of Psychiatry, 149*, 680–685.

Frierson, R. L. (1991). Suicide attempts by the old and very old. *Archives of Internal Medicine, 15*, 141–144.

Frierson, R. L., & Lippman, S. B. (1988). Suicide and AIDS. *Psychosomatics, 29*, 226–231.

Frisbie, J. H., & Kache, A. (1983). Increasing survival and changing causes of death in myelopathy patients. *Journal of American Paraplegia Society, 6*, 51–56.

Gabuzda, D. H., & Hirsch, M. S. (1987). Neurological manifestations of infection with human immunodeficiency virus: Clinical features and pathogenesis. *Annals of Internal Medicine, 197*, 383–391.

Gallant, D. M. (1987). Antidepressant overdose: Symptoms and treatment. *Psychopathology, 20* (Suppl. No. 1), 75–81.

Gamble, D. E., & Peterson, L. G. (1986). Trazodone overdose: Four years of experience from voluntary reports. *Journal of Clinical Psychiatry, 47*, 544–546.

Gardner, D. L., & Cowdry, R. W. (1995a). Alprazolam-induced dyscontrol in borderline personality disorder. *American Journal of Psychiatry, 142*, 98–100.

Gardner, D. L., & Cowdry, R. W. (1995b). Suicidal and parasuicidal behavior in borderline personality disorder. *Psychiatric Clinics of North America, 8,* 389–403.

Gardos, G., & Casey, D. (1984). *Tardive dyskinesia and affective disorders.* Washington, DC: American Psychiatric Press, Inc.

Garfinkel, B. D., Froese, A., & Hood, J. (1982). Suicide attempts in children and adolescents. *American Journal of Psychiatry, 139,* 1257–1261.

Garfinkel, H. (1967). *Studies in ethnomethodology.* Englewood Cliffs, NJ: Prentice-Hall.

Garmezy, N. (1983). Stressors of childhood. In N. Garmezy & M. Rutter (Eds.) *Stress, coping, and development in children.* New York: McGraw-Hill.

Garnefski, N. & Diekstra, R. F. (1997). Child sexual abuse and emotional and behavioral problems in adolescence: Gender differences. *Journal of the American Academy of Child and Adolescent Psychiatry, 36,* 323–329.

Garrison, C. Z. (1992). Demographic predictions of suicide. In R. W. Maris, A. L. Berman, J. T. Maltsberger, & R. I. Yufit (Eds.), *Assessment and prediction of suicide.* New York: Guilford Press.

Garrison, C. Z., McKeown, R. E., Valois, R. F., & Vincent, M. L. (1993). Aggression, substance use, and suicidal behaviors in high school students. *American Journal of Public Health, 83,* 179–184.

Gartrell, J. W., Jarvis, G. K., & Derksen, L. (1993). Suicidality among adolescent Alberta Indians. *Suicide and Life-Threatening Behavior, 24,* 366–373.

Gauthier, D. K., & Forsyth, C. J. (1999). Bareback sex, bug chasers, and the gift of death. *Deviant Behavior, 20,* 85–100.

Gay, P. (1988). *Freud: A life for our time.* New York: Norton.

Geisler, W. O., Jousse, A. T., Wynne-Jones, M., & Breithaupt, D. (1983). Survival in traumatic spinal cord injury. *Paraplegia, 21,* 364–373.

Gibbs, J. P. (1994). Durkheim's heavy hand in the sociological study of suicide. In D. Lester (Ed.), *Emile Durkheim, Le Suicide: One hundred years later.* Philadelphia: Charles Press.

Gibbs, J. P., & Martin, W. (1964). *Status of integration and suicide.* Eugene, OR: University of Oregon Press.

Gibbs, J. T. (1997). African-American suicide: A cultural paradox. *Suicide and Life-Threatening Behavior, 27,* 68–79.

Gibbs, J. T. (Ed.). (1988). *Young, black, and male in America: An endangered species.* Dover, MA: Auburn House.

Gibson, P. (1989). Gay male and lesbian youth suicide. In Alcohol, drug abuse, and mental health administration. Report of the Secretary's Task Force on Youth Suicide. Vol. 3: Prevention and interventions in youth suicide (DHHS Publication No. ADM 89–1623). Washington, DC: U.S. Government Printing Office.

Giddens, A. (1971). *The sociology of suicide: A selection of readings.* London: Frank Cass & Co.

Ginsberg, R. B. (1966). Anomie and aspirations. *Dissertation Abstracts, 27A,* 3945–3946.

Girard, C. (1988). Church membership and suicide reconsidered. *American Journal of Sociology, 93,* 1471–1479.

Girard, R., Minaire, P., Castanier, M., Berard, E., & Perrineriche, B. (1980). Spinal cord injury by falls: Comparison between suicidal and accidental cases. *Paraplegia, 6,* 381–385.

Golann, S., & Bongar, B. (1987, August). *Dangerous intersections: Systemic treatment approaches to suicide.* Paper presented at the American Psychological Association convention, New York.

Goldacre, M., Seagroatt, V., & Hawton, K. (1993). Suicide after discharge from psychiatric inpatient care. *Lancet, 342,* 283–286.

Goldberg, S. C., Schultz, S. C., Schulz, P. M., et al. (1986). Borderline and schizotypal personality disorders treated with low-dose thiothixene vs. placebo. *Archives of General Psychiatry, 43,* 680–686.

Goldblatt, M. J., & Schatzberg, A. F. (1990). Somatic treatment of the adult suicidal patient: A brief survey. In S. J. Blumenthal & D. J. Kupfer (Eds.), *Suicide over the life-cycle.* Washington, DC: American Psychiatric Press.

Goldblatt, M. J., Silverman, M. M., & Schatzerg, A. F. (1998). Psychopharmacological treatment of suicidal inpatients. In Bongar, B., Berman, A. L., Maris, R. W., Silverman, M. M., Harris,

E. A., & Packman, W. (Eds.), *Risk management with suicidal patients.* New York: Guilford Press.

Goldblum, P., & Moulton, J. (1986, November). AIDS-related suicide: A dilemma for health care providers. *Focus: A Review of AIDS Research, 2,* 1–4.

Goldman, L. G., Silverman, M. M., & Alpert, E. (1998). Violence and aggression. In L. S. Goldman, T. N. Wise, & D. S. Brody (Eds.), *Psychiatry for primary care physicians.* Chicago: American Medical Association.

Goldman, S., & Beardslee, W. R. (1999). Suicide in children and adolescents. In D. G. Jacobs (Ed.), *Guide to suicide assessment and intervention.* San Francisco: Jossey-Bass.

Goldney, R. D., Positano, S., Spence, N. D., & Rosenman, S. J. (1985). Suicide in association with psychiatric hospitalization. *Australian and New Zealand Journal of Psychiatry, 19,* 177–183.

Goldney, R. D., Winefield, A., Saebel, J., et al. (1997). Anger, suicidal ideation, and attempted suicide: A prospective study. *Comprehensive Psychiatry, 38,* 264–268.

Gomberg, E. S. (1989). Suicide risk among women with alcohol problems. *American Journal of Public Health, 79,* 1363–1365.

Goodman, P. (1960). *Growing up absurd.* New York: Random House.

Goodwin, D. W. (1973). Alcohol in suicide and homicide. *Quaterly Journal of Studies on Alcohol, 34,* 144–156.

Goodwin, D. W. (1988). *Alcohol and the writer.* Kansas City, MO: Andrews McNeel.

Goodwin, F. K., & Jamison, K. R. (1990). *Manic-depressive illness.* New York: Oxford University Press.

Gordon, R. S. (1983). An operational classification of disease prevention. *Public Health Reports, 98,* 107–109.

Goss, M., & Reed, J. (1971). Suicide and religion: A study of white adults in New York City, 1963–1967. *Life-Threatening Behavior, 1,* 163–177.

Gottschalk, L. A., & Gleser, G. C. (1960). An analysis of the verbal content of suicide notes. *British Journal of Medical Psychology, 33,* 195–204.

Gould, M. S., & Shaffer, D. (1986). The impact of suicide in television movies: Evidence of imitation. *New England Journal of Medicine, 315,* 690–694.

Gould, M. S., Shaffer, D., Fisher, P., Kleinman, M., & Morishima, A. (1992). In R. W. Maris, A. L. Berman, J. T. Maltsberger, & R. I. Yufit (Eds.), *The clinical prediction of suicide.* New York: Guilford Press.

Gould, M. S, Shaffer, D., & Kleinman, M. (1988). The impact of suicide in television movies: Replication and commentary. *Suicide and Life-Threatening Behavior, 18,* 90–99.

Gove, W. R. (1979). Sex differences in the epidemiology of mental illness: Evidence and explanations. In E. S. Gomberg & V. Franks (Eds.), *Gender and disordered behavior.* New York: Brunner/Mazel.

Grace, F., Tenke, C., Bruder, G., & Rotheran, M. J. (1996). Abnormality of EEG alpha asymmetry in female adolescent suicide attempters. *Biological Psychiatry, 40,* 706–713.

Grant, I., Atkinson, J. H., Hesselink, J. R., et al. (1987). Evidence for early central nervous system involvement in the acquired immunodeficiency syndrome (AIDS) and other human immunodeficiency virus (HIV) infections. *Annals of Internal Medicine, 197,* 828–836.

Green, A. R., Curzin, G. (1968). Decrease of 5-hydoxytryptomine in the brain provoked by hydrocotesone and its prevention by allopurinol. *Nature, 220,* 1095–1097.

Greenberg, D. F. (1974). Involuntary psychiatric commitments to prevent suicide. *New York University Law Review 49,* 227–269.

Greenblatt, M., & Robertson, M. J. (1993). Life-styles, adaptive strategies, and sexual behaviors of homeless adolescents. *Hospital and Community Psychiatry, 44,* 1177–1180.

Greenwald, D. J., Reznikoff, M., & Plutchik, R. (1994). Suicide risk and violence risk in alcoholics: Predictors of aggressive risk. *Journal of Nervous and Mental Disease, 182,* 3–8.

Grella, C. E., Anglin, M. D., & Wugalter, S. E. (1995). Cocaine and crack use and HIV risk behaviors among high-risk methadone maintenance clients. *Drug and Alcohol Dependence, 37,* 15–21.

Grinspoon, L. (1986). Suicide. *Harvard Medical School Mental Health Newsletter, 2,* 3–4.

Grossman, D. C., Milligan, B. C., & Deyo, R. A. (1991). Risk factors for suicide attempts among Navajo adolescents. *American Journal of Public Health, 81,* 870–874.

Grosz, D. E., Lipshitz, D. S., Elder, S., Finkelstein, G., Faedda, G. L., & Plutchik, R. (1994). Correlates of violence risk in hospitalized adolescents. *Comprehensive Psychiatry, 35,* 296–300.

Group for the Advancement of Psychiatry. (1989). *Suicide and ethnicity in the United States, Report No. 128.* New York: Brunner/Mazel.

Gruenewald, P., Ponicki, W., & Mitchell P. (1995). Suicide rates and alcohol consumption in the U.S., 1970–1989. *Addiction, 90,* 1063–1075.

Grunebaum, J. G., & Klerman, C. L. (1967). Wrist-slashing. *American Journal of Psychiatry, 124,* 527–534.

Guggenheim, F. G., & Weisman, A. D. (1972). Suicide in the subway. *Journal of Nervous and Mental Disease, 155,* 404–409.

Gurman, A. S. (Ed.). (1982). *Questions and answers in the practice of family therapy* (vol. 2). New York: Brunner/Mazel.

Gutheil, E. A. (1996). Dreams and suicide. In J. T. Maltsberger & M. J. Goldblatt (Eds.), *Essential papers on suicide. Essential papers in psychoanalysis.* New York: New York University Press.

Guze, S. B., & Robins, E. (1970). Suicide and primary affective disorders. *British Journal of Psychiatry, 117,* 437–438.

Haas, G. (1997). Suicidal behavior in schizophrenia. In R. W. Maris, M. M. Silverman, & S. S. Canetto (Eds.), *Review of suicidology.* New York: Guilford Press.

Haberlandt, W. (1967). *Aportacion a la genetica del suicidio Folia Clinica Internacional, 17,* 319–322.

Haddon, W., Jr., & Baker, S. P. (1981). Injury control. In D. W. Clarke, & B. MacMahon (Eds.), *Preventive and community medicine.* Boston: Little-Brown.

Haffenden, J. (1982). *The life of John Berryman.* Boston: Routledge & Kegan Paul.

Hagnell, O., & Rorsman, B. (1979). Suicide in the Lundby study: A comparative investigation of clinical aspects. *Neuropsychobiology, 5,* 61–73.

Hall, C. S., Lindzey, G., & Campbell, J. B. (Eds.). (1997). *Theories of personality* (4th ed.). New York: Wiley.

Hamilton, M. (1960). A rating scale for depression. *Journal of Neurology, Neurosurgery, and Psychiatry, 23,* 56–61.

Hammen, C. L., & Peters, S. D. (1977). Differential responses to male and female depressive reactions. *Journal of Consulting and Clinical Psychology, 45,* 994–1001.

Hammermesh, D. (1974). An economic theory of suicide. *Journal of Political Economy, 82,* 83–98.

Hanauer, G. (1989, January). No one who cares . . . no place to go. *Penthouse,* pp. 71–77.

Hankoff, L. D. (1979). Judaic origins of the suicide prohibition. In L. D. Hankoff & B. Einsidler (Eds.), *Suicide: Theory and clinical aspects.* Littleton, MA: PSG.

Hare-Mustin, R. T. (1992). Cries and whispers: The psychotherapy of Anne Sexton. *Psychotherapy, 29,* 406–409.

Harris, E. C., & Barraclough, B. M. (1994). Suicide as an outcome for medical disorders. *Medicine, 73,* 281–296.

Harris, E. C., & Barraclough, B. (1998). Suicide as an outcome for mental disorders: A meta-analysis. *British Journal of Psychiatry, 170,* 205–228.

Harris, M. (1971). *Culture, man, and nature.* New York: Thomas Y. Crowell.

Harrison, J. (1978). Warning: The male sex role may be dangerous to your health. *Journal of Social Issues, 34,* 65–86.

Harrow, M., Westermeyer, J., Kaplan, K., & Butz, C. (1992). Schizophrenia and suicide (pp. 206–208). Paper presented at the annual meeting of the American Association of Suicidology.

Harry, J. (1989). Sexual identity issues. In Alcohol, drug abuse, and mental health administration. Report of the Secretary's Task Force on Youth Suicide. Vol. 2: Risk factors for youth suicide (DHHS Publication No. ADM 89–1622). Washington, DC: U.S. Government Printing Office.

Hassan, R., & Tan, G. (1989). Suicide trends in Australia: An analysis of sex differentials. *Suicide and Life-Threatening Behavior, 19,* 362–380.

Hasselback P., Lee, K. I., Yang, M., Nichol, R., & Wigle, D. (1991). The relationship of suicide rates to sociodemographic factors in Candian census divisions. *Canadain Journal of Psychiatry, 36,* 655–659.

Hatsukami, D., Mitchell, J. E., Eckert, E. D., & Pyle, R. (1986). Characteristics of patients with bulimia only, bulimia with affective disorder and bulimia with substance abuse. *Addictive Behaviors, 11,* 399–406.

Hawton, K., Arensman, E., Townsend, E., Bremner, S., Feldman, E., Goldney, R., Gunnell, D., Hazell, P., van Heerigan, K., House, A., Owens, D., Sakinofsky, I., & Träskman-Bendz, L. (1998). Deliberate self harm: Systematic review of efficacy of psychosocial and pharmacological treatments in preventing repetition. *British Medical Journal, 317,* 441–447.

Hawton, K., Cole, D., O'Grady, J., & Osborn, M. (1982). Motivational aspects of deliberate self-poisoning in adolescence. *British Journal of Psychiatry, 141,* 286–291.

Hawton, K., Fagg, J., & McKeown, S. P. (1989). Alcoholism, alcohol and attempted suicide. *Alcohol and Alcoholism, 24,* 3–9.

Headley, L. A. (Ed.). (1983). *Suicide in Asia and the Near East.* Berkeley: University of California Press.

Healy, D. (1998). *Antidepressant era.* Cambridge, MA: Harvard University Press.

Heath, R. P. (1997, June). You can buy a thrill: Chasing the ultimate rush. *American Demographics,* pp. 47–51.

Heikkinen, M. E., & Lönnqvist, J. K. (1996). Recent life events in elderly suicide: A nationwide study in Finland. In J. L. Pearson & Y. Conwell (Eds.), *Suicide and aging: International perspectives.* New York: Springer.

Heikkinen, M. E., Aro, H. M., Henriksson, M. M., Isometsa, E. T., Satna, S. J., Kuoppasalmi, K. I., & Lönnqvist, J. K. (1994). Differences in recent life events between alcoholic and depressive nonalcoholic suicides. *Alcoholism: Clinical and Experimental Research, 18,* 1143–1149.

Heila, H., Isometsa, E. T., Henrikkson, M. M., Heikkinen, M. E., Marttunen, M. J., & Lönnqvist, J. K. (1997). Suicide and schizophrenia: A nationwide psychological autopsy study on age-and sex-specific clinical characteristics of 92 suicide victims with schizophrenia. *American Journal of Psychiatry, 154,* 1235–1242.

Helmkamp, J. C. (1996). Occupation and suicide in the US Armed Forces. *Annals of Epidemiology, 6,* 83–88.

Hemphill, E., & Thornley, F. L. (1969). Suicide pacts. *South African Medical Journal, 43,* 1335–1337.

Hendin, H. (1964). *Suicide and Scandanavia.* New York: Grune & Stratton.

Hendin, H. (1969). *Black suicide.* New York: Harper & Row.

Hendin, H. (1982). *Suicide in America.* New York: Norton.

Hendin, H. (1992). Reply to Prenzlauer et al. *American Journal of Psychiatry, 149,* 1416–1417.

Hendin, H. (1993). Review article: The suicide of Anne Sexton. *Suicide and Life-Threatening Behavior, 23,* 257–262.

Hendin, H. (1997). *Seduced by death: Doctors, patients, and the Dutch cure.* New York: Norton.

Hendrix, R. C. (1972). *Investigation of violent and sudden death.* Springfield, IL: Charles C. Thomas.

Henriksson, M. M., Aro, H. M., Marttunen, M. J., Heikkinen, M. E., Isometsa, E. T., Kueppasalmi, K. I., & Lönnqvist, J. K. (1993). Mental disorders and comorbidity in suicide. *American Journal of Psychiatry, 150,* 935–940.

Henriksson, M. M., et al. (1996). Mental disorders in elderly suicide. In J. L. Pearson & Y. Conwell (Eds.), *Suicide and aging: International perspectives.* New York: Springer.

Henriksson, M. M., Isometsa, E. T., Kueppasalmi, K. I., Heikkinen, M. E., Marttunen, M. J., & Lönnqvist, J. K. (1996). Panic disorder in completed suicide. *Journal of Clinical Psychiatry, 57,* 275–281.

Henry, A. F., & Short, J. (1954). *Suicide and homicide.* Glencoe, IL: Free Press.

Henslin, J. A. (1996). *Social problems.* Englewood Cliffs, NJ: Prentice-Hall.

Hill, H., Soriano, F., Chen, A., & La Fromboise, T. (1994). Sociocultural factors in the etiology and prevention of violence among ethnic minority youth. In L. Eron, J., Gentry, S. P., & Schlegel (Eds.), *Reason to hope: A. psychosocial perspective on violence and youth.* Washington, DC: American Psychological Press.

Hill, T. E., (1983). Self-regarding suicide: A modified Kantian view. *Suicide and Life-Threatening Behavior, 13*(4), 254–275.

Hillbrand, M. (1992). Self-directed and other-directed aggressive behavior in a forensic service. *Suicide and Life-Threatening Behavior, 23*, 333–340.

Hilliard-Lysen, J., & Riemer, J. (1988). occupational stress and suicide among dentists. *Deviant Behavior, 9*, 333–346.

Hillman, J. (1977). Suicide as the soul's choice. In J.P Carse & A. B. Dallery (Eds.), *Death and society.* New York: Harcourt Brace Jovanovich.

Himmelhoch, J. M. (1987). Lest treatment abet suicide. *Journal of Clinical Psychiatry, 48*, 44–54.

Hirschfeld, R. M. A., & Blumenthal, S. J. (1986). Personality, life events, and other psychosocial factors in adolescent depression and suicide. In G. L. Klerman (Ed.), *Suicide and depression among adolescents and young adults.* Washington, DC: American Psychiatric Press.

Hirschfeld, R., & Davidson, L. (1988). Risk factors for suicide. In A. J. Frances & R. E. Hales (Eds.), *Review of psychiatry 7*, 307–333.

Hogberg, U., & Innala, E. (1995). Maternal mortality in Sweden. *Obstetrics and Gynecology, 84*, 240–244.

Holinger, P. C. (1987). *Violent deaths in the United States.* New York: Guilford Press.

Holinger, P. C., & Kleman, E. H. (1982). Violent deaths in the U.S., 1900–1975. *Social Science and Medicine, 16*, 1929–1938.

Holinger, P. C., Offer, D., & Ostrov, E. (1987). Suicide and homicide in the U.S. An epidemiologic study of violent death, population changes, and the potential for prediction. *American Journal of Psychiatry, 144*, 215–219.

Holinger, P. C., Offer, D., Barter, J. T., & Bell, C. C. (1994). *Suicide and homicide among adolescents.* New York: Guilford Press.

Holland, J. C., & Tross, S. (1985). The psychosocial and neuropsychiatric sequellae of the acquired immunodeficiency syndrome and related disorders. *Annals of Internal Medicine, 103*, 760–764.

Holley, H. L. (1993). *Suicide mortality following first admission for a suicide attempt or psychiatric illness.* Doctoral dissertation, University of Calgary, Edmonton, Alberta, Canada.

Holmes, T. H., & Rahe, R. H. (1967). The Social Readjustment Rating Scale. *Journal of Psychosomatic Research, 11*, 213–218.

Homans, G. C. (1974). *Social behavior: Its elementary forms.* New York: Harcourt Brace Jovanovich.

Hopkins, M. T. (1971). Patterns of self-destruction among the orthopedically disabled. *Rehabilitation and Resuscitation Practice Review, 3*, 5–16.

Hornig, C. D., & McNally, R. J. (1995). Panic disorder and suicide attempt. A reanalysis of data from the Epidemiologic Catchment Area study. *British Journal of Psychiatry, 167*, 76–79.

House, J. S. (1986). Occupational stress among men and women in the Tecumseh community health study. *Journal of Health and Social Behavior, 27*, 62–77.

Huffine, C. L. (1971). Equivocal single-auto traffic fatalities. *Life-Threatening Behavior, 2*, 83–95.

Humphry, D. (1996). *Final exit: The practicalities of sef-deliverance and assisted suicide for the dying.* New York: Bantam/Doubleday Dell.

Humphry, D., & Wickett, A. (1986). *The right to die: Understanding euthanasia.* New York: Harper & Row.

Hutchinson, G., Daisely, H., Simeon, D., Simmonds, V., Shetty, M., & Lynn, D. (1999). High rates of paraquat-induced suicide in Trinidad. *Suicide and Life-Threatening Behavior, 29*, 186–191.

Huxley, J., & Brandon, S. (1961). Partnership in transsexualism, part I: Paired and non-paired groups. *Archives of Sexual Behavior, 10*, 133–141.

Hyde, J. (1985). *Half the human experience: The psychology of women.* Lexington, MA: D. C. Heath.

Hyde, J. (1990). *Understanding human sexuality.* New York: McGraw-Hill.

Hyland, P. S. (1990). Family therapy in the hospital treatment of children and adolescents. *Bulletin of the Menniger Clinic, 54*, 48–63.

Iacono, W. G., & Beiser, M. (1992). Are males more likely than females to develop schizophrenia? *American Journal of Psychiatry, 149*, 1070–1074.

Iga, M. (1993). Japanese suicide. In A. A. Leenaars (Ed.), *Suicidology: Essays in honor of Edwin S. Shneidman.* Northvale, NJ: Jason Aronson.

Iga, M., & Tatai, K. (1975). Characterisitic of suicides and attitudes toward suicide in Japan. In N. L. Farberow (Ed.), *Suicide in different cultures*. Baltimore: University Park Press.

Igra, V., & Irwin, C. E. (1996). Theories of adolescent risk-taking behavior. In R. J. DiClimente, W. B. Hansen, & L. E. Ponton (Eds.), Handbook of adolescent health risk behavior. New York: Plenum.

Inamdar, S. C., Lewis, D. O., Siomopoulos, G., Shanok, S. S., & Lamela, M. (1982). Violent and suicidal behavior in psychotic adolescents. *American Journal of Psychiatry, 139*, 932–935.

Inamdar, S. C., Oberfield, R. A., & Darrell, E. B. (1983). A suicide by self-immolation: Psychological perspectives. *International Journal of Social Psychiatry, 29*, 130–133.

Inskip, H. M., Harris, E. C., & Barraclough, B. (1998). Lifetime risk of suicide for affective disorder, alcoholism and schizophrenia. *British Journal of Psychiatry, 172*, 35–37.

Institute of Medicine. (1994). *Reducing risk for mental disorder. Frontiers for preventive intervention research*. Washington, DC: National Academy Press.

Irwin, C. E., Jr., & Millstein, S. G. (1986). Biopsychosoical correlates of risk-taking behaviors during adolescence. *Journal of Adolescent Health Care, 7*, 82S–96S.

Irwin, C. E., Jr., & Ryan, S. A. (1989). Problem behaviors of adolescence. *Pediatrics in Review, 10*, 235–246.

Isaccson, G., & Rich, C. L. (1997). Depression, antidepressants, and suicide: Pharmacoepidemiological evidence for suicide prevention. In R. W. Maris, M. M. Silverman, & S. S. Canetto (Eds.), *Review of Suicidology, 1997*. New York: Guilford Press.

Isaccson, G., Bergman, U., & Rich, C. L (1994a). Antidepressants, depression, and suicide: An analysis of the San Diego study. *Journal of Affective Disorders, 32*, 277–286.

Isaccson, G., Boethius, G., & Bergman, U. (1992). Low level of antidepressant prescription for people who later commit suicide: 15 years of experience from a population-based drug database in Sweden. *Acta Psychiatrica Scandinavica, 85*, 444–448.

Isaccson, G., Holmgren, P., Wasserman, D., et al. (1994b). Use of antidepressants among people committing suicide in Sweden. *British Journal of Medicine, 308*, 500–509.

Isaccson, G., Rich, C. L., & Bergman, U. (1996). Antidepressants and suicide prevention [letter]. *American Journal of Psychiatry, 153*, 1659.

Isometsa, E. T., Henriksson, M. M., Aro, H. M., Heikkinen, M. E., Kuoppasalmi, K. I., & Lönnqvist, J. K. (1994). Suicide in major depression. *American Journal of Psychiatry, 151*, 530–536.

Isometsa, E. T., Henriksson, M. M., Heikkinen, M. E., Aro, H. M., Marttunen, M. J., Kuoppasalmi, K. I., & Lönnqvist, J. K. (1996). Suicide among subjects with personality disorders. *American Journal of Psychiatry, 153*, 667–673.

Jacobs, D. G. (Ed.). (1992). *Suicide and clinical practice*. Washington, DC: American Psychiatric Press.

Jacobs, D. G. (Ed.). (1999). *The Harvard Medical School guide to suicide assessment and intervention*. San Francisco: Jossey-Bass.

Jacobs, D. G., & Brown, H. N. (Eds.). (1989). *Suicide: Understanding and responding*. Madison, CT: International University Press.

Jacobs, J. (1967). Phenomenological study of suicide notes. *Social Problems, 15*, 60–72.

Jacobson, A. M. (1996, May). The psychological care of patients with insulin-dependent diabetes mellitus. *New England Journal of Medicine, 334*, 1249–1253.

Jacobson, R., Jackson, M., & Berkowitz, M. (1986). Self-incineration: A controlled comparison of inpatient suicide attempts. Clinical features and history of self-blame. *Psychological Medicine, 16*, 107–116.

Jail Suicide Mental Health Update. National Center on Institutions and Alternatives. Volumes 1–8. Mansfield, MA.

Jakubascik, J., & Hubschmid, T. (1995). Aggression and depression: A reciprocal relationship? *European Journal of Psychiatry, 8*, 69–80.

James, D., & Hawton, K. (1985). Overdosers: Explanations and attitudes in self-poisoners and significant others. *British Journal of Psychiatry, 146*, 481–485.

James, J. (1980). Self-destructive behavior and adaptive strategies in female prostitutes. In N. L. Farberow (Ed.), *The many faces of suicide: Indirect self-destructive behavior.* New York: McGraw-Hill.

Jamison, K. R. (1993). *Touched with fire: Manic–depressive illness and the artistic temperament.* New York: Free Press.

Jarvis, G. K., & Boldt, M. (1980). Suicide in the later years. *Essence, 4,* 145–158.

Jeffreys, M. D. W. (1952). Samsonic suicides: Or suicides of revenge among Africans. *African Studies, 11,* 118–122.

Jensen, K., Knudsen, L., Stenager, E., & Grant, I. (Eds.). (1989). *Mental disorders and cognitive deficits in multiple sclerosis.* London: John Libbey.

Jobes, D. A. (1995). The challenge and the promise of clinical suicidology. *Suicide and Life-Threatening Behavior, 25,* 437–449.

Jobes, D. A., & Berman, A. L. (1993). Suicide and malpractice liability: Assessing and revision policies, procedures, and practice in outpatient settings. *Professional Psychology: Research and Practice, 24,* 91–99.

Jobes, D. A., Luoma, J. B., Jacoby, A. M., & Mann, R. E. (1988). *Manual for the collaborative assessment and management of suicidality (CAMS).* Washington, DC: Catholic University of America.

Jobes, D. A., & Maltsberger, J. T. (1995). The hazards of treating suicidal patients. In M. B. Sussman (Ed.), *A perilous calling: The hazards of psychotherapy practice.* New York: Wiley.

Jobes, D. A., Berman, A. L., & Josselson, A. R. (1987). Improving the validity and reliability of medical–legal certifications on suicide. *Suicide and Life-Threatening Behavior, 17,* 310–325.

Jobes, D. A., Berman, A. L., O'Carroll, P. W., Eastgard, S., & Knickmeyer, S. (1996). The Kurt Cobain suicide crisis. *Suicide and Life-Threatening Behavior, 26,* 260–271.

Jobes, D. A., Casey, J. O., Berman, A. L., & Wright, D. G. (1991). Empirical criteria for the determination of suicide manner of death. *Journal of Forensic Sciences, 36,* 244–256.

Joffe, R. T., Offord, D., & Boyle, M. H. (1988). Ontario health study: Suicidal behavior in youths 12–16 years. *American Journal of Psychiatry, 145,* 1420–1423.

Johnson, J., Weissman, M. M., & Klerman, G. (1990). Panic disorder, comorbidity and suicide attempts. *Archives of General Psychiatry, 47,* 805–808.

Johnson, R. (1992). *Elementary statistics.* Belmont, CA: Wadsworth.

Jonas, A. M., & Hearron, A. E., Jr. (1996). Alprazolam and suicidal ideation: A meta-analysis of controlled trials in the treatment of depression. *Journal of Clinical Psychopharmacology, 16,* 208–211.

Jones, G. D. (1997). The role of drugs and alcohol in urban minority adolescent suicide attempts. *Death Studies, 21,* 189–202.

Judd, S., Jobes, D. A., Arnkoff, D. B., & Fenton, W. (1999). Negative countertransference and suicide: An empirical evaluation. Unpublished manuscript.

Juel, K., Mosbech, J., & Hansen, E. S. (1997). Mortality and cause of death among Danish physicians, 1973–1992. *Ugekr Laeger, 159,* 6512–6518.

Juel-Nielsen, N., & Videbech, T. (1970). A twin study of suicide. *Acta Geneticale Medicae et Gemellologiae, 19,* 307–310.

Juon, H. S. & Ensminger, M. E. (1997). Childhood, adolescent, and young adult predictors of suicidal behaviors: A prospective study of African Americans. *Journal of Child Psychology and Psychiatry and Allied Disciplines, 38,* 553–563.

Kachur, S. P., Potter, L. B., James, S. P., & Powell, K. I. (1995). *Suicide in the United States, 1980–1992.* [Violence Summary Series, No. 1.] Atlanta: Centers for Disease Control and Prevention, National Center for Injury Prevention and Control.

Kahana, E., Leibowitz, U., & Alter, M. (1971). Cerebral multiple sclerosis. *Neurology, 21,* 1179–1185.

Kalafat, J., & Underwood, M. (1989). Responding to at-risk students' attempts and completions. In J. Kalafat & M. Underwood (Eds.), *LIFELINES: A School Based Adolescent Suicide Response Program.* IA: Kendall/Hunt.

Kammer, J., & Sayles, T. (1987, August). Hidden bodies. *Fast Lane,* 33–35.

Kant, I. (1909). *Groundwork of the metaphysics of morals.* New York: Harper & Row.

Kaplan, A. G., & Klein, R. B. (1989). Women and suicide. In D. J. Jacobs (Ed.), *Suicide: Understanding and responding.* Madison, CT: International Universities Press.

Kaplan, D. M. (1992). A life of no surprises. *Readings, 7,* 4–6.

Kaplan, H. I., & Sadock, B. J. (1995). *Comprehensive textbook of psychiatry.* Baltimore: Williams & Wilkins.

Kapur, S., Mieczkowski, T., & Mann, J. J. (1992). Antidepressant medications and the relative risk of suicide attempt and suicide. *Journal of the American Medical Association, 268,* 3441–3445.

Kastenbaum, R. (1992). Death, suicide, and the older adult. In A. A. Leenaars, R. W. Maris, J. L. McIntosh, & J. Richman (Eds.), *Suicide and the older adult* (pp. 1–14). New York: Guilford Press.

Keeve, J. P. (1984). Physicians at risk: Some epidemiological considerations of alcoholism, drug abuse, and suicide. *Jounal of Occupational Medicine, 26,* 503–508.

Keller, M. B., Lavori, P. W., Klerman, G.L., et al. (1986). Low levels and lack of predictors of somatotherapy received by depressed patients. *Archives of General Psychiatry, 43,* 458–466.

Kellerman, A. L., & Reay, D. T. (1986). Protection or peril? An analysis of firearm-related deaths in the home. *New England Journal of Medicine, 314,* 1557–1560.

Kellerman, A. L., Rivara, F. P., Somes, G., & Reay, T. (1992). Suicide in the home in relation to gun ownership. *New England Jounal of Medicine, 327,* 467–472.

Kelly, M. J., Mufson, M. J., & Rogers, M. P. (1999). Medical settings and suicide. In D. G. Jacobs (Ed.), *The Harvard Medical School guide to suicide assessment and intervention.* San Francisco: Jossey-Bass.

Kendall, P. C., & Hammen, C. (1995). *Abnormal psychology.* Boston: Houghton Mifflin.

Kendall, R. E. (1983). Alcohol and suicide. *Substance and Alcohol Actions/Misuse, 4,* 121–127.

Kenney, E. M., & Krajewski, K. T. (1980). Hospital treatment of the adolescent suicidal patient. In M. S. McIntire & C. R. Angle (Eds.), *Suicide attempts in children and youth.* Hagerstown, MD: Harper & Row.

Kessler, R. C., O'Brien, D. G., Joseph, J. G., Ostrow, D. G., Phair, J. P., Chmiel, J. S., Wortman, C. B., & Emmons, C. (1988). Effects of HIV infection, perceived health, and clinical status on a cohort at risk for AIDS. *Social Science Medicine, 27,* 569–578.

Kessler, R. C, & Stripp, H. (1984). The impact of fictional television suicide stories on American fatalities. *American Journal of Sociology, 90,* 151–167.

Kessler, R. C, Downey, G., Milavsky, J. R., & Stripp, H. (1988). Clustering of teenage suicides after television news stories about suicide: A reconsideration. *American Journal of Psychiatry, 145,* 1379–1383.

Kessler, R. C, Downey, G., Milavsky, J. R., & Stripp, H. (1989). Network television news stories about suicide and short-term changes in total U.S. suicides. *Journal of Nervous and Mental Disease, 177,* 551–555.

Kety, S. S. (1990). Genetic factors in suicide: Family, twin, and adoption studies. In S. J. Blumenthal & D. J. Kupfer (Eds.), *Suicide over the life cycle* (pp. 127–133). Washington, DC: American Psychiatric Press.

Kevorkian, J. (1991). *Prescription medicine: The goodness of planned death.* Buffalo, NY: Prometheus Books.

Khuri, R., & Akiskal, H. S. (1983). Suicide prevention: The necessity of treating contributory psychiatric disorders. *Psychiatric Clinics of North America, 6,* 193–207.

King, C. A. (1997). Suicidal behavior in adolescence. In R. W. Maris, M. M. Silverman, & S. S. Canetto (Eds.), *Review of suicidology.* New York: Guilford Press.

King, C. A., Akiyama, M. M., & Elling, K. A. (1996). Self-perceived competencies and depression among middle school students in Japan and the United States. *Journal of Early Adolescence, 16,* 192–210.

King, C. A., Hill, E. M., Naylor, M. W., Evans, T., Shain, B. (1993a). Alcohol consumption in relation to other predictors of suicidality among adolescent inpatient girls. *Journal of American Academy of Child Psychiatry, 32,* 82–88.

King, C. A., Naylor, M. W., Segal, H. G., Evans, T., & Shain, B. N. (1993b). Global self-worth, specific self-perception of competency, and depression in adolescents. *Journal of American Academy of Child Psychiatry, 32,* 745–752.

King, H. E. (1987). *Pragmatic factors in dealing with families of suicidal clients: Issues for clinicians: Suicide in the Family.* Symposium conducted at the convention of the American Psychological Association, New York.

Klatsky, A. L., & Armstrong, M. A. (1993). Alcohol use, other traits, and risk of unnatural death. *Alcoholism: Clinical and Experimental Research, 17,* 1156–1162.

Klausner, S. Z. (Ed.). (1968). *Why men take chances: Studies in stress-seeking.* Garden City, NY: Doubleday/Anchor.

Kleespies, P. M., Penk, W. E., & Forsyth, J. P. (1993). The stress of patient suicidal behavior during clinical training: Incidence, impact, and recovery. *Professional Psychology: Research and Practice, 24,* 293–303.

Kleepsies, P. M., Smith, M. R., & Becker, B. R. (1990). Interns as patient suicide survivors: Incidence, impact, and recovery. *Professional Psychology: Research and Practice, 21,* 257–263.

Klein, M. (1948). A contribution to the psychogenesis of manic–depressive states. In M. Klein (Ed.), *Contributions to psycho-analysis, 1921–1945.* London: Hogarth Press.

Knop, J., & Fischer, A. (1981). Duodenal ulcer, suicide, psychopathology and alcoholism. *Acta Psychiatry Scandinavica, 63,* 346–355.

Korn, M. L., Kotler, M., Macho, A., Botsis, A. J., Grosz, D., Chen, C., Plutchik, R., Brown, S. L., & van Praag, H. M. (1992). Suicide and violence associated with panic attacks. *Biological Psychiatry, 31,* 607–612.

Korn, M. L., Plutchik, R. & van Praag, H. M. (1997)). Panic-associated suicidal and aggressive ideation and behavior. *Journal of Psychiatric Research, 31,* 481–487.

Korndorfer, S., Krahn, L. E., Lucas, A. R., Suman, V. J., Melton, III, J. (1999). *Mortality in anorexia nervosa: A 60-year follow-up.* Paper presented at the meeting of the American Psychiatric Association, Washington, DC.

Kosky, R., Silburn, S., & Zubrick, S. R. (1990). Are children and adolescents who have suicidal thoughts different from those who attempt suicide? *Journal of Nervous and Mental Disease. 178*(1), 38–43.

Kovacs, M., Beck, A. T., & Weisman, A. (1975, Summer). Hopelessness: An indicator of suicide risk. *Suicide, 5,* 98–103.

Kovacs, M., Goldston, D., & Gatsonis, D. (1993). suicidal behaviors and childhood-onset depressive disorders: A longitudinal investigation. *Journal of American Academy of Child Psychiatry, 32,* 8–20.

Kowalski, G. S., Faupel C., & Starr, P. D. (1987). Urbanism and suicide: A study of American counties. *Social Forces, 66,* 85–101.

Kposowa, A., Breault, K. D., & Singh G. K. (1995). White male suicide in the U.S. *Social Forces, 74,* 315–323.

Kramer, P. D. (1993). *Listening to Prozac.* New York: Viking.

Kramer-Ginsberg, E., Greenwald, B. S., Aisen, P. S., et al. (1989). Hypochondriasis in the elderly depressed. *Journal of the American Geriatrics Society, 37,* 507–510.

Kreitman, N. (1976). The coal gas story: United Kingdom suicide rates, 1960–1971. *British Journal of Preventative and Social Medicine, 30,* 86–93.(Ch3,21)

Kreitman, N. (Ed.). (1977). *Parasuicide.* New York: Wiley.

Kreitman, N., & Foster, J. (1991). The construction and selection of predictionscales, with special reference to parasuicide. *British Journal of Psychiatry, 159,* 185–192.

Kreitman, N., Carstairs, V., & Duffy, J. (1991). Association of age and social class with suicide among men in Great Britain. *Journal of Epidemiology and Community Health, 45,* 195–202.

Krieger, M. J., McAnnich, J. W., & Weimer, S. R. (1980, August). *Self-inflicted genital injuries.* Paper presented at the American Psychological Association, Montreal.

Krueger, D. W., & Hutcherson, R. (1978). Suicide attempts by rock climbing falls. *Suicide and Life-Threatening Behavior, 8,* 41–45.

Kua, E. H., & Tsoi, W. F. (1985). Suicide in the Island of Singapore. *Acta Psychiatrica Scandinavica, 71,* 227–229.

Kübler-Ross, E. (1969). *On death and dying.* New York: Macmillan.

Kurdek, L. A., & Siesky, G. (1990). The nature and correlates of psychological adjustment in gay men with AIDS-related conditions. *Journal of Applied Social Psychology, 20,* 846–860.

Kushner, H. I. (1989). *Self-destruction in the promised land.* New Brunswick, NJ: Rutgers University Press.

Kushner, H. I. (1991). *American suicide: A psychocultural exploration.* New Brunswick, NJ: Rutger University Press.

La Free, G., Drass, K., & O'Day, P. (1992). Race and crime in postwar America. *Criminology, 30,* 157–188.

Labovitz, S., & Hagedorn, R. (1971). An analysis of suicide rates among occupational categories. *Sociological Inquiry, 41,* 67–72.

Lalli, M., & Turner, S. (1968). Suicide and homicide: A comparative analysis by race and occupational level. *Journal of Criminal Law, Criminology, and Police Science, 59,* 191–200.

Lamb, F., & Dunne-Maxim, K. (1987). Postvention in schools: Policy and process. In E. J. Dunne, J. L. McIntosh, & K. Dunne-Maxim (Eds.), *Suicide and its aftermath: Understanding and counseling the survivors.* New York: Norton.

Lampert, D., Bourque, L., & Kraus, J. (1984). Occupational status and suicide. *Suicide and Life-Threatening Behavior, 14,* 254–269.

Landau-Stanton, J., & Stanton, D. (1985). Treating suicidal adolescents and their families. In M. P. Mirkin & S. L. Koman (Eds.), *Handbook of adolescents and family therapy.* New York: Gardner Press.

Langevin, R., Paitich, D., & Steiner, B. (1977). The clinical profile of male transsexuals living as females vs. those living as males. *Archives of Sexual Behavior, 6,* 143–154.

Leckman, J. F., Sholomskas, D., Thompson, D., Belanger, A., & Weissman, M. (1982). Best estimate of lifetime diagnosis: A methodological study. *Archives of General Psychiatry, 39,* 879–883.

Lecrubier, Y. (1998). The impact of comorbidity on the treatment of panic disorder. *Journal of Clinical Psychiatry, 59,* 11–14.

Leenaars, A. A. (1988). *Suicide notes: Predictive clues and patterns.* New York: Human Sciences Press.

Leenaars, A. A. (1991). *Life-span perspectives of suicide: Time-lines in the suicide process.* New York: Plenum.

Leenaars, A. A. (1992). Suicide notes, communications, and ideation. In R. W. Maris, A. L. Berman, J. T. Maltsberger, & R. I. Yufit (Eds.), *Assessment and prediction of suicide.* New York: Guilford Press.

Leenaars, A. A. (1996). Suicide: A multidimensional malaise. *Suicide and Life-Threatening Behavior, 26,* 221–236.

Leenars, A. A., Berman, A. L., Cantor, P., Litman, R. L., & Maris, R. W. (Eds.) (1993). *Suicidology: Essays in honor of Edwin S. Shneidman.* Northvale, NJ: Jason Aronson.

Leenaars, A. A., Maris, R. W., McIntosh, J. L., & Richman, J. (Eds.). (1992). *Suicide and the older adult.* New York: Guilford Press.

Leenaars, A. A., Maris, R. W., & Takahashi, Y. (Eds.). (1997). *Suicide: Individual, cultural, international perspectives.* New York: Guilford Press.

Leenaars, A. A., Wenckstern, S., & Lester, D. (1999). An examination of the suicide notes of alcoholics. Submitted for publication.

Lehman, D., Ellard, J., & Wortman, C. (1986). Social support for the bereaved: Recipients and providers' perspectives on what is helpful. *Journal of Consulting and Clinical Psychology, 54,* 438–446.

Leighton, A. H., & Hughes, C. C. (1955). Notes on Eskimo patterns of suicide. *Southwestern Journal of Anthropology, 11,* 327–338.

Lemp, G. F., Jones, M., Kellogg, T. A., Nieri, G. N., Anderson, L., Withum, D., & Katz, M. (1995). HIV seroprevalence and risk behaviors among lesbians and bisexual women in San Francisco and Berkeley, California. *American Journal of Public Health, 85,* 1449–1552.

Lenski, G. E., Nolan, P., & Lenski, J. (1995). *Human societies: An introduction to macrosociology.* New York: McGraw-Hill.

Leon, A. C., Keller, M. B., Warshaw, M. G., Mueller, T. I., Solomon, D. A., Coryell, W., & Endicott,

J. (1999). Prospective study of fluoxetine treatment and suicidal behavior in affectively ill subjects. *American Journal of Psychiatry, 156,* 195–201.

Leonard, C. V. (1967). *Understanding and preventing suicide.* Springfield, IL: Charles C. Thomas.

Lepine, J. P., Chigon, J. M., & Teherani, M. (1993). Suicide attempts in patients with panic disorder. *Archives of General Psychiatry, 50,* 144–149.

Lesage, A. D., Boyer, R., Grunberg, F., Vanier, C., Morissette, R., Menard-Buteau, C., & Loyer, M. (1994). Suicide and mental disorders: A case-control study of young men. *American Journal of Psychiatry, 151,* 1063–1068.

Lesham, A., & Lesham, Y. (1976). Attitudes of college students toward men and women who commit suicidal acts. *Dissertation Abstracts International, 37,* 7042A.

Lester, D. (1971). Need for affiliation in suicide notes. *Perceptual and Motor Skills, 33*(2), 550.

Lester, D. (1983). Preventive effect of strict handgun control laws on suicide rates [letter]. *American Journal of Psychiatry, 140,* 1259.

Lester, D. (1984). Suicide. In C. Widom (Ed.), *Sex roles and psychopathology.* New York: Plenum.

Lester, D. (1988a). The perception of different methods of suicide. *Journal of General Psychology, 115,* 215–217.

Lester, D. (1988b). Why do people choose particular methods of suicide? *Activitas Nervosa Superior, 30,* 312–314.

Lester, D. (1988c). What does the study of simulated suicide notes tell us? *Psychological Reports, 62,* 962.

Lester, D. (1988d). *The biochemical basis of suicide.* Springfield, IL: Charles C. Thomas.

Lester, D. (1988e). Suicide and the menstrual cycle. In D. Lester (Ed.), *Why women kill themselves.* Springfield, IL: Charles C. Thomas.

Lester, D. (1989a). Experience of parental loss and later suicide. *Acta Psychiatrica Scandinavica, 79,* 450–452.

Lester, D. (1990). Suicide rates around the world: An IASP project. *Crisis, 11,* 82–84.

Lester, D. (1991). Suicide across the life span: A look at international trends. In A. A. Leenaars (Ed.), *Life span perspectives of suicide.* New York: Plenum.

Lester, D. (1992a). *Why people kill themselves.* Springfield, IL: Charles C. Thomas.

Lester, D. (1992b). Alcoholism and drug abuse. In R. Maris, A. Berman, T. Maltsberger, & R. Yufit (Eds.), *Assessment and prediction of suicide.* New York: Guilford Press.

Lester, D. (1992c). Alcohol consumption and personal violence in Australia. *Drug and Alcohol Dependence, 31,* 15–17.

Lester, D. (1992d). The dexamethasone suppression test as an indicator of suicide. *Pharmacopsychiatry, 25,* 265–270.

Lester, D. (1992e). Suicide and the writer. In *Proceedings of the Pavese society, 92.*

Lester, D. (1993a). War and alcohol use. *Psychological Reports, 72,* 1282.

Lester, D. (1993b). Restricting the availability of alcohol and rates of personal violence (suicide and homicide). *Drug and Alcohol Dependence, 31,* 215–217.

Lester, D. (1993c). A study of police suicide in New York City, 1934–1939. *Psychological Reports, 73,* 1395–1398.

Lester, D. (1993d). Reliability of judging genuine and simulated suicide notes. *Perceptual and Motor Skills, 77,* 882.

Lester, D. (1993e). Suicidal behavior in bipolar and unipolar affective disorders: A meta-analysis. *Journal of Affective Disorders, 27,* 117–121.

Lester, D. (1994a). A comparison of 15 theories of suicide. *Suicide and Life-Threatening Behavior, 24,* 80–88.

Lester, D. (Ed.). (1994b). *Emile Durkheim, Le Suicide: One Hundred Years Later.* Philadelphia: Charles Press.

Lester, D. (1995b). The concentration of neurotransmitter metabolites in the cerebrospinal fluid of suicidal individuals. *Pharmacopsychiatry, 28,* 45–50.

Lester, D. (1997a). *Suicide in American Indians.* Commack, NY: Nova Science.

Lester, D. (1997b). The role of shame in suicide. *Suicide and Life-Threatening Behavior, 27,* 352–361.

Lester, D. (1998). The association of alcohol use, abuse and treatment with suicide and homicide rates. *Italian Journal of Suicidology, 8,* 23–26.

Lester, D., & Beck, A. T. (1976). Early loss as a possible sensitizer to later loss in attempted suicides. *Psychological Reports, 39,* 121–122.

Lester, D., & Frank, M. L. (1989). The use of motor vehicle exhaust for suicide and the availability of cars. *Acta Psychiatrica Scandinavica, 79,* 238–240.

Lester, D., & Heim, N. (1992). Sex differences in suicide notes. *Perceptual and Motor Skills, 75,* 582.

Lester, D., & Jason, D. (1989). Suicides at the casino. *Psychological Reports, 64,* 337–338.

Lester, D., & Leenaars, A. A. (1988). The moral justification of suicide in suicide notes. *Psychological Reports, 63,* 106.

Lester, D., & Murrell, M. E. (1980). The influence of gun control laws on suicidal behavior. *American Journal of Psychiatry, 137,* 121–122.

Lester, D., & Yang, B. (1997a). *The economy and suicide.* Commack, NY: Nova Science.

Lester, D., & Yang, B. (1997b). *Unemployment and suicide: Linear or curvilinear relationship?* Paper presented at the annual meetings of the American Association of Suicidology, Memphis, TN.

Lester, D., & Yang, B. (1998). *Suicide and homicide in the 20th century.* Commack, NY: Nova Science.

Lester, D., Seiden, R. H., & Tauber, R. K. (1990). Menninger's motives for suicide in genuine, simulated, and hoax suicide notes. *Perceptual and Motor Skills, 71,* 248.

Lester, G., & Lester, D. (1971). *Suicide: The gamble with death.* Englewood Cliffs, NJ: Prentice-Hall.

Lettieri, D. J. (1974). Suicidal death prediction scales. In A. T. Beck, H. L. P. Resnik, & D. J. Lettieri (Eds.), *The prediction of suicide.* Bowie, MD: Charles Press.

Leutwyler, K. (1995). Depression's double standard: Clues emerge as to why women have higher rates of depression. *Scientific American, 272*(6), 23, 26.

Levenson, M. (1974). Cognitive Characteristics of Suicide Risk. In C. Neuringer (Ed.), *Psychological assessment of suicide risk.* Springfield, IL: Charles C. Thomas.

Levinson, D. J. (1978). *The seasons of a man's life.* New York: Knopf.

Levy, N. B. (1979). Psychological problems of the patient on hemodialysis and their treatment. *Psychotherapy and Psychosomatics, 31,* 260–266.

Lewinsohn, P. M., Rohde, P., & Seeley, J. R. (1994). Psychosocial risk factors for future adolescent suicide attempts. *Journal of Consulting and Clinical Psychology, 62,* 297–305.

Lewinsohn, P. M., Rohde, P., & Seeley, J. R. (1995). Adolescent psychopathology: III. The clinical consequences of comorbidity. *Psychiatry, 34,* 510–519.

Lewis, W., Lee, A. B., & Grantham, S. A. (1965). Jumpers syndrome. *Journal of Trauma, 5,* 812–818.

Li, F. (1971). Suicide among chemists. *Archives of Environmental Health,* 518–520.

Lidberg, L., Äsberg, M., & Sundquist-Stenmann, J. (1984, October 20). 5-hydroxyindoleacetic acid levels in attempted suicides who have killed their children. *The Lancet, 2,* 928.

Lidberg, L., Tuck, J. R., Äsberg, M., Scalia-Tomba, G. P., & Bertilsson, L. (1985). Homicide, suicide, and CSF 5-HIAA. *Acta Psychiatrica Scandinavica, 71,* 230–236.

Lifton, R. J. (1983). The broken connection: On death and the continuity of life. New York: Basic Books.

Lindekilde, K., & Wang, A. G. (1985). Train suicide in the county of Fyn. *Acta Psychiatrica Scandinavia, 72,* 150–154.

Lindeman, S., Laara, E., & Lönnqvist, J. (1997). Medical surveillance often precedes suicide among female physicians in Finland. *Journal of Occupational and Environmental Medicine, 39,* 1115–1117.

Linehan, M. M. (1973). Suicide and attempted suicide: A study of perceived sex differences. *Perceptual and Motor Skills, 37,* 31–34.

Linehan, M. M. (1986). Suicide people: One population or two? In J. J. Mann & M. Stankley (Eds.), *Psychobiology of suicidal behavior.* New York: New York Academy of Sciences.

Linehan, M. M. (1993). *Cognitive-behavioral therapy of borderline personality disorder.* New York: Guilford Press.

Linehan, M. M. (1997). Behavioral treatment of suicidal behaviors: Definitional obfuscation and treatment outcomes. *Annals of the New York Academy of Sciences, 836,* 302–328.

Linehan, M. M. (1998). Is anything effective for reducing suicidal behavior? In J. L. McIntosh (Ed.).

Proceedings of the 31st Annual Conference of the American Association of Suicidology. Washington, DC: American Association of Suicidology.

Linehan, M. M., & Laffaw, J. A. (1982). Suicidal behaviors among clients of an outpatient clinic versus the general population. *Suicide and Life-Threatening Behavior, 12,* 234–239.

Linehan, M. M., Goodstein, J. L., Neilsen, S. L., & Chiles, J. K. (1983). Reasons for staying alive when you are thinking about killing yourself: The reasons for living inventory. *Journal of Consulting and Clinical Psychiatry, 51,* 276–286.

Linkowski, P., deMaertelaer, F., & Mendlewicz, J. (1985). Suicidal behavior in major depressive illness. *Acta Psychiatrica Scandinavica, 72,* 233–238.

Linnoila, M., & Virkkunen, M. (1992). Aggression, suicidality and serotonin. *Journal of Clinical Psychiatry, 53*(Suppl.), 46–51.

Linnoila, M., Erwin, D., Ramm, D., Cleveland, P., & Brendle, A. (1980). Effects of alcohol on psychomotor performance of women. *Alcoholism, 4,* 302–305.

Linnoila, M., Virkkunen, M., Scheinin, M., Nuutila, A., Rimon, R., & Goodwin, F. K. (1983). Low cerebrospinal fluid 5-hydroxyindoleacetic acid concentration differentiates impulsive from nonimpulsive violent behavior. *Life Sciences, 33,* 2609–2614.

Linsky, A. S., Bachman, R., & Straus, M. A. (1995). *Stress, culture, and aggression.* New Haven, CT: Yale University Press.

Litman, R. E. (1967). Sigmund Freud on suicide. In E. Shneidman (Ed.), *Essays in self-destruction.* New York: Science House.

Litman, R. E. (1980). Psychodynamics of indirect self-destructive behavior. In N. L. Farberow (Ed.), *The many faces of suicide: Indirect self-destructive behavior.* New York: McGraw Hill.

Litman, R. E. (1982). Hospital suicides: Lawsuits and standards. *Suicide and Life-Threatening Behavior, 12,* 212–220.

Litman, R. E. (1988). Psychological autopsies, mental illness, and intention to suicide. In J. L. Nolan (Ed.), *The suicide case: Investigation and trial of insurance claims.* Chicago: American Bar Association.

Litman, R. E. (1989). 500 psychological autopsies. *Journal of Forensic Sciences, 34,* 638–646.

Litman, R. E. (1992). Predicting and preventing hospital and clinic suicides. In R. W. Maris, A. L. Berman, J. T. Maltsberger, & R. I. Yufit (Eds.), *Assessment and prediction of suicide.* New York: Guilford Press.

Litman, R. E. (1996). Sigmund Freud on suicide. In J. T. Maltsberger & M. J. Goldblatt (Eds.), *Essential papers on suicide. Essential papers in psychoanalysis.* New York: New York University Press.

Litman, R. E., & Tabachnick, N. (1967). Fatal one-car accidents. *Psychoanalytic Quarterly, 36,* 248–259.

Litman, R. E., Curphey, T., Shneidman, E. S., Farberow, N. L., & Tabachnick, N. (1963). The psychological autopsy of equivocal deaths. *Journal of the American Medical Association, 184,* 924–929.

Litman, R. E., Curphey, T., Shneidman, E. S., Farberow, N. L., & Tabachnick, N. (1963). Investigations of equivocal suicides. *Journal of the American Medical Association, 184,* 924–929. (ch. 13)

Litt, I., Cuskey, W., & Rudd, S. (1983). Emergency room evaluation of the adolescent at risk for suicide: Compliance with follow-up. *Journal of Adolescent Health Care, 4,* 106–108.

Long, D. D., & Miller, B. J. (1991). Suicidal tendency and multiple sclerosis. *Health and Social Work, 16,* 106–109.

Lopez-Ibor, J. J., & Carrasco, J. L. (1993). Aggression: Clinical status and future research. [Editorial]. *International Monitor.*

Louhivuori, K. A., & Hakama, M. (1979). Risk of suicide among cancer patients. *American Journal of Epidemiology, 109,* 59–65.

Lowry, M. R. (1979). Frequency of depressive disorder in patients entering home dialysis. *Journal of Nervous and Mental Disorders, 167,* 199–204.

Lucas, G. M., Hutton, J. E., & Lim, R. C. (1981). *Journal of Trauma, 21,* 612–618.

Mack, J. E., & Hickler, H. (1981). *Vivienne: The life and suicide of an adolescent girl.* Boston: Little, Brown.

Mackay, A. (1979). Self-poisoning: A complication of epilepsy. *British Journal of Psychiatry, 134,* 277–282.

Mackenzie, T. B., & Popkin, M. K. (1990). Medical illness and suicide. In S. J. Blumenthal & D. J. Kupfer (Eds.), *Suicide over the life cycle: Risk factors, assessment, and treatment of suicidal patients*. Washington, DC: American Psychiatric Press.

Maguen, S. (1991). Teen suicide. *The Advocate, 586,* 40–47.

Makela, P. (1996). Alcohol consumption and suicide mortality by age among Finnish men, 1950–1991. *Addiction, 91,* 101–112.

Malkin, M. J., & Rabinowitz, E. (1998, July). Sensation seeking and high-risk recreation. *Park and Recreation,* pp. 34–45.

Malmquist, D. (1983). The functioning of self-esteen in childhood depression. In J. E. Mack & S. L. Ablon (Eds.), *The development and sustaining of self-esteem in childhood*. New York: International Universities Press.

Malone, K. (1997). Pharmacotherapy of affectively ill suicidal patients. *Psychiatric Clinics of North America, 20,* 613–625.

Malone, K., Haas, G., Sweeney, J., & Mann, J. (1995). Major depression and the risk of attempted suicide. *Journal of Affective Disorders, 34,* 173–185.

Maltsberger, J. T. (1992). The psychodynamic formulation: an aid in assessing suicide risk. In R. W. Maris, A. L. Berman, J. T. Maltsberger, & R. I. Yufit (Eds.), *Assessment and prediction of suicide*. New York: Guilford Press.

Maltsberger, J. T. (1992). The psychodynamic formulation: An aid in assesseing suicide risk. In R. W. Maris, A. L. Berman, J. T. Maltsberger, & R. I. Yufit (Eds.), *The Assessment and prediction of suicide* (pp. 25–49). New York: Guilford Press.

Maltsberger, J. T. (1998). Pass consultation: Robert Salter: Attempted suicide by jumping from a high bridge. *Suicide and Life-Threatening Behavior, 28,* 226–333.

Maltsberger, J. T., & Buie, D. H. (1980). The devices of suicide: Revenge, riddance, and rebirth. *International Review of Psychoanalysis, 7,* 61–72.

Maltsberger, J. T., & Goldblatt, M. J. (1996). *Essential papers on suicide*. New York: New York University Press.

Mann, J. J. (1995). Violence and aggression. In F. E. Bloom & D. J. Kupfer (Eds.), *Psychopharmacology: The fourth generation of progress*. New York: Raven Press.

Mann, J. J. (1998). The neurobiology of suicide. *Nature Medicine, 4,* 25–30.

Mann, J. J., & Kapur, S. (1991). The emergence of suicidal ideation and behavior during antidepressant pharmacotherapy. *Archives of General Psychiatry, 48,* 1027–1033.

Mann, J. J., Goodwin, F. K, O'Brien, C. P., & Robinson, D. S. (1993). Suicidal behavior and psychotropic medication: accepted as a consensus statement by the ACNP council, March 2 1992. *Neuropsychopharmacology, 8,* 177–183.

Mann, J. J., McBride, P. A., Anderson, G. M., & Mieczkowski, T. A. (1992). Platelet and whole blood serotonin content in depressed inpatients: Correlations with acute and life-time psychopathology. *Biological Psychiatry, 32,* 243–257.

Mann, J. J., Stanley, M., McBride, P. A., & McEwen, B. (1986). Increased serotonin and beta-adrenergic receptor binding in the frontal cortices of suicide victims. *Archives of General Psychiatry, 43,* 954–959.

Mann, J. J., Waternaux, C., Haas, G. L., & Malone, K. M. (1999). Toward a clinical model of suicidal behavior in psychiatric patients. *American Journal of Psychiatry, 156,* 181–189.

Maris, R. W. (1961). *Ludwig Wittgenstein's philosophical investigations and the private language argument*. Unpublished master's thesis, University of Illinois (Urbana).

Maris, R. W. (1967). Suicide, status, and mobility in Chicago. *Social Forces, 46,* 246–256.

Maris, R. W. (1969). *Social forces in urban suicide*. Homewood, IL: Dorsey Press.

Maris, R. W. (1970). The logical adequacy of Homans's social theory. *American Sociological Review, 35,* 1069–1081.

Maris, R. W. (1981). *Pathways to suicide: A survey of self-destructive behaviors*. Baltimore: Johns Hopkins University Press.

Maris, R. W. (1982a). Rational suicide: An impoverished self-transformation. *Suicide and Life-Threatening Behavior, 12,* 3–16.

Maris, R. W. (1982b). A book review of Jo Roman, *Exit house. Suicide and Life-Threatening Behavior, 12,* 124–127.

Maris, R. W. (1985). The adolescent suicide problem. *Suicide and Life-Threatening Behavior, 15,* 91–109.

Maris, R. W. (1986). Basic issues in suicide prevention. *Suicide and Life-Threatening Behavior, 16,* 326–334.

Maris, R. W. (1988). *Social problems.* Belmont, CA: Wadsworth.

Maris, R. W. (1989). The social relations of suicide. In D. Jacobs & H. N. Brown (Eds.), *Suicide: Understanding and responding.* Madison, CT: International Universities Press.

Maris, R. W. (1991). Suicide. In R. Dulbecco (Ed.), *Encyclopedia of human biology.* New York: Academic Press.

Maris, R. W. (1992a). Suicide. In E. F. Borgatta (Ed.), *Encyclopedia of sociology.* New York: Macmillan.

Maris, R. W. (1992b). Forensic suicidology: Litigation of suicide cases. In B. Bongar (Ed.), *Suicide: Guidelines for assessment, management, and treatment.* New York: Oxford University Press.

Maris, R. W. (1992c). A book review of Derek Humphry, *Final exit. Suicide and Life-Threatening Behavior, 22,* 514–516.

Maris, R. W. (1992d). How are suicides different? In R. W. Maris, A. L. Berman, J. T. Maltsberger, & R. I. Yufit (Eds.), *The Assessment and prediction of suicide* (pp. 65–87). New York: Guilford Press.

Maris, R. W. (1992e). The relation of nonfatal suicide attempts to completed suicides. In R. W. Maris, A. L. Berman, J. T. Maltsberger, & R. I. Yufit (Eds.), *The Assessment and prediction of suicide* (pp. 362–380). New York: Guilford Press.

Maris, R. W. (1992f). Overview of the study of suicide assessment and prediction. In R. W. Maris, A. L. Berman, J. T. Maltsberger, & R. I. Yufit (Eds.), *The Assessment and prediction of suicide* (pp. 3–22). New York: Guilford Press.

Maris, R. W. (1993). The evolution of suicidology. In A. A. Leenaars (Ed.), *Suicidology: Essays in honor of Edwin Shneidman.* Northvale, NJ: Jason Aronson.

Maris, R. W. (1997). Social and familiar risk factors in suicidal behavior. In J. J. Mann (Ed.), *Psychiatric Clinics of North America: Suicide.* Philadelphia: Saunders.

Maris, R. W., & Connor, H. (1973). Do crisis services work: a follow-up of a psychiatric outpatient sample? *Journal of Health and Social Behavior, 14,* 311–322.

Maris, R. W., Berman, A. L., & Maltsberger, J. T. (1992). Summary and conclusions: What have we learned about suicide assessment and prediction? In R. W. Maris, A. L. Berman, J. T. Maltsberger, & R. I. Yufit (Eds.), *Assessment and prediction of suicide* (pp. 640–672). New York: Guilford Press.

Maris, R. W., Berman, A. L., Maltsberger, J. T., & Yufit, R. I. (Eds.). (1992). *Assessment and prediction of suicide.* New York: Guilford Press.

Maris, R. W., Silverman, M. M., & Canetto, S. S. (Eds.). (1997). *Review of suicidology, 1997.* New York: Guilford Press.

Marks, A. (1977). Sex differences and their effect upon cultural evaluations of methods of self-destruction. *Omega, 8,* 65–70.

Marks, A. (1980). Socioeconomic status and suicide in the state of Washington, 1950–1971. *Psychological Reports, 46,* 924–926.

Marks, A., & Abernathy, T. (1974). Towards a sociocultural perspective on means of self-destruction. *Life-Threatening Behavior, 4,* 3–17.

Markush, R. E., & Bartolucci, A. A. (1984). Firearms and suicide in the United States. *American Journal of Public Health, 74,* 123–127.

Marsella, A. J., Hirschfeld, R. M. A., & Katz, M. M. (1987). *The measurement of depression.* New York: Guilford Press.

Marshall, J. R., Burnett, W., & Brasure, J. (1983). On precipitating factors: Cancer as a cause of suicide. *Suicide and Life-Threatening Behavior, 13,* 15–27.

Marshall, J., & Hodge, R. (1981). Durkheim and Pierce on suicide and economic change. *Social Science Research, 10,* 101–114.

Martin, G., & Koo, L. (1996). Celebrity suicide: Did the death of Kurt Cobain influence young suicides in Australia? *Archives of Suicide Reasearch, 3*(3), 187–198.

Martin, R. L., Cloninger, C. R., Guze, S. B. & Clayton, P. J. (1985). Mortality in a follow-up of 500 psychiatric outpatients. *Archives of General Psychiatry, 42,* 58–66.

Marttunen, M. J., Aro, H. M., Henriksson, M. M., & Lönnqvist, J. K. (1994). Psychosocial stressors more common in adolescent suicides with alcohol abuse compared with depressive adolescent suicides. *Journal of the American Academy of Child and Adolescent Psychiatry, 33,* 490–497.

Marzuk, P. M. (1994). Suicide and terminal illness. *Death Studies, 18,* 497–512.

Marzuk, P. M., & Mann, J. J. (1988). Suicide and substance abuse. *Psychiatric Annals, 18,* 639–644.

Marzuk, P. M., Leon, A. C., Tardiff, K., & Morgan, E. B. (1992a). The effect of access to lethal methods of injury on suicide rates. *Archives of General Psychiatry, 49,* 451–458.

Marzuk, P. M., Tardiff, K., Leon, A. D., et al. (1996). Dr. Marzuk and colleagues reply (letter). *American Journal of Psychiatry, 153,* 1659.

Marzuk, P. M., Tardiff, K., Leon, A. C., Stajic, M., Morgan, E. B., & Mann, J. J. (1992b). Prevalence of cocaine use among residents of New York City who committed suicide during a one-year period. *American Journal of Psychiatry, 149,* 371–375.

Marzuk, P. M., Tardiff, K., Smyth, D., Stajic, M., & Leon, A. C. (1992c). Cocaine use, risk-taking, and fatal Russian roulette. *Journal of the American Medical Association, 267,* 2635–2637.

Marzuk, P. M., Tierney, H., Tardiff, K., Gross, E. M., Morgan, E. B., Hsu, M., Mann, J. (1988). Increased risk of suicide in persons with AIDS. *Journal of the American Medical Association, 259,* 1333–1337.

Maslow, A. H. (1963). *Motivation and personality.* New York: Harper & Row.

Massie, M. J., Holland, J. C., & Glass, E. (1983). Delirium in terminally ill cancer patients. *American Journal of Psychiatry, 140,* 1048–1050.

Matthews, W. S., & Barabas, G. (1981). Suicide and epilepsy: A review of the literature. *Psychosomatics, 22,* 515–524.

Mattson, A., Seese, L. R., & Hawkins, J. W. (1969). Suicidal behavior as a child psychiatric emergency. *Archives of General Psychiatry, 20,* 100–109.

Mauk, G. W., Gibson, D. G., & Rodgers, P. L. (1994). Suicide postvention with adolescents: School consultation practices and issues. *Education and Treatment of Children, 17,* 468–483.

Mausner, J. S., & Bahn, A. K. (1985). *Epidemiology: An introductory text.* Philadelphia: Saunders.

McCormick, R. A., Russo, A. M. Ramirez, L. F., & Tabor, J. I. (1984). Affective disorders among pathological gamblers seeking treatment. *American Journal of Psychiatry, 141,* 215–218.

McDowell, C. P., Rothberg, J. M., & Kushes, R. J. (1994). Witnessed suicides. *Suicide and Life-Threatening Behavior, 24,* 213–223.

McIntosh, J. L. (1985). *Research on suicide: A bibliography.* Westport, CT: Greenwood Press.

McIntosh, J. L. (1987). Survivor family relationships: Literature review. In E. J. Dunne, J. L. McIntosh, & K. Dunne-Maxim (Eds.), *Suicide and its aftermath: Understanding and counseling the survivors.* New York: Norton.

McIntosh, J. L. (1992). Methods of suicide. In R. W. Maris, A. L. Berman, J. T. Maltsberger, & R. I. Yufit (Eds.), *Assessment and prediction of suicide* (pp. 381–417). New York: Guilford Press.

McIntosh, J. L. (1993). Control group studies of suicide survivors: A review and critique. *Suicide and Life-Threatening Behavior, 23,* 146–161.

McIntosh, J. L. (1996). Survivors of suicide: A comprehensive bibliography update, 1986–1995. *Omega, 33,* 147–175.

McIntosh, J. L. (1998). *USA Suicide: 1996 official final data* [Mimeograph]. South Bend, IN.

McIntosh, J. L., & Jewell, B. L. (1986). Sex difference trends in completed suicide. *Suicide and Life-Threatening Behavior, 16,* 16–27.

McIntosh, J. L., & Santos, J. F. (1982). Changing patterns in methods of suicide by race and sex. *Suicide and Life-Threatening Behavior, 12,* 221–233.

McKenry, P. C., Tishler, C. L., & Kelley, C. (1982). Adolescent suicide. A comparison of attempters and nonattempters in an emergency room population. *Clinical Pediactrics, 21,* 266–270.

Meehan, P. J., Lamb, J. A., Saltzman, L. E., & O'Carroll, P. W. (1992). Attempted suicide among young adults: Progress toward a meaningful estimate of prevalence. *American Journal of Psychiatry, 149,* 41–44.

Meerloo, J. A. M. (1968). Hidden suicide. In H. L. P. Resnik (Ed.), *Suicidal behaviors and management.* Boston: Little-Brown.

Mehlum, L., Friis, S., Vaglum, P., & Karterud, S. (1994). The longitudinal pattern of suicidal behaviour in borderline personality disorder: A prospective follow-up study. *Acta Psychiatrica Scandinavica, 90,* 124–130.

Meltzer, H. Y., & Okayli, G. (1995). Reduction of suicidality during clozapine treatment of neuroleptic-resistant schizophrenia: Impact on risk-benefit assessment. *American Journal of Psychiatry,* 152, 183–190.

Mendez, M. F., Lanska, D. J., Manon-Espaillat, R., & Burnstine, T. H. (1989). Causative factors for suicide attempts by overdose in epileptics. *Archives of Neurology, 46,* 1065–1068.

Menninger, K. (1938). *Man against himself.* New York: Harcourt, Brace & World.

Menninger, W. W. (1990). Anxiety in the psychotherapist. *Bulletin of the Menninger Clinic, 54,* 384–391.

Merrill, J., Milner, G., Owens, J., & Vale, A. (1992). Alcohol and attempted suicide. *British Journal of Psychiatry, 87,* 83–89.

Metzger, E. D. (1998). Electroconvulsive therapy and suicide. In D. Jacobs (Ed.), *Harvard Medical School guide to suicide assessment and intervention.* Boston: Harvard University Press.

Middlebrook, D. W. (1992). *Anne Sexton: A biography.* Boston: Houghton Mifflin.

Miles, C. P. (1977). Conditions predisposing to suicide: A review. *Journal of Nervous and Mental Disorder, 164,* 231–246.

Milgram, S. (1974). *Obedience to authority: An experimental view.* New York: Harper & Row.

Milham, S. (1983). *Occupational mortality in Washington State.* Olympia, WA: State Department of Social and Health Services.

Miller, H. L., Coombs, D. W., Leeper, J. D., & Barton, S. N. (1984). An analysis of the effects of suicide prevention facilities on suicide rates in the United States. *American Journal of Public Health, 74,* 340–343.

Milling, L., Campbell, N. B., Bush, E., & Laughlin, A. (1996). Affective and behavioral correlates of suicidality among hospitalized preadolescent children. *Journal of Clinical Child Psychology, 25,* 454–462.

Mitchell, M. G., & Rosenthal, D. M. (1992). Suicidal adolescents: Family dynamics and the effects of lethality and hopelessness. *Journal of Youth and Adolescence, 21,* 23–33.

Mitterauer, B. (1990). A contribution to the discussion of the role of the genetic factors in suicide, based on five studies in an epidemiologically defined area (province of Salzburg, Austria). *Comprensive Psychiatry, 31,* 557–565.

Modestin, J., & Kopp, W. (1988). Study on suicide in depressed inpatients. *Journal of Affective Disorders, 15,* 157–162.

Modestin, J., Oberson, B., & Erni, T. (1997). Possible correlates of DSM-III-R personality disorders. *Acta Psychiatrica Scandinavica, 96,* 424–430.

Moir, A., & Jessel, D. (1991). *Brain sex: The real difference between men and women.* New York: Carol.

Moksony, F. (1995). Age patterns of suicide in Hungary. *Archives of Suicide Research, 1,* 217–222.

Moksony, F. (1996). *Religion and suicide in Hungary: Results from a case-control study.* Paper presented at the Sixth European Symposium on Suicide, Lund, Sweden.

Moksony, F. (1997, March 23–27). *Educational mobility and suicide in Hungary.* Paper presented at the 19th Congress of the International Association for Suicide Prevention, Adelaide, Australia.

Molcho, A., & Stanley M. (1992). Antidepressants and suicide risk: Issues of chemical and behavioral toxicity. *Journal of Clinical Psychopharmacology, 12,* 27S–31S.

Money, J., & Earhardt, A. A. (1972). *Man and woman, boy and girl.* Baltimore: Johns Hopkins University Press.

Money, J. & Wiedeking, C. (1980). Gender identity/role: Normal differentiation and its transpositions. In D. Wolman & J. Money (Eds.), *Handbook of human sexuality* (pp. 270–284). Englewood Cliffs, NJ: Prentice-Hall.

Monk, M., & Warshauer, M. E. (1974). Completed and attempted suicide in three ethnic groups. *American Journal of Epidemiology, 100,* 333–345.

Montgomery, S., & Montgomery, D. (1982). Pharmacological prevention of suicidal behaviors. *Journal of Affective Disorders, 4,* 291–298.

Montgomery, S. A., & Montgomery, D. B. (1984). The prevention of suicidal acts in high-risk patients. In E. Usden (Ed.), *Frontiers in biochemical and pharmacological research in depression*. New York: Raven Press.

Montgomery, S. A., Montgomery, D. B., Green, M., et al. (1992). Pharmacotherapy in the prevention of suicidal behavior. *Journal of Clinical Psychopharmacology, 12*, 27S–31S.

Moore, R., & Gillette, D. (1992). *The warrier within*. New York: William Morrow.

Morrison, J. R. (1982). Suicide in a psychiatric practice population. *Journal of Clinical Psychiatry, 43*, 348–352.

Moscicki, E. K. (1999). Epidemiology of suicide, in D. G. Jacobs (Ed.), *The Harvard Medical School Guide to Suicide Assessment and Intervention*. San Francisco: Jossey-Bass Publishers.

Moscicki, E. K., O'Carroll, P., & Regier, D. A. (1988). Suicide attempts in the Epidemiologic Catchment Area study. *Yale Journal of Biology and Medicine, 61*, 259–268.

Moss, H. B., Salloum I. M., & Fisher, B. (1994). Psychoactuve substance abuse. In M. Hersen, R.T. Ammerman, & L.A. Sisson (Eds.) *Handbook of aggressive and destructive behavior in psychiatric patients*. New York: Plenum.

Motto, J. A. (1967). Suicide and suggestibility. *American Journal of Psychiatry, 124*, 252–256.

Motto, J. A. (1970). Newspaper influence on suicide. *Archives of General Psychiatry, 23*, 143–148.

Motto, J. A. (1980). Suicide risk factors in alcohol abuse. *Suicide and Life-Threatening Behavior, 10*, 230–238.

Motto, J. A. (1992). An integrated approach to estimating suicide risk. In R. W. Maris, A. L. Berman, J. T. Maltsberger, & R. I. Yufit, *Assessment and prediction of suicide*. New York: Guilford Press.

Motto, J. A., Heilbron, D. C., & Juster, R. P. (1985). Development of a clinical instrument to estimate suicide risk. *American Journal of Psychiatry, 142*, 680–686.

Moyer, K. E. (1986). Biological bases of aggressive behavior. In R. Plutchik & H. Kellerman (Eds.), *Biological foundations of emotion* (vol. 3). New York: Academic Press.

Muller, R. (1949). Studies on disseminated sclerosis with special reference to symptomatology, course and prognosis. *Acta Medica Scandinavica, 222*, 1–214.

Murphy, G. E. (1992). *Suicide in alcoholism*. New York: Oxford University Press.

Murphy, G. E., & Wetzel, R. (1982). Family history of suicidal behavior among suicide attempters. *Journal of Nervous and Mental Disease, 170*, 86–90.

Murphy, G. E., Gatner, G. E., Wetzel, R. D., Katz, D., & Ernst, M. F. (1974). On the improvement of suicide determination. *Journal of Forensic Sciences, 19*, 276–283.

Murphy, G. E., & Wetzel, R. D. (1990). The lifetime risk of suicide in alcoholism. *Archives of General Psychiatry, 47*, 383–392.

Murphy, G. K. (1977). Cancer and the coroner. *Journal of the American Medical Association, 237*, 786–788.

Murray, H. A. (1938). *Explorations in personality*. New York: Oxford University Press.

Myers, J. K., Weissman, M. M., Tischler, G. L., Holzer III, C. E., Leaf, P. J., Orvaschel, H., Anthony, J. C., Boyd, J. H., Burke, J. D., Kramer, M., & Stoltzman, R. (1984). Six-month prevalence of psychiatric disorders in three communities. *Archives of General Psychiatry, 41*, 959–967.

Myers, W. C., Otto, T. A., Harris, E., Diaco, D., & Moreno, A. (1992). Acetaminophen overdose as a suicidal gesture: A survey of adolescents; knowledge of its potential for toxicity. *Journal of the American Academy of Child and Adolescent Psychiatry, 31*, 686–690.

Napier, A. (1978). *The family crucible*. New York: Harper & Row.

Narveson, J. (1983). Self-ownership and the ethics of suicide. *Suicide and Life-Threatening Behavior, 13*(4), 240–253.

National Center for Health Statistics. (1982). *Vital statistics of the United States, 1978*. Hyattsville, MD: U.S. Department of Health and Human Services.

National household survey on drug abuse. (1999, Winter). *SAMHSA News*, p. 6.

National Safety Council. (1996). *Accident Facts*. Washington, DC: Author.

Nelson, F. L., Litman, R. E., & Diller, J. (1983). Ethnic differeces in analgesic drug related deaths. *Journal of Drug Education, 13*, 15–24.

Nelson, S. H., McKinney, A., Ludwig, K., & Davis, R. (1983). An unusual death of a patient in seclusion. *Hospital and Community Psychiatry, 2*, 259.

Nemeroff, C. B. (1994). Evolutionary trends in the pharmacotherapeutic management of depression. *Journal of Clinical Psychiatry, 55,* 3–15.

Nemeroff, C. B., Ownes, M. J., Bissette, G., Andorn, A. C., & Stanley, M. (1988). Reduced corticotropin releasing factor binding sites in the frontal cortex of suicide victims. *Archives of General Psychiatry, 45,* 577–79.

Neuringer, C. (1982). Suicidal behavior in women. *Crisis, 3,* 41–49.

Neuringer, C., & Lettieri, D. J. (1982). *Suicidal women.* New York: Gardner Press.

New York Academy of Sciences. (1985). *International conference on electroconvulsive therapy (ECT): Clinical and basic research issues.* New York: New York Academy of Sciences.

New, A. S., Trestman, R. L., Mitropoulou, V., & Benishay, D. S. (1997). Serotonergic function and self-injuriousbehavior in personality disorder patients. *Psychiatry Research, 69,* 17–26.

Newman, B. (1992, October 5). Smash hits. *Sports Illustrated,* pp. 77–87.

Newman, S. C., & Bland, R. C. (1991). Suicide risk varies by subtype of affective disorder. *Acta Psychiatrica Scandinavica, 83,* 420–426.

Nichols, M. P. (1987). *The self in the system: Expanding the limits of family therapy.* New York: Brunner/Mazel.

Nichols, S. E. (1983). Psychiatric aspects of AIDS. *Psychosomatics, 24,* 1083–1089.

Nielson, D., Goldman, D., Virkkunen, M., et al. (1994). Suicidality and 5-hydroxyindoleacetic acid concentration associated with a tryptophan hydroxylase polymorphism. *Archives of General Psychiatry, 51,* 34–38.

Niemeyer, R. A., & Pfeiffer, A. M. (1994). The ten most common errors of suicide interventionists. In A. A. Leenaars, J. T. Maltsberger, & R. A. Niemeyer (Eds.), *Treatment of suicidal people* (pp. 207–224). Bristol, PA: Taylor & Francis.

Nierenberg, A. A., Ghaemi, S. N., Clancy-Colecchi, K., & Rosenbaum, J. E. (1996). Cynicism, hostility and suicidal ideation in depressed outpatients. *Journal of Nervous and Mental Disease, 184,* 607–610.

Nieto, E., Vietra, E., Gasto, C., Vallejo, J., & Cirera, E. (1992). Suicide attempts of high medical seriousness in schizophrenic patients. *Comprehensive Psychiatry, 33,* 384–387.

Nisbet, P. A. (1995). *Suicidal protective factors in black females.* Unpublished master's thesis, University of South Carolina (Columbia).

Nisbet, P. A. (1996). Protective factors for suicidal black females. *Suicide and Life-Threatening Behavior, 26,* 325–341.

Nisbet, P. A. (1998). *Interactive wealth and the opportunity for self-destructive behaviors.* Unpublished doctoral dissertation, University of South Carolina (Columbia).

Nock, M. K., & Marzuk, P. M. (1999). Murder-suicide: Phenomenology and clinical implications. In D. G. Jacobs (Ed.), *The Harvard Medical School guide to assessment and intervention* (pp. 188–209). San Francisco: Jossey-Bass.

Nolan, J. L. (Ed.). (1988). *The suicide case: Investigation and trial of insurance claims.* Chicago: American Bar Association.

Nolen-Hoeksema, S. (1990). *Sex differences in depression.* Stanford, CA: Stanford University Press.

Nordstroem, P., Schalling, M., & Äsberg, M. (1995). Temperamental vulverability in attempted suicide. *Acta Psychiatrica Scandiavica, 92,* 155–160.

Nordstrom, P., Gustavsson, P., Edman, G., & Äsberg, M. (1996). Temperamental vulnerability and suicide risk after attempted suicide. *Suicide and Life-Threatening Behavior, 26,* 380–394.

Nordstrom, P., Samuelsson, M., Äsberg, M., et al. (1994). CSF 5-HIAA predicts suicide risk after attempted suicide. *Suicide and Life-Threatening Behavior, 24,* 1–9.

Norstrom, T. (1995a). Alcohol and suicide. *Addiction, 90,* 1463–1469.

Norstrom, T. (1995b). Prevention strategies and alcohol policy. *Addiction, 90,* 515–524.

Norstrom, T. (1995c). The impact of alcohol, divorce, and unemployment on suicide. *Social Forces, 74,* 293–314.

Nowers, G. D. (1997). Suicide by jumping [a review]. *Acta Psychiatrica Scandinavica, 96,* 1–6.

Nyquist, R. H., & Bors, E. (1967). Mortality and survival in traumatic myelopathy during nineteen years, from 1946 to 1965. *Paraplegia, 5,* 22–48.

O'Carroll, P. W. (1993). Suicide causation: Pies, paths and pointless polemics. *Suicide and Life-Threatening Behavior, 12,* 27–36.

O'Carroll, P. W., Berman, A. L., Maris, R. M., Moscicki, E., Silverman, M., & Tanney, B. (1996). Beyond the Tower of Babel: A nomenclature for suicidology. *Suicide and Life-Threatening Behavior, 26,* 237–252.

Ochoa, L., Beck, A. T., & Steer, R. (1992). Gender differences in co-morbid anxiety and mood disorders. *American Journal of Psychiatry, 149,* 1409–1410.

O'Donnell, J. A. (1969). *Narcotic addicts in Kentucky.* Chevy Chase, MD: National Institute of Mental Health.

Office of Independent Counsel. (1997). *Report of the death of Vincent W. Foster.* Washington, DC:

Ogilvie, D. M., Stone, P. J., & Shneidman, E. S. (1966). Some characteristics of genuine versus simulated suicide notes. In P. J. Stone, D. C. Dunphey, M. S. Smith, & D. M. Ogilvie (Eds.), *The general inquirer: A computer approach to content analysis.* Cambridge, MA: MIT Press.

Okie, S. (1990, January 13). Sullivan cold-shoulders suicide report. *Washington Post,* p. A5.

Orbach, I. (1997). A taxonomy of factors related to suicidal behavior. *Clinical Psychology: Science and Practice, 4*(3), 208–224.

Ornstein, M. (1983). The impact of marital status, age, and employment on female suicide in British Columbia. *Canadian Review of Sociology and Anthropology, 20,* 96–100.

Osgood, C. E., & Walker, E. G. (1959). Motivation and language behavior: A content analysis of suicide notes. *Journal of Abnormal and Social Psychology, 59,* 58–67.

Osmond, D. (Ed.). (1998). *The AIDS knowledge base.* http://hivinsite.ucsf.edu/akb/.

Overbeek, T., Rikken, J., Schruers, K., & Griez, E. (1998). Suicidal ideation in panic disorder patients. *Journal of Nervous and Mental Diseases, 186,* 577–580.

Overholser, J. C., Freiheit, S. R., & DiFilippo, J. M. (1997). Emotional distress and substance abuse as risk factors for suicide attempts. *Canadian Journal of Psychiatry, 42,* 402–408.

Owen, G., Fulson, R., & Markuson, E. (1982). Death at a distance: A study of family survivors. *Omega, 13,* 191–225.

Pabis, R., Masood, M. A., & Tozman, S. (1980). A case study of autocastration. *American Journal of Psychiatry, 137,* 626–627.

Palmer, C., Revicki, D., Halpern, M., & Hatziandreu, E. J. (1995). The cost of suicide and suicide attempts in the United States. *Clinical Neuropharmacology, 18*(3), S25–S33.

Pampel, F. (1993). Relative cohort size and fertility: The socio-political context of the easterlin effect. *American Sociological Review, 58,* 496–514.

Pampel, F., & Peters, E. (1995). The Easterlin effect. *Annual Preview of Sociology, 21,* 163–194.

Parkin, R., & Dunne-Maxim, K. (1995). *Child survivors of suicide: A guidebook for those who care for them.* New Jersey: American Suicide Foundation.

Patterson, W. M., Dohn, H. H., Bird, J., & Patterson, G. A. (1983). Evaluation of suicide patients: The SAD PERSONS scale. *Psychosomatics, 24,* 343–352.

Paykel, E. S. (1972). Depressive typologies and responses to amitryptiline. *British Journal of Psychiatry, 139,* 176–181.

Paykel, E. S. (Ed.). (1992). *Handbook of affective disorders.* New York: Guilford Press.

Paykel, E. S., Prusoff, B. A., & Myers, J. K. (1975). Suicide attempts and recent life events. A controlled comparison. *Archives of General Psychiatry, 32*(3),327–333.

Pearson, J. L., & Conwell, Y. (Eds.). (1996). *Suicide aging: International perspectives.* New York: Springer.

Peck, D. L. (1986). Completed suicides: Correlates of choice of method. *Omega, 16,* 309–323.

Peipins, L., Burnett, S., & Alterman, T. (1997). Mortality patterns among female nurses: A 27 state study, 1984–1990. *American Journal of Public Health, 87,* 1539–1543.

Perlin, S. (1975). A handbook for the study of suicide. New York: Oxford University Press.

Perlmuter, L. C., Hakami, M. K., Hodgson-Harrington, C., et al. (1984). Decreased cognitive function in aging non-insulin-dependent diabetic patients. *American Journal of Medicine, 77,* 1043–1048.

Perry, S. W. (1990). Organic mental disorders caused by HIV: Update on early diagnosis and treatment. *American Journal of Psychiatry, 147,* 696–710.

Perry, S. W., Jacobsberg, L., & Fishman, B. (1990). Suicidal ideation and HIV testing. *Journal of the American Medical Association, 263,* 679–682.

Perry, S. W., & Jacobsen, P. (1986). Neuropsychiatric manifestations of AIDS-spectrum disorders. *Hospital and Community Psychiatry, 37,* 1001–1006.

Pescosolido, B. A. (1994). Bringing Durkheim into the twenty-first century: A network approach to unresolved issues in the sociology of suicide. In D. Lester (Ed.), *Emile Durkheim, Le suicide: One hundred years later.* Philadelphia: Charles Press.

Pescosolido, B. A., & Georgianna, S. (1989). Durkheim, suicide, and religion: Toward a network theory of suicide. *American Sociological Review, 54,* 33–48.

Pescosolido, B. A., & Mendelsohn, R. (1986). Social causation or social construction of suicide? *American Sociological Review, 51,* 81–100.

Peters, K. D., Kochanek, K. D., & Murphy, S. L. (1998). *Deaths: Final data for 1996. National vital statistics reports: 47(9).* Hyattsville, MD: National Center for Health Statistics (CDC).

Peterson, B. S., Zhang, H., Santa Lucia, R., & King, R. A. (1996). Risk factors for presenting problems in child psychiatric emergencies. *Journal of the American Academy of Child and Adolescent Psychiatry, 35,* 1162–1173.

Petronis, K. R., Samuels, J. F., Moscicki, E. K., & Anthony, J. C. (1990). An epidemiologic investigation of potential risk factor for suicide attempts. *Social Psychiatry and Psychiatric Epidemiology, 25,* 193–199.

Pfeffer, C. R. (1981). Parental suicide: An organizing event in the development of latency age children. *Suicide and Life-Threatening Behavior, 11,* 43–50.

Pfeffer, C. R. (1982). Interventions for suicidal children and their parents. *Suicide and Life-Threatening Behavior, 12,* 240–248.

Pfeffer, C. R. (1986). *The suicidal child.* New York: Guilford Press.

Pfeffer, C. R. (1989). *Suicide among youth.* Washington, DC: American Psychiatric Press.

Pfeffer, C. R., Conte, H. R., Plutchik, R., & Jerrett, I. (1979). Suicidal behavior in latency age children: An empirical study. *Journal of American Academy of Child Psychiatry, 18,* 679–692.

Pfeffer, C. R., Conte, H. R., Plutchik, R., & Jerrett, I. (1980). Suicidal behavior in latency age children: An empirical study. *Journal of American Academy of Child Psychiatry, 19,* 703–710.

Pfeffer, C. R., Newcorn, J., Kaplan, G., Mizruchi, M. S., & Plutchik, R. (1988). Suicidal behavior in child psychiatric inpatients. *Journal of American Academy of Child Psychiatry, 27,* 357–361.

Pfeffer, C. R., Newcorn, J., Kaplan, G., Mizruchi, M. S., & Plutchik R. (1989). Subtypes of suicidal and assaultive behaviors in adolescents and psychiatric inpatients: A research note. *Journal of Child Psychology and Psychiatry, 30,* 151–163.

Pfeffer, C. R., Plutchik, R., Mizruchi, M. S., et al. (1986). Suicidal behavior in child psychiatric inpatients and outpatients and in nonpatients. *American Journal of Psychiatry, 143,* 733–738.

Pfohl, B., Stangl, D., & Zimmerman, M. (1984). The implications of DSM-III personality disorders for patients with major depression. *Journal of Affective Disorders, 7,* 309–318.

Phillips, D. P. (1970). *Deathday and birthday.* Unpublished PhD dissertation, Princeton University, Princeton, New Jersey.

Phillips, D. P. (1974). The influence of suggestion on suicide: Substantive and theoretical implications of the Werther effect. *American Sociological Review, 39,* 340–354.

Phillips, D. P. (1979). Suicide, motor vehicle fatalities, and the mass media. Evidence toward a theory of suggestion. *American Journal of Sociology, 84,* 1150–1174.

Phillips, D. P. (1980). Airplane accidents, murder, and the mass media. *Social Forces, 58,* 1001–1024.

Phillips, D. P. (1982). The impact of fictional television stories on American adult fatalities: New evidence of the effect of mass media on violence. *American Journal of Sociology, 87,* 1340–1359.

Phillips, D. P. (1985). The Werther effect. *The Sciences, 25,* 33–39.

Phillips, D. P., & Carstensen, L. L. (1986). Clustering of teenage suicides after television news stories about suicide. *New England Journal of Medicine, 315,* 685–689.

Phillips, D. P., & Feldman, K. (1973). A dip in deaths before ceremonial occasions. *American Sociological Review, 38,* 678–696.

Phillips, D. P., & Lesyna, K. (1995). Suicide and the media: Research and policy implications. In R. Diekstra et al. (Eds.), *Preventive Strategies on Suicide.* Leiden: World Health Organization.

Phillips, D. P., Lesyna, K., & Paight, D. J. (1992). Suicide and the media. In R. W. Maris, A. L. Berman, J. T. Maltsberger, & R. I. Yufit (Eds.), *Assessment and prediction of suicide*. New York: Guilford Press.

Phillips, D. P., Welty, W. R., & Smith, M. (1997). Elevated suicide levels associated with legalized gambling. *Suicide and Life-Threatening Behavior, 27*, 373–378.

Picton, B. (1971). *Murder, suicide, or accident: The forensic pathologist at work*. London: Hale.

Pierce, A. (1967). The economic cycle and the social suicide rate. *American Sociological Review, 32*, 457–462.

Pierce, C. (1987, October). Underscore urgency of HIV counseling. *Clinical Psychiatry News*, p. 1.

Piercy, F. P., Sprenkle, D. H., & Associates. (1986). *Family therapy sourcebook*. New York: Guilford Press.

Piet, S. (1987). What motivates stunt men? *Motivation and Emotion, 11*, 195–213.

Pindyck, R. S., & Rubinfeld, D. L. (1981). *Econometric models and economic forecasts*. New York: McGraw-Hill.

Pittman, F. (1992, October). Family therapy and the death of patriarchy. *Family Therapy News*, pp. 8–10.

Pitts, G., & Winokur, G. (1964). Affective disorder: Part 3. Diagonstic correlates and incidence of suicide. *Journal of Nervous and Mental Disease, 139*, 176–181.

Platt, S. (1984). Unemployment and suicidal behavior: A review of the literature. *Social Science and Medicine, 19*, 93–115.

Platt, S. (1992). Suicide and unemployment in Italy. *Social Science and Medicine, 34*, 1191–1201.

Plutchik, R. (1980). *Emotion: A psychoevolutionary synthesis*. New York: Harper & Row.

Plutchik, R. (1994). *The psychology and biology of emotion*. New York: HarperCollins.

Plutchik, R. (1995). Outward and inward directed aggressiveness: The interaction between violence and suicidality. *Pharmacopsychiatry, 28* (Suppl.), 47–57.

Plutchik, R. (1997). The circumplex as a general model of the structure of emotions and personality. In R. Plutchik & H.R. Conte (Eds.), *The circumplex model in personality and emotions*. Washington, DC: American Psychological Press.

Plutchik, R., & Karasu, T. B. (1991). Computers in psychotherapy: An overview. *Computers in Human Behavior, 7*, 33–44.

Plutchik, R., & van Praag, H. M. (1986). The measurement of suicidality, aggressivity and impulsivity. *Clinical Neuropharmacology, 9* (Suppl. 4), 380–382.

Plutchik, R., & van Praag, H. M. (1990). Psychosocial correlates of suicide and violence risk. In: H. M. vanPraag, R. Plutchik, & A. Apter (Eds.), *Violence and suicidality: Perspective in clinical and psychobiological research*. New York: Brunner/Mazel.

Plutchik, R., & van Praag, H. M. (1994). Suicide risk: Amplifiers and attenuators. In M. Hillbrand & N.J. Pollone (Eds.), *The psychobiology of aggression*. Binghamton, NY: Harworth Press.

Plutchik, R., Botsis, A. J., & van Praag, H. M. (1995). Psychopathology, self-esteem, sexual and ego functions as correlates of suicide and violence risk. *Archives of Suicide Research, 1*, 27–38.

Plutchik, R., van Praag, H. M., & Conte, H. R. (1989) Correlates of suicide and violence risk: III. A two-stage model of countervailing forces. *Psychiatry Research, 28*, 215–225.

Poesner, J. A., LaHaye, A., & Cheifetz, P. N. (1989). Suicide notes in adolescence. *Canadian Journal of Psychiatry, 34*, 171–176.

Pokorny, A. D. (1960). Characteristics of forty-four patients who subsequently committed suicide. *Archives of General Psychiatry, 2*, 314–323.

Pokorny, A. D. (1983). Prediction of suicide in psychiatric patients. *Archives of General Psychiatry, 40*, 249–257.

Pokorny, A. D. (1992). Prediction of suicide in psychiatric patients: Report of a prospective study. In R. W. Maris, A. L. Berman, J. T. Maltsberger, & R. I. Yufit (Eds.), *Assessment and prediction of suicide* (pp. 105–129). New York: Guilford Press.

Pokorny, A. D. (1993). Suicide and prediction revisited. *Suicide and Life-Threatening Behavior, 23*, 1–10.

Pope, K. S., & Tabachnick, B. G. (1993). Therapists' anger, hate, fear, and sexual feelings: National survey of therapist responses, client characteristics, critical events, formal complaints, and training. *Professional Psychology: Research and Practice, 24*, 142–152.

Popkin, M. K., Callies, A. L., Lentz, R. D., Colon, E. A., & Sutherland, D. E. (1988). Prevalence of major depression, simple phobia and other psychiatric disorders in patients with long-standing type I diabetes mellitus. *Archives of General Psychiatry, 45,* 64–68.

Porterfield, A., & Gibbs, J. (1960). Occupational prestige and social mobility of suicides in New Zealand. *American Journal of Sociology, 66,* 147–152.

Post, R.M, Rubinow, D. R., Uhde, T. W., et al. (1989). Dysphoric mania: Clinical and biological correlates. *Archives of General Psychiatry, 46,* 353–358.

Potts, M. K., Burnam, A., & Wells, K. B. (1991). Gender differences in depression detection: A comparison of clinician diagnosis and standardized assessment. *Psychological Assessment, 3*(4), 609–615.

Pounder, D. (1985). Suicide by leaping from multistory car parks. *Medical Science and the Law, 5,* 179–188.

Practice Management Information Corporation. (1992). *ICD–9-CM. International Classification of Diseases, 9th revision, 4th edition, Clinical Modification.* Los Angeles: Author.

Prasad, A., & Lloyd, G. (1983). Attempted suicide by jumping. *Acta Psychiatrica Scandinavica, 68,* 394–396.

Prenzlauer, S., Drescher, J., & Winchel, R. (1992). Suicide among homosexual youth. *American Journal of Psychiatry, 149,* 1416.

Quitkin, F. M., Rabkin, J. G, Ross, D., et al. (1984). Duration of antidepressant drug treatment: What is an adequate trial? *Archives of General Psychiatry, 41,* 238–245.

Raczek, S. W., True, P. K., & Friend, R. C. (1989). Suicidal behavior and personality traits. *Journal of Personality Disorders, 3,* 345–351.

Rajs, J., & Fugelstad, A. (1992). Suicide related to human immunodeficiency virus in Stockholm. *Acta Psychiatrica Scandinavica, 85,* 234–239.

Ramefedi, G., Farrow, J. A., & Deiher, R. W. (1991). Risk factors for attempted suicide in gay and bisexual youth. *Pediatrics, 87,* 869–875.

Ramefedi, G., French, S., Story, M., Resnick, M. D., & Blum, B. (1998). The relationship between suicide risk and sexual orientation: Results of a population-based study. *Pediatrics, 87,* 869–875.

Range, L. M., & Goggin, W. D. (1990). Reactions to suicide: Does age of the victim make a difference? *Death Studies, 14,* 269–275.

Range, L. M., & Niss, N. M. (1990). Long-term bereavement from suicide, homicide, accidents, and natural deaths. *Death Studies, 14,* 423–433.

Range, L. M., Bright, P. S., & Ginn, P. D. (1985). Public reactions to child suicide: Effects of child's age and method used. *Journal of Community Psychology, 13,* 288–294.

Rawls, J. (1971). *Theory of justice.* Cambridge, MA: Harvard University Press.

Redlich, F. C. (1993). The death and autopsy of Adolf Hitler. In A. A. Leenaars, A. L. Berman, P. Cantor, R. E. Litman, & R. W. Maris (Eds.), *Suicidology: Essays in honor of Edwin S. Shneidman.* Northvale, NJ: Jason Aronson.

Reed, G. E., McGuire, R. J., & Boehm, A. (1990). Analysis of gunshot residue test results in 112 suicides. *Journal of Forensic Science, 35*(1), 62–68.

Reed, M. D. (1993). Sudden death and bereavement outcomes: The impact of resources on grief symptomatology and detachment. *Suicide and Life-Threatening Behavior, 23,* 203–220.

Reed, M. D. (1998). Predicting grief symptomatology among the suddenly bereaved. *Suicide and Life-Threatening Behavior, 28,* 285–301.

Reed, M. D., & Greenwald, J. Y. (1992). Survivor-status, attachment, and sudden death bereavement. *Suicide and Life-Threatening Behavior, 21,* 385–401.

Regier, C. A., Boyd, J. H., Burke, J. D., Rae, D. S., Myers, J. K., Kramer, M., Robins, L. N., George, L. K., Karmo, M., & Locke, B. Z. (1988). One month prevalence of mental disorders in the United States. *Archives of General Psychiatry, 45,* 977–986.

Reid, W. H., Mason, M., & Hogan, T. (1998). Suicide prevention effects associated with clozapine therapy in schizophrenia and schizoaffective disorder. *Psychiatric Services, 49,* 1029–1033.

Revicki, D. A., & May, H. J. (1984). Physician suicide in North Carolina. *Southern Medical Journal, 78,* 1205–1207.

Reynolds, F. M. T., & Cimbolic, P. (1988). Attitudes toward suicide survivors as a function of survivors' relationship to the victim. *Omega, 19,* 125–133.

Rich, A. R., & Bonner, R. L. (1987). Concurrent validity of a stress–vulnerability model of suicidal ideation and behavior. *Suicide and Life-Threatening Behavior, 17*(4), 265–270.

Rich, C. L., Fowler, R. C., Young, D., & Blenkush, M. (1986a). San Diego suicide study: Comparison of gay to straight males. *Suicide and Life-Threatening Behavior, 16,* 448–457.

Rich, C. L., Young, D., & Fowler, R. C. (1986b). San Diego suicide study: I. Young vs. old subjects. *Archives of General Psychiatry, 43,* 577–582.

Rich, C. L., Young, J. G., Fowler, R. C., Wagner, J., & Black, N. A. (1990). Guns and suicide: Possible effects of some legislation. *American Journal of Psychiatry, 147,* 342–346.

Rich, S., Warsradt, G., & Nemiroff, R. (1991). Suicide, stressors, and the life cycle. *American Journal of Psychiatry, 4,* 524–527.

Richman, J. (1971). Family determinants of suicide potential. In D. Anderson, & L. J. McClain (Eds.), *Identifying suicide potential.* New York: Behavioral.

Richman, J. (1979). The family therapy of attempted suicide. *Family Process, 18,* 131–142.

Richman, J. (1984). The family therapy of suicidal adolescents: Promises and pitfalls. In H. S. Sudak, A. B. Ford, & N. B. Rushforth (Eds.), *Suicide in the young.* Littleton, MA: John Wright.

Richman, J. (1986). *Family therapy for suicidal people.* New York: Springer.

Richman, J. (1991, April). *Role modeling and context in the determination of method.* Paper presented at the annual meeting of American Association of Suicidology, Boston.

Richman, J. (1992a). A rational approach to rational suicide. *Suicide and Life-Threatening Behavior, 22,* 130–141.

Richman, J. (1992b). *The management of risk and the risk of management of the family in therapy with suicidal patients.* Unpublished manuscript.

Richman, J. (1994). Psychotherapy with older suicidal adults. In A. A. Leenaars, J. T. Maltsberger, & R. Niemeyer (Eds.), *Treatment of suicidal people.* Washington, DC: Taylor & Francis.

Rimpala, A. H., Nurminen, M. M., Rimpala, M. K., & Valkonen, T. (1987). Mortality of doctors. *Lancet, 1,* 84–86.

Ringel, E. (1978). *Das Leben Wegwerfen: Reflexionen Uber Selbstmord.* Wien: Herder.

Robbins, D. R., & Alessi, N. E. (1985). Depressive symptoms and suicidal behavior in adolescents. *American Journal of Psychiatry, 142,* 588–592.

Robertson, I., & McKee, M. (1980). *Social problems* (2nd ed.). New York: Random House.

Robin, A. A., & Langley, G. E. (1964). A controlled trial of imipramine. *British Journal of Psychiatry, 110,* 419–422.

Robins, E. (1981). *The final months: A study of the lives of 134 persons who committed suicide.* New York: Oxford University Press.

Robins, E. (1986). Psychosis and suicide. *Biological Psychiatry, 21,* 665–672.

Robins, E., & O'Neal, P. (1958). Culture and mental disorders. *Human Organization, 16,* 7–11.

Robins, E., Murphy, G. E., Wilkinson, R. H., Gassner, S., & Kayes, J. (1959). Some clinical considerations in the prevention of suicide based on a study of 134 successful suicides. *American Journal of Public Health, 49,* 888–889.

Robins, L. N., West, P. A., & Murphy, G. E. (1977). A high rate of suicide in older white men. *Social Psychiatry, 12,* 1–20.

Robinson, D., & Spiker, D. (1985). Delusional depression: A one-year follow-up. *Journal of Affective Disorders, 9,* 79–83.

Roesler, T., & Deisher, R. (1972). Youthful male homosexuality. *Journal of the American Medical Association, 219,* 1018–1023.

Rogers, J. R. (1992). Suicide and alcohol. *Journal of Counseling and Development, 70,* 540–543.

Rollman, B., Mead, L., Wang, N. Y., & Klag, M. (1997). Medical specialty and the incidence of divorce. *New England Journal of Medicine, 336,* 800–803.

Roman, E., Beral, V., & Inskip, H. (1985). Occupational mortality among women in England and Wales. *Brithish Medical Journal, 291,* 194–196.

Roose, S. P., Glassman, A. H., Walsh, B. T., Woodring, S., & Vital-Herne, J. (1983). Depression, delusions and suicide. *American Journal of Psychiatry, 140,* 1159–1162.

Rose, K. D., & Rosow, L. (1973). Physicians who kill themselves. *Archives of General Psychiatry, 29,* 800–805.

Rosen, D. H. (1970). The serious suicide attempt: Epidemiological and follow-up study of 886 patients. *American Journal of Psychiatry, 127,* 764–770.

Rosenberg, M. L. et al. (1988). Operational criteria for the determination of suicide. *Journal of Forensic Sciences, 33,* 1445–1456.

Rosenberg, M. L., Smith, J. C., Davidson, L. E., & Conn, J. M. (1987). The emergence of youth suicide: An epidemiologic analysis and public health perspective. *American Review of Public Health, 8,* 417–440.

Rosenthal, M. (1981). Sexual differences in the suicidal behavior of young people. *Adolescent Psychiatry, 9,* 422–442.

Rosenthal, R., Crisafi, B. R., & Coomaraswamy, R.P, (1980). Manual extraction of a permanent pacemaker: An attempted suicide. *Pace, 3,* 229–231.

Rossow, I. (1993). Suicide, alcohol, and divorce. *Addiction, 88,* 1659–1665.

Rossow, I., & Amundsen, A. (1995). Alcohol abuse and suicide: A 40 year prospective study of Norwegian conscripts. *Addiction, 90,* 685–691.

Rothberg, J. M., & Geer-Williams, C. (1992). A comparison and review of suicide prevention scales. In R. W. Maris, A. L. Berman, J. T. Maltsberger, & R. I. Yufit (Eds.), *Assessment and prediction of suicide* (pp. 202–217). New York: Guilford Press.

Rothschild, A. J., Schatzberg, A. F., Langlais, P. J., et al. (1987). Psychotic and nonpsychotic depressions: Comparison of plasma catecholamine and cortisol measures. *Psychiatry Research, 20,* 143–153.

Roy, A. (1982). Risk factors for suicide in psychiatric patients. *Archives of General Psychiatry, 39,* 1089–1095.

Roy, A. (1983). Family history of suicide. *Archives of General Psychiatry, 40,* 971–974.

Roy, A. (1992). Genetics, biology, and suicide in the family. In R. Maris, A. L., Berman, J. T. Maltsberger, & R. I. Yufit (Eds.), *Assessment and prediction of suicide.* New York: Guilford Press.

Roy, A. (1993). Risk factors for suicide among adult alcoholics. *Alcohol Health and Research World, 16,* 133–136.

Roy, A. (1994) Affective disorders. In M. Hersen, R. T. Ammerman, & L. A. Sisson (Eds.), *Handbook of aggressive and destructive behavior in psychiatric patients.* New York: Plenum.

Roy, A., Lamparski, D., DeJong, J., et al. (1990). Cerebrospinal fluid monoamine metabolites in alcoholic patients who attempt suicide. *Acta Psychiatrica Scandinavica, 81,* 58–61.

Roy, A., & Linnoila, M. (1986). Alcoholism and suicide. *Suicide and Life-Threatening Behavior, 16,* 244–273.

Roy, A., & Linnoila, M. (1988). Suicidal behavior, impulsiveness and serotonin. *Acta Psychiatrica Scandinavica, 78,* 529–535.

Roy, A., & Linnoila, M. (1990). Monoamines and suicidal behavior. In H. van Praag (Ed.), *Monoamine regulation of aggression and impulse control.* New York: Brunner/Mazel.

Roy, A., Agren, H., Pickar, D., Linnoila, M., Doran, A., Cutler, N., & Paul, S. (1986). Reduced CSF concentration of homovanillic acid and homovanillic acid to 5-hydroxyindoleacetic acid ratios in depressed patients: Relationship to suicidal behavior and dexamethasone nonsuppression. *American Journal of Psychiatry, 143,* 1539–1545.

Roy, A., DeJong, J., & Linnoila, M. (1989). Cerebrospinal fluid monoamine metabolites and suicidal behavior in depressed patients. *Archives of General Psychiatry, 143,* 1539–1545.

Roy, A., Nutt, D., Virkkunen, M., & Linnoila, M. (1987). Serotonin, suicidal behavior and impulsivity. *Lancet, 2,* 949–950.

Roy, A., Rylander, G., & Sarchiapone, M. (1997). Genetic studies of suicidal behavior. *Psychiatric Clinics of North America, 20,* 595–611.

Roy, A., Segal, N. L., Centerwall, B. S., & Robinette, C. D. (1991). Suicide in twins. *Archives of General Psychiatry, 48,* 29–32.

Roy, A., Segal, N., & Sarchiapone, M. (1995). Attempted suicide among living cotwins of twin suicide victims. *American Journal of Psychiatry, 152,* 1075–1076.

Rudd, M. D., & Joiner, T. (1998). The assessment, management, and treatment of suicidality: Toward clinically informed and balanced standards of care. *Clinical Psychology: Science and Prac-*

tice, 5, 135–150.

Rudd, M. D., Dahm, P. F., & Rajab, M. H. (1993). Diagnostic comorbidity in persons with suicidal ideation and behavior. *American Journal of Psychiatry, 150,* 928–934.

Rudestam, K. E. (1971). Stockholm and Los Angeles: A cross-cultural study of the communication of suicidal intent. *Journal of Consulting and Clinical Psychology, 36,* 82–90.

Rudestam, K. E. (1992). Research contributions to understanding the suicide survivor. *Crisis, 13,* 41–46.

Rushing W. (1969). Suicide and the interaction of alcoholism (liver cirrhosis) with the social situation. *Quarterly Journal of Studies on Alcohol, 30,* 93–103.

Rutter, M. (1994). Family discord and conduct disorder: Cause, consquence, or correlate? *Journal of Family Psychology, 8,* 170–186.

Rutz, W., von Knorring, L., & Walinder, J. (1989). Frequency of suicide on Gotland after systematic postgraduate education of general practitioners. *Acta Psychiatrica Scandinavica, 80,* 151–154.

Rutz, W., von Knorring, L., & Walinder, J. (1992). Long-term effects of an educational program for general practitioners given by Committee for the Prevention and Treatment of Depression. *Acta Psychiatrica Scandinavica, 85,* 83–88.

Ryan, C., Vega, A., & Drash, A. (1985). Cognitive deficits in adolescents who developed diabetes early in life. *Pediatrics, 75,* 921–927.

Sabbath, J. C. (1969). The suicidal adolescent: The expendable child. *Journal of American Academic Child Psychiatry, 8,* 272–289.

Sabo, A. N. J. G., Gunderson, J. G., Najavits, L. M., Chauncey, D., & Kisiel, C. (1995). Changes in self-destructiveness of borderline patients in psychotherapy: A prospective follow-up. *Journal of Nervous and Mental Disease, 183,* 370–376.

Sadovnick, A. D., Ebers, G. C., Wilson, R. W., & Paty, D. W. (1992). Life expectancy in patients attending multiple sclerosis clinics. *Neurology, 42,* 991–994.

Sadovnick, A. D., Eisen, K., Ebers, G. C., & Paty, D. W. (1991). Cause of death in patients attending multiple sclerosis clinics. *Neurology, 41,* 1193–1196.

Saghir, M., & Robins, E. (1973). *Male and female homosexuality: A comprehensive investigation.* Baltimore: Williams & Wilkins.

Sahni, S. P. (1992). Heroin addiction and criminality. *Journal of Personality and Clinical Studies, 8,* 35–38.

Sainsbury, P. (1955). *Suicide in London.* London: Chapman & Hall.

Sainsbury, P., Jenkins, J., & Levey, A. (1980). The social correlates of suicide in Europe. In M. Farmer (Ed.), *Suicide syndrome.* London: Croom & Helm.

Salive, M. E., Smith, G. S., & Brewer, T. F. (1989). Suicide mortality in the Maryland state prison system, 1979–1987. *Journal of the American Medical Association, 262,* 365–369.

Salmons, P. (1984). Suicide in high buildings. *British Journal of Psychiatry, 154,* 469–472.

Salzman, C. (1999). Treatment of the suicidal patient with psychotropic drugs and ECT. In D. Jacobs (Ed.), *The Harvard Medical school guide to suicide assessment and intervention.* San Francisco: Jossey-Bass.

Salzman, C., Wolfson, A. N., & Schatzberg, A. (1995). Effect of fluoxetine on anger in symptomatic volunteers with borderline personality disorder. *Journal of Clinical Psychopharmacology, 15,* 23–29.

Samuels, J. F., Nestadt, G., Romanoski, A. J., Folstein, M. F., & McHugh, P. R. (1994). DSM-III personality disorders in the community. *American Journal of Psychiatry, 151,* 1055–1062.

Samy, M. H. (1995) Parental unresolved ambivalence and adolescent suicide: A psychoanalytic perspective. In B. Mishara (Ed.), *The impact of suicide.* New York: Springer.

Sanders, C. M. (1980). A comparison of adult bereavement in the death of a spouse, child, and parent. *Omega, 10,* 303–322.

Sartorius, N., & Gulbinat, W. (1994). Suicide in Eastern Europe. In M. J. Kelleher (Ed.), *Divergent perspectives on suicidal behavior.* Cork, Ireland: D. & A. O'Leary.

Schaefer, H. H. (1967). Can a mouse commit suicide? In E. S. Shneidman (Ed.), *Essays in self-destruction.* New York: Science House.

Schatzberg, A. F., Rothschild, A. J., & Stahl, J. B. (1983). The dexamethasone suppression test: Identification of subtypes of depression. *American Journal of Psychiatry, 140,* 1231–1233.

Schatzberg, A. G., Cole, J. O., Cohen, B. M., et al. (1983). Survey of depressed patients who have failed to respond to treatment. In J. M. Davis & J. W. Mass (Eds.), *The affective disorders.* Washington, DC: American Psychiatric Press.

Schein, M. M. (1976). Obstacles in the education of psychiatric residents. *Omega, 7,* 75–82.

Schifano, F., & DeLeo, D. (1991). Can pharmacological intervention aid in the prevention of suicidal behavior? *Pharmacopsychiatry, 24,* 113–117.

Schildkraut, J. J., Hirshfeld, A. J., & Murphy, J. M. (1994). Mind and mood in modern art. *Ameican Journal of Psychiatry, 151,* 482–488.

Schlesselman, J. J. (1982). *Case-control studies: Design, conduct, analysis.* New York: Oxford University Press.

Schmidt, C. W., Shaffer, J. W., Zlotowitz, H. J., & Fisher, R. (1977). Suicide by vehicular crash. *American Journal of Psychiatry, 134,* 175–178.

Schmidtke, A. (1997). Perspectives: Suicide in Europe. In A. A. Leenaars, R. W. Maris, & Y. Takahashi (Eds.), Suicide: Individual, cultural, international Perspectives. New York: Guilford Press.

Schmidtke, A., & Hafner, H. (1988). The Werther effect after television films: New evidence for an old hypothesis. *Psychological Medicine, 18,* 665–676.

Schmidtke, A., Bille-Brahe, U., Kerkhof, A. J. F. M., De Leo, D., Bjerke, T., Crepet, P., Haring, C., Hawton, K., Lönnqvist, J., Michel, K., Pommereau, X., Querejeta, I., Salander-Renberg, E., Temesvary, B., Wasserman, D., Sampaio-Faria, J. G., & Fricke, S. (1994). Sociodemographic characteristics of suicide attempters in Europe. In A. J. F. M. Kerkhof et al. (Eds.), *Attempted suicide in Europe: Findings from the multicentre study on parasuicide* (pp. 231–241). Leiden, The Netherlands: DSWO Press.

Schmidtke, A., Fricke, S., & Weinacker, B. (1994). The epidemiology of atttempted suicide in the Wuraburg area: 1989–1992. In A. J. F. M. Kerkhof et al. (Eds.), *Attempted suicide in Europe.* Leiden: DSWO Press.

Schneider, S. G., Farberow, N. L., & Kruks, G. N. (1989). Suicidal behavior in adolescent and adult gay men. *Suicide and Life-Threatening Behavior, 19,* 381–394.

Schony, W., & Grausgruber, A. (1987). Epidemiological data on suicide in Upper Austria. *Crisis, 8,* 49–52.

Schrut, A. (1964). Suicidal adolescents and children. *Journal of the American Medical Association, 188,* 1102–1107.

Schubert, D., & Foliart, R. H. (1993). Increased depression in multiple sclerosis patients. *Psychosomatics, 34,* 124–130.

Schuckit, M. A. (1985). The clinical implications of primary diagnostic groups among alcoholics. *Archives of General Psychiatry, 42,* 1043–1049.

Schuckit, M. A., & Schuckit, J. J. (1989). Substance use and abuse: A risk factor in youth suicide. *In Alcohol, drug abuse, and mental health administration. Report of the Secretary's Task Force on Youth Suicide. Vol. 2: Risk factors for youth suicide* (DHHS Publication No. ADM 89–1622). Washington, DC: U.S. Government Printing Office.

Schuckit, M. A., Tipp, J. E., Bergman, M., & Reich, W. (1997). Comparison of induced and independent major depressive disorders in 2,945 alcoholics. *American Journal of Psychiatry, 154,* 948–957.

Schulsinger, F., Kety, S., Rosenthal, D., & Wender, P. (1979). A family study of suicide. In M. Schou & E. Stromgren (Eds.), *Origin, prevention and treatment of affective disorders.* London: Academic Press.

Schuyler. (1979). Counseling suicide survivors: Issues and answers. *Omega, 4,* 313–320.

Schwartz, M. L., & Pierron, M. (1972). Suicide and fatal accidents in multiple sclerosis. *Omega, 3,* 291–293.

Scully, J. H., & Hutcherson, R. (1983). Suicide by burning. *American Journal of Psychiatry, 140,* 905–906.

Seiden, R. H. (1968). *Suicide behavior contagion on a college campus.* Paper presented at the meeting of the fourth International Conference on Suicide Prevention.

Seiden, R. H., & Gleiser, M. (1990). Sex differences in suicide among chemists. *Omega, 21,* 177–189.

Seiden, R. H., & Spence, M. C. (1982). A tale of two bridges: Comparative suicide incidence on the Golden Gate and San Francisco–Oakland Bay Bridges. *Crisis, 3,* 32–40.

Sellers, E. M., Naranjo, C. A., & Peachey, J. E. (1981). Drugs to decrease alcohol consumption. *New England Journal of Medicine, 305,* 1255–1262.

Selltiz, C., Wrightsman, L. S., & Cook, S. W. (1976). *Research methods in social relations.* New York: Holt, Rinehart & Winston.

Selye, H. (1976). *The stress of life.* New York: McGraw Hill.

Selye, H. (1982). History and present status of the stress concept. In L. Goldberge & S. Brenitz (Eds.), *Handbook of stress.* New York: Free Press.

Shaffer, D. (1974). Suicide in childhood and early adolescence. *Journal of Child Psychology and Psychiatry, 5,* 275–291.

Shaffer, D., & Fisher, P. (1981). The epidemiology of suicide in children and young adolescents. *Journal of American Academy of Child Psychiatry, 20,* 545.

Shaffer, D., Garlan, A., Gould, M., Fisher, P., & Trautman, P. (1990). Preventing teenage suicide: A critical review. In S. Chess, & M. E. Hertzig (Eds.), *Annual progress in child psychiatry and child development, 1989.* New York: Brunner/Mazel.

Shaffer, D., Gould, M. S., Fisher, P., & Trautman, P. (1985, September). *Suicidal behavior in children and young adults.* Paper presented at the Psychobiology of Suicidal Behavior Conference, New York, New York.

Shaffer, D., Gould, M. S., Fisher, Trautman, P., Moreau, D., Kleinman, M., & Flory, M. (1996). Psychiatric diagnosis in child and adolescent suicide. *Archives of General Psychiatry, 53,* 339–348.

Shafii, M., Carrigan, S., Whittinghill, R., & Derrick, A. (1985). Psychological autopsy of completed suicides in children and adolescents. *American Journal of Psychiatry, 142,* 1061–1064.

Shafii, M., Steltz-Lenarsky, J., & Derrick, A. M. (1988). Comorbidity of mental disorders and the post-mortem diagnoses of completed suicide in children and adolescents. *Journal of Affective Disorders, 15,* 227–233.

Shapiro, S. (1992). Suicidality and the sequelae of childhood victimization. In S. Shapiro & G. M. Dominiak (Eds.), *Sexual trauma and psychopathology.* New York: Lexington Books.

Shaunesey, K., Cohen, J. L, Plummer, B., & Berman, A. (1993). Suicidality in hospitalized adolescents: Relationship prior to abuse. *American Journal of Orthopsychiatry, 63,* 113–119.

Shaver, P., Schwartz, J., Kirson, D., & O'Connor, C. (1987). Emotion knowledge: Further exploration of a prototype approach. *Journal of Personality and Social Psychology, 52,* 1061–1086.

Sheperd, D., & Barraclough, B. (1980). Work and suicide: An empirical investigation. *British Journal of Psychiatry, 136,* 469–478.

Shiang, J. (1998). Does culture make a difference? Racial/ethnic patterns of completed suicide in San Francisco, CA 1987–1996 and clinical applications. *Suicide and Life-Threatening Behavior, 28(4),* 338–354.

Shiang, J., Blinn, R., Bongar, B., Stephens, B., Allison, D., & Schatzberg, A. (1997). Suicide in San Francisco, CA: A comparison of Caucasians and Asian groups, 1987–1994. *Suicide and Life-Threatening Behavior, 27(1),* 80–91.

Shneidman, E. S. (1967). Some current developments in suicide prevention. *Bulletin of Suicidology, 1,* 31–34.

Shneidman, E. S. (1968). Orientation toward death: A vital part of the study of lives. In H. L. P. Resnik (Ed.), *Suicidal behaviors and management.* Boston: Little-Brown.

Shneidman, E. S. (1971). Prevention, intervention, and postvention. *Annals of Internal Medicine, 75,* 453–458.

Shneidman, E. S. (1973). Suicide notes reconsidered. *Psychiatry, 36,* 379–395.

Shneidman, E. S. (1980a). *Voices of death.* New York: Harper & Row.

Shneidman, E. S. (1980b). Suicide. In E. S. Shneidman (Ed.), *Death: Current perspectives.* Palo Alto, CA: Mayfield.

Shneidman, E. S. (1985). *Definition of suicide.* New York: Wiley.

Shneidman, E. S. (1987). A Psychological Approach to Suicide. In G. R. VandenBos & B. K. Bryant

(Eds.), *Cataclysms, crises, and catastrophes*. Washington, DC: American Psychological Association.

Shneidman, E. S. (1992). A conspectus of the suicidal scenario. In R. W. Maris, A. L. Berman, J. T. Maltsberger, & R. I. Yufit (Eds.), *The Assessment and prediction of suicide* (pp. 50–64). New York: Guilford Press.

Shneidman, E. S. (1993). *Suicide as psychache: A clinical approach to self-destructive behavior*. Northvale, NJ: Jason Aronson.

Shneidman, E. S. (1994). Clues to suicide, reconsidered. *Suicide and Life-Threatening Behavior, 24*, 395–397.

Shneidman, E. S., & Farberow, N. L. (1957a). The logic of suicide. In E. S. Shneidman & N. L. Farberow (Eds.), *Clues to suicide*. New York: McGraw-Hill.

Shneidman, E. S., & Farberow, N. L. (1957b). *The cry for help*. New York: McGraw-Hill.

Shneidman, E. S., & Farberow, N. L. (1957c). In E. S. Shneidman & N. L. Farberow (Eds.), *Clues to suicide*. New York: McGraw-Hill.

Shneidman, E. S., & Farberow, N. L. (1957d). Some comparisons between genuine and simulated suicide notes in terms of Mowrer's concepts of discomfort and relief. *Journal of General Psychology, 56*, 251–256.

Sholders, M. A. (1981). Suicide in Indianapolis. *Sociological Focus, 14*, 221–231.

Shuckit, M. A. (1983). Alcoholism and other psychiatric disorders. *Hospital Community Psychiatry, 34*, 1022–1027.

Shuwall, M., & Siris, S. G. (1994). Suicidal ideation in postpsychotic depression. *Comprehensive Psychiatry, 35*, 132–134.

Silverman, M. M. (1997). Current controversies in suicidology. In R. W. Maris, M. M. Silverman, & S. S. Canetto (Eds.), *Review of suicidology, 1997* New York: Guilford Press.

Silverman, M. M. (1998). Clinical psychopharmacotherapy with hospitalized patients: A forensic perspective. In B. Bongar, A. L. Berman, R. W. Maris, M. M. Silverman, E. A. Harris, & W. L. Packman (Eds.), *Risk management with suicidal patients*. New York: Guilford Press.

Silverman, M. M., & Maris, R. W. (1995). The prevention of suicidal behaviors: An overview. *Suicide and Life-Threatening Behavior, 2*, 10–21.

Silverman, M., & Maris, R. W. (1995). *Suicide prevention: Toward the year 2000*. New York: Guilford Press.

Simon, F., Stierlin, H., & Wynne, L. C. (1985). *The language of family therapy: A systemic vocabulary and sourcebook*. New York: Family Process Press.

Simpson, M. A. (1980). Self-mutilation as indirect self-destructive behavior. In N. L. Farberow (Ed.), *The many faces of suicide: Indirect self-destructive behavior*. New York: McGraw-Hill.

Singh, B. L., Williams, J. S., & Ryther, B. J. (1986). Public approval of suicide: A situational analysis. *Suicide and Life-Threatening Behavior, 16*, 409–418.

Skinner, B. F. (1953). *Science and human behavior*. New York: Macmillan.

Skog, O. J. (1993). Alcohol and suicide in Denmark 1911–1924. *Addiction, 88*, 1189–1193.

Skog, O. J. (1995). Alcohol and suicide. *Addiction, 90*, 1053–1061.

Slaby, A. E. (1994a). Psychopharmacotherapy of suicide. In A. A. Leenaars, J. T. Maltsberger, & R. A. Neimeyer (Eds.), *Treatment of suicidal people*. Washington, DC: Taylor & Francis.

Slaby, A. E. (1994b). The neurobiology of suicide. In A. A. Leenaars, J. T. Maltsberger, & R. A. Neimeyer (Eds.), *Treatment of suicidal people*. Washington, DC: Taylor & Francis.

Slaby, A. E., & Dumont, L. E. (1992). Psychopharmacotherapy of suicidal ideation and behavior. In B. Bongar (Ed.), *Suicide: Guidelines for assessment, management, and treatment*. New York: Oxford University Press.

Slaby, A. E., Lieb, J., & Tancredi, L. R. (1985). *The handbook of psychiatric emergencies* (3rd ed.). New York: Elsevier.

Slater, J., & Depue, R. A. (1981). The contribution of environmental events and social support to serious suicide attempts in primary depressive disorder. *Journal of Abnormal Psychiatry, 40*, 275–285.

Smith, B. D., & Salzman, C. (1991). Do benzodiazepines cause depression? *Hospital Community Psychiatry, 42*, 1101–1102.

Smith, C., & Krohn, M. D. (1995) Delinquency and family life: The role of ethnicity. *Journal of Youth and Adolescence, 24,* 69–93.

Smith, K. (1985). An ego vulnerabilities approach to suicide prevention. *Bulletin of the Menninger Clinic, 49,* 489–499.

Smith, K., Conroy, R. W., & Ehler, B. D. (1984). Lethality of Suicide Attempt Rating Scale. *Suicide and Life-Threatening Behavior, 14,* 215–242.

Sokol, M., & Pfeffer, C. (1992). Suicidal behavior in children. In B. Bongar (Ed.), *Assessment and management of suicide in clinical practice.* Manuscript submitted for publication.

Soloff, P. H., George, A., Nathan, R. S., et al. (1986). Progress in pharmacotherapy of borderline disorders: A double blind study of amitriptyline, haloperidol, and placebo. *Archives of General Psychiatry, 43,* 691–697.

Soloff, P. H., George, A., Nathan, R. S., et al. (1987). Behavioral dyscontrol in borderline patients treated with amitriptyline. *Psychopharmacological Bulletin, 23,* 177–181.

Soloff, P. H., Lis, J. A., Kelly, T., Cornelius, J., & Ulrich, R. (1994). Risk factors for suicidal behavior in borderline personality disorder. *American Journal of Psychiatry, 151,* 1316–1326.

Sommers-Flannagan, J., & Sommers-Flannagan, R. (1996). Efficacy of antidepressant medication with depressed youth: What psychologists should know. *Professional Psychology: Research and Practice, 27,* 145–153.

Sonnad, S. R. (1992). Nonparametric statistics. In E. F. Borgatta & M. L. Borgatta (Eds.), *Encyclopedia of Sociology* (pp. 1348–1359). New York: Macmillan.

Sonneck, G., & Wagner, R. (1996). Suicide and the burnout of physicians. *Omega. 33,* 2155–2163.

Sonneck, G., Etzersdorfer, E., & Nagel-Kuess, S. (1994). Imitative suicide on the Viennese subway. *Social Sciences and Medicine, 38,* 453–457.

South, S. (1987). Metropolitan migration and social problems. *Social Science Quarterly, 68,* 3–18.

Spaulding, K. S. (1999, August). Suicide in persons served by Missouri Department of Mental Health. Conference proceeding on Creating Community Action for Suicide Prevention, Missouri Department of Health, Kansas City, MO.

Sperry, K., & Sweeney, E. S. (1989). Suicide by intravenous injection of cocaine. *Journal of Forensic Sciences, 34,* 244–248.

Spiegel, D. E., & Neuringer, C. (1963). Role of dread in suicidal behavior. *Journal of Abnormal and Social Psychology, 66,* 507–511.

Spiker, D. G., Hanin, I., Cofsky, J., et al. (1981). Pharmacological treatment of delusional depressives. *Psychopharmachology Bulletin, 17,* 201–202.

Spirito, A., Stark, L., Fristad, M., Hart, K., & Owens-Stively, J. (1987). Adolescent suicide attempters hospitalizes on a pediatric unit. *Journal of Pediatric Psychology, 12,* 171–189.

Spitz, R. A. (1946). Anaclitic depression. In D. Greenacre (Ed.), *Psychoanalytic study of the dead.* New York: International Universities Press.

Spitz, W., & Fisher, R. (Eds.). (1980). *Medicolegal investigation of death.* Springfield, IL: Charles C.Thomas.

Stack S. (1987a). Celebrities and suicide: A taxonomy and analysis, 1948–1983. *American Sociological Review, 52,* 401–412.

Stack, S. (1978). Suicide: A comparative analysis. *Social Forces, 57,* 644–653.

Stack, S. (1980). Occupational status and suicide: A relationship reexamined. *Aggressive Behavior, 6,* 223–234.

Stack S. (1982). Suicide: A decade review of the sociological literature. *Deviant Behavior, 4,* 41–66.

Stack, S. (1987b). The effect of female participation in the labor force on suicide: A time series analysis, 1948–1980. *Sociological Forum, 2,* 257–277.

Stack, S. (1988). Suicide: Media impacts in war and peace. *Suicide and Life-Threatening Behavior, 18,* 342–357.

Stack, S. (1989). The impact of divorce on suicide in Norway. *Journal of Marriage and the Family, 51,* 229–238.

Stack, S. (1990a). The effect of divorce on suicide in Denmark. *Sociological Quarterly, 31,* 359–370.

Stack, S. (1990b). New micro level data on the impact of divorce on suicide: A test of two theories. *Journal of Marriage and the Family, 52*, 119–127.

Stack, S. (1995a). Suicide risk among laborers: A multivariate anaylsis. *Sociological Focus, 28,* 197–199.

Stack, S. (1995b). Gender and suicide risk among laborers. *Archives of Suicide Research, 1,* 19–26.

Stack, S. (1995c). Country music and suicide: Individual, indirect, and interaction effects. *Social Forces, 74,* 331–335.

Stack, S. (1996a). Suicide risk among dentists. *Deviant Behavior, 1,* 107–117.

Stack, S. (1996b). Gender and suicide risk among artists: A multivariate analysis. *Suicide and Life-Threatening Behavior, 26,* 374–379.

Stack, S. (1997). The impact of relative cohort size on national suicide trends, 1950–1980: A comparative analysis. *Archives of Suicide Research, 3,* 213–222.

Stack, S. (1998a). Education and risk of suicide: An analysis of African Americans. *Sociological Focus, 31,* 295–302.

Stack, S. (1998b). *Suicide risk among physicians: A multivariate analysis.* Paper presented at the annual meetings of the American Association of Suicidology, Bethesda.

Stack, S. (1999a, March). *Occupational risk and suicide: An analysis of national data, 1990.* Paper presented at the annual meeting of the Michigan Academy of Science, Arts, and Letters, Grand Rapids, Michigan.

Stack, S. (1999b). Suicide risk among carpenters: A multivariate analysis. *OMEGA: Journal of Death and Dying, 38*(3), 229–232.

Stack, S., & Gundlach, J. (1992). The effect of country music on suicide. *Social Forces, 71,* 211–218.

Stack, S., & Haas, A. (1984). The effect of unemployment duration on national suicide rates. *Sociological Focus, 17,* 17–29.

Stack, S., & Kelley, T., (1995). Police suicide: An analysis. *American Journal of Police, 13,* 73–90.

Stack, S., & Wasserman, I. (1995). Effect of marriange, family, and religious ties on African American suicide ideology. *Journal of Marriage and the Family, 57,* 215–222.

Stahl, S. M. (1996). *Essential psychopharmacology.* New York: Cambridge University Press.

Stall, R. D., Coates, T. J., & Hoff, C. (1988). Behavioral risk reduction for hiv infection among gay and bisexual men. *American Psychologist, 43,* 878–885.

Stanley, M., & Mann, J. J. (1983). Increased serotonin-W binding sites in frontal cortex of suicide victims. *Lancet, 1,* 214–216.

Stanley, M., & Mann, J. J. (1988). Biological factors associated with suicide. In A. J. Frances & R. E. Hales (Eds.), *Review of psychiatry* (vol. 7, pp. 334–352). Washington, DC: American Psychiatric Press.

Stanley, M., & Stanley, B. (1990). Postmortem evidence of serotonin's role in suicide. *Journal of Clinical Psychiatry, 51,* 22–28.

Stanley, M., Mann, J., & Cohen, L. (1986). Serotonin and serotonergic receptors in suicide. *Annals of the New York Academy of Sciences, 487,* 122–127.

Stanley, M., Virgilio, J., & Gershon, E. S. (1982). Titrated imipramine binding sites are decreased in the frontal cortex of suicides. *Science, 216,* 1337–1339.

Statistical Abstract of the United States. (1997). Washington, DC: U.S. Government Printing Office.

Stearns, S. (1959). Self-destructive behavior in young patients with diabetes mellitus. *Diabetes, 8,* 379–382.

Steele, C. M., & Joesph, R. A. (1990). Alcohol myopia. *American Psychologist, 45,* 921–933.

Steele, D. (1998). *His bright light.* New York: Delacorte Press.

Stefansson, C. G., & Wicks, S. (1991). Health care occupations and suicide in Sweden, 1961–1985. *Social Psychiatry and Psychiatric Epidemiology, 26,* 259–264.

Steiger, B., & Hewes, H. (1997). *Inside Heaven's Gate: The UFO cult leaders tell their story in their own words.* New York: Penguin Putnam Books.

Stein, D. J., Trestman, R. L., Mitropoulou, V., & Coccaro, E. F. (1996). Impulsivity and serotonergic function in compulsive personality disorder. *Journal of Neuropsychiatry and Clinical Neurosciences, 8,* 393–398.

Stein, D., Apter, A., Ratzoni, G., Har-Even, D., & Avidan, G. (1998). Association between multiple suicide attempts and negative affects in adolescents. *Journal of the American Academy of Child and Adolescent Psychiatry, 37,* 488–494.

Stenager, E., Koch-Henricksen, N., Brønnum-Hansen, H., Hyllested, K., Jensen, K., & Bille-Brahe, U. (1992). Suicide and multiple sclerosis: An epidemiological investigation. *Journal of Neurology and Neurosurgical Psychiatry, 55,* 542–545.

Stengel, E. (1964). *Suicide and attempted suicide.* Baltimore: Penguin Books.

Stensman, R., & Sundqvist-Stensman, U. B. (1988). Physical disease and disability among 416 suicide cases in Sweden. *Scandinavia Journal of Social Medicine, 16,* 149–153.

Stephens, B. J. (1985). Suicidal women and their relationships with husbands, boyfriends, and lovers. *Suicide and Life-Threatening Behavior, 15*(2), 77–89.

Stephens, B. J. (1987). Cheap thrills and humble pie: The adolescence of female suicide attempters. *Suicide and Life-Threatening Behavior, 17,* 107–118.

Steward, I. (1960). Suicide: The influence of organic disease. *Lancet, 2,* 919–920.

Stillion, J. M., McDowell, E. E., & May, J. H. (1989). *Suicide across the life span—premature exits.* New York: Hemisphere.

Stoddard, F. J., Pahlavan, K., & Cahners, S. S. (1985). Suicide attempted by self-immolation during adolescence. *Adolescent Psychiatry, 12,* 251–263.

Stoff, D. M., & Mann, J. J. (Eds.). (1997). Neurobiology of suicide: From the bench to the clinic. *Annals of the New York Academy of Sciences, 836,* 1–363.

Stoff, D. M., Breiling, J., & Maser, J. D. (1997). *Handbook of antisocial behavior.* New York: Wiley.

Stone, G. (1999). *Suicide and attempted suicide.* New York: Carroll & Graf.

Stone, I. C. (1987). Observations and statistics relating to suicide weapons. *Journal of Forensic Sciences, 32,* 711–716.

Stone, M. H., Hurt, S. W., & Stone, D. K. (1987). The PI 500: Long-term follow-up of borderline inpatients meeting DSM-III criteria. I. Global outcome. *Journal of Personality Disorders, 1,* 291–298.

Storm, H. H., Christiensen, N., & Jemsen, O. M. (1992). Suicides among Danish patients with cancer, 1971 to 1986. *Cancer, 69,* 1507–1512.

Stowe, R. (1994). Impulse control disorder. In M. Hersen, R. T. Ammerman, & L. A. Sisson (Eds.), *Handbook of aggressive and destructive behavior in psychiatric patients.* (New York: Plenum.

Strakowski, S. M., McElroy, S. L., Keck, P. E., & West, S. A. (1996). Suicidality among patients with mixed and manic bipolar disorder. *American Journal of Psychiatry, 153,* 674–676.

Straus, M., Gelles, R. J., & Steinmetz, S. (1981). *Behind closed doors: Violence in the American family.* New York: Anchor-Doubleday.

Styron, W. (1990). *Darkness visible.* New York: Random House.

Suokas, J., & Lönqvist, J. (1995). Suicide attempts in which alcohol is involved. *Acta Psychiatica Scandinavica, 91,* 36–40.

Suominen, K., & M. Henriksson. (1996). Mental disorders and comorbidity in attempted suicide. *Acta Psychiatrica Scandinavica, 94,* 234–240.

Suter, B. (1976). Suicide and Women. In B. B Wolman (Ed.), *Between survival and suicide.* New York: Gardner Press.

Suyemoto, K. L., & McDonald, M. L. (1995). Self-cutting in female adolescents. *Psychotherapy, 32,* 162–171.

Swift, W., Copeland, J., & Hall, W. (1996). Characteristics of women with alcohol and other drug problems. *Addiction, 91,* 1141–1150.

Sym, J. (Ed.). (1988/1637). *Lifes preservatives against self-killing* (with an introduction by M. MacDonald). London: Routledge.

Szadoczky, E., & Fazekas, I. (1994). The role of psychosocial and biological variables in separating chronic and non-chronic major depression and early/late-onset dysthymia. *Journal of Affective Disorders, 32,* 1–11.

Szasz, T. (1977). *The theology of medicine.* New York: Harper & Row.

Szasz, T. (1985, February). *Suicide: What is the clinician's responsiblity?* Unpublished paper presented at the Harvard Medical School.

Tabachnick, N. (1973). *Accident or suicide? Destruction by automobile.* Springfield, IL: Charles C. Thomas.

Tabachnick, N., Gussen, J., Litman, R. E., Peck, M., Tiber, N., & Wold, C. (1973). *Accident or suicide? Destruction by automobile.* Springfield, IL: Charles C. Thomas.

Takahashi, Y. (1988). *Aokigahara-jukai:* Suicide and amnesia in Mt. Fuji's Black Forest. *Suicide and Life-Threatening Behavior, 18,* 164–175.

Takahashi, Y. (1989). Mass suicide by members of the Japanese Friend of the Truth Church. *Suicide and Life-Threatening Behavior, 19,* 289–296.

Takahashi, Y. (1997). Culture and suicide: From a Japanese psychiatrist's perspective. *Suicide and Life-Threatening Behavior, 27,* 137–145.

Tanney, B. (1995b). Handout. Assessment and therapy with suicidal adults. AAS Summer Institute, Santa Fe, NM.

Tanney, B. L. (1986). Electroconvulsive therapy and suicide. In R. Maris (Ed.), *Biology of suicide.* New York: Guilford Press.

Tanney, B. L. (1992). Mental disorders, psychiatric patients, and suicide. In R. W. Maris, A. L. Berman, J. T. Maltsberger, & R. I. Yufit (Eds.), *Assessment and prediction of suicide.* New York: Guilford Press.

Tanney, B. L. (1992). Mental disorders, psychiatric patients, and suicide. In R. W. Maris, A. L. Berman, J. T. Maltsberger, & R. I. Yufit (Eds.), *The Assessment and prediction of suicide* (pp. 277–320). New York: Guilford Press.

Tanney, B. L. (1995a). After a suicide: A helper's handbook. In B. L. Mishara (Ed.), *The impact of suicide.* New York: Springer.

Tardiff, K. (1981). The risk of assaultive behavior in suicidal patients: I. I. An inpatient survey. *Acta Psychiatrica Scandinavice, 64,* 295–300.

Tardiff, K., Gross, E., Wu, J., Stajic, M., & Millman, R. (1989). Analysis of cocaine-related fatalities. *Journal of Forensic Sciences, 34,* 53–63.

Taylor, M. C., & Wicks, J. W. (1980). The choice of weapons: A study of methods of suicide by sex, race, and region. *Suicide and Life-Threatening Behavior, 10,* 142–149.

Teicher, M. H., Glod, C., & Cole, J. O. (1990). Emergence of intense suicidal preoccupation during fluoxetine treatment. *American Journal of Psychiatry, 147,* 207–210.

Teutsch, S. M., Herman, W. H., Dwyer, D. M., et al. (1984). Mortality among diabetic patients using continuous subcutaneous insulin-infusion pumps. *New England Journal of Medicine, 310,* 361–368.

Thornberry, T. P., & Krohn, M. D. (1997). Peers, drug use, and delinquency. In D.M. Stoff, J. Breiling, & J. D. Maser (Eds.), *Handbook of antisocial behavior.* New York: Wiley.

Tollefson, G. D., Rampwy, A. H., Beaseley, C. M., et al. (1994). Absence of a relationship between adverse effects and suicidality during pharmacotherapy for depression. *Journal of Clinical Psychopharmology, 14,* 163–169.

Tondo, L., Jamison, K. R., & Baldessarini, R. J. (1998). Effect of lithium maintenance on suicidal behavior in major mood disorders. *Annals of the New York Academy of Science, 836,* 339–351.

Toolan, J. M. (1975). Suicide in children and adolescents. *American Journal of Psychotherapy, 29,* 339–344.

Toolan, J. M. (1980). Depression and suicidal behavior. In P. Sholevar (Ed.), *Treatment of emotional disorders in children and adolescents.* New York: Spectrum.

Träskman, L., Äsberg, M., Bertilsson, L., & Sjostrand, L. (1981). Monoamine metabolites in CSF and suicide behavior. *Archives of General Psychiatry, 38,* 631–636.

Träskman-Bendz, L., Äsberg, M., & Schalling, D. (1990). Serotonergic function and suicidal behavior in personality disorders. *Annals of the New York Academy of Science, 487,* 168–174.

Trautman, P. D. (1995). Cognitive behavior therapy of adolescent suicide attempters. In J. K. Zimmerman, & G. M. Asnis (Eds.), *Treatment approaches with suicidal adolescents.* New York: Wiley.

Trautman, P. D., Stewart, N., & Morishima, A. (1993). Are adolescent suicide attempters noncompliant with outpatient care? *Journal of the American Academy of Child and Adolescent Psychiatry, 32,* 89–94.

Troisi, A., & Marchetti, M. (1994) Epidemiology. In M. Hersen, R.T. Ammerman, & L. A. Sisson (Eds.), *Handbook of aggressive and destructive behavior in psychiatric patients.* New York: Plenum.

Trovato, F. (1986). A time series analysis of international immigration and suicide mortality in Canada. *International Journal of Social Psychiatry, 32,* 38–46.

Trovato, F., & Vos, R. (1990). Domestic/religious individulaism and youth suicide in Canada. *Family Perspective, 24,* 69–82.

Tsuang, M. (1983). Risk of suicide in the relatives of schizophrenics, manic depressives and controls. *Journal of Clinical Psychiatry, 44,* 396–400.

Tuckman, J., & Youngman, W. F. (1968). A scale of assessing suicide risk of attempted suicides. *Journal of Clinical Psychology, 24,* 179–180.

Tuckman, J., & Ziegler, R. (1968). A comparison of single and multiple note writers among suicides. *Journal of Clinical Psychology, 24,* 179–180.

Tuckman, J., Kleiner, R., & Lavell, M. (1959). Emotional content of suicide notes. *American Journal of Psychiatry, 116,* 59–63.

Tuckman, J., Youngman, W., & Kreizman, G. (1964). Occupations and suicide. *Industrual Medicine and Surgery, 33,* 818–820.

Tunving, K. (1988). Fatal outcome in drug addiction. *Acta Psychiatrica Scandinavica, 77,* 551–566.

Turgay, A. (1989). An integrative treatment approach to child and adolescent suicidal behavior. *Psychiatric Clinics of North America, 12,* 971–985.

Turnbridge, W. M. (1981). Factors contributing to deaths of diabetics under fifty years of age. *Lancet, 2,* 569–572.

Turner, J. H. (1998). *The structure of sociological theory* (6th ed.). Belmont, CA: Wadsworth.

Tylor, E. B. (1871). *Primitive culture.* London: J. Murray.

U.S. Department of Health and Human Services. (1989). *Alcohol, drug abuse, and mental health administration. Report of the Secretary's Task Force on Youth Suicide. Vol. 1: Overview and recommendations* (DHHS Publication No. ADM 89-1621). Washington, DC: U.S. Govenment Printing Office.

U.S. Public Health Service. (1999). *The Surgeon General's call to action to prevent suicide 1999.* Washington, DC: U.S. Government Printing Office.

Vaillant, G. E., & Blumenthal, S. J. (1990). Introduction—suicide over the life-cycle: Risk factors and life-span development. In S. J. Blumethal & D. J. Kupfer (Eds.), *Suicide over the life cycle.* Washington, DC: American Psychiatric Press.

Valdisserri, R. O., Lyeter, D., Leviton, L. C., Callahan, C. M., Kingsley, L. A., & Rinaldo, C. R. (1988). Variables influencing condom use in a cohort of gay and bisexual men. *American Journal of Public Health, 78,* 801–805.

Valente, S. M. (1994). Psychotherapist reactions to the suicide of a patient. *American Journal of Orthopsychiatry, 64,* 614–621.

van der Kolk, B. A., Perry, J. C., & Lewis-Herman, J. (1991). Childhood origins of self-destructive behavior. *American Journal of Psychiatry, 146,* 1665–1671.

Van Dogen, C. (1993). Social context of postsuicide bereavement. *Death Studies, 17,* 125–141.

van Hooff, A. J. L. (1998). The image of ancient suicide, *Syllecta Classica* (Department of Classics, University of Iowa), *9,* 47–69.

van Praag, H. M. (1982). Biological and psychopathological predictors of suicidality. *Biological Psychiatry, 16,* 42–60.

van Praag, H. M. (1983). CSF 5-HIAA and suicide in nondepressed schizophrenics. *Lancet, 2,* 977–978.

van Praag, H. M. (1986). Affective disorders and aggressive disorders. *Suicide and Life-Threatening Behavior, 16,* 102–132.

van Praag, H. M., & Plutchik, R. (1984). Depression type and depression severity in relation to risk of violent suicide attempt. *Psychiatry Research, 12,* 333–338.

van Praag, H. M., Plutchik, R., & Apter, A. (Eds.). (1990). *Violence and suicidality: Perspectives in chemical and psychobiological research.* New York: Brunner/Mazel.

van Reekum, R., Links, P. S., & Heslegrave, R. J. (1997). Impulsivity and suicide: Research issues. *CPA Bulletin, 29*, 75–76.

VanGastel, A., Schotte, C., & Maes, M. (1997). The prediction of suicidal intent in depressed patients. *Acta Psychiatrica Scandinavica, 96*, 254–259.

Varah, C. (1981). Letter to the the editor. *Crisis*, p. 2.

Vega, W. A., Gil, A., Warheit, G., Apospori, E., & Zimmerman, R. (1993). The relationship of drug use to suicide ideation and attempts among African American, Hispanic, and white non-Hispanic male adolescents. *Suicide and Life-Threatening Behavior, 23*, 110–119.

Velirt, J. C., & Rollins, D. E. (1988). A comparison of the frequency and severity of poisoning cases for ingestion of acetaminophen, aspirin, and ibuprofen. *American Journal of Emergency Medicine, 6*, 104–107.

Velting, D. M., & Gould, M. S. (1997). Suicide contagion. In R. W. Maris, M. M. Silverman, & S. Canetto (Eds.), *Review of suicidology, 1997*. New York: Guilford Press.

Velting, D. M., Rathus, J. H., & Asnis, G. M. (1998). Asking adolescents to explain discrepancies in self-reported suicidality. *Suicide and Life-Threatening Behavior, 28*, 187–196.

Viale-Val, G., & Rattenbury, F. (1994, June). *Substance abuse, prostitution, suicidal behavior and running away in delinquent girls*. Paper presented at national conference on Risk-Taking Behaviors among Children and Adolescents, Washington, DC.

Vietra, E., Nieto, E., Gasto, C., & Cirera, E. (1992). Serious suicide attempts in affective patients. *Journal of Affective Disorders, 24*, 147–152.

Virkkunen, M., & Alha, A. (1971). On suicides committed under the influence of alcohol in Finland in 1967. *British Journal of Addiction, 65*, 317–323.

Virkkunen, M., Goldman, D., Nielsen, D. A., & Linnoila, M. (1995). Low brain serotonin turnover rate (low CSF 5-HIAA) and impulsive violence. *Journal of Psychiatry and Neuroscience, 20*, 271–275.

Viskum, K. (1975). Ulcer, attempted suicide and suicide. *Acta Psychiatrica Scandinavica, 51*, 221–227.

Vlasak, G. J. (1975). Medical sociology. In S. Perlin (Ed.), *A handbook for the study of suicide*. London: Oxford University Press.

Waern, M., Beskow, J., Allebeck, P., & Spak, F. (1997). Suicidal thoughts in women—A general population survey. Proceedings of the 19th Congress of the International Association for Suicide Prevention, Adelaide, Australia.

Wagner, B. M. (1997). Family risk factors for child and adolescent suicidal behavior. *Psychological Bulletin, 121*, 246–298.

Wahl, C. W. (1957). Suicide as a magical act. In E. S. Shneidman, & N. L. Farberow (Eds.), *Clues to suicide*. New York: McGraw-Hill.

Waldron, I. (1976). Why do women live longer than men? *Journal of Human Stress, 2*, 1–13.

Wallace, L. J. D, Calhoun, A. D., Powell, K. E., O'Neil, J., & James, S. P. (1996). *Homicide and suicide among Native Americans, 1979–1992* [Violence Surveillance Summary Series, No. 2]. Atlanta, GA: Centers for Disease Control and Prevention, National Center for Injury Prevention and Control.

Walsh, B. W., & Rosen, P. M. (1988). *Self-mutilation*. New York: Guilford Press.

Wardle, J. (1995). Cholesterol and psychological well-being. *Journal of Psychosomatic Research, 39*, 549–562.

Warshaw, M. G., Massion, A. O., Peterson, L. G., Pratt, L. A., & Keller, M. B. (1995). Suicidal behavior in patients with panic disorder: Retrospective and prospective data. *Journal of Affective Disorders, 34*, 235–247.

Washer, G. F., Schroter, G. P., Starzl, T. E., & Weill, R. (1983). Causes of death after kidney transplantation. *Journal of the American Medical Association, 250*, 49–54.

Wassenaar, D. R. (1987). Brief strategic family therapy and the management of adolescent Indian parasuicide patients in the general hospital setting. *South African Journal of Psychology, 17*, 93–99.

Wasserman, D., Varnik, A., & Eklund, G. (1994). Male suicides and alcohol consumption in the former USSR. *Acta Psychiatrica Scandinavica, 89*, 306–313.

Wasserman, I. (1983). Political business cycles, presidential elections, and suicide mortality patterns. *American Sociological Review, 48,* 771–720.

Wasserman, I. (1984). Imitation and suicide: A reexamination of the Werther effect. *American Sociological Review, 49,* 427–436.

Wasserman, I. (1989a). The effects of war and alcohol consumption patterns on suicide: United States, 1910–1933. *Social Forces, 68,* 513–530.

Wasserman, I. (1989b). Age, period, and cohort effects in suicide behavior in the U. S. and Canada in the 20th century. *Journal of Aging Studies, 3,* 295, 311.

Wasserman, I. (1992a). Economy, work, occupation, and suicide. In R. Maris, A. L. Berman, J. T. Maltsberger, & R. I. Yufit, (Eds.), *Assessment and prediction of suicide,.* New York: Guilford Press.

Wasserman, I. (1992b). The impact of epidemic, war, prohibition, and media on suicide: United States, 1910–1920. *Suicide and Life-Threatening Behavior, 22,* 240–254.

Watterson, O., Simpson, D., & Sells, S. (1975). Death rates and causes of death among opioid addicts in community drug treatment programs during 1970–1973. *American Journal of Drug and Alcohol Abuse, 2*(1), 99–111.

Way, B. B., Allen, M. H., Mumpower, J. L., Stewart, T. R., & Banks, S. M. (1998). Interrater agreement among psychiatrists in psychiatric emergency assessments. *American Journal of Psychiatry, 155,* 1423–1428.

Webb, J. P., & Willard, W. (1975). Six American Indian patterns of suicide. In N. L. Farberow (Ed.), *Suicide in different cultures* (pp. 17–34). Baltimore: University Park Press.

Weber, M. (1925). *Wirtschaft und Gesellschaft* (2nd ed.). Tubingan: J. C. B. Mohr.

Webster's New World Dictionary. (1966). Cleveland: World Publishing Company.

Weishaar, M. E., & Beck, A. T. (1990). Cognitive approaches to understanding and treating suicidal behavior. In S. J. Blumenthal & D. J. Kupfer (Eds.), *Suicide over the life cycle: Risk factors, assessment, and treatment of suicidal patients.* Washington, DC: American Psychiatric Press.

Weishaar, M. E., & Beck, A. T. (1992). Clinical and cognitive predictors of suicide. In R. W. Maris, A. L. Berman, J. T. Maltsberger, & R. I. Yufit (Eds.), *Assessment and prediction of suicide.* New York: Guilford Press.

Weisman, A. (1967). Self-destruction and sexual perversion. In E. S. Sheidman (Ed.), *Essays in self-destruction.* New York: Science House.

Weisman, A., & Worden, J. W. (1974). Risk–rescue rating in suicide assessment. In A. T. Beck, H. L. P. Resnick, & D. J. Lettieri (Eds.), *The prediction of suicide.* Bowie, MD: Charles Press.

Weiss, D., & Coccaro, E. F. (1997). Neuroendocrine challenge studies of suicidal behavior. *Psychiatric Clinics of North America, 20,* 563–579.

Weissman, M. M. (1974). The epidemiology of suicide attempts, 1960–1971. *Archives of General Psychiatry, 30,* 737–746.

Weissman, M. M., & Klerman, G. L. (1973). Psychotherapy with depressed women: An empirical study of content themes and reflection. *British Journal of Psychiatry, 123*(572), 55–61.

Weissman, M. M., & Klerman, G. L. (1977). Sex differences and the epidemiology of depression. *Archives of General Psychiatry, 34,* 98–111.

Weissman, M. M., Klerman, J. L., Markowitz, J. S., & Ouellette, R. (1989). Suicidal ideation and suicide attempts in panic disorder and attacks. *New England Journal of Medicine, 321,* 1209–1214.

Weissman, M. M., Myers, J. K., & Harding, R. S. (1980). Prevalence and psychiatric heterogeneity of alcoholism in a U.S. urban community. *Journal of Studies on Alcohol, 41,* 672–681.

Wellman, M. M., & Wellman, R. J. (1986). Sex differences in peer responsiveness to suicide ideation. *Suicide and Life-Threatening Behavior, 16,* 360–378.

Welte, J., Abel, E., & Wieczorek, W. (1988). The role of alcohol in suicides in Erie County, NY, 1972–1984. *Public Health Reports, 103,* 648–652.

Wender, P., Kety, S., Rosenthal, D., & Schulsinger, F. (1986). Psychiatric disorders in the biological and adoptive families of adopted individuals with affective disorders. *Archives of General Psychiatry, 43,* 923–929.

Werth, J. L., Jr. (1996). *Rational suicide? Implications for mental health professionals.* Washington, DC: Taylor & Francis.

West, D. J. (1966). *Murder followed by suicide*. Cambridge, MA: Harvard University Press.

Westin, A., Engstroem, G., Ekman, R., & Traeskmna-Bendz, L. (1998). Correlated between plasmo-neuropeptides and temperament dimensions differ between suicidal patients and healthy controls. *Journal of Affective Disorders, 49*, 45–54.

Wetli, C. V. (1983). Changing patterns of methaqualone abuse. *Journal of the American Medical Association, 249*, 621–626.

White, H., & Stillion, J. M. (1988). Sex differences in attitudes toward suicide: Do males stigmatize males? *Psychology of Women Quarterly, 12*, 257–272.

Whitlock, F. A. (1986). Suicide in physical illness. In A. Roy (Ed.), *Suicide*. Baltimore: Williams & Wilkins.

Whittemore, K. (1970). *Ten centers*. Atlanta: Lullwater Press.

Wickett, A. (1989). *Double exit: When aging couples commit suicide together*. Eugene, OR: Hemlock Society.

Wihelmsen, L., Elmfeldt, D., & Wedel, J. (1983). Causes of death in relation to social and alcohol problems among Swedish men aged 35–44 years. *Acta Medica Scandinavica, 213*, 263–268.

Wilcox, N. E., & Stauffer, E. S. (1972). Follow-up of 423 consecutive patients admitted to the spinal cord center, Rancho Los Amigos Hospital, 1 January to 31 December 1967. *Paraplegia, 10*, 115–122.

Wilens, T. E., Stern, T..A., & O'Gara, P. T. (1990). Adverse cardiac effects of combined neuroleptic ingestion and tricyclic antidepressant overdose. *Journal of Clinical Psychopharmacology, 10*, 51–54.

Windle, M. (1994). Characteristics of alcoholics who attempted suicide: Co-occurring disorders and personality differences with a sample of male Vietnam era veterans. *Journal of Studies on Alcohol, 55*, 571–577.

Wirshing, C., van Putten, T., Rosenberg, J., et al. (1992). Fluoxetine, akathisia, and suicidality: Is there a causal connection? *Archives of General Psychiatry, 49*, 581–582.

Wittgenstein, L. (1953). *Philosophical investigations*. New York: Macmillan.

Wold, C. (1971). Subgroupings of suicidal people. *Omega, 2*, 19–29.

Wolfersdorf, M., Keller, F., Steiner, B., & Hole, G. (1987). Depressional depression and suicide. *Acta Psychiatrica Scandinavica, 76*, 359–363.

Woodruff, R. A., Clayton, P. J., & Guze, S. B. (1972). Suicide attempts and psychiatric diagnosis. *Diseases of the Nervous System, 33*, 617–621.

Workman, M., & Beer, J. (1992). Depression, suicide intention and aggression among high school students whose parents are divorced and use alcohol at home. *Psychological Reports, 70*, 504–511.

World Health Organization. (1992). *The ICD-10 classification of mental and behavioral disorders: Clinical descriptions and diagnostic guidelines*. Geneva: Author.

World Health Organization. (1999). *Global AIDS surveillance*. Geneva: Author.

Wulfert, E., Safren, S., Brown, I., & Wan, C. K. (1999). Cognitive, behavioral, and personality correlates of hiv-positive persons' unsafe sexual behavior. *Journal of Applied Social Psychology, 29*, 223–244.

Yadlowsky, J. M. (1980). Suicide by snake venom injection. *Journal of Forensic Sciences, 25*, 760–764.

Yampey, N. (1975). Suicide in Buenos Aires: Social and cultural influences. In N. L. Farberow (Ed.), *Suicide in different cultures*. Baltimore: University Park Press.

Yang, B., & Lester, D. (1994). Crime and unemployment. *Journal of Socio-Economics, 23*, 215–222.

Yap, P. M. (1958). *Suicide in Hong Kong*. Hong Kong: Hong Kong University Press.

Yates, G. L., MacKenzie, R., & Pennbridge, J. (1988). A risk profile comparison of runaway and non-runaway youth. *American Journal of Public Health, 78*, 820–821.

Yonkers, K. A., Kando, J. C., Cole, J. O., & Blumenthal, S. (1992). Gender differences in pharmacokinetics and pharmacodynamics of psychotropic medications. *American Journal of Psychiatry, 149*, 587–595.

Young, M. A., Fogg, L. F., Scheftner, W. A., & Fawcett, J. A. (1994). Interactions of risk factors in predicting suicide. *American Journal of Psychiatry, 151*, 434–435.

Young, S. E., Mikulich, S. K., Goodwin, M. B., & Hardy, J. (1995). Treated delinquent boys' substance use: Onset, pattern, relationship to conduct and mood disorders. *Drug and Alcohol Dependence, 37,* 149–162.

Yuen, N., Androde, N., Nahulu, L., & Makine, G. (1996). The rate and characteristics of suicide attempters in the native Hawaiian adolescent population. *Suicide and Life-Threatening Behavior, 26,* 27–36.

Yufit, R. I., & Bongar, B. (1992). Suicide, stress, and coping with life-cycle events. In R. W. Maris, A. L. Berman, J. T. Maltberger, & R. I. Yufit (Eds.), *Assessment and prediction of suicide.* New York: Guilford Press.

Zair, K. (1981). A suicidal family. *British Journal of Psychiatry, 139,* 68–69.

Zemishlany, Z. (1987). An epidemic of suicide attempts by burning in a psychiatric hosptal. *British Journal of Psychiatry, 150,* 703–706.

Zhang, J. (1996). Suicides in Beijing, China 1992–1993. *Suicide and Life-Threatening Behavior, 26,* 176–180.

Zich, J., & Temoshok, L. (1987). Perceptions of social support in men with AIDS and ARC: Relationships with distress and hardiness. *Applied Social Psychology, 17,* 193–215.

Zimmerman, S. (1987). States' public welfare expenditures as predictors of state suicide rates. *Suicide and Life-Threatening Behavior,* 271–287.

Zinner, E. S. (1985). Group survivorship: A model and case study application. *New Directions for Student Services, 31,* 51–68.

Zinner, E. S. (1990). Survivors of suicide: Understanding and coping with the legacy of self-inflicted death. In P. Cimblic & D. A. Jobes (Eds.), *Youth suicide: Issues, assesment, and intervention.* Springfield, IL: Charles C. Thomans.

Zuckerman, M. (1979). *Sensation seeking: Beyond optimal level of arousal.* Hillsdale, NJ: Erlbaum.

Author Index

Author Index

Subject Index